CHANGING THE
U.S. HEALTH CARE SYSTEM

CHANGING THE U.S. HEALTH CARE SYSTEM

Key Issues in Health Services Policy and Management

4TH EDITION

Gerald F. Kominski

Editor

JB JOSSEY-BASS™

A Wiley Brand

Published by Jossey-Bass
A Wiley Brand
One Montgomery Street, Suite 1200, San Francisco, CA 94104-4594—www.josseybass.com

Jossey-Bass books and products are available through most bookstores. To contact Jossey-Bass directly call our Customer Care Department within the U.S. at 800-956-7739, outside the U.S. at 317-572-3986, or fax 317-572-4002.

Wiley publishes in a variety of print and electronic formats and by print-on-demand. Some material included with standard print versions of this book may not be included in e-books or in print-on-demand. If this book refers to media such as a CD or DVD that is not included in the version you purchased, you may download this material at http://booksupport.wiley.com. For more information about Wiley products, visit www.wiley.com.

Library of Congress Cataloging-in-Publication Data
Changing the U.S. health care system : key issues in health services policy and management / Gerald F. Kominski, editor. —4th ed.
    p. ; cm.
Includes bibliographical references and index.
ISBN 978-1-118-12891-6 (cloth)—ISBN 978-1-118-41890-1 (pdf)—
ISBN 978-1-118-41640-2 (epub)
I. Kominski, Gerald F.
[DNLM: 1. Health Care Reform—United States. 2. Delivery of Health Care—United States. 3. Health Policy—United States. WA 540 AA1]
RA395.A3
362.10973—dc23
                                                                                2013013537

Printed in the United States of America
FOURTH EDITION
HB Printing   10 9 8 7 6 5 4

CONTENTS

PART FIVE: DIRECTIONS FOR CHANGE   621

22 Public Health and Clinical Care 681

23 Strengthening the Safety Net 703

FIGURES AND TABLES

Figures

Tables

FOREWORD TO THE THIRD EDITION

The book you hold in your hand is a gift. With his wife, Audrey, the late Samuel J. Tibbitts gave generously to the Department of Health Services in the UCLA School of Public Health to commission a study of key issues in health policy and management challenging the U.S. health care system. The leadership, scholarship, and charity that Sam exhibited in making this gift typified his life in a number of ways.

Sam changed the health care system in California and the nation, perhaps as much as anyone else of his generation. After receiving a B.S. in public health from the University of California, Los Angeles, in 1949 and an M.S. in public health and hospital administration from the University of California, Berkeley, in 1950, he pioneered the development of integrated health care delivery and financing systems. His career course trajectory led in 1988 to the creation of the nonprofit UniHealth America, where he was chairman of the board until his death in 1994.

Along the way, Sam founded and chaired both PacifiCare Health Systems, one of the first major health maintenance organizations, and American Health Care Systems, a group of thirty-two hospital systems across the country that organized the nation's first preferred provider system, PPO Alliance. Both a leader and a scholar, he served as chairman of the board of trustees of the American Hospital Association and published more than one hundred articles. Sensing the need to establish a corporate conscience in a changing health care environment, he was founding chairman of Guiding Principles for Hospitals, the first program to delineate ethical and quality principles in the industry.

Even while he entered the twilight of a long and storied career, his concern for the future of health care remained. For this reason, he invested in the school that had nurtured him and asked its faculty to address the challenges that are crucial to the future of health care in the United States: those relating to cost, quality, and access.

To achieve Sam Tibbitts's vision, the editors sought to gather, in a single book, "a comprehensive, yet readable" account of these issues. We believe that they succeeded remarkably in the first two editions, published in 1996 and 2001, as well as in their efforts to update those issues in this new edition. In particular, the addition of four new chapters covering such issues as disparities in health and health care, the nursing shortage, and information technology make the volume especially useful in confronting key issues for the new millennium and beyond.

We commend this volume to you, sharing the hope of Sam and Audrey Tibbitts that training and discourse shall result, in turn leading to innovations in policy and management that enable the gift of health to be shared by all.

January 2007

Abdelmonem A. Afifi
dean emeritus and professor of biostatistics
UCLA School of Public Health

Linda Rosenstock
dean, UCLA School of Public Health

FOREWORD TO THE FOURTH EDITION

Our health and that of our family members and friends has as profound an impact on the quality of our daily lives as any experience. Given the importance of health to all our lives, it should come as no surprise that access to medical care and preventive public health measures are fundamental rights captured in the Universal Declaration of Human Rights. Moreover, one hundred countries guarantee or aspire to the right to medical care services in their constitutions. Yet, despite this widespread agreement on the importance of health, the United States has struggled.

The United States does not have a constitutional provision guaranteeing access to health care services and has been an outlier when it comes to health care coverage. A recent study of nineteen Organisation for Economic Co-operation and Development (OECD) countries demonstrated that the United States had fallen to last place in addressing deaths amenable to health care. At least as disturbing as the overall health picture in the United States are the disparities. Men and women with less than a high school diploma can expect to live nearly a decade less than those with a bachelor's degree or higher, and the life-expectancy gap has been widening. Not only are Americans with less education and lower incomes more likely to die, but they are more likely to live with a chronic condition or disability.

The United States is failing to address preventable conditions adequately—from cancer to heart disease, from diabetes to infections. Better population and public health measures could help reduce the hundreds of thousands of deaths linked to preventable causes—overweight and obesity contributed to 216,000 deaths in one year, physical inactivity contributed to 191,000 deaths, and tobacco smoking was linked to 467,000. At the same time, medical care that is accessible and affordable to all, including early interventions, would help reduce the 395,000 deaths linked to high blood pressure and the 190,000 linked to high blood sugar, among others.

Public health insurance has been available in most affluent countries for decades. In 1966, Canada passed the Medical Care Act to ensure all Canadians had access to acute hospital services, and in 1984 the Canada Health Act guaranteed access to a wide range of outpatient care. Canada was hardly the first; social health insurance in Germany began in 1893. Physician services have been covered in Norway since 1912. The United Kingdom created its National Health Service to cover medical services in 1948. Sweden followed suit shortly thereafter in 1955. The spread of health insurance across the globe is not limited to Europe and Canada; Chile passed legislation in the 1950s, Japan has had public health insurance since 1961, and the United Arab Emirates since 1971.

So what happened in the United States? It is not that no one tried to pass health insurance. In fact, a century ago Theodore Roosevelt made health insurance a part of his campaign. Health care was debated as an element for inclusion in FDR's New Deal in the 1930s, but was ultimately omitted due to the fear that it would sink Social Security. In 1945, Truman sought to add health insurance to Social Security, but failed. Finally, in 1965 the Johnson administration succeeded in establishing health insurance for older and poor Americans through Medicare and Medicaid. While there were multiple subsequent attempts to expand coverage, it took nearly fifty years to pass a plan for near-universal expansion. Proposals by Nixon for comprehensive health insurance, which included an employer mandate, and by Carter for universal care funded by payroll taxes, failed. Clinton's initial efforts for universal coverage could not make it through Congress; an expansion of care for children was all that passed.

This edition of *Changing the U.S. Health Care System* comes out at an extraordinary moment in American history. After more than a century of repeated efforts, the United States is taking a major step closer to universal health coverage. The Affordable Care Act is expected to cover twenty-nine million more Americans and improve the coverage of many others. With tens of millions of Americans uncovered or poorly covered by health insurance and with a national debt that many have argued cannot be addressed without improving the efficiency and effectiveness of U.S. health care expenditures, the need is urgent.

Leaders in their fields, the contributors to *Changing the U.S. Health Care System* lay out foundational information for the generation who will lead us at this critical stage and address the issues central to transforming American health care. The contributors examine crucial questions including: Are we supporting the social conditions and providing the services needed to prevent illness and injuries? Once people become sick, do Americans have access to the care they need? Is the medical care provided affordable to the individuals and communities receiving it, and to society as a whole? Are we providing the best quality of care we can? Is the same quality of medical care accessible to poor and marginalized populations? Each of these questions is covered from many angles.

In looking at access to care, the book begins with an in-depth look at the Affordable Care Act, the greatest transformation in access to medical care the United States has seen in generations. Other chapters investigate what can be done to extend overall coverage, coverage through private insurers, as well as coverage through the largest public system, Medicare. In examining quality, chapters in the book focus on how we can successfully measure outcomes that will lead to improving quality of life—the ultimate outcome—and change health care delivery systems. Improving health care is covered with particular attention to addressing disparities, be they due to age, ethnicity, social class, or position. Similarly broad and deep in its attention to costs, the book examines cost trends, the best ways to measure expenses, approaches to containing costs, and new drivers of costs, including expansion in pharmaceutical access and the implications for pricing; it also addresses issues looming large on the horizon, like long-term care. Importantly, as health care is only half of the equation, commonly coming into play only after people become sick or injured, *Changing the U.S. Health Care System* examines how social conditions shape health in the first place.

In striving to ensure that we all understand the opportunities and challenges the United States faces in transforming health and health care, the contributors to and readers of *Changing the U.S. Health Care System* could not be taking on a more important task.

August 2013   Jody Heymann
                                  dean, UCLA Fielding School of Public Health

THE EDITOR

Gerald F. Kominski is a professor of health policy and management and director of the UCLA Center for Health Policy Research in the UCLA Fielding School of Public Health. He also currently serves as an associate director of the California Medicaid Research Institute (CaMRI), a multicampus organizational unit that brings together University of California researchers to collaborate with the California Department of Health Services on issues related to the Medi-Cal program.

Dr. Kominski's research interests focus on evaluating the costs and cost-effectiveness of health care programs and interventions, with a special emphasis on public insurance programs, including Medicare, Medicaid, and Workers' Compensation. He is principal investigator at UCLA of a joint project with the UC Berkeley Center for Labor Research and Education to develop and apply the California Simulation of Insurance Markets (CalSIM) model. CalSIM is currently being used to develop estimates for the California Health Benefit Exchange Board to determine eligibility and likely enrollment in the subsidized exchange starting in 2014.

Prior to joining the faculty at UCLA in 1989, Dr. Kominski worked for three and a half years as a staff member for the agency now known as the Medicare Payment Advisory Commission (MedPAC), which develops recommendations for Congress regarding updates to Medicare payment policy. Dr. Kominski is a fellow of Academy Health and a member of the National Academy of Social Insurance. Dr. Kominski received his PhD in public policy analysis from the University of Pennsylvania Wharton School in 1985 and his AB in chemistry from the University of Chicago in 1978.

THE AUTHORS

John L. Adams is a senior statistician in the health program at RAND. His current work focuses on improved quantitative methods in quality assessment. His interests include statistical methods for profiling managed care organizations, provider groups, and providers. With Elizabeth McGlynn, he has worked on the QA Tools quality measurements system. He is currently involved in the development of a quality measurement system for cancer care and the validation of patient self-reports of quality of care.

Ronald M. Andersen is the Wasserman Professor Emeritus in the UCLA Departments of Health Policy and Management and Sociology. Previously he chaired the Department of Health Services at UCLA and was professor at the University of Chicago, serving for ten years as director of the Center for Health Administration Studies and the Graduate Program in Health Administration. Dr. Andersen has studied health behavior and access to medical care for his entire professional career of almost fifty years. He developed the Behavioral Model of Health Services Use that has been used extensively nationally and internationally as a framework for utilization studies including special studies of minorities, low-income persons, children, women, the elderly, oral health, and the homeless.

Lisa Arangua is senior research analyst in the Department of Family Medicine, David Geffen School of Medicine at UCLA. She has been a health services researcher and policy analyst for more than a decade. She is a National Woodrow Wilson Public Policy and International Affairs Fellow. Prior to her appointment at UCLA, she was on the research staff at UC Data Archive and Technical Assistance at the University of California, Berkeley, where she evaluated health and welfare programs for the state and federal government. Her professional activities include social justice and health, epidemiology, clinical trials, women and child/adolescent health, cancer research, mental health research, illicit drug use and treatment research, and concurrent behavior change research of severely underserved health populations. She received her M.P.P. from UCLA in 1999.

Roshan Bastani is professor in the Department of Health Policy and Management in the Fielding School of Public Health at UCLA. She is a social and health psychologist and her research interests are in chronic disease prevention and control among disadvantaged groups, with a focus on testing the efficacy of patient, community, and health care system–directed interventions to improve access and reduce disparities. Dr. Bastani leads a number of research centers, including the UCLA Kaiser Permanente Center for Health Equity, the UCLA/RAND Prevention Research Center, and the Center for Cancer Prevention and Control Research, all of which are focused on addressing health disparities.

Sebastian E. Baumeister, is a senior epidemiologist and a member of the faculty at the University of Greifswald. As head of the statistics unit of the Study of Health in Pomerania, a large population-based cohort study, he is primarily responsible for statistical analyses and consulting. Previously he worked on other large-scale epidemiological studies, including the German Epidemiological Survey of Substance Abuse and the WHO MONICA Surveys. He teaches graduate courses in epidemiology and biostatistics. He has published and worked on various research projects in epidemiology, health care access, health economics, and substance use. Currently, he is working on consortia investigating the role of genetic background on social science phenotypes.

Jeanne T. Black received her PhD in health services research from UCLA and currently is manager of Health Policy Research at Cedars-Sinai Health System in Los Angeles. Her research interests include the effect of health reform incentives on academic medical centers and the cross-cultural validity of health outcomes measures. She was formerly associate director of the Health Policy Institute at the University of Pittsburgh's Graduate School of Public Health, where she conducted research on employer-sponsored health insurance. Dr. Black received an MBA from the Kellogg School of Management at Northwestern University in 1977, and she has extensive experience in strategic planning and management of health services organizations.

The late *Lester Breslow* received his MD from the University of Minnesota in 1938 and his MPH from the University of Minnesota in 1941. Before coming to UCLA in 1968, he was director of the California Department of Health. He served as dean of the UCLA School of Public Health from 1972 to 1980 and was professor emeritus until his death in 2012. He was a past president of the American Public Health Association, the International Epidemiological Association, and the Association of Schools of Public Health. Dr. Breslow received the American Public Health Association's Sedgwick Memorial Medal and was a member of the Institute of Medicine and recipient of its Lienhard Award.

The late *E. Richard Brown* was professor in the Department of Health Policy and Management in the UCLA Fielding School of Public Health, developer and principal investigator of the California Health Interview Survey, Director of the National Network of State and Local Health Surveys, and the Founding Director Emeritus of the UCLA Center for Health Policy Research prior to his death in 2012. He served on numerous study committees of the Institute of Medicine and was a past president of the American Public Health Association, from which he received the Sedgwick Memorial Medal. He received his PhD in sociology of education from the University of California, Berkeley.

Arturo Vargas Bustamante is assistant professor, Department of Health Policy and Management, UCLA Fielding School of Public Health. His research focuses on population groups that are overwhelmingly uninsured or that have poor access to health care, predominantly among Hispanics or Latinos and immigrants. He specializes in the statistical analyses of disparities in health care access, utilization, quality, and insurance coverage. The outcomes of his research have had direct policy applications, particularly since they estimate the share of disparities that can be attributed to socioeconomic and demographic factors and the corresponding part associated to health system variables, such as usual source of care and insurance status.

William S. Comanor is professor of health policy and management at UCLA and also professor of economics at UC Santa Barbara. At UCLA, he is director of the Research Program in Pharmaceutical Economics and Policy. His doctoral dissertation at Harvard was entitled *The Economics of Research and Development in the Pharmaceutical Industry*, and this subject remains a primary topic of his research. He has written many articles on facts of the pharmaceutical industry and lectured throughout the world on related issues.

William E. Cunningham, MD, is a professor in the Department of Health Policy and Management, UCLA Fielding, School of Public Health, and in the Division of General Internal Medicine, Department of Medicine, UCLA Geffen School of Medicine. He was trained as a Robert Wood Johnson Foundation Clinical Scholar. He has led numerous federally funded research projects. He has authored more than 110 scientific papers, many of which address access to care, barriers to medical care, linkage and retention in care, use of HIV services, racial disparities, HIV prevention, and health outcomes. He teaches courses on health services organization and effectiveness and outcomes research.

Pamela L. Davidson is the director of the UCLA Clinical and Translational Science Institute (CTSI) Evaluation Program and associate professor in the Schools of Public Health and Nursing. Her expertise is in health services research and evaluation design and methods. She teaches graduate courses in evaluation research and health systems and organizations. Methodologically her research involves conceptualizing and analyzing individual and contextual variables to predict access and access outcomes. Her research and professional interests include leadership and organizational development, and a systems perspective to investigate the effectiveness of policy and the performance of the health care delivery system.

Linda Delp is director of the UCLA Labor Occupational Safety and Health Program (UCLA-LOSH) and teaches in the Community Health Sciences Department of the Fielding School of Public Health. Her research focuses on home care workers in California; occupational health disparities of teenage, low-wage, and immigrant workers; the effectiveness of worker education and empowerment programs to change workplace and public policy; and the integration of occupational health and health promotion programs. She is chairperson of the Occupational Health and Safety Section of the American Public Health Association.

Jonathan E. Fielding, MD, is director of public health and health officer for Los Angeles County. He is also vice-chair and commissioner of the First 5 LA Commission, and distinguished professor at the UCLA Geffen School of Medicine and Fielding School of Public Health. He chaired the national 2020 Healthy People Project, chairs the U.S. Community Preventive Services Task Force, is editor of the Annual Review of Public Health, and serves on the federal Advisory Group on Prevention, Health Promotion, and Integrative and Public Health. He earned medical and public health degrees from Harvard and his MBA from the Wharton School of Business.

Paul Fu Jr., MD, is associate professor of pediatrics and health policy and management at the David Geffen School of Medicine at UCLA and UCLA Fielding School of Public Health. He is director, clinical informatics, and director of general pediatrics inpatient service at Harbor-UCLA Medical Center. He was previously chief medical information officer at the Los Angeles County Department of Health Services, one of the largest public health service delivery systems in the country. Dr. Fu also leads the Center for Biomedical and Public Health Informatics at the Los Angeles Biomedical Research Institute. Dr. Fu is a graduate of Boston University School of Medicine and completed postgraduate medical training in pediatrics.

Patricia A. Ganz, MD, is professor of health policy and management at the UCLA Fielding School of Public Health and professor of medicine at the David Geffen School of Medicine at UCLA. Dr. Ganz is a medical oncologist and health outcomes researcher who teaches courses on public health ethics and evidence-based medicine. Dr. Ganz was elected to the Institute of Medicine in 2007 and serves as vice-chair of its National Cancer Policy Forum. Her major research interests include cancer survivorship and late effects of cancer treatment, cancer in the elderly, and quality of care for cancer patients.

Lillian Gelberg is a family physician, health services researcher, and professor in UCLA's Department of Family Medicine and Fielding School of Public Health and the VA Greater Los Angeles Healthcare System. She is an elected member of the Institute of Medicine of the National Academy of Sciences and associate director of the UCLA Primary Care Research Fellowship. Her current research focuses on clinical trials to promote healthy lifestyle change in low-income populations using leading behavior change methodologies supported by wireless technology. Over the past two decades, Dr. Gelberg has conducted community-based health services research to improve the health of our nation's most vulnerable populations and has developed the art and science of collecting data under the most difficult field conditions, including the shelters, meal programs, parks, streets, and busy community health centers of Los Angeles County.

Beth A. Glenn is adjunct assistant professor in the Department of Health Policy and Management at the UCLA Fielding School of Public Health and assistant researcher in the UCLA Division of Cancer Prevention and Control Research. Her main research interests are in the area of cancer prevention and control among ethnic minority and underserved populations. She has been involved in a variety or research projects since she joined UCLA in 2001, including surveys focused on understanding factors that predict cancer prevention behaviors and intervention studies aimed at promoting cancer screening and lifestyle changes. She received her PhD in clinical health psychology from Finch University of Health Sciences and the Chicago Medical School in 2001.

Erin G. Grinshteyn is a PhD candidate in the Department of Health Policy and Management at the UCLA Fielding School of Public Health. In addition to HIV, her research interests include aging across the life and violence and injury prevention. She is currently finishing a dissertation that examines the link between fear of neighborhood crime and mental health outcomes and service utilization among adolescents.

Neal Halfon, MD, is director of the UCLA Center for Healthier Children, Families, and Communities and the National Center for Infant and Early Childhood Health Policy. He is also professor of pediatrics in the David Geffen School of Medicine at UCLA, health policy and management in the UCLA Fielding School of Public Health, and policy studies in the UCLA School of Public Affairs. Dr. Halfon was a member of the Board on Children, Youth, and Families of the National Research Council and Institute of Medicine from 2001 to 2006. In 2006, the ambulatory Pediatric Association awarded him its annual Research Award in recognition of his lifetime achievement in the field of pediatric research.

Ron D. Hays is a professor of medicine in the UCLA Department of Medicine and an adjunct researcher at RAND. He specializes in research and teaching courses in health-related quality of life, patient evaluations of care, and health-related behavior. He is a principal investigator for the

Consumer Assessment of Healthcare Providers and Systems (CAHPS®) project. Hays was editor-in-chief of *Quality of Life Research* and is a former deputy editor of *Medical Care*. He is a member of the *Journal of General Internal Medicine* special methodology panel. Dr. Hays has published 451 peer-reviewed articles and thirty-six book chapters.

Moira Inkelas is associate professor in the Department of Health Policy and Management, UCLA Fielding School of Public Health, and assistant director of the UCLA Center for Healthier Children, Families, and Communities. She received her MPH in 1993 and her doctorate in public policy analysis at the Frederick S. Pardee RAND Graduate School in 2000. Here research interests include systems of care for children with special health care needs, tailoring managed care and health care financing policies to the needs of children with chronic illness, impact of systems on quality and performance, measuring quality of care, and quality improvement.

Robert M. Kaplan is NIH associate director for behavioral and social sciences (Office of the Director) and director of the Office of Behavioral and Social Sciences Research (OBSSR). Prior to working for NIH, Kaplan was distinguished professor of health services and medicine at UCLA. His nearly five hundred publications have been cited in more than 25,000 papers, and the ISI includes him in the listing of the most cited authors in his field (defined as above the 99.5th percentile). In 2005 he was elected to the Institute of Medicine of the National Academies of Sciences.

Kathryn G. Kietzman is a research scientist at the UCLA Center for Health Policy Research and assistant researcher in the Department of Community Health Sciences, UCLA Fielding School of Public Health. Her primary research projects are concerned with the health and social care needs of community-dwelling older adults and their families. Kietzman was a Health and Aging Policy Fellow (2008–2010) in the office of United States Senator Debbie Stabenow of Michigan. She currently serves on the board of directors for the American Society on Aging and for the Center for Health Care Rights in Los Angeles County.

Kenneth W. Kizer is a distinguished professor in the University of California, Davis, School of Medicine and the Betty Irene Moore School of Nursing, and the director of the Institute for Population Health Improvement in the UC Davis Health System. His previous positions have included president, CEO, and chairman, Medsphere Systems Corporation; founding president and CEO, National Quality Forum; undersecretary for health, U.S. Department of Veterans Affairs; and director, California Department of Health Services. He is a member of the Institute of Medicine, National Academy of Sciences, and the National Academy of Public Administration.

Michelle Ko, MD, holds a joint appointment as a postdoctoral fellow in the Department of Medicine and the Philip R. Lee Institute of Health Policy Studies at UCSF. Her general areas of research interest include disparities in health and health care, health care safety net systems, and diversity in the health professions workforce. Her work particularly focuses on the intersection of health care delivery and social context, and how this leads to the production of disparities.

Ellen T. Kurtzman is assistant research professor in the School of Nursing at the George Washington University. In the past, she has worked for the National Quality Forum, American Health Care, and National PACE Associations, and American Red Cross and has served as a senior examiner for the Malcolm Baldrige National Quality Award. Ms. Kurtzman holds a bachelor's degree in nursing from the University of Pennsylvania and master's degree in public health from Johns Hopkins University. She and is a fellow of the American Academy of Nursing and a member of Sigma Theta Tau International.

Shana Alex Lavarreda is a research scientist at the UCLA Center for Health Policy Research. As the center's director of health insurance studies, she works with numerous projects, including the State of Health Insurance in California, the California Health Benefits Review Program, and the California Health Interview Survey. Her research focuses on discontinuous health insurance and access to care, underinsurance, and political issues surrounding health care reform. She received her master's degree in public policy from the UCLA Luskin School of Public Affairs and her PhD in health services from the UCLA Fielding School of Public Health.

Mark S. Litwin teaches in the UCLA Geffen School of Medicine and Fielding School of Public Health and practices urologic oncology at UCLA, where he specializes in the surgical management of patients with testicular, bladder, prostate, kidney, and penile cancer. He is a translational population scientist who has authored numerous original articles, reports, reviews, and book chapters in urologic oncology and health services research. Dr. Litwin published the first validated quality-of-life instrument to track outcomes in men with prostate cancer and has been an international leader in this area. Dr. Litwin's research includes medical outcomes assessment, quality of care, health-related quality of life, epidemiology, costs and resource utilization, patient preferences, and health care access for malignant and benign diseases in urology.

Jeff Luck is associate professor of health management and policy at the College of Public Health and Human Sciences, Oregon State University, and adjunct associate professor of health policy and management at the UCLA Fielding School of Public Health. His informatics research focuses on aggregation, analysis, and dissemination of data to support research, management, and policy analysis in public health, quality measurement, cancer research, and integrated health care systems. He received his MBA from the Anderson Graduate School of Management at UCLA and his PhD in public policy analysis from the Frederick S. Pardee RAND Graduate School of Policy Studies.

Elizabeth A. McGlynn is the director of Kaiser Permanente's Center for Effectiveness and Safety Research (CESR). She is responsible for the strategic direction and scientific oversight of CESR. Dr. McGlynn is an internationally known expert on methods for evaluating the appropriateness, quality, and efficiency of health care delivery. She has conducted research in the United States and in other countries. Dr. McGlynn has also led major initiatives to evaluate health reform options under consideration at the federal and state levels. She is a member of the Institute of Medicine and serves on several boards and national advisory committees.

Leo S. Morales is a physician-investigator at the Group Health Research Institute and associate professor of health services at the University of Washington. He received his MD and MPH from the University of Washington and his PhD in policy studies from the RAND Graduate School. Dr. Morales's research areas include health services, disparities in health and health care, and measurement of patient-reported outcomes. In addition to his research activities, Dr. Morales is a practicing general internist in the Group Health delivery system.

Jack Needleman is professor in the Department of Health Policy and Management at the UCLA Fielding School of Public Health. His research on nurse staffing and patient outcomes in hospitals and business case for nursing received the AcademyHealth Health Services Research Impact

Award in 2006. Other research has examined the performance of quality improvement programs, safety net hospitals, and nonprofit and public hospital conversions to for-profit status. He is a member of the Institute of Medicine.

Alexander N. Ortega is professor of health policy and management in the UCLA Fielding School of Public Health, he is the principal investigator of the UCLA Center for Population Health and Health Disparities, and he is the associate director of the UCLA Chicano Studies Research Center. He conducts research on health disparities with a particular focus on Latino children and families. Prior to joining the UCLA faculty, he was assistant professor of health policy and administration at Yale University and associate professor of public health at the Ohio State University. At UCLA, he teaches graduate courses in research methods, health services organization, and health care inequities.

Ninez A. Ponce is a professor in the Department of Health Policy and Management at the UCLA Fielding School of Public Health, and senior research scientist at the UCLA Center for Health Policy Research, where she is the principal investigator of the California Health Interview Survey. Trained as a health economist, her research focuses on understanding the intersection of race or ethnicity, immigration status, gender, and socioeconomic status with health care systems to improve access to health insurance, and health care in the United States. Dr. Ponce received her BS degree at UC Berkeley, MPP at Harvard University, and PhD at UCLA.

Nadereh Pourat is professor of health policy and management at the UCLA Fielding School of Public Health and director of research at the UCLA Center for Health Policy Research. Her research interests and publications include diverse topics ranging from disparities in access to health care to primary care redesign—including implementation and outcomes of patient-centered medical home—to safety-net system integration and care delivery challenges, long-term care services, and oral health care. She received her PhD in health services at UCLA.

Thomas H. Rice is distinguished professor, Department of Health Policy and Management, in the UCLA Fielding School of Public Health. He is a health economist, with a doctorate in economics from the University of California, Berkeley. His areas of interest include health insurance, competition, physicians' economic behavior, and Medicare. The third edition of his book, *The Economics of Health Reconsidered*, was published in 2009. He served as editor of the journal *Medical Care Research and Review* from 1994 to 2000. Dr. Rice was elected to the Institute of Medicine of the National Academy of Sciences in 2006.

Dylan H. Roby is assistant professor of Health Policy and Management in the UCLA Fielding School of Public Health and director of health economics and evaluation research in the UCLA Center for Health Policy Research. Dr. Roby studies access to care, care delivery in the safety net, and chronic illness management and quality. He is also an expert on the Affordable Care Act and modeling its potential impacts. He teaches courses in health policy and health services in the Fielding School. Dr. Roby earned his BA in geography from UCLA and his PhD in public policy from the George Washington University.

Hector P. Rodriguez is associate professor of health policy and management at the UC Berkeley School of Public Health. His research focuses on clarifying the organizational influences on medical care quality and public health system effectiveness, performance measurement, and patients' experiences of ambulatory care. Dr. Rodriguez earned his PhD in health policy and medical sociology from Harvard University, MPH in health administration from University of California, Berkeley, and BA in urban studies and planning from University of California, San Diego. He is the 2011 recipient of the Thompson Prize for Young Investigators from the Association of University Programs in Health Administration.

The late *Ruth Roemer* joined the UCLA faculty in 1962 and was professor emerita in the Department of Health Services (now Health Policy and Management) in the UCLA School of Public Health from 1980 until her death in 2005. She taught courses in health law, ethical issues, tobacco control, and public policy. In a career spanning more than sixty years, her research involved studies of mental hospital admission law, education and legal regulation of health personnel, laws governing abortion and family planning, organization of health services, and legislation for tobacco control. Roemer received her JD degree from Cornell University Law School in 1939.

Pauline Vaillancourt Rosenau is a professor at the University of Texas School of Public Health. She has authored or edited eight books and authored or coauthored more than seventy professional peer-reviewed articles and book chapters. She wrote *The Competition Paradigm: America's Romance with Conflict, Contest, and Commerce* (Rowman & Littlefield, 2003) and *Post-Modernism in the Social Sciences* (Princeton, 1992), which has been translated into Chinese, Korean, and Turkish. She does research on the topics of national and comparative international health policy, public-private policy partnerships, competition, the implications of investor status for the provision of health services, pharmacy policy, long-term care, and postmodernism.

Linda Rosenstock was dean of the UCLA School of Public Health from 2000 to 2012 and currently serves at UCLA as professor in the Departments of Health Policy and Management, Environmental Health Sciences, and Medicine. Prior to joining UCLA, Dr. Rosenstock served for seven years as the director of the National Institute for Occupational Safety and Health (NIOSH). Dr. Rosenstock is a recognized authority in environmental and occupational health as well as global public health and science policy. In 2011 she was also appointed by President Barack Obama to the Advisory Group on Prevention, Health Promotion, and Integrative and Public Health.

Stuart O. Schweitzer is a professor in the Department of Health Policy and Management at the UCLA Fielding School of Public Health. He teaches courses in health economics, health systems, and pharmaceutical policy. He served as senior staff at The Urban Institute, the National Institutes of Health, and President Carter's Commission for a National Agenda for the Eighties. He has held visiting appointments at universities in Oxford, Paris, and Shanghai, and is currently a visiting professor of economics at the University of Ferrara (Italy). His research interests are in industrial policy, health policy pertaining to pharmaceuticals, and genetics. He codirects the UCLA Research Program in Pharmaceutical Economics and Policy.

Steven M. Teutsch, MD, is the chief science officer, Los Angeles County Public Health. He is retired from Merck and CDC, where most recently he was responsible for assessing the effectiveness, safety, and cost-effectiveness of disease and injury prevention strategies and developing CDC's quantitative policy analysis capacity and the *Guide to Community Preventive Services*. He served on the U.S. Preventive Services Task Force, IOM panels, MEDCAC, and on subcommittees of the Secretary's Advisory Committee on Healthy People 2020. He chaired the Secretary's Advisory Committee on Genetics

Health and Society. Dr. Teutsch has published over 190 articles and eight books.

Leah J. Vriesman is director of executive education programs in the Department of Health Policy and Management and faculty in UCLA's Fielding School of Public Health. She teaches strategic management, international health systems, and health care financial management. Dr. Vriesman is also an adjunct professor at the University of Colorado Denver, teaching international pharmaceutical marketing. As a 2010–2011 U.S. Fulbright grant recipient, Dr. Vriesman lived in Bavaria while analyzing German HIT initiatives at the University of Applied Sciences, Neu Ulm. Dr. Vriesman is also president and founder of Excel Research, LLC, a strategic leadership consulting firm specializing in the pharmaceutical and biotechnology industry.

Steven P. Wallace is professor and chair of the Department of Community Health Sciences at the UCLA Fielding School of Public Health and associate director of the UCLA Center for Health Policy Research. Wallace is a leading scholar nationally on aging in communities of color. He has published research on access to long-term care by diverse elderly, disparities in the consequences of health policy changes on racial or ethnic minority elderly, and the politics of aging. Wallace is a fellow of the Gerontological Society of America and received his doctorate in sociology from the University of California, San Francisco.

David Lee Wood MD, MPH, Clinical Professor of Pediatrics, University of Florida, is board certified in Pediatrics and in Preventive Medicine and Public Health and completed a health services research fellowship at RAND/UCLA. For over twenty years his research and advocacy efforts have focused on improving health systems for underserved children and adults. He has served on the American Academy of Pediatrics Council on Community Pediatrics and Committee on Psychosocial Aspects of Child and Family Health. He is the past President of the North East Florida Pediatric Society. Since 2007 he has directed the Jacksonville Health and Transition Services (JaxHATS) program. He is also codirector of the University of Florida College of Medicine-Jacksonville Center for Health Equity and Quality Research.

The late *Antronette K. (Toni) Yancey*, MD, was professor in the Department of Health Policy and Management and codirector of the UCLA Kaiser

Permanente Center for Health Equity in the UCLA Fielding School of Public Health. Prior to her death in 2013, she served in public health practice, first as director of Public Health for Richmond, Virginia, and then as founding director of chronic disease prevention for Los Angeles County. Dr. Yancey served on the boards of directors of Action for Healthy Kids and the Partnership for a Healthier America, the nonprofit supporting First Lady Michelle Obama's Let's Move campaign. Dr. Yancey was also a published poet and spoken word artist.

Frederick J. Zimmerman is a professor in the Department of Health Policy and Management in the UCLA Fielding School of Public Health. He holds a PhD in economics from the University of Washington and has written extensively about the economic factors that impinge on individual decision making and their effects on population health. Dr. Zimmerman teaches the ethics course in the department's MPH program.

*This volume is dedicated to the memory of
my esteemed colleagues who made contributions to this edition
but who are no longer with us—Lester Breslow, Ruth Roemer,
Rick Brown, and, most recently, Antronette (Toni) Yancey. May your
good work continue to inspire the next generation of public
health professionals. And, to my wife, Laurie, who inspires me daily and
who has shared with me the most wonderful journey I could
ever have imagined.*

INTRODUCTION AND OVERVIEW

The Patient Protection and Affordable Care Act of 2010, now more commonly known simply as the Affordable Care Act (ACA), is the most significant piece of U.S. health legislation since the enactment of Medicare and Medicaid in 1965. At the time of its enactment, the ACA was expected to extend health insurance coverage to thirty-two million uninsured U.S. citizens and permanent residents by 2016, reducing the portion of uninsured legal residents from 17 percent to 5 percent.

How did this major piece of legislation get enacted after several failed attempts to expand health insurance to all Americans during the forty-five years between the enactment of Medicare and Medicaid in 1965 and the ACA's enactment in 2010? And will the ACA finally achieve the goal of providing (nearly) universal access to health insurance in the United States while promoting higher-quality care at an affordable and sustainable rate of growth in health care expenditures into the future? These are fundamental questions that will be explored throughout this book.

Since the first edition was published in 1996, just a few short years after the failed effort of President Clinton to enact universal health insurance, this book's major goal has been to discuss the fundamental challenges facing the U.S. health care system and to provide readers with both conceptual frameworks and the most current empirical evidence necessary to formulate effective strategies for innovation. At the time of this writing, the United States stands poised to undertake a fundamental reform of health care financing in almost five decades. It goes without saying that the ACA will have profound effects on health care financing and delivery in the United States for decades to come. My coauthors and I believe this book will continue to be a valuable tool for understanding not only the expected impacts of the ACA over the next decade, but for understanding the impacts of the other significant trends in health care that have been occurring independently of the ACA.

This fourth edition follows the general format of the first three. The goal of this book is still to examine in a comprehensive and careful manner current issues in health care policy and management. This edition, in contrast to earlier editions, is intended to reach a broader audience by serving also as an introduction to current issues and challenges facing the U.S. health care system. I have asked authors of revised chapters in this edition both to emphasize recent developments in their area of expertise and to address the implications of the ACA for their topic areas. Further, to make the fourth edition more comprehensive, I have added new chapters on the ACA, multilevel social determinants of health, health delivery system innovations, and efforts to strengthen the safety net.

This book continues to aim at providing, in a single source, a comprehensive and readable account of the issues facing the United States in health care policy and management. I intend for it to continue to benefit a variety of audiences:

- Students, who will benefit from having a comprehensive and up-to-date introduction to the core subject areas in health care policy and management
- Health service researchers and policy analysts, who will find it useful to have ready access to the state of the art in research, as well as analysis of policy options relevant to many aspects of the health care market
- Health care managers, who will benefit from having a single source of information on how to promote quality and better health outcomes while controlling expenditures
- Practitioners and providers, especially doctors and nurses, who will find issues of special interest addressed in various chapters

Organization and Summary of the Volume

This volume, like the previous editions, is divided into five parts. Each section contains three or more chapters relevant to that particular topic. The first three parts are on the three key components of health care policy: access, costs, and quality. In each section, there are chapters on measurement and trends, as well as chapters on policy options. The fourth part addresses special populations, with individual chapters on long-term care and the elderly, HIV/AIDS, children's health, and the homeless. The fifth and final part concerns proposals for reform, with chapters on delivery system innovation, Medicare reform, public and personal health, strengthening the safety net, and ethical issues in public health and health services management.

Access to Health Care

It is particularly appropriate to start with this topic. Understanding access is essential to addressing major challenges to our health care system today: health and health care disparities. Despite the tremendous attention they have received, both in research and in policy, there are more uninsured people in the country now than in previous decades. The United States holds the dubious distinction of being the only developed country that does not ensure access to health care through guaranteed coverage. Furthermore, many analysts believe that one of the major barriers to controlling health care costs is exactly this lack of universal coverage. This is not only because it is difficult for poor and sick people to seek preventive care but also because it fragments the financing system, requiring the existence of an expensive safety net as well as aggravating the problem of cost shifting. The ACA promises to address many of the negative consequences of a fragmented delivery and financing system, but expanded access to health insurance may not be sufficient to guarantee improved health and reduced disparities.

Chapter One, by Gerald F. Kominski, is new to this edition and describes in detail the provisions of the ACA dealing with insurance expansion. The chapter first describes the political environment leading to the eventual passage of the ACA, and argues that the managed competition model first outlined by Alain Enthoven in the late 1970s served as a crucial blueprint not only for the ACA, but also for the failed health reform effort of President Clinton and the successful effort enacted by Massachusetts in 2006. The chapter then goes on to describe the major components of the health insurance expansion contained in the law, including the expansion of state Medicaid programs, the establishment of state-based insurance exchanges, the standardization of insurance policies and plans sold in the exchanges, and the provision of federal subsidies for low- and middle-income families and individuals to purchase insurance in the exchanges. The chapter concludes by discussing the likely impacts of the

ACA on major stakeholders in the health care system, including payers, providers, employers, and the uninsured.

Chapter Two, by Ronald M. Andersen, Pamela L. Davidson, and Sebastian E. Baumeister, is a comprehensive examination of access to health care. The authors argue that understanding access is the key to understanding health policy because the access framework (1) predicts and measures health service use, (2) can be used to promote social justice, and (3) can be used to promote health outcomes. The chapter explains the multiple dimensions of access using a revised version of the behavioral model that emphasizes contextual as well as individual determinants of health services utilization. It goes on to discuss how access can be measured and presents data on the levels of access and trends in the United States. Certain trends emerge from this analysis: though an increasing number of people are being covered by Medicaid, there has been a decline in the number covered by private insurance in the last twenty years and an overall increase in the proportion without any health insurance coverage, and low-income and African American populations appear to have achieved equity of access according to gross measures of hospital and physician utilization, not taking into account their greater need for medical care in the United States. Minorities and those with low income continue to lag considerably in receipt of dental care, and equity has certainly not been achieved according to health insurance coverage, what with the proportion of uninsured 50 percent higher for blacks and more than twice as high for Hispanics and the low-income population compared to the uninsured rate for non-Hispanic whites.

Chapter Three, by Antronette K. Yancey, Roshan Bastani, and Beth A. Glenn, describes current health status disparities, reviews the potential determinants of observed disparities, and outlines future directions for policy and practice, with specific emphasis on the contribution of chronic diseases. They show socioeconomic status is a major contributor to ethnic disparities in health. However, income inequality may also be an important contributor to poorer health, and economic indicators demonstrate that the gap between rich and poor is increasing dramatically while opportunities for upward social mobility are decreasing. They suggest that discrimination is the primary social environmental contribution to health disparities. Health services policy and health care organizations must reach beyond their accustomed boundaries of medical care delivery to address the physical, social, and economic environmental conditions underlying health disparities.

Chapter Four, by Arturo Vargas Bustamante, Leo S. Morales, and Alexander N. Ortega, adds another perspective on racial and ethnic disparities, switching the focus from health to health care disparities. They begin by defining disparities in care and reviewing some of the historical factors that have contributed to the pattern of disparity we observe today. In the next sections, they summarize some of the evidence documenting racial and ethnic disparities in the treatment of specific disease diseases and discuss some ongoing initiatives to reduce disparities in care. They show that disparities in health care are prevalent, with racial and ethnic minorities receiving lower-quality care in a variety of health care settings and across a range of medical conditions. A variety of factors contributes to disparities in care, among them legal and structural factors as well as patient and provider factors. The authors discuss multiple, ongoing efforts to address racial and ethnic disparities in care. They conclude that if current care disparities are not overcome, minority patients can be expected to continue to have suboptimal health status, which will in turn negatively affect labor market productivity and increase national health care spending.

Chapter Five, by Ninez A. Ponce and Michelle Ko, is new to this edition and discusses the social determinants of health. The authors first present and discuss two conceptual models for the social determinants of health—the World Health Organization's Commission on Social Determinants of Health model and the Robert Wood Johnson Foundation's Commission to Build a Healthier America framework. They then focus on five contextual-level social determinants that have been conceptualized as generating the social processes that lead to health and health inequities. They conclude that several of these factors—income, income inequality, racial or ethnic composition, and residential segregation—produce inequities in health care and may ultimately undermine population health.

Chapter Six, by Shana Alex Lavarreda and E. Richard Brown, examines the significant role of public insurance programs for covering the uninsured and improving access for populations who are not well served by private insurance markets. The authors discuss the successes and failures of Medicare, Medicaid, and the Children's Health Insurance Program (CHIP), with regard to giving their beneficiaries access to affordable, high-quality coverage. They also provide a detailed historical discussion of the difficult road to universal health insurance in the United States and the political circumstances leading to the major expansion of health insurance enacted as part of the ACA.

Chapter Seven, by Nadereh Pourat and Gerald F. Kominski, discusses the private insurance markets, including employment-based group insurance markets and the nongroup market for individually purchased insurance. The authors provide data describing private markets in detail and define a number of key terms and concepts relevant to private insurance markets. The chapter describes the various models of managed care that have evolved from the traditional model of prepaid group practice. It then summarizes the growth in managed care during the past three decades and the factors that have contributed to its growth, as well as the managed care backlash that began in the late 1990s. They conclude that the ACA will fundamentally change the individual (nongroup) market for private insurance and may in the longer term accelerate changes in the large-group market in which the majority of Americans obtain health insurance coverage.

Costs of Health Care

Health care costs have been a major policy concern since the 1970s, when health expenditures began to outpace growth in gross domestic product and thus became an ever-growing share of the nation's economy. There is no shortage of culprits, although most analysts identify a variety of factors—especially the movement away from heavy-handed managed care and continued development of expensive medical and pharmaceutical technologies. At the same time, more Americans than ever lack insurance coverage, and concerns about overall quality persist. It is the trade-offs between costs on the one hand and access and quality on the other that will continue to be the major tension in health care policy for the foreseeable future. The expansion of health insurance coverage associated with the ACA could result in a new round of health care expenditure growth, putting further pressure on policymakers and providers and payers to identify more effective mechanisms for improving quality while controlling cost growth.

Chapter Eight, by Thomas H. Rice, focuses on measuring health care costs and presenting their trends. With regard to measurement, the chapter distinguishes between expenditures and costs, focusing thereafter on the more easily measured concept of expenditures. It also discusses the advantages and disadvantages of various measures of alternative health care prices and expenditures, and the reliability of the data sources that are used to measure expenditures in the United States and throughout the world. The chapter also lays out a discussion of the need for better data in the United States, concluding that requiring private insurers to collect and release data on expenditures is essential for making sensible policy decisions about alternative types of health care reform. As a lead-in to Chapter Nine, it concludes with a look at the reasons that cost control is important and is likely to be on the forefront of health policy for years to come.

Chapter Nine, by Thomas H. Rice and Gerald F. Kominski, focuses on alternative ways of containing health care costs. It begins by developing a conceptual framework that allows cost-containment methods to be divided into two categories: those based on fee for service and those based on capitation. Within fee for service, strategies fall into one of three groups: price controls, volume controls, and expenditure controls. Most of the remainder of the chapter reviews the literature and experiences, both in the United States and in other developed countries, regarding the success and failure of the many strategies employed to contain costs: hospital rate-setting programs, diagnosis-related groups, certificate-of-need programs, utilization review, technology controls, physician fee controls, practice guidelines, expenditure controls, health maintenance organizations, patient cost sharing, and managed competition. Although no conclusions are warranted as to the best way to control costs, the chapter indicates that it is important to continually assess the domestic and international experience regarding the success and failure of both market and government strategies to control health care costs.

Chapter Ten, by Stuart O. Schweitzer and William S. Comanor, examines a particular aspect of health care costs: pharmaceuticals. The costs of pharmaceuticals have been an important policy issue for decades, with concern among many consumer advocates that they are too high and should be controlled. The authors analyze the causes of increasing pharmaceutical costs by critiquing studies conducted by others and then by conducting their own review of drug prices and expenditures over time in the United States and in other countries, adjusting for improvements in quality. They review the many public policies that have been employed to control these costs, which have been aimed at consumers, physicians, and manufacturers. They also discuss current trends, including recent data on the impact of Medicare's Part D pharmacy benefit, which has been newly implemented since the last edition of this book. Although the authors do not reach any definitive conclusion about which policy levers are best, they are particularly concerned whether success can be achieved without sacrificing the vitality and viability of the industry, whose hallmark is a large investment in research and development for new products.

Quality of Health Care

There is little question that establishing and preserving quality in health care has become the leading issue for health care managers. With tremendous competitive pressures to control health care costs, managers are faced with the task of formulating financial incentives and other mechanisms that will help ensure that a high-quality, cost-effective product is provided to patients. The advent of health care report cards and wider dissemination of information on health care quality, especially over the Internet, symbolize consumers' need for easily digestible information on the relative quality of their alternative insurance choices. This interest is paralleled on the research front, where a great deal of effort is being expended to produce reliable measures of health care outcomes.

Chapter Eleven, by Patricia A. Ganz, Ron D. Hays, Robert M. Kaplan, and Mark S. Litwin, examines the measurement of health outcomes and quality of life. After providing a historical perspective on the health outcomes movement, the authors present an overview of the concept of health-related quality of life (HRQL), which focuses on the patient's own perception of health and the ability to function as a result of health status or disease experience. Much of the remainder of the chapter is devoted to the challenging goal of measuring HRQL and to presenting health services research studies that have attempted to measure it. An important conclusion is that patients are most concerned not with prolonging their lives per se, but rather with improving the quality of their remaining years. Therefore, the authors argue, consumers are anxious to have information about the HRQL impact of new treatments. What is needed is careful and appropriate inclusion of HRQL outcomes in traditional health services.

Chapter Twelve, by Elizabeth A. McGlynn, focuses on ensuring quality of care. The chapter begins by considering criteria for selecting topics for quality assessment. Next, it presents a conceptual framework useful for organizing evaluations of the quality. The definitions, methods, and state of the art in assessing the structure, process, and outcomes of care are then discussed. The essential message of this chapter is that scientifically sound methods exist for assessing quality and that they must be employed systematically in the future to guard against deterioration in quality that might otherwise occur as an unintended result of organizational and financial changes in the health services system.

In Chapter Thirteen, Elizabeth A. McGlynn and John L. Adams observe that routine public reports on the quality of health care are being demanded thanks to changes in the organization and financing of care. In the unrestricted-choice model characterized by fee for service, individual providers were accountable for ensuring the delivery of high-quality health care. However, as third parties began to use financial incentives to control costs and restrict choices, the perception (if not the reality) was that physicians could no longer act solely in the patient's interest. Routine reports to the public on the quality of health care are one response to concerns about accountability. This chapter describes the type of information that is currently being publicly released; it discusses some of the methodological issues that arise in producing information for public release and summarizes what is known about the use of information on quality for consumer choice and quality. The authors conclude that the evidence to date on use of report cards by various audiences—consumers, purchasers, providers—suggests that the information is not widely used and appears to have only a small effect on performance. However, it is premature to declare these efforts a failure. Increased attention to the methods that are used to construct report cards, better use of communication techniques known to be effective, and more formal evaluations of such efforts are required before we have the information necessary to draw conclusions about the utility of public reporting.

Chapter Fourteen, by Jeff Luck, Leah Vriesman, and Paul Fu Jr., carries out a crucial examination of the emerging role of health care information systems. The authors argue that such systems have the potential to boost both the efficiency and the quality of the health care system. The chapter begins by defining and presenting examples of the many types of health insurance systems. It goes on to examine how these systems can be applied to public health systems. The chapter also discusses several emerging applications of health insurance systems: imaging, telemedicine, and bioinformatics. It ends with recognition of the increasing importance being placed on privacy and security with the advent of electronic medical records.

Chapter Fifteen, by Jack Needleman, Ellen T. Kurtzman, and Kenneth W. Kizer, reviews recent efforts and issues involved in identifying a set of nursing-sensitive performance measures. It examines the scope of nursing's contribution to hospital care, priorities for measuring nursing care, and current initiatives to develop and implement systems for measuring nursing care, with special emphasis on the National Quality Forum's endorsement of national voluntary consensus standards. The authors conclude that developing effective performance measurement systems will enable stakeholders to better understand and monitor the degree to which nursing care influences patient safety and quality. They also argue that the implementation of value-based payment methods by Medicare and private payers and implementation of the ACA will lead to increased assessment of nursing performance.

Special Populations

The problems of access, cost, and quality have varied historically for segments of the U.S. population because of their special needs and the ways the health care system has responded to those needs. It is likely that the nature of the problems faced by numerous groups will continue to change in the face of major alterations in how health services are organized and financed. All of the authors in Part Four have suggestions for health services research and policy implementation that might improve the prognosis for these vulnerable populations.

Chapter Sixteen, by Steven P. Wallace, Nadereh Pourat, Linda Delp, and Kathryn G. Kietzman, is a comprehensive overview of the long-term care system as a response to the rapidly increasing number of elderly in the United States and their needs for treatment of chronic and disabling illness. This chapter reviews the recent literature on long-term care, showing how financial considerations have framed the dominant policy debates and research agenda. It offers up-to-date information on nursing homes, the range of community-based care, informal long-term care, and workers in the long-term care system. The authors emphasize that long-term care includes social as well as medical services, is furnished overwhelmingly by family and friends, and is financed primarily by Medicaid and out-of-pocket payments. Policymakers frequently view nursing homes as a low-cost alternative to hospitals and consider community services and family care as less expensive substitutes for nursing homes, neglecting quality-of-life issues. The chapter concludes that the limited financial resources of many older persons, especially racial and ethnic minorities, widows, and the working class, create a need for a universal Medicare type of social insurance.

In Chapter Seventeen, Erin G. Grinshteyn and William E. Cunningham argue that the characteristics of HIV/AIDS—contagious, chronically disabling, fatal, and emerging in epidemic proportions—will increasingly force health care policymakers and managers to reevaluate the organization, delivery, and financing of health services for the HIV population. They state that as of 2008, global HIV infections had reached approximately 60 million. More than 33 million people were living with HIV infection, and more than 25 million had died of AIDS. In the United States, an estimated 1.5 million Americans are living with HIV infection, and there have been 524,060 deaths from AIDS. The authors review what is known and the research needs concerning the changing epidemiology and treatment of AIDS, including use of new and expensive antiretroviral drugs; measures of access, costs, and quality; and the range of services needed to treat AIDS, including not only formal medical services but also prevention, psychosocial services, and community-based health and social services. They discuss the growing challenges in providing and paying for services as the HIV/AIDS epidemic spreads from its initial geographic epicenters of Caucasian, homosexual men to much broader communities of socially and economically disadvantaged populations of women, children, adolescents, and minority groups.

Chapter Eighteen, by Moira Inkelas, Neal Halfon, and David Lee Wood, examines the key issues underlying the incongruities between the needs of children and families and the current and evolving structure of the health services organization in the United States. The authors review the health needs of children and families by examining children's unique vulnerabilities, current health risks and conditions, and service needs. Next, they describe the characteristics of the health care system that influence children's access to care and the overall efficiency of health care for children. They find the organization of services to be disjointed, with multiple financial and structural barriers to children's receipt of care, despite recent enactment of the federally supported SCHIP. They note that the movement to manage care to rationalize delivery of personal medical services may substantially improve children's access to basic medical care, but many of their health needs—especially for complex medical or socially based health problems—may not be sufficiently addressed. The authors conclude that adequate response to the health care needs of at-risk children requires greater effort to expand coverage for the uninsured, including greater effort to enroll eligible children in current programs and development of multidisciplinary coordination that integrates the fragmented child health system.

In Chapter Nineteen, Lisa Arangua and Lillian Gelberg describe the sociodemographic characteristics of homeless adults and children as well as their health status, risk factors for illness, barriers to care, quality of care, and current medical programs available to homeless individuals. They estimated that 3.5 million in the United States are currently without a home and that 14 percent of the U.S. population (26 million people) have been homeless at some time in their lives. The homeless constitute a heterogeneous population that includes families, runaway youths, the physically and mentally ill, and substance abusers. The homeless population experiences a high rate of acute and chronic illness but has limited access to medical care as reflected by high inpatient utilization and low ambulatory service use relative to their level of need. The medical care they do receive is limited in terms of availability, continuity, and comprehensiveness. The authors find the homeless particularly vulnerable in the policy arena because of the absence of strong advocates, a tendency on the part of the public to accept large-scale homelessness as inevitable, and commonly held beliefs that the homeless are responsible for their status. Still, their plight could be improved by stabilizing funding for health care, funding respite care, medical education reform, and more affordable housing options. They conclude that the best way to help the homeless is for the United States to address more fundamental issues concerning alleviation of poverty.

Directions for Change

The enactment of the ACA will lead to the largest expansion of health insurance coverage since the passage of Medicare and Medicaid in 1965. But not everyone will be covered, and other significant challenges to improving health care delivery remain. In Part Five, some of these fundamental challenges facing health care researchers, policymakers, and managers are examined in detail.

Chapter Twenty, by Nadereh Pourat and Hector P. Rodriguez, is new to this edition and focuses specifically on the core issue raised in the title of the book—delivery system change and innovation. The authors first present a conceptual model for assessing changes in the delivery system. They then describe various efforts aimed at patients or at providers for changing health care delivery to improve quality and outcomes. They argue that regardless of which innovations prove to be most effective, efforts to improve integration of care delivery and to enhance accountability are now a permanent part of the health care landscape. Therefore, even if current models don't survive, continued innovation is essential for the delivery system to meet what is now commonly referred to as the triple aims of improved health and quality at an affordable cost.

Chapter Twenty-One, by Gerald F. Kominski, Jeanne T. Black, and Thomas H. Rice, examines the federal government's largest health insurance program, Medicare, and the challenges facing its future. The authors review the political conditions leading to enactment of Medicare, which was widely viewed as a compromise on the road to national health insurance when it was enacted in 1965. Fifty years later, Medicare faces several significant challenges, including ongoing cost increases and an expanding eligible population that threaten its public support. These challenges have led to a gradual transformation of Medicare during the past two decades toward greater reliance on private markets and managed care. The authors examine the nature of the "crisis" in Medicare and efforts to reform the program, including the introduction of the Part D prescription drug benefit. This major expansion of benefits and ongoing concerns about the future financial viability of this essential public insurance program are likely to lead to calls for further modification in the future.

In Chapter Twenty-Two, Jonathan E. Fielding, Lester Breslow, and Steven M. Teutsch reexamine the significant role of public health agencies in delivery of personal health services in the United States. They find that these agencies have a vital interest in health care delivery because a substantial portion of the population has inadequate access to services or unstable health benefits. Public health has traditionally been directed at ensuring a safe environment and at addressing behavioral influences on health. Access to quality personal health services made available by the public health system, they argue, is also an important determinant of health. The ability of public health agencies to perform all their core public health functions, however, requires greater commitment to public health and health promotion.

Chapter Twenty-Three, by Dylan H. Roby, is new to this edition and underscores the essential role of the safety net in providing care to the underinsured and the uninsured. The author describes the elements of the safety net and contrasts the differences between a narrow and broad definition of safety-net providers that provide services to vulnerable populations. Under the broader definition, about one-third of the U.S. population relies on the safety net to some extent. Despite the expectation that the ACA will significantly reduce demand for safety net services, there is ample reason to believe that the safety net will still be an essential component of the health care delivery system. As many as twenty million may remain uninsured despite the ACA, and even among those newly insured, many may continue to seek care from safety-net providers. The author concludes that the safety net will need to evolve into coordinated and integrated delivery systems much like the rest of the health care system.

Finally, Chapter Twenty-Four, by Pauline Vaillancourt Rosenau, Ruth Roemer, and Frederick J. Zimmerman, deals with the ethics of public health and health care services. The cardinal principles of medical ethics—autonomy, beneficence, and justice—apply in public health ethics, but in a somewhat altered form. The authors contrast these principles as usually applied in medical ethics (where individual rights and autonomy prevail) with a broader social perspective in which individual rights may be subsumed by consideration of social welfare. At a time when we continue moving toward market-based solutions, the authors construct a framework for reexamining some of the ethical and social issues related to resource development, economic support, organization, management, delivery, and quality of care. Ethical issues in public health and health services management are likely to become increasingly complex in the future. The authors conclude, however, that even in the absence of agreement on ethical assumptions and in the face of diversity and complexity that prohibit easy compromise, mechanisms for resolving ethical dilemmas in public health do exist.

Conclusion

I asked the authors of this edition to provide a comprehensive review of key policy and management issues regarding problems of access, costs, and quality, as well as problems of serving special populations and assessing strategies for reform. Those authors whose chapters appeared in previous editions of this book have met this challenge by updating their chapters with advances in the field since the last edition was published in 2007 and by addressing the possible implications of the ACA in their topic area, where relevant. Those authors who contributed new chapters to this edition have further enhanced the relevance and usefulness of this book for anyone seeking a single source of information about the challenges facing the U.S. health care system. Although the authors of this volume may not have answers for all the major challenges facing our health care system, I believe readers of this edition will find that the authors have delineated the critical questions clearly and proposed informed, innovative solutions.

ACKNOWLEDGMENTS

The authors of this volume have once again met their obligations effectively and brought their considerable expertise to the presentation of the information and analyses contained within these pages. Their rewards for substantial contributions to this fourth edition are largely the intangible ones of providing service to the students and practitioners of health services policy and research. I am particularly thankful to the new authors who have contributed to this edition; they have expanded the scope of topics in a meaningful and valuable way.

Michael E. Begay, LaVonne Downey, Janice L. Dreachslin, Xiaoxing He, Alan M. Preston, and Eric R. Wright provided valuable feedback on the third edition and revision plan. Christine Brough and Betsy Eastwood provided thoughtful and constructive comments on the complete fourth edition draft manuscript.

Hala Douglas, administrative assistant in the UCLA Center for Health Policy Research, deserves a special thanks for assisting me in communication with my coauthors and the publisher and for tracking the progress of all the pieces needed to assemble an edited volume.

The late Andy Pasternak, who oversaw production of the earlier editions of this book, and who will be sorely missed.

Finally, Seth Schwartz, associate editor at Wiley, was outstanding in his support during this revision. The advances in publishing technology since the first edition of this book have made the production process much more efficient, but the process of managing so many coauthors still requires lots of virtual hand holding, and Seth provided just the right amount of tea and sympathy throughout.

December 2013   Gerald F. Kominski
Los Angeles

CHANGING THE
U.S. HEALTH CARE SYSTEM

PART ONE

ACCESS TO HEALTH CARE

CHAPTER ONE

THE PATIENT PROTECTION AND AFFORDABLE CARE ACT OF 2010

Gerald F. Kominski

Learning Objectives

- Understand the political circumstances leading to the enactment of the Patient Protection and Affordable Care Act (ACA) in 2010
- Learn the major components of the ACA and the timetable for their implementation
- Examine the expected impacts of the ACA on major stakeholders in the U.S. health care system

The Patient Protection and Affordable Care Act of 2010 is the most significant piece of U.S. health legislation since the enactment of Medicare and Medicaid in 1965. The law is now more commonly known simply as the Affordable Care Act (ACA) and will be referred to throughout this book as the ACA. It has also been referred to pejoratively by opponents as Obamacare, at least until the 2012 presidential campaign, when President Obama embraced that label to describe the most significant legislative achievement of his first term. At the time of its enactment, the ACA was expected to extend health insurance coverage to thirty-two million uninsured U.S. citizens and permanent residents by 2016 (Congressional Budget Office [CBO], 2011), thus reducing the portion of uninsured legal residents from 17 percent to 5 percent.

How did this major piece of legislation get enacted after several failed attempts to expand health insurance to all Americans during the forty-five years between the enactment of Medicare and Medicaid in 1965 and the enactment of the ACA in 2010? And will the ACA finally achieve the goal of providing (nearly) universal access to health insurance in the United States while promoting higher quality care at an affordable and sustainable rate of growth in health care expenditures into the future? These are fundamental questions that will be explored throughout this book.

Since the first edition of this book was published in 1996, just a few short years after the failed effort of President Clinton to enact universal health insurance, the book's major purpose has been to discuss the fundamental challenges facing the U.S. health care system and to provide readers with both conceptual frameworks and the most current empirical evidence necessary to formulate effective strategies for innovation. At the time of this writing, the United States stands poised to undertake a fundamental reform of health care financing in almost five decades. It goes without saying that the ACA will have profound effects on health care financing and delivery in the United States for decades to come. My coauthors and I believe this book will continue to be a valuable tool for understanding not only the expected impacts of the ACA over the next decade, but for understanding the impacts of the other significant trends in health care that have been occurring independently of the ACA.

The likely consequences of the ACA will be addressed in varying degrees of depth in every chapter of this volume. Therefore, to set the stage for the rest of this book, the remainder of this chapter describes the major components of the law and discusses its likely impacts on major stakeholders in the health care system. But before dealing with the content of the law and its impacts, it is worth briefly reviewing how this law came to be after so many years of failed efforts to expand health insurance coverage to virtually all Americans.

Events Leading to the Enactment of the ACA

The evolution of the unique mix of private and public health insurance in the United States is discussed in more detail in Chapters Six, Seven, and Twenty-One of this volume and is summarized in two recent articles by Oberlander (2010; 2012). Briefly, the origins of the Affordable Care Act can be traced most directly to three significant events that occurred since the enactment of Medicare:

- The growth of managed care in the 1970s and the formulation of a proposal for national health care reform based on "managed competition" among insurers
- The failure of the Clinton Administration's proposal for health reform based on managed competition among managed care plans in 1993 and 1994
- The enactment of significant health reform in Massachusetts in 2006 based on managed competition, including subsidies for low- and middle-income individuals and families to purchase private insurance in regulated market places

Managed competition was first proposed by Professor Alain Enthoven of the Stanford Business School in the late 1970s (Enthoven, 1978). It was designed to build on the strengths of private insurance markets, but to correct their weaknesses through regulated competition. Enthoven's model of managed competition was based on the Federal Employees Health Benefits Program (FEHBP), which provides health insurance benefits to more than three million federal employees nationally through a regulated marketplace that offers employees multiple plan choices. In the political context of the 1970s, managed competition was viewed as a private-market alternative to liberal proposals for a single-payer health care system through, for example, the expansion of Medicare to all ages.

Enthoven proposed to standardize insurance policies to promote price comparison among similar products, so consumers could make "apples-to-apples" comparisons. He also proposed to address inefficiencies in the demand (the buyers') side of the market by pooling small companies and individual (nongroup) purchasers into larger groups known as health insurance purchasing cooperatives (HIPCs) and by providing vouchers (subsidies) for low-income individuals to purchase private insurance. HIPCs were a central feature of President Clinton's national health reform proposal and were the template for both the Massachusetts Insurance Connector established in 2006 and the American Health Benefit and Small Business Health Options Program (SHOP) exchanges included in the ACA.

After the recession of 1990 through 1991, millions of Americans lost their employment-based insurance, and the number of uninsured rapidly jumped from 35 million to 40 million between 1991 and 1993 nationally (DeNavas-Walt, Proctor, & Smith, 2011). President Clinton was elected in 1992 in part because he campaigned on a platform that proposed major health care reform with universal access. Although the Clinton plan, known as the Health Security Act, was based on many of the principles of managed competition, it went further to include federal controls on premiums, national budgets, and perhaps most controversial of all to many Americans, a requirement that employers enroll their employees in managed care plans. This last element was very controversial because millions of those with employment-based insurance would be required to give up their insurance to join health maintenance organizations (HMOs), the most common form of managed care in the early 1990s.

After the failure of the Clinton plan to even move forward for a vote in Congress in 1994, major health reform seemed out of the question for the foreseeable future, and the first edition of this book contained language to that effect. Nevertheless, two significant expansions of health insurance occurred over the decade following the Clinton plan. One was the creation of the State Children's Health Insurance Program (SCHIP) in 1997, to be discussed further in Chapters Six and Eighteen. The other was the enactment in 2003 of Medicare Part D, the pharmaceutical drug benefit, which is discussed further in Chapter Twenty-One.

What caught many health policy analysts by surprise at the national level was the enactment of significant health reform in Massachusetts in 2006 based on an innovative combination of Medicaid expansion, subsidies for purchase of private insurance in a regulated market known as the Insurance Connector, and employer and individual mandates. Of course, this approach did not simply appear overnight; as explained by McDonough, Rosman, Phelps, and Shannon (2006), the road to reform in Massachusetts started in 2001 and represented the "third wave" of reform efforts that began under Governor Dukakis in 1988, just prior to his unsuccessful run for the presidency. One of the major forces driving the 2006 reform, however, was the threatened loss of almost $400 million dollars in funds under the state's Medicaid waiver with the Centers for Medicare and Medicaid Services (CMS), the federal agency that runs these programs, unless the state provided expanded coverage for the uninsured (Holahan & Blumberg, 2006). These diverse, concurrent pressures within Massachusetts in the early 2000s led to a unique compromise approach to reform, forged by Republican Governor Mitt Romney and Democratic legislative leaders, combining both conservative and liberal elements to achieve the goal of nearly universal access for all legal residents of the state. But the core of the Massachusetts reform reflected key elements of managed competition.

The successful enactment of significant health reform in Massachusetts in 2006—and the fact that it represented a genuine compromise between conservative and liberal proposals—immediately elevated the Massachusetts model as a template for feasible reform for the rest of the nation. Governor Schwarzenegger in early 2007 proposed legislation to implement a Massachusetts-style reform for California, perhaps hoping to replicate the bipartisan support for health reform. Although California's effort was ultimately unsuccessful, the attempt to enact such a reform in the nation's largest state virtually ensured that health reform would be a central issue in the 2008 presidential election.

The role of health reform in the 2008 election, the difficult path to eventual enactment of the ACA in March 2010, and the Supreme Court's decision to uphold the constitutionality of the individual mandate provision in June 2012 are discussed in more detail in Chapter Six. But, for the remainder of this chapter, it is important to remember that the major elements of the ACA were based directly on the following components of the 2006 Massachusetts reform: (1) expansion of Medicaid for those with the lowest income, (2) subsidies for low- to middle-income individuals and families to buy private health insurance in regulated markets, (3) and mandates for employers to offer insurance and for individuals who are legal residents to acquire insurance.

Major Provisions of the ACA

This section provides an overview of the major elements of the ACA. The final version of the law is over nine hundred pages in print and includes ten significant sections, or titles. Thousands of additional pages of federal regulations have been issued since the law's enactment on March 23, 2010, as part of the administrative rule-making process by which federal laws are implemented. This section cannot provide a comprehensive review of the entire law, so it focuses primarily on the small-group and individual (nongroup) market reforms and expansion of Medicaid contained in Titles I and II, respectively, of the law. More complete summaries of all the provisions of the law are available at www.healthcare.gov, which also includes the complete text version of the law, and at kff.org/health-reform.

Medicaid Expansion

Since the enactment of Medicaid in 1965, low-income individuals qualify for this program based on what is known as *categorical eligibility*. In effect, this means that eligibility is based on both low-income status and having a qualifying medical condition or need. As a result, simply being poor has never been a sufficient condition to qualify individuals for Medicaid. The ACA fundamentally changes Medicaid eligibility by establishing a uniform, national eligibility standard based solely on income. Starting in 2014, Medicaid eligibility will be available to everyone with income up to and including 138 percent of the federal poverty level (FPL), which varies according to family size. For example, in 2013, 138 percent of the FPL is equal to $15,856 for an unmarried individual and $32,500 for a family of four. Because federal rules permit an offset of 5 percent of income in determining eligibility, the 133 percent FPL limit for Medicaid eligibility identified in the law is effectively 138 percent in practice (Angeles, 2011).

The ACA changes the federal matching assistance percentages (FMAPs) available to states for newly eligible Medicaid populations. As of 2013, states receive FMAPs that range from 50 to 77 percent for their existing Medicaid programs. Under the ACA, states will receive a 100 percent FMAP to cover their newly eligible Medicaid beneficiaries from 2014 through 2016, 95 percent in 2017, 94 percent in 2018, 93 percent in 2019, and 90 percent from 2020 onward. As a result, after 2014, states will receive a "regular" FMAP for individuals who would have qualified for their Medicaid programs as of 2013 and a separate, more generous FMAP for their newly eligible Medicaid population (Heberlein, Guyer, & Rudowitz, 2010).

Despite the ACA's effort to create Medicaid expansions in every state and the District of Columbia, the one component of the ACA found to be unconstitutional by the Supreme Court in June 2012 was the mandatory aspect of the law's Medicaid expansion. Specifically, the court found the provision of the law penalizing a state that did not expand their Medicaid program by eliminating all federal funding to the state for Medicaid was excessively punitive and struck down that provision of the law. Therefore, Medicaid expansion is now voluntary on the part of states, although states that choose to expand Medicaid must expand to 133 percent of FPL (or 138 percent of FPL accounting for the 5 percent offset). As of February 2013, twenty-four states are committed to Medicaid expansion in 2014, and another four are leaning toward expansion. The impact of the voluntary expansion of Medicaid will be discussed later in this chapter. More detail on Medicaid can be found in Chapter Six.

Subsidies to Purchase Private Insurance

For individuals and families between 139 and 400 percent of FPL who are above the Medicaid income eligibility threshold, the ACA will provide subsidies to purchase private health insurance in regulated markets known in the law as American Health Benefit Exchanges, or now simply known as exchanges. For marketing purposes, individual states may rename their exchanges to a more consumer-friendly title; for example, California's exchange is known as Covered California, while Oregon's is Cover Oregon.

Eligibility for subsidies will be processed by the exchanges through income verification with the Internal Revenue Service. Income determination will be based on modified adjusted gross income (MAGI) from the most recent tax return, which is essentially the adjusted gross income from a tax filing unit's return plus any foreign or tax-exempt interest income (Angeles, 2011). Of course, exceptions will be made for those whose financial circumstances have changed, for example, through loss of employment. The amount of the subsidy is based on a sliding proportion of income (the MAGI) and the cost of the second-lowest-cost Silver plan (defined next) offered in the exchange. The personal share of the premium is determined by this sliding scale:

- 100 to 133 percent of FPL: 2 percent of income
- 133 to 150 percent of FPL: 3 to 4 percent of income
- 150 to 200 percent of FPL: 4 to 6.3 percent of income
- 200 to 250 percent of FPL: 6.3 to 8.05 percent of income
- 250 to 300 percent of FPL: 8.05 to 9.5 percent of income
- 300 to 400 percent of FPL: 9.5 percent of income

To illustrate, for a family of four in 2013, 400 percent of FPL is $94,200. Such a family would have a maximum contribution for health insurance of $8,949 (that is, 9.5 percent of $94,200). If the second-lowest-cost Silver plan in this family's exchange cost $12,000, they would be eligible for a subsidy of $3,051. The family is not required to buy a Silver plan, but their subsidy remains the same regardless of whether they buy a more or less expensive plan than the second-lowest-cost Silver plan.

In addition to premium subsidies, low-income individuals and families from 100 to 250 percent of FPL also qualify for subsidies to reduce their out-of-pocket expenses due to cost sharing (deductibles and copayments). However, to qualify for this additional assistance, qualifying individuals and families must purchase a Silver plan sold in their exchange.

The ACA intends for all individuals below 139 percent of FPL to be eligible for mandatory Medicaid expansions. The premium limit listed earlier for those from 100 to 133 percent of FPL is intended only to apply only for those legal residents with less than five years of residency who are not eligible for Medicaid. However, because the Supreme Court overturned mandatory Medicaid expansion, those with income from 100 to 133 percent FPL will now be eligible for subsidies if their state has rejected the Medicaid expansion. Those with incomes below 100 percent of FPL in such states will continue to be without insurance, unless Congress finds another solution, which seems unlikely in the current polarized political environment.

Finally, subsidies in the form of tax credits are available to small employers to assist with their health insurance costs. For tax years 2014 and later, small businesses with fewer than twenty-five employees that purchase coverage through the state exchange can receive a tax credit of up to 50 percent of the employer's contribution toward health insurance premiums if the employer contributes at least 50 percent of the total premium cost. The full credit will be available to employers with ten or fewer employees and average annual wages of less than $25,000, and it phases out as firm size (maximum twenty-five) and average wage (maximum $50,000) increase. Tax-exempt small businesses meeting these requirements are eligible for tax credits of up to 35 percent of the employer's contribution toward health insurance premiums. The employer tax credit will be available for a maximum of two years to any individual firm. As described in the next section, because these firms employ less than twenty-five employees, they are exempt from the employer mandate under the ACA either to provide insurance or pay a tax penalty.

Mandates for Individuals and Employers

Perhaps the most controversial aspect of the ACA, at least in the period immediately following its enactment in 2010, was the so-called individual mandate, or minimum coverage requirement. The rationale for an individual mandate is that individuals will have no incentive to buy or enroll in insurance that requires them to pay a premium if insurers cannot deny insurance to anyone who seeks it and cannot charge higher premiums based on health status. In fact, the incentive in such a market is to sit on the sidelines until insurance is absolutely necessary. These circumstances can lead to adverse selection in the insurance market, where only those with high-use or severe illnesses seek insurance, while those who are relatively healthy avoid insurance until necessary. When adverse selection occurs, premiums spiral because only the sickest individuals seek insurance. To prevent this sort of market disruption, the Massachusetts reform and the ACA included an individual mandate requiring all legal residents to demonstrate that they have minimal acceptable coverage or pay a penalty as part of their income tax return.

The constitutionality of the individual mandate was upheld by the Supreme Court in June 2012. Specifically, the court found that the mandate is constitutional because failure to comply with the mandate results in a tax, which is constitutional under Congress's taxation authority. Therefore, starting in 2014, legal residents will need to demonstrate that they have minimal acceptable coverage through either public insurance (Medicare, Medicaid, SCHIP, military insurance, or Veterans Administration coverage), employment-based coverage, coverage purchased through the exchange, or a grandfathered plan certified as acceptable by the Department of Health and Human Services and already in effect on the date the ACA was signed into law. Those who fail to demonstrate that they have such coverage will be required to pay a tax equal to:

- In 2014, $95 per adult and $47.50 per child, up to a family maximum of $285 or 1.0 percent of family income, whichever is greater
- In 2015, $325 per adult and $162.50 per child, up to a family maximum of $975 or 2.0 percent of family income, whichever is greater
- In 2016, $695 per adult and $347.50 per child, up to a family maximum of $2,085 or 2.5 percent of family income, whichever is greater

There are various exemptions from the tax: individuals who have religious objections, are members of an American Indian tribe, have income below the threshold required to file income taxes, are incarcerated, have to pay more than 8 percent of income for insurance, or are undocumented. The undocumented are generally excluded from all requirements and benefits under ACA, including the ability to purchase insurance inside the exchanges with their own funds. The ACA does include additional funding from safety net clinics, which serve a large portion of the undocumented population; further discussion of the undocumented and the role of the safety net under the ACA can be found in Chapter Twenty-Three.

In addition to the individual mandate, the ACA requires employers with fifty or more full-time equivalent (FTE) employees to provide affordable health insurance coverage or pay a penalty to the federal government, although this provision of the law has been delayed until January 1, 2015. This type of "pay-or-play" employer mandate was tried by several states over the past two decades, but in 2013 the only states with employer mandates are Massachusetts, which implemented its mandate in 2006, and Hawaii, which was the first state to enact an employer mandate in 1974 (Buchmueller, DiNardo, & Valetta, 2011). Employer requirements under the ACA are illustrated in a useful flow chart that can be found at http://kff.org/infographic/employer-responsibility -under-the-affordable-care-act.

Under the ACA, affordable coverage is defined as insurance where the employer share of the premium is at least 60 percent and no employee pays more than 9.5 percent of his or her income toward the employee share of the premium. For firms that do not offer insurance, the penalty is $2,000 annually times the number of full-time employees, but excluding the first thirty employees. For firms that offer insurance, but either pay less than 60 percent of the cost or have at least one employee who seeks an exchange subsidy because he or she has to pay more than 9.5 percent of their salary for the premium, the penalty is $3,000 times the number of full-time employees receiving a subsidy in the exchange, up to a maximum of $2,000 times the number of full-time employees minus thirty. These penalties are increased each year by the growth in insurance premiums.

Creation of Regulated Markets for Purchasing Private Insurance with Subsidies

The ACA requires individuals and families who qualify for subsidies, as well as small firms receiving tax credits starting in 2014, to purchase standard insurance policies and plans in regulated markets knows as exchanges. This section describes these marketplaces, the requirements for the standard health policies sold in these markets, and other reforms that apply both in and outsides the new exchanges. It is worth noting that the market reforms introduced by the ACA represent the first comprehensive federal regulation of private health insurance in U.S. history.

Individual Market Exchanges. The ACA requires states to establish individual (nongroup) market exchanges in time to begin enrolling new members by October 1, 2013. Because of ongoing efforts by conservatives to overturn and delay implementation of the ACA, as of February 2013, only eighteen states had declared their intention to establish an exchange, and seven others declared their intention to establish an exchange in partnership with the federal government. By default, the twenty-six remaining states will have exchanges operated by the federal government. Despite the potential for ongoing conflict over the ACA that federally run exchanges present, every state is expected to have an operating exchange in time for enrollment starting in October.

The role of the exchanges is to offer qualified health plans (QHPs) with essential health benefits (EHBs) (defined next), to offer four "metal" tiers (defined next) of QHPs that vary according actuarial value (AV) but that all offer minimum acceptable coverage, and to provide customer-friendly methods for purchasers to both determine if they are eligible for subsidies and to comparison-shop for competing health plans and policies all having the same EHBs. Exchanges can operate as active purchasers, in which they negotiate on premium prices or contract with only selected insurers, or as passive clearinghouses, in which they accept all qualified health plans into the exchange. State-run exchanges were eligible for federal funds to support their development from 2011 through 2013, and over $1.5 billion was awarded in 2013 to assist eleven states to finish building their exchanges. Exchanges will ultimately need to be self-sufficient, with the most likely source of revenue being a small surcharge on all policies and plans sold through the exchange. States that are relying on federally operated exchanges can apply to develop state-run exchanges in the future, but the availability of start-up funds is uncertain.

Small Business Health Options Program Exchanges. States are also required by the ACA to establish a small-group market exchange, known in the law as Small Business Health Options Program (SHOP) exchanges, and have the authority to sell affordable insurance to small employers with up to one hundred employees. States have the flexibility to establish SHOP exchanges using definitions of small employers below the statutory definition of one hundred employees. For example, California's SHOP exchange will initially be available only to employers with up to fifty employees. Small firms that qualify for tax credits must purchase insurance in the SHOP Exchange, but firms with fifty to one hundred employees are not required to buy insurance in the SHOP exchange to satisfy the employer mandate.

Qualified Health Plans with Essential Health Benefits. One of the major functions of exchanges is to certify qualified health plans (QHPs) for sale within the exchange. QHPs are health plans or policies with essential health benefits (EHBs), which were defined in the ACA to includes services in each of the following ten categories: outpatient, emergency, inpatient hospital, laboratory, maternity and newborn, mental health and substance abuse, prescription drugs, rehabilitative, preventive, and pediatric oral and vision. EHBs can vary across states and can be based on actual benchmark health policies or plans currently offered in each state, but must comply with federal guidelines and must be expanded to include all ten categories of benefits just described if they don't currently cover such services. States have the option of designating an existing health insurance policy within the state to serve as its EHB benchmark, or, by default, the health policy with the largest enrollment in the small-group market will be designated as the EHB benchmark for that state. As of December 2012, nineteen states and the District of Columbia had designated a small-group plan as their EHB benchmark, four had selected a managed care plan, three had selected a state employee health plan, and twenty-four had the default small-group plan as their benchmark EHB.

In addition to providing coverage for EHBs, QHPs must comply with a number of other significant market reforms discussed in the next section.

Other Market Reforms. The ACA includes significant federal requirements affecting private health insurance markets for the first time. These requirements affect not only health plans and policies sold in the individual and SHOP exchanges starting in 2014, but all markets, including the large-group and self-insured employment-based insurance markets. These requirements include:

- Coverage for adult children up to their twenty-sixth birthday
- Prohibition on rescissions
- Prohibition of preexisting condition exclusions
- Elimination of annual and lifetime dollar limits on benefits
- Preventive services with no copays
- Medical loss ratio thresholds
- Premiums based on modified community rating
- Metal tiers of coverage based on actuarial value (AV)
- Minimum AV requirement
- Annual out-of-pocket limits

These requirements, their effective dates, and the insurance markets to which they apply are summarized in Table 1.1.

Large-group plans and policies will generally continue to operate outside of exchanges, unless a state decides to open its exchange to the large-group market after 2017. The additional requirements such a decision would impose on large employers are shown in Table 1.1. Grandfathered plans are exempt from most of the requirements listed earlier, as shown in Table 1.1. Such plans cannot be offered to new customers in the individual (nongroup) market, but can be offered to new

TABLE 1.1. SUMMARY OF MAJOR ACA REGULATIONS AFFECTING PRIVATE INSURANCE

ACA Regulations	Nongroup	Small Group	Large Group	Self-Insured	Grandfathered
After September 23, 2010					
Adult child coverage up to age 26	X	X	X	X	1
Rescissions prohibited	X	X	X	X	X
Preexisting conditions covered for ages <19	X	X	X	X	2
No lifetime dollar limits on benefits	X	X	X	X	X
Phased elimination of annual dollar limits on benefits by 2014	X	X	X	X	2
Preventive services without cost sharing[3]	X	X	X	X	
After January 1, 2011					
Medical loss ratio (MLR) thresholds	X	X	X		X
After January 1, 2014					
Modified community rating	X	X	4		
Essential health benefits (EHBs)	X	X	5		
Metal tiers of coverage	X	X	5		
Annual limits on out-of-pocket spending	X	X	X	X	
Subsidies to buy qualified health plans (QHPs)	6				
Minimum actuarial value of coverage	X	X	X	X	
Preexisting conditions covered for all ages	X	X	X	X	2

Small group = up to 100 full-time equivalent (FTE) employees; large group = more than 100 FTE employees.

[1]Until 2014, grandfathered group policies are exempt for adult children eligible for other employer-based coverage, such as through their own job.

[2]Policies in the nongroup (individual) market are exempt from this requirement.

[3]Additional preventive services for women required after August 1, 2012.

[4]Applies only in states that allow large employers to purchase in the exchange after 2017.

[5]Applies inside and outside the exchange for large employers in states that allow large employers to purchase in the exchange after 2017.

[6]For citizens and legal residents of fewer than five years who qualify for subsidies based on income, or who have unaffordable insurance or insurance that fails to meet the 60 percent minimum actuarial value requirement through their job.

Source: Adapted from Linder, Moore, & Udow-Phillips, 2012.

employees within firms that continue to offer grandfathered plans in the small-group market.

The requirement to provide coverage for adult children up to (but not including) age twenty-six has had the largest impact to date. An estimated 3.1 million young adults have become newly insured as a result of this provision of the ACA (Sommers, 2012). Prior to the ACA, employers often permitted adult children to stay on their parents' health insurance policies, but this practice usually applied only to children who were still financially dependent on their parents, usually because of college enrollment. Under the ACA, adult children no longer need to be financially dependent to remain on their parents' policy. Employers are not required to offer family coverage to employees under the ACA, but if they do, they must offer coverage for adult children.

The prohibitions on rescissions and on preexisting condition exclusions are related. Rescission refers to the practice of cancelling the insurance policy of someone after coverage is granted because of alleged omission of information about preexisting conditions on the application for insurance. Insurers have been accused of employing rescission to cancel the policies of policyholders who develop high-cost illnesses as a way to avoid paying for expensive claims. Preexisting condition exclusions allow insurers to issue insurance policies with specific exclusions for conditions that exist at the time someone applies for insurance or that are part of an applicant's medical history. They generally specify a time period during which the insurer is not required to provide benefits for the preexisting condition, although in some cases the exclusion is permanent (Georgetown University Health Policy Institute, 2012). Depending on the state, health insurers can also employ *medical underwriting* to avoid offering insurance, or to charge higher premiums, to those with preexisting conditions.

The federal Health Insurance Portability and Accountability Act (HIPAA) of 1996 imposed limits on the look-back period (six months) and the duration of preexisting condition exclusions in the group market, but these protections don't extend to individuals in the nongroup market unless they had at least eighteen months of continuous coverage in the group market. Therefore, the ACA will provide significant new protections, particularly for those with preexisting conditions in the individual market. Preexisting condition exclusions were eliminated for children up to nineteen years of age for policy years starting after September 23, 2010; they are eliminated for all ages effective January 1, 2014, except for grandfathered plans in the individual market.

The elimination of lifetime and annual dollar limits on benefits provides catastrophic protection. Lifetime limits were prohibited for new and existing policy years starting on or after September 23, 2010. Annual limits are eliminated for all health plans and policies as of January 1, 2014, except grandfathered plans in the individual market.

Approved preventive services must be provided at no cost to the insurer member. Insurers cannot charge a copayment for preventive services, and those services must be exempt from deductibles. Preventive services that must be covered without cost sharing by insurers include all services graded as A or B by the U.S. Preventive Services Task Force (USPSTF), an independent panel of primary care providers that rates or grades the scientific evidence concerning the clinical effectiveness of various preventive services, including screening tests and immunizations. Services are graded A or B by the USPSTF when there is high certainty of substantial (A) or moderate (B) net benefit of performing the service. This ACA requirement was effective for all policy years on or after September 23, 2010, except for grandfathered plans, which are exempt. As of 2013, there are sixteen recommended preventive services for adults, twenty-two for women, and twenty-seven for children under age eighteen.

Medical loss ratio (MLR) thresholds require insurers to meet minimum payout requirements on the premiums they collect. Insurers in the large-group market must spend at least 85 percent of their premium revenue on medical expenses, while small-group and individual market insurers must spend at least 80 percent. The law requires insurers to issue rebates to employers or individual purchases by August 1 of the following year if they do not meet these minimum standards; the rebates must be sufficient to bring the insurer into compliance with the threshold. In 2012, insurer rebates were estimated $1.3 billion nationally (Cox, Levitt, & Claxton, 2012). Only self-insured employers are exempt from the MLR requirement.

On January 1, 2014, when the exchanges open for business, the small-group and individual markets are required to meet the following requirements both inside and outside of the exchanges (1) use of modified community rating to set premiums, (2) all policies must include essential health benefits (EHBs), (3) all policies must be one of four "metal" tiers, and (4) all policies must include limits on out-of-pocket spending by policyholders (this also applies to large and self-insured employers).

Modified community rating refers to the use of a limited set of demographic characteristics in setting insurance premiums. Under pure community rating, insurers charge a single premium to everyone. Under the ACA's modified community rating requirements, insurers can use only the following characteristics in setting premiums:

- Age, limited to no more than a 3-to-1 ratio between the highest- and lowest-cost age group
- Tobacco use, limited to no more than a 1.5-to-1 ratio between smokers and nonsmokers
- Family size
- Geographic regions within a state

Perhaps most important, insurers are now prohibited from using health status as a basis for setting premiums. In addition, they are also required to comply with *guaranteed issue* and *guaranteed renewal* requirements—they must issue insurance to anyone willing to pay for it and renew any policyholder who wishes to continue with the same company. Furthermore, for insurers selling the same policy both inside and outside the exchange, they must charge the same premium for that policy in each market.

Metal tiers refer to the provision requiring insurers to offer standard health policies and plans in one or more of four coverage tiers based on actuarial value (AV). The Bronze tier must have an AV of 60 percent, meaning the premium should cover 60 percent of the costs for EHBs, while out-of-pocket spending by policyholders should cover the remaining 40 percent of costs. Bronze plan holders, therefore, pay less in monthly premiums, but have higher copayments or deductibles when they use health care services. The remaining tiers are Silver (70 percent AV), Gold (80 percent AV), and Platinum (90 percent AV). The law requires insurers to offer at least one Silver and one Gold plan to participate in the exchange, but as with other aspects of the law, states have the right to require insurers to offer three or four metal tiers, or to offer plans outside the exchange, as a condition for participating in the exchange.

In addition to the four metal tiers, insurers can also offer catastrophic policies with AVs below 60 percent that can be sold only to young adults under thirty years of age, or those who are exempted from the individual mandate because of financial hardship or lack of affordable coverage. Catastrophic plans have deductibles equal to the annual limit on out-of-pocket spending, discussed next, but must cover preventive services and three primary care visits at no cost to the policyholder.

It is important to note that all four tiers and catastrophic policies must include the same exact EHBs; what differs between the tiers is the relative share of costs covered by premiums versus policyholder out-of-pocket spending. Because all tiers must have the same EHBs, and within each tier all policies must have the same AV, consumers should be able to make more informed choices between comparable policies. Within each metal tier, policies can still differ with regard to their schedule of copayments or coinsurance; there are many possible combinations to achieve the target AV. For example, one Bronze plan might require $500 copayments for each inpatient hospital day, while another plan might require a 30 percent coinsurance rate per day, but both plans cover 365 days of care per year. In theory, these market changes will promote greater price competition between insurers. To further promote "apples-to-apples" comparison shopping, some states, such as California, have gone beyond the ACA requirements, and are requiring insurers to offer standardized QHPs all having the same copayment or coinsurance schedules within a metal tier. Such standardization further promotes price competition among essentially identical insurance policies, down to the precise out-of-pocket requirements for copayments or coinsurance rates for each service.

Insurance in the large-group and self-insured markets does not need to comply with the metal tiers or EHB requirements, but must offer at least one plan that satisfies the 60 percent AV requirement. In these markets, whatever benefits are offered, the employer must either verify that they offer coverage with at least a 60 percent AV, or if self-insured, verify that they pay at least 60 percent of the total claims cost of the covered benefits.

Annual limits on out-of-pocket spending by policyholders are also required. All insurance policies, including large-group policies and self-insured employer plans, but excluding grandfathered policies, must comply with the federal out-of-pocket limits that apply to high-deductible health plans (HDHPs) approved for purchase in combination with health savings accounts (HSAs). For 2013, these limits are $6,250 for individuals and $12,500 for families, and are adjusted annually for inflation. The ACA provides for lower limits for individuals and families with incomes 100 to 250 percent of FPL who purchase Silver plans in the exchanges; the limits are one-third of the HSA limits for those 100 to 199 percent of FPL, and one-half of the HSA limits for those 200 to 250 percent of FPL. These lower limits, combined with additional federal subsidies to insurers for those from 100 to 250 percent of FPL who buy Silver plans, result in the higher AVs (that is, lower out-of-pocket spending) for those with the lowest incomes in the Exchange: 94 percent AV for those with incomes from 100 to 149 percent of FPL, 87 percent AV for those 150 to 199 percent of FPL, and 73 percent AV for those 200 to 250 percent of FPL. Finally, the ACA limits deductibles for policies and plans in the small-group market to $2,000 for individuals and $4,000 for families.

Future Directions

The ACA will have profound effects on health care financing and on reducing the number of uninsured legal residents and citizens in the United States. It may also serve as a catalyst for changing the organization and delivery of health care services by encouraging the development of new models of managed care known as accountable care organizations (ACOs). The remainder of this chapter briefly discusses the expected impacts of the ACA on each of the major stakeholders in the U.S. health care system for the remainder of this decade.

The Uninsured

Obviously, a primary goal of the ACA is to reduce significantly the number of uninsured in the United States. Specifically, the ACA was targeted at (1) those who were too poor to buy insurance but who didn't qualify for Medicaid because they lacked categorical eligibility or because they lived in a state with low income eligibility thresholds and (2) those who did not receive health insurance through their place of employment, largely because they worked for small employers who were less likely to offer health insurance benefits.

The Congressional Budget Office (CBO) estimated in 2010 that the ACA would extend coverage to 32 million uninsured nationally by 2019, including 16 million through the Medicaid expansion and another 16 million through the exchanges (CBO, 2010). Despite ongoing efforts by many states since 2010 to avoid complying with Obamacare, every state and the District of Columbia is expected to have exchanges operating by October 1, 2013. Therefore, CBO's estimate of 16 million fewer uninsured as a result of subsidies to purchase insurance in the exchanges is still relevant.

Because the Supreme Court found the mandatory expansion of Medicaid unconstitutional, conservatives are using opposition to the Medicaid expansion as a rallying cry in what appears to be a last stand against Obamacare. For the poor in states refusing to expand their Medicaid programs, there are few good alternatives at the time of this writing. The drafters of the ACA did not anticipate low-income individuals below 133 percent of FPL being excluded from Medicaid, because Medicaid expansion was mandatory in the legislation. However, the law does allow subsidies for individuals with incomes from 100 to 133 percent of FPL who don't qualify for Medicaid, mostly legal residents who have lived in the United States for fewer than five years, so applying for exchange subsidies is an option for these individuals in states that don't expand Medicaid. But purchasing insurance will require these individuals to pay 2 percent of their income for insurance, while Medicaid would have been available at no cost. For individuals below 100 percent of FPL, there are no options for insurance if their state foregoes the Medicaid expansion.

As discussed earlier in this chapter, twenty-two states have announced as of February 2013 their intention not to expand their Medicaid programs, although eight Republican governors are pursuing the expansion. Clearly, political opposition to Obamacare may ebb in the future in states that refuse the Medicaid expansion, and the economic reality of forgoing hundreds of millions or billions of dollars in federal support for the uninsured may accelerate the erosion of current political opposition to Medicaid expansion. Until then, it is truly devastating from a public health perspective that as many as six million poor Americans (CBO, 2012a), mostly in the South and West, will be denied access to health insurance through Medicaid in 2014 and for the foreseeable future because of ongoing political opposition by well-insured voters in those states.

Employers

With regard to employers, some of the major questions regarding the impact of ACA are whether firms will (1) drop coverage if they offered it prior to 2015, (2) add coverage if they didn't prior to 2015, or (3) reduce the number of full-time employees (those averaging thirty hours per week) to avoid having to offer insurance benefits (Merlis, 2011).

Large employers with more than one hundred employees currently offer insurance to virtually all employees, and estimates are that 98 percent of large firms currently are in compliance with the ACA requirement to offer affordable insurance of with at least 60 percent actuarial value to their employees (Blumberg, 2010; Yong, Bertko, & Kronick, 2011). Therefore, there is little reason to believe that the large-group market will change in any measurable way as a result of the ACA.

There is speculation that employers in general will drop insurance coverage in favor of letting their employees buy insurance in the exchange. Employers who drop insurance and pay penalties could save significantly on employee benefits by pursuing such a strategy, but this strategy ignores the fact that employers were not required to offer insurance prior to 2015, so they could have chosen this cost-saving strategy at any time. Most large employers don't choose to drop coverage, because in a competitive labor market health insurance benefits have considerable value in recruiting and retaining employees, particularly higher-income employees, who receive the most advantage from the tax-exempt status of health insurance benefits. Furthermore, companies that simply drop health insurance benefits without compensating their employees for the economic value of lost benefits should experience significant disadvantages in a competitive labor market.

CBO (2012b) estimates the net loss of employment-based insurance due to the ACA will be as much as five million individuals per year by 2019. This includes eleven million losing coverage because their employer stops offering coverage, three million who switch to receiving coverage through the exchange because their employment-based insurance is unaffordable, and nine million gaining insurance because their employer now offers insurance.

Regarding negative impacts of the ACA on employment, there are good reasons based on economic theory to be concerned. Some employers may hire fewer workers because the cost of employment has been increased for those firms. Employers may also reduce employee hours so that fewer workers qualify as full-time and thus are ineligible for health insurance benefits. However, the most relevant evidence is from Massachusetts, and the experience there suggests that these negative employment impacts were largely avoided (Dubay, Holahan, Long, & Lawton, 2012).

Hospitals

The hospital industry supported the ACA primarily because of the prospect of some thirty-two million newly insured individuals who would no longer require free care. But the ACA will reduce special subsidy payments to hospitals, known as disproportionate share hospital (DSH) payments, under both the Medicare and Medicaid programs, that compensate hospitals for the higher costs of serving a large portion of uninsured and low-income patients. The rationale for reducing these DSH subsidies is that as the number of uninsured patients declines under ACA, the need for DSH payments should also decline. Although the industry supported this rationale, there are clearly some safety-net hospitals that may fare worse under ACA. For example, public hospitals in Los Angeles County, where more than a million residents are likely to remain uninsured because they are undocumented or don't sign up for Medicaid, may not experience a significant increase in their share of patients with insurance (Lucia et al., 2012). As a result, traditional safety-net providers see the ACA as a potential mixed blessing, particularly if newly insured patients begin seeking care at other, non-safety-net hospitals.

Physicians

Physicians are largely unaffected by the ACA. However, the substantial increase in the number of people with insurance has raised concerns about the adequacy of the supply of physicians to meet the expected increase in demand for physician services. For individuals with exchange insurance plans, access should be less of an issue, because they will be privately insured. The Medicaid expansion population is more likely to have access problems, particularly in states such as California where Medicaid payment rates are so low that physicians are reluctant to treat Medicaid patients.

There are several options in the short term to meet the increased demand for primary care services. One is to expand state scope-of-service laws, allowing nonphysicians to legally provide certain primary care services. Another is to increase the availability of care at community clinics, including federally qualified health centers (FQHCs), which serve low-income and uninsured populations. The ACA includes increased funding for FQHCs for this reason. Another is to increase payments for primary care services under Medicaid, which is also a provision under the ACA. The federal government paid states to raise their Medicaid payment rates for primary care services to Medicare levels, but only for 2013 and 2014. Lack of access to specialty care services has been a long-standing concern for Medicaid beneficiaries and may be worse under the ACA (Kaiser Commission on Medicaid and the Uninsured, 2011). As discussed in Chapters Two, Three, Four, and Five, access to adequate care requires more than access to health insurance.

Payers

The ACA will significantly affect all major payers of health care, largely because of the increased funding for federal subsidies to purchase private insurance and the Medicaid expansion. To achieve savings in federal expenditures so that the overall legislation was budget-neutral, the ACA also included significant reductions in Medicare expenditures over the next ten years.

Private Insurers. The private insurance industry is one of the biggest winners under the ACA, primarily because of the tens of millions of individuals who will be newly insured. In exchange for allowing federal regulation of their business, private insurers stand to gain almost $1 trillion in additional revenue during the next decade as a result of the ACA. Even the Medicaid expansion benefits private insurers, because many states use private managed care plans to provide care to their Medicaid beneficiaries. In 2010, about 70 percent of the sixty million Medicaid beneficiaries nationally were enrolled in managed care (Sparer, 2012).

One fundamental issue that will unfold over the next decade is whether the increased reliance by government on private insurers will lead to significant innovations in health care delivery systems and control of costs. Or will significant additional reforms be necessary within the next ten years because the ACA has created subsidies and an expansion of Medicaid that prove to be unsustainable? The private insurance industry was largely supportive of the ACA because of the appeal of significant additional revenues, but will private insurers fully engage in vigorous price competition or increase lobbying efforts seeking a relaxation of federal regulations as ACA implementation moves forward? The next decade will provide a fascinating and once-in-a-lifetime opportunity to determine whether regulated competition of private health insurers at the state level can produce a more efficient, high-performance health care system.

Medicare. Medicare is largely unaffected by the ACA, with a few notable exceptions. CBO (2012c) estimates that Medicare savings will amount to $716 billion from 2013 through 2022, mostly due to lower inflation allowances for payments to hospitals and other facilities, lower payments to Medicare managed care plans, and lower DSH payments to hospitals. In addition, Medicare revenues will increase starting in 2013 due to a higher withholding tax rate (2.35 percent for the employee share only) for those with income greater than $200,000 for single and head of household tax filers or income greater than $250,000 for married taxpayers filing jointly. A new Medicare tax of 3.8 percent went into effect on unearned income starting in 2013. Although these savings and additional revenues in Medicare do not directly support the federal funding available for ACA, they did count toward the CBO "scoring" of the ACA's federal budgetary impacts and led CBO to conclude that the ACA would not increase the federal budget deficit during the decade from 2013 through 2022 (CBO, 2010).

The ACA includes two other provisions related to Medicare that could have broader significance for the U.S. delivery system. One is the creation of the Center for Medicare and Medicaid Innovation (CMMI). CMMI is supporting the development of new mechanisms for coordinating care under the Medicare program known as accountable care organizations (ACOs). More information on ACOs can be found in Chapter Twenty. The other provision is the creation of a new agency known as the Independent Payment Advisory Board (IPAB). In contrast to the Medicare Payment Advisory Commission (MedPAC), which advises Congress on changes to the Medicare program, IPAB has the authority to implement changes in Medicare payment policies to reduce the growth of Medicare expenditures if those expenditures exceed targeted growth rates. However, because IPAB's fifteen members must be appointed by the president and approved by the Senate, as of this writing in early 2013, no IPAB board members have been appointed. IPAB continues to face considerable opposition from conservative groups as well as from medical professionals, so its future remains uncertain.

Medicaid. The fact that the Medicaid expansion is now voluntary obviously reduces the effectiveness of this option for reducing the number of uninsured who are poor. Medicaid has been successful over the past four decades in improving access to health care and the health status of beneficiaries, as discussed in Chapters Two, Three, and Six. By increasing the federal commitment to Medicaid, the ACA builds on both the strengths and weaknesses of that program and allows for existing variation between states in the effectiveness of their Medicaid programs to continue (Kaiser Commission on Medicaid and the Uninsured, 2011). The success of the Medicaid expansions may in fact be crucial to future public support for the ACA. Because the ACA significantly increases our nation's federal commitment to fund health insurance for the poor, evidence that the expansions are not working smoothly or that government funds are not being well utilized will be used to fan the flames of ongoing opposition and as "proof" that the law was ill conceived. Supporters of universal access to care and equality for the poor cannot afford to squander this once-in-a-lifetime opportunity to dramatically increase access and health status for our uninsured population.

SUMMARY

The ACA is likely to change the landscape of health care financing in the United States as dramatically as Medicare and Medicaid did in 1965. Political opposition to the law is diminishing, but remains active, particularly in southern and western states with Republican governors and Republican majorities in the state legislatures. Whether this opposition will diminish more rapidly after the major provisions of the law discussed in this chapter go into effect in 2014 remains an open question. There is no question, however, that tens of millions of Americans will have access to more affordable insurance starting in 2014. Sustaining political and taxpayer support for the ACA throughout the next decade will be an enormous challenge. If the Medicare and Medicaid programs have taught us anything over the last five decades, it is that federal health insurance programs have to evolve and innovate to remain viable.

KEY TERMS

Actuarial value (AV) the portion of a health insurance policy's total costs for covered benefits covered by the premium, as opposed to the portion of costs paid for directly by policyholders at the time of service in the form of out-of-pocket deductibles and copayments. A policy's AV is based on the average experience of everyone who is covered by that particular insurance policy.

Essential health benefits (EHBs) ACA provision that requires insurers to offer health policies or plans with benefits in ten categories of services: outpatient, emergency, inpatient hospital, laboratory, maternity and newborn, mental health and substance abuse, prescription drugs, rehabilitative, preventive, and pediatric oral and vision. EHBs can vary across states, and can be based on actual benchmark health policies or plans currently offered in each state, but must comply with federal guidelines and must be expanded to include all ten categories of benefits described above if they don't currently cover such services.

Exchanges regulated private health insurance marketplaces where individuals receiving subsidies under the ACA can purchase qualified health plans (QHPs).

Federal poverty level (FPL) amount of income needed according to the U.S. Census Bureau to avoid living in poverty. The FPL depends on family size and is updated annually, but does not vary geographically, despite significant differences in the cost of living across the United States. For 2013, the FPL is $11,490 for a single individual and $23,550 for a family of four.

Guaranteed issue requires insurers to issue a policy to anyone able to pay for it, regardless of their health status or medical history.

Guaranteed renewal requires insurers to renew the existing policy of any policyholder as long as they are able to pay for it, regardless of their claims history, health status, or medical history.

Managed competition a model for health care reform proposed by Alain Enthoven in the late 1970s based on the Federal Employees Health Benefits Program. Its key elements are (1) price competition in regulated insurance markets between insurers based on standard insurance policies and (2) pooling of small companies and individual purchasers into larger groups known as health insurance purchasing cooperatives. Enthoven's managed competition model is the conceptual basis for the market reforms adopted under the ACA.

Medical loss ratio (MLR) thresholds require insurers to meet minimum payout requirements on the premiums they collect. Insurers in the large-group market must spend at least 85 percent of their premium revenue on medical expenses, while small-group and individual market insurers must spend at least 80 percent. The law requires insurers to issue rebates to employers or individual purchasers by August 1 of the following year if they do not meet these minimum standards; the rebates must be sufficient to bring the insurer into compliance with the threshold.

Medical underwriting insurer practice of using information about an applicant's medical history health status and preexisting conditions to establish premiums or to deny coverage for those with high-cost medical conditions. The ability of insurers to engage in medical underwriting varied according to state law prior to the ACA, which essentially outlaws the practice as of January 1, 2014.

Metal tiers ACA provision that requires insurers to offer standard health policies and plans in one or more of four coverage tiers based on actuarial value (AV). The Bronze tier must have an AV of 60 percent, meaning the premium should cover 60 percent of the costs for covered benefits, while out-of-pocket spending by policyholders should cover the remaining 40 percent of costs. Bronze plan holders, therefore, pay less in monthly premiums, but have higher copayments or deductibles when they use health care services. The remaining tiers are Silver (70 percent AV), Gold (80 percent AV), and Platinum (90 percent AV). It is important to note that all four tiers must include the same exact EHBs.

Modified community rating   ACA provision that permits insurers to set premiums for qualified health plans (QHPs) inside exchanges as well as policies outside exchanges in the small-group and individual markets after January 1, 2014, based on only a limited set of personal factors, specifically, age, tobacco use, family size, and geographic area. Health status and medical history may not be considered in setting premiums.

Qualified health plans (QHPs)   health insurance policies or health plans approved for sale within exchanges under the ACA. QHPs must offer the essential health benefits (EHBs) package approved within a particular state.

DISCUSSION QUESTIONS

1. The ACA represents a political compromise by providing subsidies to purchase private insurance in regulated markets to those who don't qualify, can't afford, or aren't offered health insurance through their job, rather than, for example, an expansion of eligibility for Medicare. Do you think the ACA will stabilize employment-based insurance in the future? Or will further government intervention be necessary to further "fix" the private market for health insurance? In your opinion, is the ACA too much or not enough reform? Why?

2. The exchanges will be offering standard health insurance plans and policies, all with EHBs and all fitting into one of four metal tiers based on their AVs. Do you believe standard benefits and standard tiers will both increase transparency and increase price competition between insurance policies? If price competition doesn't increase, is that because it is impossible to create competitive markets for health insurance, or is the ACA flawed in its design?

3. Because the implementation of the ACA allows for some significant variation across states in how to comply with the law's requirements, discuss the status of the state in which you are currently residing. Given your state's choices regarding EHBs, type of exchange (state-run, state-federal partnership, or federally run), Medicaid expansion efforts, and so forth, how would you assess the impact of the ACA in your state to date? Specifically, has the exchange in your state gained broad market recognition, and does it appear to be operating effectively?

FURTHER READING

Kaiser Family Foundation website on health reform: http:// kff.org/health-reform

This website contains numerous valuable documents explaining the components of the Affordable Care Act, including a detailed summary of the law, timeline for implementation, and flow charts showing employer and individual responsibilities (or mandates) under the law.

Oberlander, J. (2012). Unfinished journey: A century of health care reform in the United States. *New England Journal of Medicine, 367,* 585–590.

An excellent account of the long road to health reform and universal access in the United States.

Official federal government website on health reform: http://www.healthcare.gov

This website contains valuable information on various elements of the Affordable Care Act, including a consumer-friendly format and presentation style intended to explain various aspects of the law to the general public.

REFERENCES

Angeles, J. (2011). *Explaining health reform: The new rules for determining income under Medicaid in 2014* (Policy Brief, Publication #8194). Washington, DC: Kaiser Commission on Medicaid and the Uninsured. Retrieved from http://kff.org/health-reform/issue-brief/explaining-health-reform-the-new-rules-for/

Blumberg, L. J. (2010). *How will the Patient Protection and Affordable Care Act affect small, medium, and large businesses?* Washington, DC: The Urban Institute. Retrieved from http://www.urban.org/uploadedpdf/412180-ppaca-businesses.pdf

Buchmueller, T. C., DiNardo, J., & Valetta, R. G. (2011). The effect of an employer health insurance mandate on health insurance coverage and the demand for labor: Evidence from Hawaii (Working Paper 2009–08). San Francisco: Federal Reserve Bank of San Francisco. Retrieved from http://www.frbsf.org/publications/economics/papers/2009/wp09-08bk.pdf

Congressional Budget Office (CBO). (2010, March 20). Letter to Speaker Nancy Pelosi regarding the effects of an amendment to H.R. 4872, the Reconciliation Act of 2010. Washington, DC: Author. Retrieved from http://www.cbo.gov/sites/default/files/cbofiles/ftpdocs/113xx/doc11379/amendreconprop.pdf

Congressional Budget Office (CBO). (2011). *CBO estimate of the effects of the insurance coverage provisions contained in P.L. 111–148 and 111–152: March 2011.* Retrieved from http://www.cbo.gov/sites/default/files/cbofiles/attachments/HealthInsurance Provisions.pdf

Congressional Budget Office (CBO). (2012a, March). *CBO and JCT's estimates of the effects of the Affordable Care Act on the number of people obtaining employment-based health insurance.* Washington, DC: CBO. Retrieved from http://cbo.gov/sites/default/files/cbofiles/attachments/03–15-ACA_and_Insurance_2.pdf

Congressional Budget Office (CBO). (2012b, July). *Estimates for the insurance coverage provisions of the Affordable Care Act updated for the recent Supreme Court decision.* Washington, DC: Author. Retrieved from http://www.cbo.gov /sites/default/files/cbofiles/attachments/43472–07–24–2012-Coverage Estimates.pdf

Congressional Budget Office (CBO). (2012c, July 24). Letter to Speaker John Boehner regarding the direct revenue and spending effects of H.R. 6079, Repeal of Obamacare Act. Washington, DC: Author. Retrieved from http://www.cbo.gov /sites/default/files/cbofiles/attachments/43471-hr6079.pdf

Cox, C., Levitt, L., & Claxton, G. (2012). *Insurer rebates under the medical loss ratio: 2012 estimates* (Publication #8305). Menlo Park, CA: Kaiser Family Foundation. Retrieved from http://www.kff.org/healthreform/upload/8305.pdf

DeNavas-Walt, C., Proctor, B. D., & Smith, J. C. (2011). *Income, poverty, and health insurance coverage in the United States: 2010* (Current Population Reports, P60–239). Washington, DC: U. S. Census Bureau. Retrieved from http://www .census.gov/prod/2011pubs/p60–239.pdf

Dubay, L., Holahan, J., Long, S. K., & Lawton, E. (2012). *Will the Affordable Care Act be a job killer?* Washington, DC: The Urban Institute. Retrieved from http://www.urban.org/UploadedPDF/412684-Will-the-Affordable-Care-Act-Be-a -Job-Killer.pdf

Enthoven, A. C. (1978). Consumer choice health plan: A national health insurance proposal based on regulated competition in the private sector. *New England Journal of Medicine, 298,* 709–720.

Georgetown University Health Policy Institute. (2012). *Health insurance market reforms: Pre-existing condition exclusions* (Publication #8356). Menlo Park, CA: Kaiser Family Foundation. Retrieved from http://kff.org/health-reform/fact-sheet/health-insurance-market-reforms-pre-existing-condition/

Heberlein, M., Guyer, J., & Rudowitz, R. (2010). *Financing new Medicaid coverage under health reform: The role of the federal government and states* (Publication #8072). Menlo Park, CA: Kaiser Family Foundation. Retrieved from http://ccf.georgetown.edu /ccf-resources/financing-new-medicaid-coverage-under-health-reform-the-role-of-the-federal-government-and-states/

Holahan, J., & Blumberg, L. (2006). Massachusetts health care reform: A look at the issues. *Health Affairs, 25*(6), w432–w443.

Kaiser Commission on Medicaid and the Uninsured. (2011). *Ensuring access to care in Medicaid under health reform* (Publication #8187). Menlo Park, CA: Kaiser Family Foundation. Retrieved from http://kff.org/health-reform/issue-brief/ensuring-access-to-care-in-medicaid-under/

Linder J., Moore, J., & Udow-Phillips, M. (2012). *The Affordable Care Act and its effect on health insurance market segments.* Ann Arbor, MI: Center of Healthcare Research and Transformation. Retrieved from http://www.chrt.org/assets/policy-briefs/CHRT-Policy-Brief-August-2012.pdf

Lucia, L., Jacobs, K., Dietz, M., Graham-Squire, D., Pourat, N., & Roby, D. H. (2012). *After millions of Californians gain health coverage under the Affordable Care Act, who will remain uninsured?* San Francisco and Los Angeles: UC Berkeley Labor Center and UCLA Center for Health Policy Research. Retrieved from http:// healthpolicy.ucla.edu/publications/Documents/PDF/aca_uninsured12.pdf

McDonough, J. E., Rosman, B., Phelps, F., & Shannon, M. (2006). The third wave of Massachusetts health care access reform. *Health Affairs, 25*(6), w420–w431.

Merlis, M. (2011). *The Affordable Care Act and employer-sponsored insurance for working Americans.* Washington, DC: AcademyHealth. Retrieved from http://www.academyhealth.org/files/nhpc/2011/AH_2011AffordableCareReport FINAL3.pdf

Oberlander, J. (2010). Long time coming: Why health reform finally passed. *Health Affairs, 29*(6), 1112–1116.

Oberlander, J. (2012). Unfinished journey: A century of health care reform in the United States. *New England Journal of Medicine, 367,* 585–590.

Sommers, B. D. (2012). *Number of young adults gaining insurance due to the Affordable Care Act now tops 3 million* (Issue Brief). Washington, DC: Department of Health and Human Services, Office of the Assistant Secretary for Planning and Evaluation. Retrieved from http://aspe.hhs.gov/aspe/gaininginsurance/rb.pdf

Sparer, M. (2012). *Medicaid managed care: Costs, access, and quality of care* (Research Synthesis Report No. 23). Princeton, NJ: Robert Wood Johnson Foundation. Retrieved from http://www.rwjf.org/content/dam/farm/reports/reports/2012 /rwjf401106

Yong, P. L., Bertko, J., & Kronick, R. (2011). *Actuarial value and employer sponsored insurance* (Research Brief). Washington, DC: Department of Health and Human Services, Office of the Assistant Secretary for Planning and Evaluation. Retrieved from http://aspe.hhs.gov/health/reports/2011/av-esi/rb.pdf

CHAPTER TWO

IMPROVING ACCESS TO CARE

Ronald M. Andersen
Pamela L. Davidson
Sebastian E. Baumeister

Learning Objectives

- Learn about the behavioral model as a conceptual framework for analyzing access and equity in health care
- Understand how contextual and individual characteristics influence health behaviors and outcomes of care
- Examine how the dimensions of access can be used to improve utilization and health outcomes
- Describe how access has changed over time using nationally standardized indicators that measure potential access (health insurance coverage and regular source of care), realized access (use of hospital, physician, and dental services), and equitable access (providing services according to need for all income and racial and ethnic groups)
- Predict how the 2010 Affordable Care Act might improve health care access

This chapter presents basic trends as well as research and policy issues related to monitoring and evaluating health care access. We define *access* as actual use of personal health services and everything that facilitates or impedes their use. It is the link between health services systems and the populations they serve. Access means not only visiting a medical care provider but also getting to the right services at the right time to promote improved health outcomes. Conceptualizing and measuring access is the key to understanding and making health policy. Monitoring and evaluating access allows us to (1) predict use of health services, (2) promote social justice, and (3) improve effectiveness and efficiency of health service delivery.

This chapter presents a conceptual framework for understanding the multiple dimensions of access to medical care. The sixth revision of the behavioral model in this edition is expanded to include (1) genetic susceptibility as an individual predisposing factor and (2) quality of life as an outcome factor. Consequently, the description of these factors is somewhat more detailed than that of the other factors in the model. The various types of access are considered and related to their policy purposes. Examples of access indicators are provided, including potential, realized, equitable, inequitable, effective, and efficient access indicators. Trend data are used to track changes that have occurred over time in these access indicators. The chapter addresses these questions: Are access, indicators of the U.S. health care system improving or declining? For whom? According to what indicators? How might access be improved?

Understanding Access to Health Care

This section presents a conceptual framework based on a behavioral model of health services use that emphasizes contextual as well as individual determinants of access to medical care. Dimensions of access are defined according to components of the framework, and we examine how access might be improved for each dimension.

Conceptual Framework

Figure 2.1 stresses that improving access to care is best accomplished by focusing on contextual as well as individual determinants (Andersen, 1995, 2008; Andersen & Davidson, 2007). By *contextual*, we mean the circumstances and environment of health care access. Context includes health organization and provider-related factors as well as community characteristics (Davidson, Andersen, Wyn, & Brown, 2004; Robert, 1999). Contextual factors are measured at the aggregate rather than the individual level.

FIGURE 2.1. A BEHAVIORAL MODEL OF HEALTH SERVICES USE—6TH REVISION

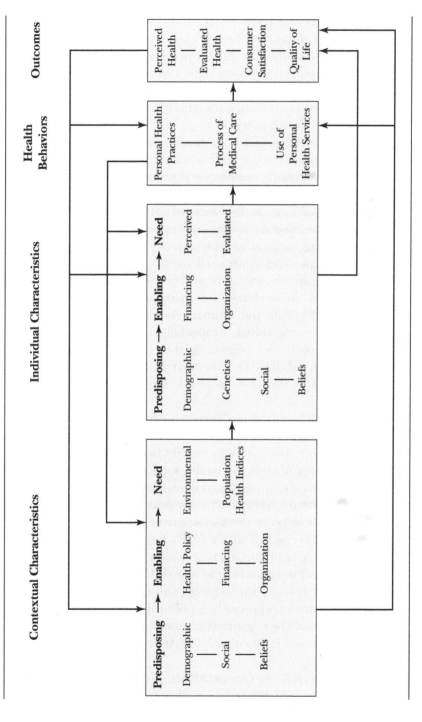

These aggregate levels range from units as small as the family to those as large as a national health care system. In between are work groups, provider organizations, health plans, neighborhoods, local communities, and metropolitan statistical areas. Individuals are related to these aggregate units through membership (family, work group, provider institutions, or health plan) or residence (neighborhood, community, metropolitan area, or national health system).

The model suggests the major components of contextual characteristics are divided in the same way as individual characteristics determining access: (1) existing conditions that predispose people to use or not use services even though these conditions are not directly responsible for use, (2) enabling conditions that facilitate or impede use of services, and (3) need or conditions that laypeople or health care providers recognize as requiring medical treatment (Andersen, 1968; Andersen, 1995). The model emphasizes contextual factors in recognition of the importance of community, the structure and process of providing care (Donabedian, 1980), and the realities of a managed care environment (Bindman & Gold, 1998). Still, the ultimate focus of the model remains on health behavior of individuals (especially their use of health services) and resulting outcomes regarding their health, satisfaction with services, and quality of life. We now turn to brief consideration of each major component of the model shown in Figure 2.1.

Contextual Predisposing Characteristics. Demographic characteristics of a community include its age, gender, and marital status composition. Thus, a community populated primarily by older persons might well have a different mix of available health services and facilities from one in which the majority are younger parents and children.

Social characteristics at the contextual level describe how supportive or detrimental the communities where people live and work might be to their health and access to health services. Relevant measures include educational level, ethnic and racial composition, measures of spatial segregation, employment level, and crime rate (White, Haas, & Williams, 2012).

Beliefs refer to underlying community or organizational values and cultural norms and prevailing political perspectives regarding how health services should be organized, financed, and made accessible to the population (Andersen & Smedby, 1975; Andersen, Smedby, & Anderson, 1970).

Contextual Enabling Characteristics. Health policies are authoritative decisions made pertaining to health or influencing the pursuit of health

(Longest, 1998). They can be public policies made in the legislative, executive, or judicial branch of government, at all levels from local to national, such as the Affordable Care Act (ACA). Policies in both the private and public sectors influence access, such as those made by executives of managed care organizations concerning product lines, pricing, marketing, or by accrediting agencies such as the Joint Commission on Accreditation of Health Care Organizations (JCAHO) or quality assessment organizations such as the National Committee for Quality Assurance (NCQA).

Financing characteristics are described by an array of contextual measures that suggest resources potentially available to pay for health services, including per capita community income and wealth. Other financial characteristics are incentives to purchase or provide services, such as the relative price of medical care and other goods and services, and the method of compensating providers. Also included here are per capita expenditures for health services and the rate of health insurance coverage.

Organization at the contextual level includes the amount and distribution of health services facilities and personnel as well as how they are structured to offer services. Structure includes supply of services in the community, such as the ratios of physicians and hospital beds to population. Structure also includes how medical care is organized in a particular institution or delivery system where people receive care, as with office hours and location of service, provider mix, utilization and quality control, oversight, and outreach and education programs.

Contextual Need Characteristics. Environmental need characteristics include health-related measures of the physical environment, among them the quality of housing, water, and air, (for example, residing in a county that meets national ambient air quality standards throughout the year) (National Center for Health Statistics & U.S. Department of Health and Human Services, 1999). Other measures suggesting how healthy the environment might be are injury or death rate, such as rate of occupational injury and disease and related deaths, as well as death rates from motor vehicle accidents, homicides, and firearms.

Population health indices are more general indicators of community health that may or may not be associated with the physical environment. These indices include general and condition-specific rates of mortality (for example, infant mortality; age-adjusted mortality; and mortality rates for heart disease, cancer, stroke, and HIV); morbidity (incidence of preventable childhood communicable diseases and AIDS, and prevalence of cancer, hypertension, and untreated dental caries); and disability

(disability days due to acute conditions and limitation of activity due to chronic conditions).

The arrows in Figure 2.1 leading from the contextual characteristics indicate they can influence health behaviors and outcomes in multiple ways. They can work through individual characteristics, as when increased generosity of a state Medicaid program leads to an increase in insured low-income children and health insurance and subsequent increases in their health services use. Contextual characteristics can also influence health behaviors and outcomes directly, as when the presence of community health clinics in a metropolitan statistical area leads to increased use of primary care services by low-income persons independent of personal income or other individual characteristics.

Individual Predisposing Characteristics. Demographic factors such as sex and age of the individual represent biological imperatives suggesting the likelihood that people will need health services (Hulka & Wheat, 1985). Genetic susceptibility also potentially influences need, by increasing disease incidence. Genetic testing for rare, monogenetic diseases involves testing single genes (such familial hypercholesterolemia, fragile X syndrome, Duchenne muscular dystrophy, Huntington's disease, and BRCA1 and BRCA2 mutations for breast cancer). However, more prevalent conditions such as cardiovascular diseases, age-related macular degeneration, type 2 diabetes, depression, and many types of cancer have a multifactorial and polygenetic etiology involving hundreds or thousands of genetic variants, making the development of relevant genetic susceptibility measures extremely challenging (Becker et al., 2011). In the case of multifactorial conditions, family history can serve as an adequate source of risk differentiation (Thanassoulis & Vasan, 2010).

Social factors determine the status of a person in the community as well as his or her ability to cope with presenting problems and command resources to deal with those problems. Traditional measures include an individual's education, occupation, and ethnicity. Expanded measures include people's social networks, such as presence of family and friends and affiliations with religious and other community organizations that can potentially facilitate (or impede) access to services (Bass & Noelker, 1987; Guendelman, 1991; Pescosolido, Wright, Alegria, & Vera, 1998; Portes, Kyle, & Eaton, 1992). Health beliefs are attitudes, values, and knowledge people have about health and health services that can influence their subsequent perception of need and use of health services (Andersen, 1968).

Individual Enabling Characteristics. Financing of health services for the individual involves the income and wealth available to the individual to pay for services. Financing also includes the effective price of health care to the patient, determined by having insurance and cost-sharing requirements. Social support may also be considered an enabling variable. It is the actual amount of emotional, informational, tangible, and affectionate support generated through the social network (a predisposing variable) (Seeman & Berkman, 1988).

Organization of health services for the individual describes whether or not the individual has a regular source of care or medical home and the nature of that source (private doctor, community clinic, or emergency room). It also includes means of transportation, reported travel time, and waiting time for care.

Individual Need Characteristics. Perceived need is how people view their own general health and functional status. Also included here is how they experience and emotionally respond to symptoms of illness, pain, and worry about their health condition. Perceptions about the importance and magnitude of a health problem or symptom lead to a decision to seek medical care (or not to do so). Perceived need is a social phenomenon that, when appropriately modeled, should itself be largely explainable by the severity and discomfort of the symptoms, such as pain, predisposing and social characteristics (such as gender, age, ethnicity, or education) and health beliefs (health attitudes, knowledge about health care, and so on).

Evaluated need represents professional judgment and objective measurement about a patient's physical status and need for medical care (blood pressure readings, temperature, and blood cell count, as well as diagnoses and prognoses for particular conditions the patient experiences). Of course, evaluated need is not simply, or even primarily, a valid and reliable measure from biological science. It also has a social component and varies with the changing state of the art and science of medicine, clinical guidelines and protocols, and prevailing practice patterns, as well as the training and competency of the professional expert doing the assessment.

Logical expectations of the model are that perceived need helps us to better understand the care-seeking process and adherence to a medical regimen, while evaluated need is more closely related to the kind and amount of treatment that is given after a patient has presented to a medical care provider.

Health Behaviors. Health behaviors are personal practices performed by the individual that influence health status. They include diet and nutrition, exercise, stress reduction, alcohol and tobacco use, self-care, and adherence to medical regimens. The process of medical care is the behavior of providers interacting with patients in the process of care delivery (Donabedian, 1980). General process measures might relate to patient counseling and education, test ordering, prescribing patterns, and quality of provider-patient communication. Process measures might also describe the specifics of caregiving for particular conditions, such as whether a provider checks a CD4 cell count in a person with HIV disease or reviews the patient's record of home glucose monitoring in a diabetic.

Use of personal health services is the essential component of health behaviors in a comprehensive model of access to care. The purpose of the original behavioral model was to predict health services use, measured rather broadly as units of physician ambulatory care, hospital inpatient services, and dental care visits. We hypothesized that predisposing, enabling, and need factors would have differential ability to explain use, depending on what type of service was examined (Andersen, 1968). Hospital services used in response to more serious problems and conditions would be primarily explained by need and demographic characteristics, while dental services (considered more discretionary) would more likely be explained by social conditions, health beliefs, enabling resources, and severity of symptoms such as oral pain (Davidson & Andersen, 1997; Davidson, Rams, & Andersen, 1997).

We expected all the components of the model to explain ambulatory physician use because the conditions stimulating care seeking would generally be viewed as less serious and demanding than those resulting in inpatient care but more serious than those leading to dental care. More specific measures of health services use are now being employed to describe a particular medical condition or type of service or practitioner, or they are linked in an episode of illness to examine continuity of care (Andersen, 1995). For example, a longitudinal study of rheumatoid arthritis measures patient visits to various types of providers, treatment used, level of patient compliance with treatment, and associated changes in functional status and pain over time. Although specific measures are in many ways likely to be more informative, the more global ones (number of physician visits, self-rated general health status) still have a role to play. In addition, these global measures are used to assess the overall effects of health policy changes over time.

Outcomes. The patient's perceived health status is influenced by health behavior, personal health services use, and individual characteristics, as well as the contextual environment. Perceived health status indicates the extent to which a person can live a functional, comfortable, and pain-free existence. Outcome measures include reports of general perceived health status, activities of daily living, and disability.

Evaluated health status is dependent on the judgment of the professional, on the basis of established clinical standards and state-of-the-art practices. Measures include biomarkers and tests of patient physiology and function as well as diagnosis and prognosis regarding their condition. Outcome measures of perceived and evaluated health may appear suspiciously like perceived and evaluated need measures. Indeed, they are. The ultimate outcome validation of improved access is to reduce individual needs previously measured and evaluated.

Consumer satisfaction is how individuals perceive the health care they receive. It can be judged by patient ratings of travel time, waiting time, communication with providers, and technical care received. From a health plan perspective, an ultimate outcome measure of patient satisfaction might be whether or not enrollees choose to switch plans (Cunningham & Kohn, 2000).

We have added quality of life to the model as an outcome because health behaviors affect more than an individual's health, and quality of life measures are increasingly employed by health policymakers, managers, providers, payers, patients, and researchers both as outcomes of health care delivery and subsequent determinants of need and health status (Guyatt, Feeny, & Patrick, 1993; Kaplan & Ries, 2007). One reason for this increasing attention to quality of care is the patient-centered care movement (Lambert et al., 1997; Patient-Centered Outcomes Research Institute, 2013). The components of quality of life include the following broad domains: physical health, psychological health, social relationships, and environment that the individual perceives as important to his or her well-being or happiness (Skevington, Lotfy, & O'Connell, 2004). Ideally, the individual determines not only the particular conditions to be satisfied for his or her quality of life but also the relative importance of each condition and the extent to which the condition is realized (Locker & Allen, 2007; Nordenfelt, 1993).

Central to the model shown in Figure 2.1 is feedback, depicted by the arrows from outcomes to health behaviors, individual characteristics, and contextual characteristics. Feedback allows insights about how access might come to be improved. Feedback can occur at the national level, as illustrated by the apparent affirmation of the ACA through the Supreme Court ruling in support of health care reform in 2012. Feedback can also occur at the community or institutional level. Certainly there are expectations that feedback to hospitals and other health care providers from accrediting institutions such as the Joint Commission and the National Commission for Quality Assurance to policies such as the Health Insurance Portability and Accountability Act (HIPAA) that result in contextual changes in the organization and processes of care for their patients.

Dimensions of Access: Measurement, Trends, and Strategies for Improvement

Access to medical care is a relatively complex multidimensional phenomenon. Over several decades, the behavioral model has been used as a tool to help define and differentiate these dimensions (Andersen & Davidson, 1996). In this section, we define dimensions of access and suggest how *improvement* is measured in those dimensions (see Figure 2.2).

Trends are examined according to several dimensions of access. We consider changes over time in potential access (health insurance coverage), realized access (use of hospital, physician, and dental services), and equitable access (health insurance and regular source of care) according to income and race. In addition, we examine some key research findings concerning effective and efficient access. Finally, we consider strategies for improving trends in access.

Potential Access. Potential access is measured by the enabling variables of the behavioral model both at the contextual level (health policy and financing) and individual level (regular source of care, health insurance, and income). More enabling resources constitute the means for use and increase the likelihood that it will take place. Depending on the national, state, or local context, policies can be formed to increase potential access for minority populations or to decrease potential access to contain rising health care costs. Potential access measures, such as having a regular source of care and health insurance and a medical or dental home, are used as indicators of greater access.

The proportion of population eighteen to forty-four years who were uninsured increased during the 1980s and 1990s, reaching 25 percent in 2011 (see Table 2.1). The proportion covered by private insurance decreased for every age group between 1984 and 2011. Between 1984 and

FIGURE 2.2. THE POLICY PURPOSES OF ACCESS MEASURES

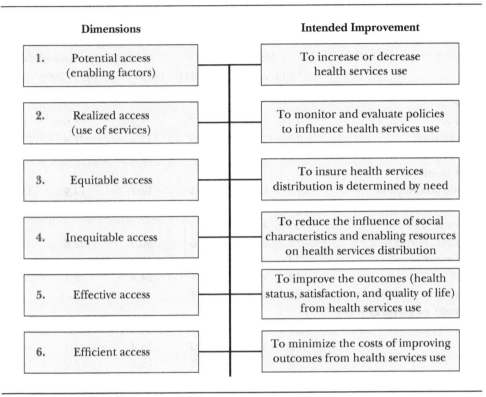

Dimensions	Intended Improvement
1. Potential access (enabling factors)	To increase or decrease health services use
2. Realized access (use of services)	To monitor and evaluate policies to influence health services use
3. Equitable access	To insure health services distribution is determined by need
4. Inequitable access	To reduce the influence of social characteristics and enabling resources on health services distribution
5. Effective access	To improve the outcomes (health status, satisfaction, and quality of life) from health services use
6. Efficient access	To minimize the costs of improving outcomes from health services use

2011, the proportion of all children covered under Medicaid increased from 12 to 38 percent. This increase reflected the expanded Medicaid income eligibility enacted by Congress in the mid-1980s and the State Children's Health Insurance Program (SCHIP), first implemented in the late 1990s.

About one-fifth of the population does not report having a regular source of medical care, another important potential access measure (see Table 2.1). Since the mid-1990s, the percentage of children without a regular source of care has declined to less than 5 percent, while it has actually increased to over 25 percent for adults eighteen to forty-four years. The results overall leave little doubt that a decline in potential access has occurred for the U.S. adult population since the early 1980s because of diminution in private health insurance coverage, while it has expanded for children due to increased Medicaid coverage.

TABLE 2.1. PERCENT OF THE U.S. POPULATION UNDER SIXTY-FIVE WITH NO HEALTH INSURANCE COVERAGE AND REGULAR SOURCE OF MEDICAL CARE BY AGE, RACE OR ETHNICITY, AND POVERTY LEVEL

	No Insurance				No Regular Source of Care		
	1984	2002	2009	2011	1993–1994	1999–2000	2010
Age							
<18 years	14%	13%	10%	7%	7.7%	6.9%	9.9%
18–44 years	17	22	24	25	21.7	21.4	25.2
45–64 years	10	13	13	15	12.8	10.9	11.8
Race or ethnicity[d]							
White, non-Hispanic	12	12	12	13	17.1	14.9	15.8
Black, non-Hispanic	20	19	18	19	19.7	19.2	22.1
Hispanic, Mexican[b]	34	40	38	33 ⎫			
Hispanic, Puerto Rican[b]	18	16	21	16 ⎬	30.3	32.6	33.3
Hispanic, Cuban[b]	22	25	23	26 ⎭			
Asian[a]	18	18	17	17	24.8	22.1	20.8
American Indian/ Alaskan Native[a]	22	38	35	34	-	-	-
Percent of poverty level[c, d]							
Below 100	34	34	32	28	29.5	29.6	32.8
100–199	22	31	29	30	25.4	27.1	30.4
200–299	8	15	16	17	15.6	17.2	19.3
300 and more	3	6	6	5	13.4	11.6	9.7
Total	14	17	17	17	17.9	17.8	19.6

Note: Table 2.1 reports a critical potential access measure: health care coverage for persons under sixty-five years of age from 1984 to 2011. The uninsured proportion of the population increased from 14 to 17 percent in that time period. Medicaid coverage actually increased (from 7 to 18 percent), but the overall decline in coverage resulted from a drop in the proportion covered by private insurance, from 77 to 62 percent (data not shown).

[a]Includes persons of Hispanic and non-Hispanic origin.

[b]Persons of Hispanic origin may be white, black, Asian, Pacific Islander, or American Indian/Alaskan Native.

[c]Poverty level is based on family income and family size, using Bureau of the Census poverty thresholds.

[d]Age-adjusted by U.S. Census 2000 data.

Source: National Center for Health Statistics, *Health United States, 2011* (Hyattsville, MD: National Center for Health Statistics, 2011). Updated tables 138, 140, 141.

Realized Access. Realized access is the actual use of services. Realized access indicators include utilization of physician, hospital, dental, and other health services. Historically, the United States experienced improving trends in access as measured by increasing health services utilization rates.

Increased realized access to health services was considered an end goal of policy change. Progressive policies designed to increase realized access were implemented in the 1950s and 1960s through workforce, policy, and structural interventions, such as increasing physician supply, the enactment of Medicare and Medicaid legislation in the mid-1960s, and prior to that augmenting hospital beds in rural communities through the Hill-Burton Act of 1946.

Table 2.2 presents current data from the late 1990s through 2011 on realized access for three types of services: those in response to serious illness (hospital admissions), services for a combination of primary and secondary care (physician visits), and services for conditions that are rarely life-threatening and generally considered discretionary but still have an important bearing on people's functional status and quality of life (dental visits).

Historically, the hospital admission rate for the U.S. population doubled between 1930 (six admissions per one hundred persons per year) and the early 1950s (twelve admissions) (Andersen & Davidson, 2007). A rising standard of living, the advent of voluntary health insurance, the increasing legitimacy of the modern hospital as a place to deliver babies and treat acute illness, and the requirements necessary for developing sophisticated medical technology all contributed to expanded use of the acute care hospital. Hospital admissions further increased in the 1960s and early 1970s (reaching fourteen admissions per hundred persons per year in 1974), reflecting continued growth in medical technology, private health insurance, and the advent of Medicare coverage for the elderly and Medicaid coverage for the low-income population in 1965.

However, beginning in the mid-1970s, use of the acute care hospital began to decline, dropping to twelve admissions per hundred population by 2002 (Andersen & Davidson, 2007). There was also a substantial decrease in average length of stay per admission during this period, from 7.5 days in 1980 to 6.5 days in 1990 and 4.9 days in 2002 (National Center for Health Statistics, 2004). Those declines accompanied an increasing effort to contain health care costs by shifting care from the more expensive inpatient setting to less expensive outpatient settings, a shift from fee for service to prospective payments by Medicare, reduced coverage and benefits with increasing coinsurance and deductibles for health insurance, and a shift in certain medical technology and styles of practice that meant reduced reliance on the inpatient settings. Contributing to the decline of inpatient volume since 1980 has been the significant growth of managed care. This growth of managed care, with its emphasis on

TABLE 2.2. PERCENT OF THE U.S. POPULATION WITH HOSPITAL ADMISSIONS, PHYSICIAN VISITS, AND DENTAL VISITS BY POVERTY LEVEL

	1997	2011	1997	2011
Acute Hospital Admissions in a Year[b]	**One or More**		**Two or More**	
Percent of poverty level[a]				
<100	10.0%	8.5%	2.8%	2.9%
100–199	7.2	6.6	1.7	1.8
200–399	6.0	5.3	1.2	1.2
400 or more	4.7	4.4	0.7	0.8
Total	7.8	7.1	1.8	1.9
Physician Visits in a Year[b]	**No Visits**		**Ten or More Visits**	
Percent of poverty level[a]				
<100	21%	19%	20%	17%
100–199	20	21	15	14
200–399	17	16	13	12
400 or more	13	11	13	12
Total	17	16	14	13
Dental Visits in a Year[b]	**No Visits**		**One or More Visits**	
Percent of poverty level[a]				
<100	49%	48%	51%	52%
100–199	49	48	51	52
200–399	34	35	66	65
400 or more	21	19	79	81
Total	35	34	65	66

[a]Poverty level is based on family income and family size, using the census poverty thresholds.

[b]Age-adjusted by U.S. Census 2000 data.

Source: National Center for Health Statistics, *Health United States, 2011* (Hyattsville, MD: National Center for Health Statistics, 2011), Updated tables 102, 83, 98.

utilization review and cost containment, contributed to reduction in hospital admissions and the length of hospital stays.

Physician visits, like inpatient services, increased substantially from 1930 (2.6 visits per person per year) to the early 1950s (4.2 visits), for many of the same reasons hospital admissions were increasing in this period (Andersen & Davidson, 2007). However, unlike hospital admissions, the number of physician visits continued to increase, reaching 4.9 visits in 1974 and 5.8 in 1996 (National Center for Health Statistics & U.S. Department of Health and Human Services, 1999). By 2011, 13 percent of the population had ten or more physician visits per year (Table 2.2). In part, the continued growth of managed care, with its relative deemphasis of the inpatient setting and greater focus on outpatient settings, may account for the divergence in trends of hospital inpatient versus physician outpatient realized access measures.

Twenty-one percent of the population visited a dentist in 1930, and the proportion increased consistently, reaching one-half of the population in 1974 (Andersen & Davidson, 2007). Further increases in the next three decades resulted in 65 percent of the population visiting a dentist in 1997 (Table 2.2). There was no significant increase in the proportion seeing a dentist from 1997 to 2011 (66 percent).

Equitable and Inequitable Access. Equity of access is determined by which predisposing, enabling, and need variables are dominant in predicting potential and realized access. Equity is in the eye of the beholder. Value judgments about which components of the model should explain utilization in an equitable health care system are crucial to the definition. We choose to follow a traditional public health approach where *equitable access* has been defined as occurring when predisposing demographic variables (age and gender), and especially need variables, account for most of the variance in utilization. Inequitable access occurs when predisposing social structure variables (education and ethnicity) and enabling variables (insurance, regular source of care, and income) determine who has access. Whether increasing use of genetic testing and the associated health services to address discovered needs is equitable is an emerging concern that will require broader societal discussion, taking into consideration the needs and resources of patients and the financial cost to government and private insurers (Bunnik, Schermer, & Janssens, 2011).

Potential Access: Equitable or Inequitable?

Table 2.1 presents health insurance coverage and regular source of care (potential access measures) by ethnicity and income for the U.S. population for selected years. Recall that we have suggested *equitable access* is indicated by similar levels of insurance coverage and having a regular source of medical care by various income and ethnic groups.

Inequitable access is indicated by discrepancies in coverage and source of care for these groups.

Health Insurance. Table 2.1 suggests considerable inequity in insurance coverage in 1984 continuing to the present time. Minorities are generally less likely to have health insurance than non-Hispanic whites, although the differences are declining. However, there are also considerable differences among minority groups in 2011. American Indians/Alaskan Natives (34 percent) and Mexican Americans (33 percent) are least likely to have coverage, while Puerto Ricans (16 percent) and Asian Americans (17 percent) are much closer to non-Hispanic whites (13 percent). Trends in insurance coverage according to income level since 1984 show considerable inequity in every time period (Table 2.1). For example, in 2011 28 percent of the lowest-income group was uninsured, compared to only 5 percent of the highest-income group. However, the difference between the lowest-income group and the rest actually declined. Between 1984 and 2011, the proportion of uninsured for persons below the 100 percent of the federal poverty level declined from 34 percent to 28 percent, while the proportion of uninsured for all higher-income groups actually increased between 1984 and 2011. For example, the proportion of uninsured in the relatively low-income group (100 to 199 percent of the poverty level) increased from 22 percent to 30 percent.

Regular Source of Care. Inequity exists based on people's reports about whether or not they have a regular source of medical care or medical home. It appears that inequity has increased between the mid-1990s and 2010 (Table 2.1). While the proportion of non-Hispanic whites without a regular source decreased in that time period, the proportion for blacks, Hispanics, and American Indians/Alaskan Natives increased. Similarly, while the proportion of the highest-income group (400 percent or more of the poverty level) without insurance decreased, the proportion for all the other income groups increased.

Realized Access: Equitable or Inequitable?

In this section we consider the realized access measures: hospital admissions, physician visits, and dental visits. To what extent has equity for realized access been achieved for ethnic and income groups?

Hospital Admissions. Historic data suggest equity in hospital admissions according to income has been more than achieved. The low-income

Americans' hospital admission rate compared to the rest of the population has grown relatively consistently since 1930, when population data were first collected. Today, it is much higher than that for any other income group (Table 2.2) (Andersen & Davidson, 2007). However, such a general conclusion about improvement in equity needs to be qualified in important ways that we will discuss after presenting the trends in admission rates by income. In 1928 to 1931 the highest-income group had the highest admission rate (Andersen & Davidson, 2007). By the 1950s, the rate equalized. In subsequent years, rate by income diverged, with the lowest-income group increasing relative to those with higher incomes so that by 2002 the lowest income had a rate (sixteen per hundred) twice that of the highest income group (eight per hundred). And in 2011, 8.9 percent of those with incomes less than 100 percent of the poverty level had one or more hospitalizations, compared to 4.4 percent of those with incomes of 400 percent or more of the poverty level (Table 2.2).

Do these findings indicate the low-income group has more than achieved equity with respect to hospital admissions? Most probably not. First, the needs of the low-income group for acute hospital care (or other realized access measures) are often much greater than the needs of higher-income groups. Table 2.3 shows rates of selected needs by poverty level. For four of the five selected need measures (self-reported health status, activity limitation, dental carries, and psychological distress) for which we have income data, the level of need is two to seven times greater for the people below 100 percent poverty than for those 400 percent or more above poverty. Only for joint pain is the difference of less magnitude. Studies directly taking into account the need for medical care suggest that greater use among low-income persons can be largely accounted for by their higher rates of disease and disability (Davis & Rowland, 1983).

Second, higher use of inpatient hospital care, rather than indicating good access to hospital care, suggests that limited access to preventive and primary services at an earlier time might increase subsequent need for inpatient hospital services for serious acute and uncontrolled chronic disease problems (Bindman et al., 1995).

Turning to ethnicity, the hospital admission rate at an earlier time in 1964 for whites (eleven per hundred) was still considerably higher than that for blacks (eight per hundred) (Andersen & Davidson, 2007). However, by the 1980s the rate for blacks exceeded that for whites, and the higher rate for blacks continued through 2011 (Table 2.4) suggesting achievement of equity by blacks. That conclusion is greatly tempered by the findings that the higher hospital admission rate for blacks, similar to

TABLE 2.3. SELECTED MEASURES OF NEED BY RACE OR ETHNICITY AND POVERTY LEVEL

	Infant Death per 1,000 Births per Year	Age-Standardized Death Rate per Year	Fair or Poor Self-Reported Health	Any Basic Action Difficulty or Complex Activity Limitation	Untreated Dental Caries (20–64)	Any Joint Pain (18 and Over)	Serious Psychological Distress in 30 Days
	2006–2008	2007–2009	2011	2011	2005–2008	2010	2009–10
Race or Ethnicity							
White, non-Hispanic	5.6	7.6	8.4%[a]	32.4%[a]	19.3%	32.6%	3.1%
Black, non-Hispanic	13.1	9.4	15.0	33.3	39.7	32.0	3.8
Hispanic, Mexican[b]			14.0		35.2	25.0	2.8
Hispanic, Puerto Rican[b]	5.5	5.3	13.2	24.4	*	25.4	3.6
Hispanic, Cuban[b]			*		*	*	*
Asian[a]	4.6	4.1	8.7	19.0	*	20.4	1.6
American Indian/Alaskan Native[a]	8.6	6.1	14.4	40.8	*	38.1	5.2
Percent of Poverty Level[c]							
Below 100	*	*	21.5%	41.0%	41.9%	35.6%	8.4%
100–199	*	*	15.0	40.0	37.7	34.0	4.8
200–399	*	*	8.7	31.4	24.3	32.2	2.8
400 and up	*	*	4.3	21.7	24.3	30.5	1.2
Total	*	*	9.8	31.9	11.1	32.1	3.2

[a]Includes persons of Hispanic and non-Hispanic origin.

[b]Persons of Hispanic origin may be white, black, Asian, Pacific Islander, or American Indian/Alaskan Native.

[c]Poverty level is based on family income and family size, using Bureau of the Census poverty thresholds.

*Not reported.

Source: National Center for Health Statistics, Health United States, 2011 (Hyattsville, MD: National Center for Health Statistics, 2011), Updated tables 15, 24, 25, 56, 54, 57, 76, 53, 59.

that for low-income people, can be largely accounted for by greater level of medical need (Manton, Patrick, & Johnson, 1987). And Table 2.3 shows blacks have high levels of need, with significantly higher age-adjusted mortality and infant mortality, and are ranked number one in percent reporting fair or poor health compared to all other ethnic groups.

Unlike blacks, the admission rate for Hispanics in 2011 (4.9 percent) with one or more admissions is less than that for non-Hispanic whites (5.8 percent). However, there is considerable variation among Hispanic subgroups (Table 2.4). The rates for Mexicans and Cubans tends to be below that for Non-Hispanic whites, while those for Puerto Ricans exceed the white rate (Hajat, Lucas, & Kington, 2000). While the proportion with one or more admissions in a year decreased for all ethnic groups between 1997 and 2011, the largest declines were for Hispanics (6.8 percent to 4.9 percent) and American Indians/Alaskan Natives (7.6 percent to 4.9 percent) (Table 2.4).

Physician Visits. Long-term trends suggest increasing equity for physician visits according to income. In 1928 to 1931, the lowest-income group averaged only one-half as many visits to the doctor (2.2 visits) as the highest-income group (4.3 visits) (Andersen & Davidson, 2007). Over time, the gap narrowed. By 1974, the lowest-income group was actually visiting a physician more often than the higher-income groups, and the difference increased after that. In 2011, 17 percent of persons below 100 percent of poverty had ten or more physician visits per year, compared to 12 percent of persons with incomes 400 percent or more above poverty (Table 2.2). However, the poverty group also had the highest percent of persons with no physician visits in the year (19 percent), versus 11 percent for the highest-income group. Again, research suggests that the apparent equity in physician visits achieved by the low-income population must be tempered by remembering their greater level of medical need (Davis & Rowland, 1983) (Table 2.3).

The movement toward equity in physician visits for minority groups is a more complex picture than for the low-income population. Parity with the white population in the proportion seeing a doctor did not take place for the black population until the early 1980s, and the proportion seeing a doctor has remained about the same for blacks and whites since (Andersen & Davidson, 2007) (Table 2.4). The proportion of Hispanics not seeing the doctor in 2011 (23 percent) continues to be considerably above the non-Hispanic whites (13 percent). Considerable variation exists among Hispanic groups, with Mexicans and Cubans less likely to see

TABLE 2.4. PERCENT OF THE U.S. POPULATION WITH HOSPITAL ADMISSIONS, PHYSICIAN VISITS, AND DENTAL VISITS BY RACE OR ETHNICITY

	1997	2011	1997	2011
Acute Hospital Admissions in a Year[c]	**One or More**		**Two or More**	
Race or Ethnicity				
White, non-Hispanic	6.1%	5.8%	1.2%	1.3%
Black, non-Hispanic	7.5	6.8	1.9	2.2
Hispanic[b]	6.8	4.9	1.2	1.2
Asian[a]	3.9	3.4	0.5	0.6
American Indian/Alaskan Native[a]	7.6	4.9	-	-
Total	7.8	9.3	1.3	2.0
Physician Visits in a Year[c]	**None**		**Ten or More**	
Race or Ethnicity				
White, non-Hispanic	15%	13%	14%	14%
Black, non-Hispanic	17	15	14	13
Hispanic[b]	25	23	13	10
Asian[a]	23	20	9	8
American Indian/Alaskan Native[a]	17	19	21	12
Total	17	16	14	13
Dental Visits in a Year[c]	**None**		**One or More**	
Race or Ethnicity				
White non-Hispanic	32%	31%	68%	69%
Black non-Hispanic	41	38	59	62
Hispanic[b]	46	43	54	57
Asian[a]	37	34	63	66
American Indian/Alaskan Native [a]	45	38	55	62
Total	35	34	65	66

[a]Includes persons of Hispanic and non-Hispanic origin.

[b]Persons of Hispanic origin may be white, black, Asian, Pacific Islander, or American Indian/Alaskan Native.

[c]Age-adjusted by U.S. Census data 2000.

Source: National Center for Health Statistics, *Health United States, 2011* (Hyattsville, MD: National Center for Health Statistics, 2011). Updated tables 102, 83, 98.

the doctor than whites, but with Puerto Ricans more likely to do so (Hajat et al., 2000). In 2011, the proportion of Asians (20 percent) and American Indians/Alaskan Natives (19 percent) without visits also exceeded the non-Hispanic white proportion (13 percent) (Table 2.4). Taking some measures of need into account (Table 2.3), one could argue that all minority groups still experience some inequity with respect to physician visits, but some experience more inequity than others. American Indians/Alaskan Natives may experience most inequity, as their use rates appear lower than whites, but show significantly more need on most measures. Blacks show high utilization, but also high levels of need. Hispanics seem to be somewhere in the middle regarding the inequity they experience. Regarding physician use, their use rates are lower than whites, but they also score better on the majority of the need measures (an exception is their higher reporting of self-rated health status as fair or poor). Among the minority groups, the Asians probably show the least inequity as their use rates tend to be lower than whites, but overall they have the best scores of any ethnic group on the need measures in Table 2.3.

Dental Visits. A major inequity in dental visits has existed according to income for many years. In 1928 to 1931, 10 percent of the lowest-income group saw a dentist within a year, compared to 41 percent of the highest-income group (Andersen & Davidson, 2007). The proportion seeing a dentist increased considerably for all income groups in the following decades, but inequities continue to exist. By 2011, 52 percent of persons with income below 100 percent of the poverty level visited a dentist during the year, compared to 81 percent of those with incomes 400 percent or more of the poverty level (Table 2.4). And the level of need remains much higher for the below-poverty group, as suggested by their proportion with untreated dental caries of 41.9 percent, compared to 11.1 percent for those with incomes of 400 percent or more of the poverty level (Table 2.3).

Considerable inequities in dental care among ethnic groups have also existed for many decades and continue to the present day, though to a lesser extent. In 1981 to 1983, 57 percent of whites saw a dentist within a year, compared to 42 percent of Hispanics and 39 percent of blacks (Andersen & Davidson, 2007). By 2011, the percentage for whites had reached 69 percent, and while still less likely to see a dentist—57 percent for Hispanics and 62 percent for blacks (Table 2.4)—the inequities were substantially less than in 1981. In 2011, the percent seeing a dentist by other minorities—66 percent for Asians and 62 percent for American Indians/Alaskan Natives—were also less than for whites but greater than for Hispanics. It is very likely that if dental need were taken into account, the inequities by ethnicity would be greater than suggested by Table 2.3. Table 2.3 shows that the percent with untreated caries was about twice as high for blacks (39.7 percent) and Mexican Americans (35. 2 percent) as for whites (19.7 percent).

Effective Access

In the late 1980s and 1990s, health services research began to measure the impact of health services utilization on health outcomes. Accordingly, the IOM Committee on Monitoring Access to Medical Care defined *effective access* as the timely use of personal health services to achieve the best possible health outcomes (Committee on Monitoring Access to Personal Health Care Services & Institute of Medicine, 1993). Measures of effective access examine the effect of potential access (health insurance and regular source of care) and realized access (health services utilization) on outcomes (health status, quality of life, and patient satisfaction with health services). Researchers conducting effectiveness and outcomes research have developed strategies for risk adjustment to control for the effects of medical need (severity of illness, number of symptoms, and comorbidities) before intervention, as well as other predisposing and enabling factors (Iezzoni, 2003). Other health behaviors (besides health services) can also influence outcomes and should be taken into account when measuring effective access. These include health practices (such as diet, exercise, and stress management) and the process of medical care (such as the quality of communication between physician and patient).

Substantial improvements have been accomplished in conceptualizing and analyzing international comparisons regarding health system effective access (Smedby & Andersen, 2010). Although both strengths and weaknesses have been identified in the Organization for Economic Cooperation and Development (OECD) data source for estimating international comparisons, it is probably the best data source available for international comparisons (Reinhardt, Hussey, & Anderson, 2002).

Quality and performance vary widely across the United States: overall, the United States appears less effective than several other industrialized countries (Squires, 2011). Over the decades, system innovation and system reforms have led to improvements in effective access. For example, in the late 1980s the effectiveness-and-outcomes movement was initiated (Heithoff & Lohr, 1990). The Health Care Financing Administration (HCFA) proposed the Effectiveness Initiative, stimulated by its need to (1) ensure quality of care for thirty million Medicare beneficiaries, (2) determine which medical practices worked best, and (3) aid policymakers in allocating Medicare resources. At approximately the same time an Outcomes Research Program was authorized by Congress, largely inspired by the work of John Wennberg and associates in small-area variations in utilization and outcomes of medical interventions (Wennberg, 2004). More current analyses show that high-performing states within the United States can serve as models for improving effective access. In one study, high-performing states have been characterized as having (1) a history of continuous reform and government leadership, (2) a culture of collaboration among stakeholders, (3) transparency of price and quality information, and (4) a congruent set of policies that focus on system improvement (Silow-Carroll & Moody, 2011).

A third major development that stimulated the effectiveness movement emerged from efforts led by Robert Brook and associates to determine whether medical interventions within the normal practice setting were being used appropriately (Brook, 2009). Within the same time period, the Agency for Health Care Policy and Research (AHCPR), renamed the Agency for Healthcare Research and Quality (AHRQ), was created, with responsibility for overseeing development of medical practice guidelines—practical application of the outcomes-and-effectiveness research movement. In the late 1990s, AHRQ conceived the Evidence-Based Practice Center Program, designed to encourage private organizations (health plans and professional societies) to improve practice through clinical guidelines, quality initiatives, and coverage decisions (Iglehart, 2005). Centers produced evidence reports and technology assessments, and a National Guideline Clearinghouse was created (Eddy, 2005). By the end of the 1990s, it was widely accepted that guidelines should be based on evidence, and that consensus-based methods were acceptable only if there was insufficient evidence to support an evidence-based approach (Eddy, 2005).

Effective Access: Equitable or Inequitable?

Despite advances in effective access, ethnic minorities and low-income adults in the United States continue to experience significant health and health care inequities when compared with white non-Hispanic and higher-income individuals. However, dramatic changes are occurring with the implementation of the 2010 Patient Protection and Affordable Care Act (ACA). The ACA represents the most sweeping change to address health care disparities since the passage of Medicare and Medicaid more than forty-five years ago. The ACA is designed to improve effective access to health care for low-income and minority populations, who often receive poorer-quality care, suffer from a higher burden of chronic and infectious diseases, have worse perceptions of their overall health, and die younger than more advantaged population subgroups (Table 2.3).

Table 2.5 shows select measures of effectiveness from the National Healthcare Disparities Report 2011 according to race or ethnicity and income level (U.S. Department of Health and Human Services, 2012). The first measure concerning cancer control (every person fifty and over should have received at least one colonoscopy, sigmoidoscopy, or proctoscopy) shows considerable inequity. Every minority group was less likely to have had one of those procedures (ranging from 35.3 percent for American Indians/Alaskan Natives) to 50.4 percent for non-Hispanic blacks) than non-Hispanic whites (58.4 percent). The inequities according to poverty level were even greater. While 36.7 percent of the group with incomes below 100 percent poverty had one or more procedures, 65.1 percent of those with incomes of 400 percent or more of the poverty level did so.

The second measure of effectiveness, deaths per one thousand hospital admissions for acute myocardial infarction for persons eighteen and over, does not show such inequities. Black non-Hispanics actually had the lowest rate (48.4 deaths per one thousand) while the white non-Hispanic rate of 59.9 exceeded the rate for all admissions (58.7) (Table 2.5).

The final effectiveness measure concerning diabetes control recommends every person age forty and over with diagnosed diabetes should receive each of four recommended procedures each year. Table 2.5 shows inequities, though possibly not as consistently as for the cancer measure; 22.7 percent of whites received all four procedures within a year, compared to 18.7 percent of Hispanics and 16.6 percent of blacks. Income differences ranged from a high 27.8 percent of the 400 percent or more of the poverty level to a low 16.2 percent for persons with incomes of less than 100 percent of the poverty level (Table 2.5).

Efficient Access

Concerns about cost containment combined with concerns about improving health outcomes have produced measures of efficient access. Like effective access, efficient access measures the impact of potential access (enabling resources like health insurance) and realized access (health services utilization) on outcomes (health status, quality of life,

TABLE 2.5. SELECTED MEASURES OF EFFECTIVENESS AND EFFICIENCY BY RACE OR ETHNICITY AND INCOME

	Effectiveness			Efficiency	
	Cancer (Age 50 and over Who Received Colonoscopy, Sigmoidoscopy, or Proctoscopy)	Cardiovascular Disease Deaths per 1,000 Hospital Admissions for Acute Myocardial Infarction (18 and over)	Diabetes (Age 40 and over with Diagnosed Diabetes Who Received All Four Recommended Services in a Calendar Year)	Potentially Avoidable Hospitalizations per 1,000 Population (18 and over)	Adults Aged 65 and over with at Least One Prescription from 33 Medications Potentially Inappropriate for Older Adults
	2008	2008	2008	2008	2008
Race and Ethnicity					
White, non-Hispanic	58.4%	59.9%	22.7%	12.6%	13.5%
Black, non-Hispanic	50.4	48.4	16.6	25.7	15.6
Hispanic[b]	38.8	59.0	18.7	13.8	15.4
Asian[a]	48.1	61.1	*	13.8	8.3
American Indian/ Alaskan Native[a]	35.3	*	*	*	*
Percent of Poverty Level[c]					
Below 100	36.7	*	16.2	*	16.8
100–199	45.5	*	17.9	*	14.8
200–399	53.3	*	17.0	*	14.4
400 and up	65.1	*	27.8	*	11.6

(continued)

TABLE 2.5. SELECTED MEASURES OF EFFECTIVENESS AND EFFICIENCY BY RACE OR ETHNICITY AND INCOME (*Continued*)

	Effectiveness				Efficiency
	Cancer (Age 50 and over Who Received Colonoscopy, Sigmoidoscopy, or Proctoscopy)	Cardiovascular Disease Deaths per 1,000 Hospital Admissions for Acute Myocardial Infarction (18 and over)	Diabetes (Age 40 and over with Diagnosed Diabetes Who Received All Four Recommended Services in a Calendar Year)	Potentially Avoidable Hospitalizations per 1,000 Population (18 and over)	Adults Aged 65 and over with at Least One Prescription from 33 Medications Potentially Inappropriate for Older Adults
	2008	2008	2008	2008	2008
Median Income of Patient Zip Code					
First quartile	*	61.6	*	20.5	*
Second quartile	*	60.1	*	13.9	*
Third quartile	*	56.1	*	12.0	*
Fourth quartile	*	56.2	*	10.7	*
Total	55.4	58.7	21.0	14.2	13.7

[a]Includes persons of Hispanic and non-Hispanic origin.

[b]Persons of Hispanic origin may be white, black, Asian, Pacific Islander, or American Indian/Alaskan Native.

[c]Poverty level is based on family income and family size, using Bureau of the Census poverty thresholds.

*Not reported.

Source: AHRQ, National Health Care Disparity Report 2011 (AHRQ Publication No. 12–0006). 2012. Retrieved from http://www.ahrq.gov/research/findings/nhqrdr/nhqrdr11. Appendix data Tables 1_3_2, 2_2_2.2, 4_1_1, 17_2_1, 17_2_2, 15_1_2.

and satisfaction). The difference is that efficient access values the input (potential or realized access) so that the cost of producing one unit of the outcome can be calculated (such as one person-year of life saved, reduction of one disability day per person per year). Thus, different combinations of enabling resources and services can be compared as to the cost of producing one unit of outcome. Lower cost equals greater efficiency. Aday and colleagues describe efficiency as producing the combination of goods and services with the highest attainable total value, given limited resources and technology (Aday, Begley, Lairson, & Slater, 1998).

International comparative studies suggest the U.S. health care system is "less efficient" (Squires, 2011; Squires, 2012). It far outspends other countries on medical care, and many outcomes are lower than they are for these countries. For example, an OECD study comparing per capita health care expenditures in major industrialized countries found that the United States spent about 40 percent more than Canada and almost three times more than the countries with the lowest expenditures. The large expenditure gap for the United States was not offset by health outcome advantages, which raised concerns that resources were being misallocated to services with low benefit relative to cost (Aday et al., 1998). Possible reasons for this apparent "inefficiency" include population aging, economic development, and basic packages of services provided by social health insurance programs (Polikowski & Santos-Eggimann, 2002; Reinhardt et al., 2002). However, research suggests the higher spending cannot simply be attributed to higher consumer income, an older population, or greater supply or utilization of hospitals and doctors. In fact, a recent study suggests major contributors to higher spending in the United States are greater access to technology and greater obesity of patients (Squires, 2012; Tchouaket, Lamarche, Goulet, & Contandriopoulos, 2012).

Efficient Access: Equitable or Inequitable?

The question can be addressed by examining the relationship between the efficient access measures and the income level or race or ethnicity of the population. As illustration, we have selected two measures of efficiency from the *National Healthcare Disparities Report 2011* (U.S. Department of Health and Human Services, 2012) (Table 2.5). The report's measures of efficiency are based on an AHRQ-commissioned report by RAND Corporation, which systematically reviewed efficiency measures, assessed their tracking potential, and provided a typology that emphasizes the multiple perspectives on health care efficiency (McGlynn, 2009).

The first efficiency measure in Table 2.5 shows potentially avoidable hospital admission rates for adults. Preventing avoidable hospitalizations can improve the efficiency of health care delivery. Not all avoidable hospitalization admissions can be prevented. But some could be prevented if good outpatient care had been provided to prevent the need for hospitalization or for which early ambulatory intervention would have prevented complications or more severe disease subsequently requiring hospitalization. Considerable inequity is shown for both race/ethnicity and income. The black rate of potentially avoidable hospitalizations per one thousand population (25.7) is more than twice the rate for non-Hispanic whites (12.6). And the rate decreases from 20.5 percent for persons in the lowest-income quartile to 10.7 percent for high-income persons (fourth quartile).

The second efficiency measure in Table 2.5 shows inappropriate medication use for persons sixty-five and older. Some drugs are potentially harmful for older patients, but are still prescribed to them (Zhan et al., 2001). Using inappropriate medications can be life-threatening and may result in expensive avoidable hospitalizations (Lau, Kasper, Potter, Lyles, & Bennett, 2005). The inappropriate medication use measure shown in Table 2.5 uses the Beers criteria, which have been generally accepted by the medical community. Inequity is not demonstrated according to race or ethnicity, as the percent of non-Hispanic white elderly prescribed one or more potentially inappropriate medications (13.5 percent) is actually higher than the Asian percent (8.3 percent) and is not so different from the black rate (15.6 percent) or the Hispanic rate (15.4 percent). However, some inequity is suggested according to income level, as the percent with one or more potentially inappropriate medications prescribed declined from 18.3 percent for the lowest-income group (below 10 percent of the poverty level) to 11.6 percent for the highest-income group (400 percent or more of the poverty level).

Future Directions

Is access improving or declining in the United States according to its various dimensions? How equitable is access according to person's race or ethnicity and income level? What is the likely impact of implementation of ACA on access to care for people in the United States?

Potential Access

A key potential access measure, health insurance, reveals that although a growing number of people are being covered by Medicaid, there has been a decline in the number covered by private insurance in the last twenty-five years and an overall increase in the proportion without any health insurance coverage. ACA will make health insurance more affordable to populations at particular risk of being uninsured or underinsured. The ACA will extend Medicaid coverage to millions of low-income Americans, make improvements to both Medicaid and SCHIP, and offer federal assistance to states that choose to establish affordable insurance exchanges (Brook, 2012; Parente & Feldman, 2013).

Realized Access

Although we have documented continuing increases in some realized access measures—notably physician and dental visits—inpatient hospital admissions and length of stay have been declining for thirty years. However, the declining hospital use rate reflects not so much a reduction in access to appropriate care, but a shift to outpatient services and greater emphasis on primary care and ambulatory outpatient care, reducing the need for acute inpatient services.

Equitable and Inequitable Access

Low-income and black populations appear to have achieved equity of access according to gross measures of hospital and physician utilization, but continue to lag considerably in receipt of dental care. Hispanics continue to lag in all of these gross measures of access. However, if the generally greater needs of all the minority groups are taken into account, inequities continue to exist for all minorities.

Equity has not been achieved regarding the potential access measure of health insurance coverage. The proportion of uninsured is higher for all minorities than for non-Hispanic whites, and the proportion of uninsured for the poverty population (28 percent) is five times higher than that for the highest-income group (5 percent). Further, numerous investigations have noted great inequity in access for low-income and minority populations regarding not having a regular source of care; not getting preventive care; delay in obtaining needed care; and higher rates of morbidity, hospitalization, and mortality that could have been avoided with appropriate access to care. The impact of ACA on equity of potential and realized access for low-income and minority populations could be substantial, particularly if components of the ACA design and implementation employ those that are found to be most effective and efficient (Mussey, 2010; Parente & Feldman, 2013).

Effective Access

Overall we might assume that the effectiveness of access is making progress over time. However, comparisons of mortality and morbidity rates between the United States and other developed countries call into question the relative effectiveness of the U.S. health care system. Also, some measurements of the treatments and outcomes for particular diseases suggest inequities in effectiveness for some minority and low-income groups.

Implementation of the ACA might lead to improvement in effectiveness, for example through newborn screening recommended by the Uniform Screening Panel to detect severe monogenetic diseases (Stark, 2012). However, genetic tests for common polygenetic diseases provide little additional information beyond clinical risk factors (Lieb, Völzke, Pulley, Roden, & Kroemer, 2012; Thanassoulis & Vasan, 2010; Völzke et al., 2013). Thus, use of genetic information will most likely not improve genetic screening for common conditions and improve access and equity in health care in the foreseeable future.

Efficient Access

Major concerns continue in the United States about the lack of efficiency in the U.S. health care system. It is by far the most costly system in the world, with continually spiraling prices and little evidence that the system is generating the kinds of outcomes that might be expected from such a costly system. There is evidence that some types of health care organization and finance (enabling resources) within the system are more efficient than others, but these forms have not been adopted on a scale to greatly influence the national concerns. We have also observed some inequities according to race or ethnicity and income, suggesting that in important ways our system may be even more inefficient for low-income and minority people than for the rest of the population.

With the enactment of the ACA, and the proposed expansion of Medicaid services, limitations in access are predicted based on inadequate supply of primary care physicians. However, these physician shortages may be offset by the increased use of advanced practice nurses and physician assistants. A recent report from the Institute of Medicine suggests that expanding the scope of practice performed by advanced practice nurses will improve efficient access without compromising quality (Institute of Medicine, 2010). New workforce development initiatives that optimize the competencies and appropriate scope of practice of all health care professionals may be required for both medical and dental care to expand efficient access, particularly for lower-income populations (Davidson et al., 2011).

SUMMARY

This chapter presented basic trends as well as research and policy issues related to monitoring and evaluating health care access. We defined access as actual use of personal health services and everything that facilitates or impedes their use. We showed how monitoring and evaluating access allows us to (1) predict use of health services, (2) promote social justice, and (3) improve effectiveness and efficiency of health services delivery.

The behavioral model provides a systematic framework of contextual and individual factors for analyzing access and health care outcomes. We expanded the model by emphasizing two new aspects: genetics as a predisposing factor and quality of life as an input and outcome of health care. Examples of access indicators were examined, including health care needs, potential access, utilization, effectiveness, and efficiency measures. Trend data were used to track changes that have occurred over time in these indicators. We concluded with observations on access, the present status and emerging promise of improving access through the ACA, the most sweeping legislation to improve access since the enactment of Medicare and Medicaid almost fifty years ago.

KEY TERMS

Access use of personal health services and everything that facilitates or impedes their use.

Effective access realized access that improves health outcomes.

Efficient access realized access that improves health outcomes while minimizing costs.

Enabling characteristics facilitate or impede use of services.

Equitable access is predicted by need, demographics, and genetic susceptibility.

Inequitable access is predicted by enabling and social characteristics.

Need characteristics laypeople and/or professionals recognize these as requiring medical treatment.

Potential access presence of enabling characteristics.

Predisposing characteristics incline people to use or not use services.

Realized access use of services.

DISCUSSION QUESTIONS

1. "Improving access to care of individuals depends more on contextual than on individual determinants." What is the rationale for this statement? Do you agree or disagree?
2. What is meant by the observation "Equity of access is in the eyes of the beholder"? How equitable is the U.S. health care system according to your definition of equity?
3. A health policy might promote "realized access" but not "effective access" or "efficient access." The majority of the U.S. population believes the U.S. system has a "major problem." Is the most important problem the system faces one of realized access, effective access, or efficient access?
4. As the United States moves increasingly toward evidenced-based medicine, what dimensions of access become increasingly important? What particular measures of access and what health services research studies would you propose to support this movement?
5. What is the good news and what is the bad news when we examine the trends in various measures of access over time? What might enable us to continue the good news and change the bad news to good?

FURTHER READING

Andersen, R. M. (2008). National health surveys and the behavioral model of health services use. *Medical Care, 46*(7), 647–653.

The article reviews the development of the behavioral model through several versions prior to the one presented in this chapter and the use of population health surveys to track changes in access and inequalities.

Andersen, R. M. (2010). *Access to health care.* Oxford Bibliographies. Available at http://www.oxfordbibliographies.com/view/document/obo-9780199756797/obo -9780199756797–0001.xml

A comprehensive annotated bibliography focusing on access to health care from contrasting international perspectives, improving access from a management perspective, and increasing equitable access for low-income Americans.

Barton, P. L. (2010). *Understanding the U.S. health services system.* Chicago: Health Administration Press.

An up-to-date introduction to the U.S. health services system, with a chapter devoted to access to care.

Mullner, R. (2009). *Encyclopedia of health services research.* Thousand Oaks, CA: Sage.

This comprehensive reference captures the diversity and complexity of the field. With more than four hundred entries, it investigates the relationship between the factors of cost, quality, and access to health care and their impact on medical outcomes such as death, disability, disease, discomfort, and dissatisfaction with care.

U.S. Department of Health and Human Services. (2012). *National healthcare disparities report 2012* (AHRQ Publication No. 12–0006). Available at http://www.ahrq.gov/research/findings/nhqrdr/nhdr12/index.html

This report provides a compendium of health disparity statistics, including multiple measures of and trends in access to care, equity, effectiveness, and efficiency.

REFERENCES

Aday, L. A., Begley, C. E., Lairson, D. R., & Slater, C. H. (1998). *Evaluating the healthcare system: effectiveness, efficiency, and equity* (2nd ed.). Chicago: Health Administration Press.

Andersen, R. M. (1968). A behavioral model of families' use of health services (Vol. 25). Chicago: Center for Health Administration Studies, University of Chicago.

Andersen, R. M. (1995). Revisiting the behavioral model and access to medical care: Does it matter? *Journal of Health and Social Behavior, 36*(1), 1–10.

Andersen, R. M. (2008). National health surveys and the behavioral model of health services use. *Medical Care, 46*(7), 647–653.

Andersen, R. M., & Davidson, P. L. (1996). Measuring access and trends. In R. Andersen, T. Rice, & G. F. Kominski (Eds.), *Changing the U.S. health care system* (1st ed., pp. 13–40). San Francisco: Jossey-Bass.

Andersen, R. M., & Davidson, P. L. (2007). Improving access to care in America: Individual and contextual indicators. In R. Andersen, T. Rice, & G. F. Kominski (Eds.), *Changing the U.S. health care system* (pp. 3–32). San Francisco: Jossey-Bass.

Andersen, R. M., & Smedby, B. (1975). Changes in response to symptoms of illness in the United States and Sweden. *Inquiry, 12*(2), 116–127.

Andersen, R. M., Smedby, B., & Anderson, O. W. (1970). *Medical care use in Sweden and the United States: A comparative analysis of systems and behavior.* Chicago: Center for Health Administration Studies.

Bass, D. M., & Noelker, L. S. (1987). The influence of family caregivers on elder's use of in-home services: An expanded conceptual framework. *Journal of Health and Social Behavior, 28*(2), 184–196.

Becker, F., van El, C. G., Ibarreta, D., Zika, E., Hogarth, S., Borry, P., . . . Cornel, M. C. (2011). Genetic testing and common disorders in a public health framework: How to assess relevance and possibilities. Background Document to the ESHG recommendations on genetic testing and common disorders. *European Journal of Human Genetics, 19*(Suppl. 1), S6–44.

Bindman, A. B., & Gold, M. R. (Eds.). (1998). Measuring access through population-based surveys in a managed care environment: A special supplement to HSR. *Health Services Research, Vol. 33.*

Bindman, A. B., Grumbach, K., Osmond, D., Komaromy, M., Vranizan, K., Lurie, N., Stewart, A. (1995). Preventable hospitalizations and access to health care. *Journal of the American Medical Association, 274*(4), 305–311.

Brook, R. H. (2009). Assessing the appropriateness of care: Its time has come. *Journal of the American Medical Association, 302*(9), 997–998.

Brook, R. H. (2012). Two years and counting: How will the effects of the Affordable Care Act be monitored? *Journal of the American Medical Association, 307*(1), 41–42.

Bunnik, E. M., Schermer, M. H., & Janssens, A. C. (2011). Personal genome testing: Test characteristics to clarify the discourse on ethical, legal and societal issues. *BMC Medical Ethics, 12,* 11.

Committee on Monitoring Access to Personal Health Care Services & Institute of Medicine. (1993). *Access to health care in America.* Washington, DC: National Academies Press.

Cunningham, P. J., & Kohn, L. (2000). Health plan switching: Choice or circumstance? *Health Affairs (Millwood), 19*(3), 158–164.

Davidson, P. L., & Andersen, R. M. (1997). Determinants of dental care utilization for diverse ethnic and age groups. *Advances in Dental Research, 11*(2), 254–262.

Davidson, P. L., Andersen, R. M., Wyn, R., & Brown, E. R. (2004). A framework for evaluating safety-net and other community-level factors on access for low-income populations. *Inquiry, 41*(1), 21–38.

Davidson, P. L., Nakazono, T. T., Carreon, D. C., Gutierrez, J. J., Shahedi, S., & Andersen, R. M. (2011). Reforming dental workforce education and practice in the USA. *European Journal of Dental Education, 15*(2), 73–79.

Davidson, P. L., Rams, T. E., & Andersen, R. M. (1997). Socio-behavioral determinants of oral hygiene practices among USA ethnic and age groups. *Advances in Dental Research, 11*(2), 245–253.

Davis, K., & Rowland, D. (1983). Uninsured and underserved: Inequities in health care in the United States. *Milbank Memorial Fund Quarterly: Health and Society, 61*(2), 149–176.

Donabedian, A. (1980). *Exploration in quality assessment and monitoring: The definition of quality and approaches to its assessment.* (Vol. 1). Ann Arbor, MI: Health Administration Press.

Eddy, D. M. (2005). Evidence-based medicine: A unified approach. *Health Affairs (Millwood), 24*(1), 9–17.

Guendelman, S. (1991). Health care users residing on the Mexican border: What factors determine choice of the U.S. or Mexican health system? *Medical Care, 29*(5), 419–429.

Guyatt, G. H., Feeny, D. H., & Patrick, D. L. (1993). Measuring health-related quality of life. *Annals of Internal Medicine, 118*(8), 622–629.

Hajat, A., Lucas, J. B., & Kington, R. (2000). Health outcomes among Hispanic subgroups: Data from the National Health Interview Survey, 1992–95. *Advance Data, (310),* 1–14.

Heithoff, K. A., & Lohr, K. N. (Eds.). (1990). *Effectiveness and outcomes in health care: Proceedings of an invitational conference.* Washington, DC: National Academies Press.

Hulka, B. S., & Wheat, J. R. (1985). Patterns of utilization: The patient perspective. *Medical Care, 23*(5), 438–460.

Iezzoni, L. I. (2003). *Risk adjustment for measuring health care outcomes* (3rd ed.). Chicago: Health Administration Press.

Iglehart, J. K. (2005). The new imperative: Producing better evidence. *Health Affairs, 24*(1), 7–7.

Institute of Medicine. (2010). *The future of nursing: Leading change, advancing health.* Princeton, NJ: Robert Wood Johnson Foundation Initiative on the Future of Nursing.

Kaplan, R. M., & Ries, A. L. (2007). Quality of life: Concept and definition. [Review]. *Journal of Chronic Obstructive Pulmonary Disease, 4*(3), 263–271.

Lambert, B. L., Street, R. L., Cegala, D. J., Smith, D. H., Kurtz, S., & Schofield, T. (1997). Provider-patient communication, patient-centered care, and the mangle of practice. *Health Communication, 9*(1), 27–43.

Lau, D. T., Kasper, J. D., Potter, D. E., Lyles, A., & Bennett, R. G. (2005). Hospitalization and death associated with potentially inappropriate medication prescriptions among elderly nursing home residents. *Archives of Internal Medicine, 165*(1), 68–74.

Lieb, W., Völzke, H., Pulley, J. M., Roden, D. M., & Kroemer, H. K. (2012). Strategies for personalized medicine-based research and implementation in the clinical workflow. *Clinical Pharmacology and Therapeutics, 92*(4), 443–445.

Locker, D., & Allen, F. (2007). What do measures of "oral health-related quality of life" measure? *Community Dentistry and Oral Epidemiology, 35*(6), 401–411.

Longest, B. B. (1998). *Health policymaking in the United States.* Chicago: Health Administration Press.

Manton, K. G., Patrick, C. H., & Johnson, K. W. (1987). Health differentials between blacks and whites: Recent trends in mortality and morbidity. *Milbank Quarterly, 65*(Suppl. 1), 129–199.

McGlynn, E. (2009). *Identifying, categorizing, and evaluating health care efficiency measures.* (Publication No. 08–0030). Rockville, MD: *Agency for Healthcare Research and Quality.* Retrieved from http://ahrq.gov/qual/efficiency

Mussey, S. M. (2010). Estimated effects of the Patient Protection and Affordable Care Act as amended, on the year of exhaustion for the Part A trust fund, Part B premiums, and Part A and Part B coinsurance amounts. Retrieved from http://www.cms.gov/Research-Statistics-Data-and-Systems/Research/ActuarialStudies/downloads/PPACA_Medicare_2010-04-22.pdf

National Center for Health Statistics. (2004). *Health United States, 2004* (August 11, 2010, ed.). Hyattsville, MD: Author.

National Center for Health Statistics & U.S. Department of Health and Human Services. (1999). *Health, United States, 1999: With health and aging chartbook.* Hyattsville, MD: Author.

Nordenfelt, L. (1993). *Quality of life, health and happiness.* Aldershot, U.K.: Avebury Ashgate.

Parente, S. T., & Feldman, R. (2013). Microsimulation of private health insurance and Medicaid take-up following the U.S. Supreme Court decision upholding the Affordable Care Act. *Health Services Research, 48*(2), 826–849.

Patient-Centered Outcomes Research Institute. (2013). Patient-Centered Outcomes Research Institute. Retrieved from www.PCORI.org

Pescosolido, B. A., Wright, E. R., Alegria, M., & Vera, M. (1998). Social networks and patterns of use among the poor with mental health problems in Puerto Rico. *Medical Care, 36*(7), 1057–1072.

Polikowski, M., & Santos-Eggimann, B. (2002). How comprehensive are the basic packages of health services? An international comparison of six health insurance systems. [Comparative Study]. *Journal of Health Services Research and Policy, 7*(3), 133–142.

Portes, A., Kyle, D., & Eaton, W. W. (1992). Mental illness and help-seeking behavior among Mariel Cuban and Haitian refugees in south Florida. *Journal of Health and Social Behavior, 33*(4), 283–298.

Reinhardt, U. E., Hussey, P. S., & Anderson, G. F. (2002). Cross-national comparisons of health systems using OECD data, 1999. *Health Affairs (Millwood), 21*(3), 169–181.

Robert, S. A. (1999). Socioeconomic position and health: The independent contribution of community socioeconomic context. *Annual Review of Sociology, 25*(1), 489–516.

Seeman, T. E., & Berkman, L. F. (1988). Structural characteristics of social networks and their relationship with social support in the elderly: who provides support. *Social Science and Medicine, 26*(7), 737–749.

Silow-Carroll, S., & Moody, G. (2011). Lessons from high- and low-performing states for raising overall health system performance. *Issue Brief (Commonwealth Fund), 7,* 1–11.

Skevington, S. M., Lotfy, M., & O'Connell, K. A. (2004). The World Health Organization's WHOQOL-BREF quality of life assessment: Psychometric properties and results of the international field trial. A report from the WHOQOL group. Quality of Life Research, *13*(2), 299–310.

Smedby, B., & Andersen, R. M. (2010). International comparisons of health care systems: Conceptual and methodological developments over half a century. *Socialmedicinsk tidskrift, 5–6,* 439–452.

Squires, D. A. (2011). The U.S. health system in perspective: A comparison of twelve industrialized nations. *Issue (Commonwealth Fund), 16,* 1–14.

Squires, D. A. (2012). Tracking trends in health system performance: Issues in international health policy. Explaining high health care spending in the United States: An international comparison of supply, utilization, prices, and quality. *Issue Brief (Commonwealth Fund), 10,* 1–14.

Stark, E. (2012). The Affordable Care Act is upheld: A great day for babies! Retrieved from http://www.babysfirsttest.org/newborn-screening/blog/the-affordable-care -act-is-upheld-a-great-day-for-babies

Tchouaket, E. N., Lamarche, P. A., Goulet, L., & Contandriopoulos, A. P. (2012). Health care system performance of 27 OECD countries. *International Journal of Health Planning and Management, 27*(2), 104–129.

Thanassoulis, G., & Vasan, R. S. (2010). Genetic cardiovascular risk prediction: Will we get there? *Circulation, 122*(22), 2323–2334.

U.S. Department of Health and Human Services. (2012). *National healthcare disparities report 2011* (AHRQ Publication No. 12–0006). Retrieved from http://www.ahrq .gov/qual/nhdr11/nhdr11.pdf

Völzke, H., Schmidt, C. O., Baumeister, S. E., Ittermann, T., Fung, G., Krafcyk-Korth, J., . . . Kroemer, H. K. (2013). Personalized cardiovascular medicine: Concepts and methodological considerations. *Nature Reviews Cardiology*. Retrieved from http://www.nature.com/nrcardio/journal/vaop/ncurrent/abs/nrcardio.2013.35.html

Wennberg, J. E. (2004). Practice variation: Implications for our health care system. *Managed Care, 13*(9 Suppl.), 3–7.

White, K., Haas, J. S., & Williams, D. R. (2012). Elucidating the role of place in health care disparities: The example of racial/ethnic residential segregation. *Health Services Research, 47*(3 Pt 2), 1278–1299.

Zhan, C., Sangl, J., Bierman, A. S., Miller, M. R., Friedman, B., Wickizer, S. W., & Meyer, G. S. (2001). Potentially inappropriate medication use in the community-dwelling elderly: Findings from the 1996 Medical Expenditure Panel Survey. *Journal of the American Medical Association, 286*(22), 2823–2829.

CHAPTER THREE

RACIAL AND ETHNIC DISPARITIES IN HEALTH STATUS

Antronette K. Yancey
Roshan Bastani
Beth A. Glenn

Learning Objectives

- Describe racial and ethnic disparities in health status in the United States, measured across a number of indicators
- Define the pressing health concerns affecting the four most populous minority groups in the United States—African Americans, Latinos, Asian American/Pacific Islanders, and American Indian/Alaskan Natives—with a focus on chronic disease
- Understand a prominent model by Evans and Stoddart that has been used to conceptualize factors that influence health status at the community level
- Understand key factors that underlie current racial and ethnic differences in health status based on recent data and including behavioral risk factors

During the past one hundred years, dramatic gains have been made in the overall health of the U.S. population. One common, albeit gross, indicator of the general health of a population is life expectancy, which increased by thirty years during the twentieth century (National

Center for Health Statistics, 2004). Although life expectancy has increased overall, racial and ethnic minorities (particularly African Americans and American Indian/Alaskan Natives) have not experienced the same gains as whites. At the start of the twentieth century, the life expectancy of African Americans lagged substantially behind that of whites, which was largely due to the extremely adverse social conditions attendant to slavery followed by the continuing injustices of Reconstruction and subsequent Jim Crow legislation. However, it is unconscionable that, although the gap has narrowed in some areas, racial and ethnic health disparities that existed at the turn of the twentieth century persist as we enter the twenty-first century.

There is ample evidence that racial and ethnic minorities experience higher rates of morbidity and mortality across many disease states (Braveman, Cubbin, Egerter, Williams, & Pamuk, 2010). Historically, the ideals of social justice and equality have served as the impetus for eliminating health disparities (Smith, 2005). Although these factors remain compelling, the growing diversification of the U.S. population is an additional rationale for eliminating inequity. Figure 3.1 presents data on the racial and ethnic distribution of the U.S. population in 2000 and projections for 2100. According to the 2000 census, slightly more than 70 percent of the population was white, with the remaining 30 percent made up of racial

FIGURE 3.1. U.S. POPULATION (2000 CENSUS) AND PROJECTIONS FOR 2100

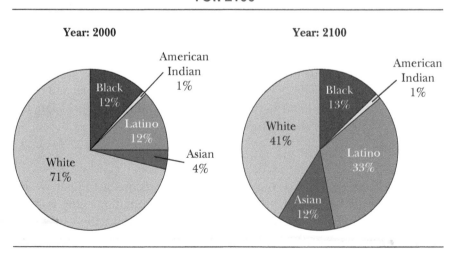

and ethnic minorities (less than 5 percent Asian, more than 10 percent African American, more than 10 percent Latino or Latina). Racial and ethnic minorities are projected to constitute more than 50 percent of the total population by 2060, with the largest growth expected to occur among Latinos and Asians. In addition, the relative youth of racial and ethnic minority populations currently will magnify existing disparities in the future, as the average age of the entire population advances, particularly among minority groups. Therefore, today, and increasingly in the future, the overall health and economic well-being of the U.S. population as a whole can only be maintained and enhanced by addressing racial and ethnic disparities in health status and their determinants.

Because the disease burden over the past century has shifted from communicable to chronic diseases, inequality in chronic disease burden represents one of the most critical areas of health disparities today. Chronic diseases account for over 70 percent of deaths and approximately 85 percent of health care expenditures annually (Anderson, 2010; Kung, Hoyert, Xu, & Murphy, 2008). This is in contrast to the early 1900s, when chronic disease accounted for less than one-quarter of all deaths (Population Reference Bureau, 2001). Despite steady improvement in the health of all Americans, racial and ethnic minorities continue to experience poorer health status, especially with regard to chronic disease. In fact, the current obesity epidemic threatens to end the steady rise in overall life expectancy of the past two centuries and contributes disproportionately to chronic disease disparities (Stewart, Cutler, & Rosen, 2009). Therefore, this chapter describes current health status disparities, reviews the potential determinants of observed disparities, and outlines future directions for policy and practice, with specific emphasis on the contribution of chronic disease.

Epidemiology of Health Disparities

In this section, we review the evidence related to racial and ethnic disparities in major health indicators.

Life Expectancy

Life expectancy is one of the summary statistics most commonly used to describe the health of a population. During the past century, we have seen a dramatic increase in life expectancy, from less than forty-seven years in the early 1900s to seventy-eight years in 2010 (U.S. Census Bureau,

FIGURE 3.2. LIFE EXPECTANCY BY RACE, ETHNICITY, AND GENDER

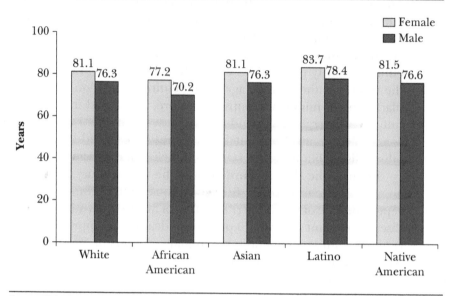

Source: U.S. Census Bureau, 2008.

Population Division, 2008). Although increased life expectancy has been observed for all racial and ethnic groups, racial and ethnic disparities in life expectancy remain fairly constant. Figure 3.2 shows the average life expectancy by race, ethnicity, and gender according to population-based data projected for 2010 (U.S. Census Bureau, Population Division, 2008). Within each racial and ethnic group, women have a higher life expectancy than men. However, substantial differences are found among racial and ethnic groups regardless of gender. The longest average life expectancy is seen among Latino women (83.7 years) and the shortest among African American men (70.2 years), a difference of more than thirteen years.

Major Causes of Mortality

Although life expectancy provides global information about disparities, it does not inform us about the underlying causes. Table 3.1 shows the top ten causes of mortality for all adults living in the United States in 2007 and separately for five racial and ethnic groups, the relative rank of each cause within racial and ethnic groups, and age-adjusted death rate

TABLE 3.1. LEADING CAUSES OF DEATH BY ETHNICITY

Causes of Death	Total Rank %	*Death Rate	White Rank %	Death Rate	African American Rank %	Death Rate	American Indian Rank %	Death Rate	Asian/Pacific Rank %	Death Rate	Latino Rank %	Death Rate
Heart disease	1 25.4	190.9	1 25.9	191.4	1 24.6	247.3	1 18.4	127.3	2 23.2	101.2	1 21.4	136.0
All cancers	2 23.2	178.4	2 23.5	182.3	2 22.2	215.5	2 17.8	117.8	1 27.0	106.7	2 20.4	116.2
Cerebrovascular diseases	3 5.6	42.2	4 5.6	40.7	3 5.9	60.3	7 4.1	29.8	3 7.9	34.3	4 5.2	32.7
Chronic lower respiratory diseases	4 5.3	40.8	3 5.9	44.9	8 2.7	28.1	6 4.3	30.9	7 2.9	13.4	7 2.6	17.5
Unintentional injuries	5 5.1	40.0	5 4.9	43.0	4 4.7	36.6	3 11.8	55.7	4 4.8	17.0	3 8.7	30.1
Alzheimer's disease	6 3.1	22.7	6 3.4	24.1					10 1.6	8.1		
Diabetes mellitus	7 2.9	22.5	7 2.6	19.8	5 4.3	42.8	4 5.5	37.2	5 3.8	16.2	5 4.7	28.9
Influenza and pneumonia	8 2.2	16.2	8 2.2	16.2			10 1.9	13.8	6 2.9	13.6	10 2.0	13.1
Nonmalignant kidney diseases	9 1.9	14.5	9 1.8	13.1	7 2.9	29.4	9 2.0	14.3	9 2.0	8.6		
Septicemia	10 1.4	11.0			10 2.2	21.7						
Suicide			10 1.5	13.5			8 2.7	11.5	8 2.0	6.1		
Homicide					6 3.1	21.1					8 2.6	6.9
HIV/AIDS disease					9 2.2	17.3						
Chronic liver disease							5 4.9	24.8			6 2.9	13.8
Certain conditions originating in the perinatal period											9 2.2	3.9

*Age-adjusted death rates per 100,000.

Source: National Center for Health Statistics, 2010a.

(National Center for Health Statistics, 2010a). For the overall population, chronic diseases comprise seven of the top ten causes of death. Heart disease ranks number one for all racial and ethnic groups except Asian Americans. However, the age-adjusted mortality rate from heart disease is not equal among the groups. African Americans rank the highest, followed by non-Latino whites, Latinos, American Indians, and Asian Americans. Cancer is the second leading cause of death for all groups except Asian Americans, for whom it ranks first. The cancer mortality rate is highest among African Americans, followed by non-Latino whites, American Indians, Latinos, and Asian Americans and Pacific Islanders. The death rate for the most common cancers (breast, lung, prostate, and colorectal) varies by race and ethnicity in a pattern similar to overall cancer mortality. African Americans and whites are most likely to die of these cancers, followed by Latinos and Asian Americans and Pacific Islanders. However, for some less common cancers, such as stomach and liver, Asian Americans and Latinos have the highest observed death rate. Cerebrovascular diseases constitute the third leading cause of death overall. African Americans are most likely to die of cerebrovascular disease, followed by whites, Asian Americans and Pacific Islanders, Latinos, and American Indians. The death rate for chronic lower respiratory disease, the fourth leading cause overall, is highest among whites and lowest among Asian Americans and Pacific Islanders. Unintentional injuries are the fifth leading cause of death overall but third for American Indians and Latinos. American Indians have a substantially higher frequency of death from unintentional injury than all other groups. Several causes of death, although not among the top ten for the overall population or whites, pose a significant health risk to racial and ethnic minorities. For example, African Americans, Latinos, and American Indians have substantially higher death rates from homicide than whites and Asian Americans. Similarly, HIV/AIDS ranks higher among African Americans and Latinos than for the other racial and ethnic groups.

Years of Potential Life Lost

Examining the years of potential life lost from specific causes of death is another way of assessing health status. Figure 3.3 presents data regarding the years of potential life lost for all racial and ethnic groups in 2007 (National Center for Health Statistics, 2010b). YPLL-75, or the years of potential life lost before age seventy-five, indicates the average per 100,000 persons, assuming that each person would otherwise live to age seventy-five.

FIGURE 3.3. YEARS OF POTENTIAL LIFE LOST BY RACE AND ETHNICITY (PER 100,000)

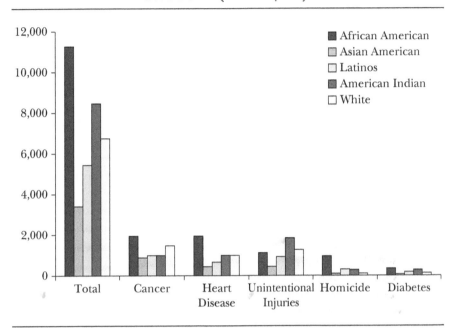

Source: National Center for Health Statistics, 2010b.

Similar to the pattern observed for life expectancy, significant health disparities remain, despite improvement in this health indicator across all racial and ethnic groups during the past several decades. Across all causes of death, African Americans have the highest average YPLL, followed by American Indians and Alaskan Natives, whites, Latinos, and Asian Americans and Pacific Islanders. The YPLL for African Americans is more than three times that of Asian Americans and Pacific Islanders, and over 1.5 times higher than the YPLL for whites. The two largest contributors to the disproportionately high YPLL rate among African Americans are cancer (17.5 percent of all YPLL) and heart disease (17 percent). Among American Indians and Alaskan Natives, the most important contributors to YPLL are unintentional injury (22 percent) and cancer (12 percent). For whites, cancer (22 percent) and unintentional injury (19 percent) account for the highest proportion of YPLL. Cancer is the most important contributor to YPLL among Latinos, accounting for 18 percent of all YPLL, followed by unintentional injury (17 percent).

Morbidity

It is important to examine morbidity in addition to mortality as an indicator of health status. This indicator incorporates the observation that some common diseases markedly impairing quality of life often do not result in shortened lifespan or in death. Arthritis and rheumatism are a common cause of disability in the United States, accounting for 19 percent of cases of disability among individuals 18 years or older (Brault, Hootman, Helmick, Theis, & Armour, 2009). The second most common cause of disability is back or spinal problems (17 percent). It should be noted that neither disability appears as a common cause of death. Four of the remaining top ten causes of disability can be considered chronic diseases: heart problems (7 percent), lung or respiratory problems (5 percent), diabetes (4.5 percent), and stroke (2.4 percent).

Figure 3.4 presents data regarding limitation of activity caused by chronic conditions, by race and ethnicity (National Center for Health Statistics, 2007). Approximately 18 percent of American Indians and Alaskan Natives report experiencing a limitation of activity caused by a chronic condition, including limitation in personal care activities such as dressing or showering (aka activities of daily living), limitation in activities to fulfill routine needs such as personal shopping and housework

FIGURE 3.4. LIMITATION OF ACTIVITY CAUSED BY CHRONIC CONDITIONS, UNITED STATES, 2006

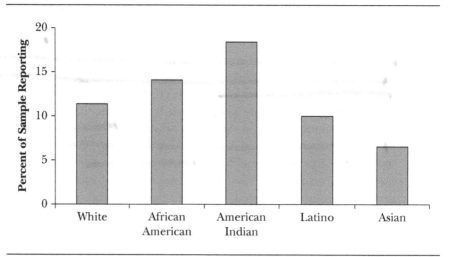

Source: National Center for Health Statistics, 2007.

(aka instrumental activities of daily living), and other limitations. African Americans have the second highest rate, with 14 percent reporting such limitation. About 11 percent of non-Latino whites and a similar proportion of Latinos (10 percent) report a limitation of activity. Asian Americans have the lowest rate of activity limitation (around 7 percent).

Epidemiology of Health Disparities: Summary

Across all the indicators of health status mentioned here, African Americans are the most disadvantaged. This is a reflection of four centuries of exploitation and oppression—forced immigration, enslavement, and brutal subjugation during the majority of their tenure in the United States. The advances of the civil rights movement, heralding greater (but far from equal) educational, housing, and employment opportunities, encompass less than 10 percent of their history in this country. They experience the highest mortality rates for heart disease, cancer, type 2 diabetes mellitus, and cerebrovascular disease. In addition, homicide and HIV/AIDS emerge as leading causes of death among African Americans, but not for the overall population. Other significant health issues that affect African Americans in particular are high incidence rates of obesity, infant and maternal mortality, and smoking among middle-aged men. Infant mortality is a particularly critical health concern for African Americans. In 2006, the African American infant mortality rate (13.4 infant deaths per thousand live births) was more than two times the rate for Latinos, whites, and Asian Americans and Pacific Islanders (each fewer than 6 per thousand live births; National Center for Health Statistics, 2010a), and the gap has widened appreciably during the past two decades (Frisbie, Song, Powers, & Street, 2004). Although the infant mortality rate decreases with higher education, the rate for African Americans exceeds that for all other racial and ethnic groups at every level of education (National Center for Health Statistics, 2008). The infant mortality rate for African American women with the highest level of education is greater than the rates for women from other racial and ethnic groups with the lowest level of education.

Latinos as a group have lower mortality rates from most of the leading causes of death. This is despite the fact that they exhibit many of the socioeconomic characteristics consistently associated with poor health status, such as lower income and level of education. This phenomenon has been labeled the "Latino or Hispanic paradox" (Hayes-Bautista et al., 2002), and it is far more pronounced for mortality than morbidity statistics (for example, type 2 diabetes mellitus). Several hypotheses have been advanced to explain this paradox, although the root causes remain largely unknown. Among the explanations for the paradox are lack of reliable data, the possibility that many older Latinos return to their native country when they become ill or are close to death (aka the "salmon bias hypothesis"), difference in risk factors for the major causes of death, protective cultural factors, and the suggestion that migration to the United States occurs principally among the healthiest individuals from the home country (aka the "healthy migrant effect"). It is also important to note that data on Latinos are often aggregated across a diverse group of people of differing nationalities, ethnicities, and races, as well as varying migration history (which may mask disparities among subgroups). Data comparing health outcomes among Latino subgroups is limited. Future research is needed to generate data that will allow for subgroup-specific estimates of key health indicators such as life expectancy, mortality, and disease burden. Furthermore, although Latinos experience a lower death rate from all cancers combined as well as for the most common cancers (lung, colon, and prostate), they have higher incidence rates of stomach, liver, gallbladder, and cervical cancer than whites and the general population (American Cancer Society, 2009). Finally, Latinos are the fasting-growing population in the United States, amplifying the importance of more fully understanding the health of this group. Recent data on the effect of acculturation on health status among Latinos indicate that health status declines and disease risk increases with acculturation (Guendelman & Abrams, 1995), illustrated by the rise of obesity and type 2 diabetes mellitus in this group. (Perez-Escamilla, 2011).

In terms of overall mortality, the rate for American Indians and Alaskan Natives is lower than for African Americans but higher than for whites, Latinos, and Asian Americans (National Center for Health Statistics, 2010a). American Indians and Alaskan Natives are the most disadvantaged with regard to activity limitation due to a chronic condition, and the second most disadvantaged when health status is measured by potential years of life lost. Research on the health of American Indians and Alaskan Natives has been hampered by lack of data. When data are collected on race and ethnicity, American Indians and Alaskan Natives are often coded as "other" and combined with other groups. Even when studies specifically recruit samples of American Indians, as in the Behavioral Risk Factor Surveillance System, small sample size can make a population estimate unreliable and unstable, and the methods used to collect data (such as telephone interviews) often fail to reach a representative sample of this small and unique population (Denny, Holtzman, & Cobb, 2003).

The health of American Indians was negatively affected originally when European settlers brought diseases that were previously unknown to native populations. Since that time, American Indians have endured substantial hardship and oppression, negatively affecting their health status. Two of the top ten health threats for American Indians are not among the top ten for the total U.S. population: chronic liver disease (fifth) and suicide (eighth). In addition, unintentional injury ranks third as a cause of death in this group, with substantially higher rates than any other racial and ethnic group (National Center for Health Statistics, 2010a). Alcohol abuse is considered a key underlying cause for the higher mortality from these three causes of death. Data from the 2009 Behavioral Risk Factor Surveillance System found that binge drinking (consuming five or more drinks on one occasion in the past month for men or four drinks for women) was quite prevalent for American Indians and Alaskan Natives. The rate for this group was 15.4 percent, compared to 17.5 percent for whites, 10.4 percent for African Americans, 14.4 percent for Latinos, and 7.8 percent for Asians (Kanny, Liu, & Brewer, 2011). Among respondents who reported at least one binge-drinking episode, American Indians and Alaskan Natives had the highest reported number of episodes per month (6.7), compared to whites (3.9), African Americans (3.8), Latinos (3.8) and Asians (3.4). The average number of drinks per episode was also highest in American Indians and Alaskan Natives, 8.4 drinks per episode on average, compared to 6.7 drinks for whites, 6.1 drinks for African Americans, 6.5 drinks for Latinos, and 5.6 drinks for Asians. Type 2 diabetes mellitus also ranks relatively high as a cause of death within this racial and ethnic group (fourth) compared to the overall population (seventh) and has been previously documented as pervasive among such tribes as the Pima and Zuni (Ritenbaugh & Goodby, 1989).

The Asian American and Pacific Islander population has been referred to as the "model minority," given their wealth and better health status as reflected in a variety of indicators. However, there are a number of critical issues to consider in understanding the health of this population. As with Latinos, immigration may select for the healthiest individuals. The category Asian American and Pacific Islander encompasses an extraordinarily diverse group of people originating from many countries with widely varying socioeconomic characteristics, immigration history, culture, and social standing in the United States. Unfortunately, the majority of research studies to date have collapsed all individuals of Asian descent into one category. This aggregation masks considerable subgroup differences for general indicators such as mortality as well as for incidence of particular diseases. For example, Asian Indian women have the highest life expectancy (88.1 years), whereas Pacific Islander men have a life expectancy among the lowest, at 70.5 years, a difference of over 17 years (Johnson & Hayes, 2004). In California (one of the only states reporting disaggregated Asian data), Vietnamese and Korean women experience higher cervical cancer incidence rates compared to non-Latino whites, whereas Chinese, Japanese, and South Asian women have lower rates of the disease (Bates, Hofer, & Parikh-Patel, 2008). In addition, as observed among other immigrant groups, increasing acculturation has been linked to diminished health status (Deapen, Liu, Perkins, Bernstein, & Ross, 2002; Gomez, Kelsey, Glaser, Lee, & Sidney, 2004). In fact, Asian Americans as a group present a unique opportunity to examine the effect of acculturation by examining the incidence of certain conditions across groups with more recent immigration history (for example, Koreans) compared to those who have lived in the United States for many generations (Japanese). An illustration of this effect can be found in data showing that Japanese women residing in Los Angeles County have higher rates of breast cancer incidence than white women, although breast cancer rates in Japan are among the lowest in the world (Deapen et al., 2002).

Factors Underlying Chronic Disease-Related Disparities

Paralleling our focus on the major disease states in describing the epidemiology of racial and ethnic disparities in health status, in this section we emphasize the underlying factors responsible for the majority of morbidity, disability, and mortality. McGinnis and Foege's classic article (1993) identified the actual causes of more than 80 percent of "preventable" mortality as diet, physical inactivity, tobacco, and alcohol. Thus we highlight these behavioral risk factors in presenting the underlying contributors to a broad spectrum of health status disparities. It is important to keep in mind that the actual cause of more than half of all deaths is not known, and thus identified determinants or risk factors generally explain only a modest amount of the variance in most disease processes.

Of the many theoretical models of determinants of health, we have elected to use the Evans-Stoddart model to depict the broad categories of variables contributing to health (see Figure 3.5) and as an organizing framework for our discussion of those most closely linked to disparities

FIGURE 3.5. THEORETICAL FRAMEWORK

Determinants of Health: Evans-Stoddart Model

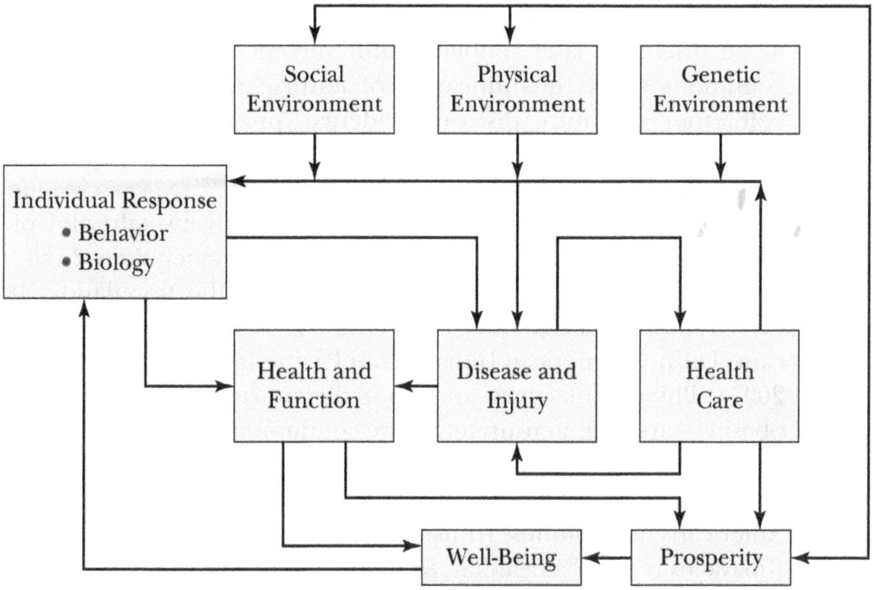

(Evans & Stoddart, 1994). We have selected several categories of determinants to be highlighted in detail, on the basis of the malleability of the determinant and the availability of data.

Specifically, we discuss behavioral, socioeconomic, and physical and social environmental factors that influence individual response, focusing especially on current areas of scientific investigation in public health. Although we recognize that behavioral and biological responses often overlap, we focus on the behavioral variables. The genetic contribution to observed racial and ethnic variation in health is considered minor and consequently is not examined here. Race and ethnicity are essentially sociocultural and ideological constructs, as reflected in the considerable genetic variation within racial groups and relatively little consistent between-group variation (consider the general failure of efforts to link racial phenotypes to biological typologies; Mays, Ponce, Washington, & Cochran, 2003). Disparities in health care access and utilization are also associated with health status disparities but are not discussed in this chapter; they are the subject of another chapter in this text.

Behavioral Risk Factors

Individual behaviors are the final common pathway through which genetic, economic, physical, and social-environmental factors influence health. They are symptomatic of the major contributors to health disparities, to be discussed later. Public health surveillance of these behaviors or conditions allows quantification of adverse exposure and disease as a bellwether of future disease incidence, providing an opportunity for targeted intervention.

Obesity is increasingly recognized as a major driver of chronic disease disparities (Braveman, 2009). Rates of being overweight and of obesity (defined as a body mass index [BMI] at or greater than $25 \, \text{kg/m}^2$ and $30 \, \text{kg/m}^2$, respectively) are increasing across the population, but even more rapidly in certain racial and ethnic groups: including African Americans, Latinos, American Indians, and Pacific Islanders (Wang & Beydoun, 2007). Physical inactivity and poor dietary quality—the antecedents of obesity—are commensurately more common in ethnic minority groups in general except Asian Americans, though certain healthful dietary components are more often consumed in these groups (legumes among African Americans and Latinos, fruits and vegetables among Latinos; Bermudez, Ribaya-Mercado, Talegawkar, & Tucker, 2005; Popkin, Siega-Riz, & Haines, 1996). Asian Americans as a group have lower incidence of overweight or obesity (Wang & Beydoun, 2007). However, the negative health effects of being overweight begin to occur at a lower BMI among Asian Americans compared to individuals of other ethnicities. Lower socioeconomic status is associated with obesity, but higher socioeconomic status is less protective against obesity for African Americans than for Latinos and whites (Williams, 2002).

Tobacco use varies in form and prevalence among racial and ethnic groups. In 2010, 19.3 percent of U.S. adults were currently smokers, with slightly higher rates among men (21.5 percent) than women (17.3 percent) (King, Dube, Kaufmann, Shaw, & Pechacek, 2011). Tobacco use among African Americans is slightly higher than among the total population (20.6 percent compared to 19.3 percent). Compared to whites, African Americans tend to start smoking at a later age and are more inclined to attempt to quit smoking, but less likely to succeed. The later age at initiation of smoking among African American women is reflected in a lower relative risk of obstructive lung disease compared to white women (Williams, 2002). The smoking rate among Latinos (12.5 percent) is lower than for the general population and is especially low among

Latinas (9.0 percent; King et al., 2011). American Indians and Alaskan Natives have the highest tobacco use of all racial and ethnic groups, at 31.4 percent overall. A higher proportion of American Indian and Alaskan Native tobacco users use smokeless tobacco products compared to the general population. Asian Americans and Pacific Islanders smoke at the lowest rate (9.2 percent overall), although it has been observed that use for Asians varies widely among Asian subgroups and between genders, and it may increase with acculturation. Tobacco consumption among adolescents from all racial and ethnic minority groups appears to be on the rise.

Alcohol use patterns also vary considerably across racial and ethnic groups. In general, men have a higher rate of alcohol use and heavy drinking than women. Whites have more alcohol use across all age groups; however, problem-related drinking and the negative consequences of alcohol are more prevalent among African Americans, American Indians and Alaskan Natives, and Latinos than whites. Research has found that American Indians and Latinos of Mexican origin may be particularly likely to abuse or be dependent on alcohol (Chartier & Caetano, 2010). Alcohol use among Asians, although lower than for other racial and ethnic groups, has been found to vary widely within racial and ethnic groups, and a higher rate is seen among U.S.-born people than in immigrant populations.

Racial and ethnic disparities in health status have traditionally been ascribed to poor health behaviors, primarily those described here, and to limited access to health care. It has become increasingly clear, however, that individual-level behavioral variables are closely linked with environmental-level variables that govern the ease or difficulty of access to healthy or unhealthy options and choices. These environmental exposures are further examined in the upcoming discussion of socioeconomic, physical, and social environmental influences.

Socioeconomic Status

Poverty is one of the most powerful determinants of health (Braveman et al., 2010), with African Americans and Latinos substantially overrepresented among households in poverty (U.S. Census Bureau, 2010). Children of color are also more likely to live in poverty compared to non-Latino whites—for example, 38 percent of African Americans and 35 percent of Latino children live at or below the poverty level, compared with 12 percent of whites (U.S. Census Bureau, 2010).

However, higher income inequality, rather than absolute deprivation, may also have an adverse influence on health (Kawachi, 2000). Several theories have been advanced to explain the relationship between income inequality and adverse health outcomes (Lynch, Davey Smith, Kaplan, & House, 2000). The psychosocial pathway theory postulates that inequality affects health through individual perceptions of low position in the social hierarchy, which in turn can have an effect on biological response (for instance, blood pressure) or maladaptive behavior (smoking or homicide). The material deprivation pathway theory proposes that inequality affects health through an accumulation of negative exposures and lack of resources held by individuals at the bottom of a social hierarchy. There is substantial evidence that income inequality is growing in the United States (Heathcote, Perri, & Violante, 2010; Kawachi, 2000; Saez, 2009; 2012). Between 1993 and 2007, the income of the upper 1 percent of the population grew at a much faster rate than the rate in the rest of the population (5.9 percent versus 1.3 percent per year), resulting in a 122 percent increase over this period among the top 1 percent and only 20 percent increase in the remaining 99 percent. In fact, over half of the overall economic growth over this time period was the result of income increases among the top 1 percent (Saez, 2009). More recent data show this trend is continuing following the Great Recession of 2007 to 2009. In 2010, the income of the top 1 percent increased by 11.6 percent, whereas the income of the remainder of the population increased by only 0.2 percent (Saez, 2012).

Researchers often use singular indicators of socioeconomic status (SES) such as income, education, or occupational attainment interchangeably. However, the interaction among these indicators may differ by racial and ethnic group. For example, formal education does not have the same socioeconomic return for African Americans as for whites (Lillie-Blanton & LaVeist, 1996). At the same level of education, research has found, whites have higher income and occupational attainment as compared to African Americans. Furthermore, there is evidence to indicate that, at an individual level, increasing SES does not have the same benefits on the health of African Americans compared to whites (Anderson & Armstead, 1995, Farmer & Ferraro, 2005). Data indicate that even at a higher level of education, African Americans experience poorer physical health outcomes such as increased infant mortality compared to whites (National Center for Health Statistics, 2010b).

Finally, community-level socioeconomic measures have not been adequately captured in most analyses examining the effect of SES on health.

Research has shown that socioeconomic characteristics of the neighborhood in which an individual lives (average income and percentage of unemployment) predict morbidity and mortality above and beyond individual characteristics (Diez Roux et al., 2001). It has been well documented that racial and ethnic minorities are significantly more likely to live in disadvantaged or resource-poor communities relative to whites (see Mohai, Pellow, & Roberts, 2009, for a review). An analysis of a fairly socioeconomically homogeneous multiethnic sample controlled for twelve community-level variables (among them robbery arrests and income inequality). However, disparities persisted in coronary heart disease risk, obesity, and hypertension among African American women compared to white women (Finkelstein, Khavjou, Mobley, Haney, & Will, 2004). Pathways by which these community-level variables influence health are elaborated later in this section and in another chapter in this text.

Physical Environmental Influences

Many tobacco control efforts implemented over the past two decades have focused on creating changes in the physical environment. The success of these efforts in reducing smoking speaks to the powerful influence of the physical environment on health behaviors. Some of the most effective tobacco control efforts have included federal laws prohibiting tobacco sales to minors, state smoking bans in public places, and federal and state policies that encourage a smoke-free workplace among grant recipients. Although many policies and laws have been enacted, adherence to and enforcement of these controls is lower in communities of color. In addition, the shift in focus of tobacco marketing to the developing world, where few such controls have been implemented, results in the addiction of many Asian American and Latino men who later immigrate to the United States.

Researchers are now beginning to elucidate the link between ecological factors, such as access to high-quality or poor-quality food, and the onset of such conditions as cardiovascular disease and diabetes (Diez Roux et al., 2001). Studies show that minority neighborhoods have fewer supermarkets and fewer high-quality food options (Morland, Wing, Diez Roux, & Poole, 2002). Other studies demonstrate that African American neighborhoods have a disproportionate number of fast food restaurants (Block, Scribner, & DeSalvo, 2002). In addition, diners in lower-income, minority neighborhoods have fewer healthy options available to them in restaurants, in both food selection and preparation (Lewis et al., 2005). These areas have been termed ''food deserts'' by English researchers (Whelan,

Wrigley, Warm, & Cannings, 2002). Numerous studies demonstrate that regular consumption of fast food can lead to higher BMI, contributing to obesity and related illnesses (Thompson et al., 2004). Studies also link periodic food insecurity to overconsumption, obesity, and poor mental health (Heflin, Siefert, & Williams, 2005).

Product consumption preferences and purchasing behaviors are also influenced by commercial advertising, marketing, and promotion. There is increasing evidence of concentrated media marketing and advertising of a range of commercial products targeted to specific racial and ethnic groups that may contribute to health risk behavior disparities, especially tobacco, alcohol, and nutrient-poor food consumption (Hackbarth, Silvestri, & Cosper, 1995). Severely constraining billboard and television advertising and counteradvertising campaigns (adolescent-targeted social marketing to counter the claims of tobacco industry advertising) are credited with contributing to decreased tobacco use. However, the decrease in tobacco billboard advertising, for example, has been accompanied by more advertising of other unhealthy products. For example, billboards in predominantly African American and Latino neighborhoods in Chicago were found to advertise alcohol five times as frequently as those in predominantly white areas (Hackbarth et al., 1995). A recent study conducted in four major U.S. cities found that the advertising density was highest in African American neighborhoods, with white neighborhoods having the lowest density (Yancey et al., 2009). Similarly, fewer advertisements for healthier food and beverage products are found in magazines and television shows targeting African Americans compared to those targeting "general audiences," and a significantly greater number of advertisements for unhealthy products are found (Pratt & Pratt, 1995; Tirodkar & Jain, 2003). Studies have also documented substantially more point-of-sale advertising and promotions, with many more for unhealthy than healthy foods, in restaurants in lower-income African American and Latino communities in Los Angeles County than in its more affluent white communities (Lewis et al., 2005). This commercial marketing is also likely to influence physical activity and sedentary behavior patterns (automobile and other private transportation usage and audiovisual electronic media consumption), and work is beginning in this area to elucidate these relationships.

The influence of physical surroundings on physical activity patterns has also recently received much attention. Lower-income and minority neighborhoods have fewer recreational facilities, private or community gardens, less safety (perceived and actual), insufficient lighting, and urban design with few concessions to pedestrians (Estabrooks, Lee, & Gyurcsik, 2003; Powell, Slater, & Chaloupka, 2004). Interestingly, the major difference is that lower-income neighborhoods have fewer free recreational facilities (such as parks) compared to higher-income neighborhoods, although minimal differences have been observed for frequency of paid usage facilities (such as gyms). In addition to these environmental stressors or disincentives (which also include noise, traffic congestion, and information overload), environmental psychologists point to neighborhood disorder (less "defensible space" and incivility) exerting a negative influence on physical activity and restorative features such as foliage, water, and spatial vistas that reduce stress positively influencing physical activity (King, Stokols, Talen, Brassington, & Killingsworth, 2002).

Health-compromising physical characteristics of workplace and residential environments are well characterized elsewhere and are only summarized here. Workplace and residential environmental characteristics have been found to influence multiple health outcomes, in particular intentional and unintentional injury, disability, chronic disease morbidity, and mortality. Potential exposures occurring in these environments include noise, toxic chemical or biological hazards (tobacco smoke, lead, asbestos, dioxin, tuberculosis, or vehicle emissions), hazardous equipment, hazardous natural elements (ionizing and nonionizing radiation, heights, bodies of water, or heat), poor ergonomic design of equipment, lack of adherence to safety protocols or safety equipment usage, traffic hazards, poorly maintained streets and sidewalks, and firearms. People of racial and ethnic minority background are more likely to work and live in an environment that can have a detrimental effect on health.

Social-Environmental Influences

As has been illustrated here, socioeconomic position explains many, but not all, of the racial and ethnic differences in health status. Recent evidence points to additional explanations for the more adverse effect of poverty on the health of people of color:

- Cumulative effects of prolonged exposure to individual stressors.
- Long-term effects of an early childhood or prenatal environment of deprivation (Population Reference Bureau, 2001; Halfon & Hochstein, 2002).
- Reaction to macrosocial factors: in today's world, social comparisons extend beyond what was formerly possible only at the neighborhood

level. Marketing by mass media to children and adolescents fosters a desire for goods and services (enjoyed by affluent whites) that are beyond the means of working and middle-class families.

Racial and ethnic discrimination is the primary social environmental influence cited, given that negative attitudes toward individuals from racial and ethnic minority groups are still commonplace (Williams & Jackson, 2005); racism may also interact with other forms of discrimination based on gender, sexual orientation, disability, or age (Fiscella & Williams, 2004; Cochran, Mays, & Sullivan, 2003); and social experiences are translated and transformed into biological responses ("embodied"), enhancing or eroding health (Krieger, 2005a). Thus social disparities mediate gene expression, which is the greater contributor to health disparities than gene frequency (genotype; Krieger, 2005b). A full explication of this topic is beyond the scope of this chapter. Here we briefly summarize the major issues attendant to investigation of the association between discrimination and health outcomes.

Epidemiological investigation of the health effects of discrimination has used three main approaches (Krieger, 2000):

1. Indirect, individual-level, inferring discrimination, when established risk factors do not fully explain racial and ethnic differences in health outcomes; for example, formal education does not produce the same returns in improved health for African Americans as whites, similar to its lesser return in wealth and income (Robert & House, 2000; Farmer & Ferarro, 2005).
2. Direct, individual-level, examining association between self-reported discrimination and particular individual health outcomes (blood pressure and peptic ulcer disease).
3. Institutional, population-level, examining association between group-level measures of discrimination and population health outcomes.

The major mediators of the relationship between discrimination and health are economic and social deprivation (for instance, diminished access to goods and services, substandard education, and poor health care); exposure to hazardous physical, chemical, and biological agents (lead-based paint and parasites); socially inflicted trauma (mental, physical, or sexual abuse or neglect); and targeted marketing of legal and illegal health-compromising substances (tobacco and energy-dense but nutrient-poor foods; Fiscella & Williams, 2004). These mediators exert their influence through psychological and physiological responses to perceived or internalized discrimination among those discriminated against, and individual and institutional policies and practices by those perpetrating discrimination that produce socioeconomic disadvantage or personal injury. One common example of the latter is work-related stress. Relegation to a position not commensurate with one's talents or to certain types of lower-status jobs increases the likelihood of an individual being subjected to high psychological demands with little decisional latitude or control or social support, an independent contributor to coronary heart disease risk (Theorell, 2000). Another example is reflected in the political expedience of the generalized stigmatization of people of Middle Eastern and South Asian descent following the 2001 terrorist attacks in the United States carried out by Islamic radicals—presenting an interesting parallel to the stigmatization of Asians following the Japanese attack on Pearl Harbor.

Factors and Influences: Summary

Socioeconomic status (SES) is a major contributor to racial and ethnic disparities in health. In fact, race and ethnicity are frequently a proxy for SES in public health research and surveillance, because the dramatic skew in the income distribution of African Americans and Latinos compared to whites and acculturated subgroups of Asian Americans precludes appropriate SES matching. Lower SES is responsible for increased exposure to many of the physical and sociocultural environmental conditions contributing to health risk behaviors and compromising health status, among them long-term effects of the early childhood or prenatal environment.

However, income inequality may also be an important contributor to poorer health, and economic indicators demonstrate that the gap between rich and poor is increasing dramatically while opportunities for upward social mobility are declining. This disproportionately disadvantages racial and ethnic minority populations and likely contributes to racial and ethnic health disparities. In addition to absolute or relative economic deprivation, recent evidence suggests that the health of racial and ethnic minorities may be negatively affected by macrosocial factors such as the social comparisons beyond what can be observed at the neighborhood level made possible through mass and social media.

Racial and ethnic discrimination is the primary social environmental contributor to health disparities, exerting both acute or immediate effects (anger and hostility) and cumulative effects of prolonged exposure to individual stressors. Discrimination also influences the physical environment, through institutional policies and practices on the part of those perpetrating discrimination that produce socioeconomic disadvantage or personal injury.

Future Directions

Our ability to identify, understand, and monitor progress in addressing disparities is severely limited by the underrepresentation of people of racial and ethnic minority and low-income backgrounds in surveillance and research (Yancey, Ortega, & Kumanyika, 2006). The paucity of data from public health practice surveillance, observational epidemiological research, and in particular policy and programmatic intervention evaluation or research constitutes a major concern in this or any discussion of disparities. In both surveillance and research, data must be disaggregated and sufficiently "local" (beyond city or county to zip code and census tract, to really reach communities or neighborhoods) if we are to accurately capture and monitor disparities and assess and refine intervention efforts.

The existence of positive racial and ethnic disparities (rate of disease and risk behavior in racial and ethnic minority populations lower than for whites) or attenuation of disparities in relation to the severity of socioeconomic disadvantage is noteworthy. A number of sociocultural protective factors may create resilience and mitigate the effects of adversity and may provide guidance for interventions to improve health equity. Such factors within the Mexican and Central American Latino communities may include the effect of strong identification with the culture of origin on healthy food choices (Smith, 2005) and family and neighborhood cohesion creating optimal birth outcomes (Lara, Gamboa, Kahramanian, Morales, & Bautista, 2005). The lower level of nonmalignant lung disease among African American women and lower smoking rate among African American adolescents may reflect a protective response to discrimination manifested in active resistance to tobacco company exploitation of the black community, as in organizing to prevent introduction of the Uptown cigarette brand. Having role models and mentors has been associated with such positive outcomes as racial and ethnic identity, academic achievement, physical activity, and self-esteem in adolescence (DuBois & Silverthorn, 2005; Yancey, Siegel, & McDaniel, 2002). Also, a lower level of overweight self-perception may protect against eating disorders, poor body image, and sedentary behavior in Latinos, Pacific Islanders, and African Americans (Yancey, Simon, et al., 2006). The sociocultural environment may in fact be as important as the physical environment in supporting physical activity participation (Stahl et al., 2001), as reflected in the comparable physical activity of Pacific Islanders and whites (Lucas, Schiller, & Benson, 2004). The fact that, for example, dancing or movement to music is normative throughout adulthood in African American, Latino, and other communities of color along with their collectivist rather than individualist values are cultural assets that may increase receptivity to intervention approaches reintegrating brief bouts of physical activity into organizational (that is, workplace) routines (Yancey, Ory, & Davis, 2006).

In addition, the relative health advantages observed for Asian Americans and Latinos are likely to dissipate over time, given the negative effect of acculturation on health status. Also, the health indicators that show the greatest benefit for Latinos and Asian Americans—life expectancy and death rate—do not yet reflect significant changes in risk factor status occurring over the past ten years. For example, among immigrants, obesity and tobacco use, poorer dietary quality, and lower level of physical activity have been correlated with increased length of stay in the United States (Kaplan, Huguet, Newsom, & McFarland, 2004). "Softer" measures, such as self-reported disability and lower perceived health status, are already more common in these groups than among whites, a harbinger of excess future disease and death.

The Affordable Care Act (ACA), assuming it is enacted as intended, has a number of provisions aimed at reducing health status disparities. Many of the ACA initiatives are aimed at increasing access to health care and reducing health care disparities, including the health insurance exchanges, requirements that Medicare and private insurance plans waive deductibles for preventive services, and efforts to enhance the cultural competency of health care systems. However, some of the initiatives extend outside of the traditional bounds of care delivery, including the use of community health teams designed to bridge the gap between the clinic and community. This approach shows promise in reducing disparities, particularly in the areas of chronic disease management and infant mortality.

Health services policy and health care organizations must extend beyond their accustomed boundaries of medical care delivery to address the physical, social, and economic environmental conditions undergirding health disparities. Changes in the health care system will have a diminishing influence on the health status of the population without immediate, careful, and considerable attention to eliminating health disparities.

SUMMARY

In summary, substantial evidence has documented the existence of racial and ethnic disparities in health status across a wide variety of indicators, with African Americans tending to fare the worst, followed by American Indians and Alaskan Natives. Latinos and Asian Americans appear to have a relative advantage, at least for more distal health outcomes such as life expectancy, although rising rates of obesity and chronic diseases suggest this advantage will diminish in the coming decades. Factors that underlie these disparities are many, with health behaviors, socioeconomic status, and the physical and social environment prominent among them. Population demographic shifts, including both aging and racial and ethnic diversification, will further increase attention to and need for programmatic and policy intervention to eliminate health disparities. In particular, as the obesity epidemic strains the health care system and otherwise increases the societal economic burden, there is clearly a need for a shift in health policy focus, and ultimately the health services funding focus, from treatment to disease prevention and health promotion. The increasing contribution of obesity-related disparities to overall health disparities and burden of disease will also drive this necessary shift; a range of sectors must engage in structural and systemic change to stem the epidemic.

KEY TERMS

Chronic disease a condition that is prolonged in duration, does not often resolve spontaneously, and is rarely cured completely

Evans and Stoddart Framework of Determinants of Health a conceptual framework that attempts to explain how some of the most important determinants of health (social, physical, and genetic) influence health of the population at the community and individual level

Immigrant health the health of racial and ethnic population subgroups who are immigrants to the United States

Minority health the health of racial and ethnic minority groups, including African Americans, Latinos, Asian Americans and Pacific Islanders, and American Indians and Alaskan Natives

Racial and ethnic disparities differences in the incidence, prevalence, mortality, and burden of diseases and other adverse health conditions that exist among specific racial and ethnic population groups

Social determinants of health the complex and overlapping social and economic influences (social environment, physical environment, and structural and societal factors) that contribute to observed disparities in health

DISCUSSION QUESTIONS

1. A number of different health indicators have been used to provide evidence of racial and ethnic disparities in health status. What are the advantages and disadvantages of using specific indicators such as life expectancy versus years of life lost? Which provide the most compelling evidence of health disparities? Which indicators have the most negative consequences for society?

2. African Americans and Native Americans have the poorest health status. What factors do you believe are most important in causing disparities among these groups? What is the relative importance of historical factors versus present conditions in accounting for the relatively poor health status of these groups?

3. What factors do you believe account for the relatively better health of Latinos and Asian Americans and Pacific Islanders currently living in the United States? Why are decreases in health status correlated with increases in acculturation? What, if anything, can be done to prevent decreasing health status among these immigrant populations?

4. Socioeconomic status has been found to be one of the most powerful single determinants of health. Why is this? How does socioeconomic status interact with other known determinants of health? How can we understand the relative contribution of socioeconomic status versus other important potential determinants?

5. The importance of community-level variables versus individual factors in determining health status has been increasingly recognized. Through what pathways do community-level factors influence health status?

6. It is increasingly clear that focusing on improving health care delivery is not sufficient to reduce health disparities. How can we as a society begin to affect the broader factors that underlie racial and ethnic disparities in health?

FURTHER READING

Braveman, P. A., Cubbin, C., Egerter, S., Williams, D. R., & Pamuk, E. (2010). Socioeconomic disparities in health in the United States: What the patterns tell us. *American Journal of Public Health, 100*, S186–S196.

Dubay, L. C., & Lebrun, L. A. (2012). Health, behavior, and health care disparities: Disentangling the effects of income and race in the United States. *International Journal of Health Services, 42*(4), 607–625.

Evans, R. G., & Stoddart, G. L. (2003). Consuming research, producing policy? *American Journal of Public Health, 93*(3), 371–379.

Kaiser Family Foundation. Webcasts devoted to health and health care disparities. http://www.kff.org/minorityhealth/todaystopics.cfm

Krieger, N. (2005). Stormy weather: Race, gene expression, and the science of health disparities. *American Journal of Public Health, 95*(12), 2155–2160.

LaVeist, T. A., & Isaac, L. A. (Eds.). (2012). *Race, ethnicity, and health: A public health reader*. San Francisco: Jossey-Bass.

National Center for Health Statistics. http://www.cdc.gov/nchs

National Institute on Minority Health and Health Disparities. http://www.nimhd.nih.gov

Williams, D. R., Mohammed, S. A., Leavell, J., & Collins, C. (2010). Race, socioeconomic status, and health: Complexities, ongoing challenges, and research opportunities. *Annals of the New York Academy of Sciences, 1186*(1), 69–101.

Williams, D. R., & Jackson, P. B. (2005). Social sources of racial disparities in health. *Health Affairs, 24*(2), 325–334.

REFERENCES

American Cancer Society. (2009). *Cancer facts and figures for Hispanics/Latinos 2009–2011*. Atlanta: American Cancer Society.

Anderson, G. (2010). Chronic care: Making the case for ongoing care. *Princeton*, NJ: Robert Wood Johnson Foundation. Retrieved from http://www.rwjf.org/pr/product.jsp?id=50968

Anderson, N. B., & Armstead, C. A. (1995). Toward understanding the association of socioeconomic status and health: A new challenge for the biopsychosocial approach. *Psychosomatic Medicine, 57*, 213–225.

Bates, J. H., Hofer, B. M., Parikh-Patel, A. (2008). Cervical cancer incidence, mortality, and survival among Asian subgroups in California. *Cancer, 113* (10 Suppl), 2955–2963.

Bermudez, O. I., Ribaya-Mercado, J. D., Talegawkar, S. A., & Tucker, K. L. (2005). Hispanic and non-Hispanic white elders from Massachusetts have different patterns of carotenoid intake and plasma concentrations. *Journal of Nutrition, 135*(6), 1496–1502.

Block, J. P., Scribner, R. A., & Desalvo, K. B. (2002). Poverty, race, and fast food: A geographical analysis. *Journal of General Internal Medicine, 17*(S1), 151.

Brault, M. W., Hootman, J., Helmick, C. G., Theis, K. A., & Armour, B. S. (2009). Prevalence and most common causes of disability among adults: United States, 2005. *Morbidity and Mortality Weekly Report, 58*(16), 421–426.

Braveman, P. (2009). A health disparities perspective on obesity research. *Preventing Chronic Disease, 6*(3), A91. Retrieved from http://www.cdc.gov/pcd/issues/2009 /jul/09_0012.htm

Braveman, P. A., Cubbin, C., Egerter, S., Williams, D. R., & Pamuk, E. (2010). Socioeconomic disparities in health in the United States: What the patterns tell us. *American Journal of Public Health, 100*, S186–S196.

Chartier, K., & Caetano, R. (2010). Ethnicity and health disparities in alcohol research. *Alcohol Research in Health, 33*(1–2), 152–160.

Cochran, S. D., Mays, V. M., & Sullivan J. G. (2003). Prevalence of mental disorders, psychological distress, and mental health services use among lesbian, gay, and bisexual adults in the United States. *Journal of Consulting and Clinical Psychology, 71*(1), 53–61.

Deapen, D., Liu, L., Perkins, C., Bernstein, L., & Ross, R. K. (2002). Rapidly rising breast cancer incidence rates among Asian-American women. *International Journal of Cancer, 90*, 747–750.

Denny, C. H., Holtzman, D., & Cobb, N. (2003). Surveillance for health behaviors of American Indians and Alaska Natives: Findings from the behavioral risk factor surveillance system, 1997–2000. *Morbidity and Mortality Weekly Report, 52*, 1–13.

Diez Roux, A. V., Merkin, S. S., Arnett, D., Chambless, L., Massing, M., Nieto, F. J., . . . Watson, R. L. (2001). Neighborhood of residence and incidence of coronary heart disease. *New England Journal of Medicine, 345*, 99–106.

DuBois, D.L., & Silverthorn, N. (2005). Natural mentoring relationships and adolescent health: Evidence from a national study. *American Journal of Public Health, 95*, 518–524.

Estabrooks, P. A., Lee, R. E., & Gyurcsik, N. C. (2003). Resources for physical activity participation: Does availability and accessibility differ by neighborhood socioeconomic status? *Annals of Behavioral Medicine, 25*, 100–104.

Evans, R. G., & Stoddart, G. L. (1994). Producing health, consuming health care. In R. G. Evans, M. L. Barer, & T. R. Marmor (Eds.), *Why are some people healthy and others not? The determinants of health of populations.* New York: de Gruyter.

Farmer, M. M., & Ferraro, K. F. (2005). Are racial disparities in health conditional on socioeconomic status? *Social Science & Medicine, 60*, 191–204.

Finkelstein, E. A., Khavjou, O. A., Mobley, L. R., Haney, D. M., & Will, J. C. (2004). Racial/ethnic disparities in coronary heart disease risk factors among WISEWOMAN enrollees. *Journal of Women's Health, 13*(5), 503–518.

Fiscella, K., & Williams, D. R. (2004). Health disparities based on socioeconomic inequities: Implications for urban health care. *Academic Medicine, 79*(12), 1139–1147.

Frisbie, W. P., Song, S. E., Powers, D. A., & Street, J. A. (2004). The increasing racial disparity in infant mortality: respiratory distress syndrome and other causes. *Demography, 41*(4), 773–800.

Gomez, S. L., Kelsey, J. L., Glaser, S. L., Lee, M. M., & Sidney, S. (2004). Immigration and acculturation in relation to health and health-related risk factors among specific Asian subgroups in a health maintenance organization. *American Journal of Public Health, 94*(11), 1977–1984.

Guendelman, S., & Abrams, B. (1995). Dietary intake among Mexican American women: Generational differences and a comparison with white non-Hispanic women. *American Journal of Public Health, 85*(1), 20–25.

Hackbarth, D. P., Silvestri, B., & Cosper, W. (1995). Tobacco and alcohol billboards in 50 Chicago neighborhoods: Market segmentation to sell dangerous products to the poor. *Public Health Reports, 16*(2):213–230.

Halfon, N., & Hochstein, M. (2002). Life course health development: An integrated framework for developing health, policy, and research. *Milbank Quarterly, 80*(3), 433–479.

Hayes-Bautista, D. E., Hsu, P., Hayes-Bautista, M., Iniguez, D., Chamberlin, C. L., Rico, C., & Solorio, R. (2002). An anomaly within the Latino epidemiological paradox: The Latino adolescent male mortality peak. *Archives of Pediatric and Adolescent Medicine, 156*(5), 480–484.

Heathcote, J., Perri, F., & Violante, G. L. (2010). Unequal we stand: An empirical analysis of economic inequality in the United States, 1967–2006. *Review of Economic Dynamics, 13*, 15–51.

Heflin, C. M., Siefert, K., & Williams, D. R. (2005). Food insufficiency and women's mental health: Findings from a 3-year panel of welfare recipients. *Social Science & Medicine 61*, 1971–1982.

Johnson, H. P., & Hayes, J. M. (2004). The demographics of mortality in California: Population trends and profiles. *California Counts, 5*(4).

Kanny, D., Liu, Y., & Brewer, R. D. (2011). Binge drinking: United States, 2009. *Morbidity and Mortality Weekly Report, 60*, 101–104.

Kaplan, M. S., Huguet, N., Newsom, J. T., & McFarland, B. H. (2004). The association between length of residence and obesity among Hispanic immigrants. *American Journal of Preventive Medicine, 27*(4), 323–326.

Kawachi, I. (2000). Income inequality and health. In L. Berkman & I. Kawachi (Eds.), *Social epidemiology.* New York: Oxford University Press.

King, A. C., Stokols, D., Talen, E., Brassington, G. S., & Killingsworth, R. (2002). Theoretical approaches to the promotion of physical activity: Forging a transdisciplinary paradigm. *American Journal of Preventive Medicine, 23*(2 Suppl), 15–25.

King, B., Dube, S., Kaufmann, R., Shaw, L., & Pechacek, T. (2011). Vital signs: Current cigarette smoking among adults aged ≥ 18 years—United States, 2005–2010. *Morbidity and Mortality Weekly Report, 60*(35), 1207–1212.

Krieger, N. (2000). Discrimination and health. In L. Berkman & I. Kawachi (Eds.), *Social epidemiology.* New York: Oxford University Press.

Krieger, N. (2005a). Embodiment: A conceptual glossary for epidemiology. *Journal of Epidemiological Community Health, 59*(5), 350–355.

Krieger, N. (2005b). Stormy weather: Race, gene expression, and the science of health disparities. *American Journal of Public Health, 95*(12), 2155–2160.

Kung, H. C., Hoyert, D. L., Xu, J. Q., & Murphy, S. L. (2008). Deaths: final data for 2005. *National Vital Statistics Reports, 56*(10). Retrieved from http://www.cdc.gov/nchs/data/nvsr/nvsr56/nvsr56_10.pdf

Lara, M., Gamboa, C., Kahramanian, M. I., Morales, L. S., & Bautista, D. E. (2005). Acculturation and Latino health in the United States: A review of the literature and its sociopolitical context. *Annual Review of Public Health, 26*, 367–397.

Lewis, L. B., Sloane, D. C., Nacimento, L. M., Diamant, A. L., Guinyard, J. J., Yancey, A. K., & Flynn, G. (2005). African Americans' access to healthy food options in South Los Angeles restaurants. *American Journal of Public Health, 95*(4), 668–673.

Lillie-Blanton, M., & LaVeist, T. (1996). Race/ethnicity, the social environment and health. *Social Science Medicine, 43*, 83–91.

Lucas, J. W., Schiller, J. S., & Benson, V. (2004). Summary health statistics for U.S. adults: National Health Interview Survey, 2001. *Vital Health Statistics, 10*(218), 1–134.

Lynch, J. W., Davey Smith, G., Kaplan, G. A., & House, J. S. (2000). Income equality and mortality: Importance to health of individual income, psychosocial environment, or material conditions. *British Medical Journal, 200*(320), 1200–1204.

Mays, V. M., Ponce, N. A., Washington, D. L., & Cochran, S. D. (2003). Classification of race and ethnicity: Implications for public health. *Annual Review of Public Health, 24*, 83–110.

McGinnis, J. M., & Foege, W. H. (1993). Actual causes of death in the United States. *Journal of the American Medical Association, 270*(18), 2207–2212.

Mohai, P., Pellow, D., & Roberts, J. T. (2009). Environmental justice. *Annual Review of Environment and Resources, 34*, 405–430.

Morland, K., Wing, S., Diez Roux, A., & Poole, C. (2002). Neighborhood characteristics associated with the location of food stores and food service places. *American Journal of Preventive Medicine, 22*, 23–29.

National Center for Health Statistics. (2004). *Health, United States, 2004.* Hyattsville, MD: Author.

National Center for Health Statistics. (2007). *Health, United States, 2007.* Hyattsville, MD: Author.

National Center for Health Statistics. (2008). *Health, United States, 2008, with special feature on the health of young adults.* Hyattsville, MD: Author.

National Center for Health Statistics. (2010a). Deaths: Final data for 2007 (Table 25). *National Vital Statistics Reports, 58*(19).

National Center for Health Statistics. (2010b). *Health, United States, 2010, with special feature on death and dying.* Hyattsville, MD: Author.

Periz-Escamilla, R. (2011). Acculturation, nutrition, and health disparities in Latinos. *American Journal of Clinical Nutrition, 93*(Suppl), 1163S–1167S.

Popkin, B. M., Siega-Riz, A. M., & Haines, P. S. (1996). A comparison of dietary trends among racial and socioeconomic groups in the United States. *New England Journal of Medicine, 335*(10), 716–720.

Population Reference Bureau. (2001). *Major causes of death in the United States and Peru.* Retrieved from http://www.prb.org/Educators/TeachersGuides/Human Population/Health.aspx

Powell, L. M., Slater, S., & Chaloupka, F. J. (2004). The relationship between community physical activity settings and race, ethnicity, and SES. *Evidence-Based Preventive Medicine, 1*(2), 135–144.

Pratt, C. A., & Pratt, C. B. (1995). Comparative content analysis of food and nutrition advertisements in *Ebony, Essence,* and *Ladies' Home Journal. Journal of Nutrition Education, 27*(1), 128–133.

Ritenbaugh, C., & Goodby, C. S. (1989). Beyond the thrifty gene: Metabolic implications of prehistoric migration into the New World. *Medical Anthropology, 11*(3), 227–236.

Robert, S. A., & House, J. S. (2000). Socioeconomic inequalities in health: Integrating individual-, community-, and societal-level theory and research. In G. L. Abrecht (Ed.), *Handbook of social studies in health and medicine*. New York: Sage.

Saez, E. (2009). *Striking it richer: The evolution of top incomes in the United States—update with 2007 estimates* (Working Paper Series). Berkeley, CA: Institute for Research on Labor and Employment, UC Berkeley. Retrieved from http://escholarship.org/uc/item/8dp1f91x

Saez, E. (2012). *Striking it richer: The evolution of top incomes in the United States—updated with 2009 and 2010 estimates*. Berkeley, CA: Institute for Research on Labor and Employment, UC Berkeley. Retrieved from http://elsa.berkeley.edu/˜saez

Smith, D. B. (2005). Racial and ethnic health disparities and the unfinished civil rights agenda. *Health Affairs, 24*(2), 317–324.

Stahl, T., Rutten, A., Nutbeam, D., Bauman, A., Kannas, L., Abel, T., . . . Van der Zee, J. (2001). The importance of the social environment for physically active lifestyle: Results from an international study. *Social Science and Medicine, 52*(1), 1–10.

Stewart, S. T., Cutler, D. M., & Rosen, A. B. (2009). Forecasting the effects of obesity and smoking on the U.S. life expectancy. *New England Journal of Medicine, 361*(23), 2252–2260.

Theorell, T. (2000). Working conditions and health. In L. Berkman & I. Kawachi (Eds.), *Social epidemiology*. New York: Oxford University Press.

Thompson, O. M., Ballew, C., Resnicow, K., Must, A., Bandini, L. G., Cyr, H., & Dietz, W. H. (2004). Food purchased away from home as a predictor of change in BMI z-score among girls. *International Journal of Obesity and Related Metabolic Disorders, 24*, 282–289.

Tirodkar, M. A., & Jain, A. (2003). Food messages on African American television shows. *American Journal of Public Health, 93*(3), 439–441.

U.S. Census Bureau, Population Division. (2008). *Projected life expectancy at birth by sex, race, and Hispanic origin for the United States: 2010 to 2050*. Washington, DC: Author.

U.S. Census Bureau. (2010). Income, poverty, and health insurance coverage in the United States, 2009 (current population reports, series P60-238). Retrieved from http://wwww.census.gov/hhes/www/poverty/poverty.html

Wang, Y., & Beydoun, M. A. (2007). The obesity epidemic in the United States: Gender, age, socioeconomic, racial/ethnic, and geographic characteristics—a systematic review and meta-regression analysis. *Epidemiological Reviews, 29*, 6–28

Whelan, A., Wrigley, N., Warm, D., & Cannings, E. (2002). Life in a food desert. *Urban Studies, 39*, 2083–2100.

Williams, D. R. (2002). Racial/ethnic variations in women's health: The social embeddedness of health. *American Journal of Public Health, 92*(4), 588–597.

Williams, D. R., & Jackson, P. B. (2005). Social sources of racial disparities in health. *Health Affairs, 24*(2), 325–334.

Yancey, A. K., Cole, B. L., Brown, R., Williams, J. D., Hillier, A., Kline, R. S., . . . McCarthy, W. J. (2009). A cross-sectional prevalence study of ethnically targeted and general audience outdoor obesity-related advertising. *Milbank Quarterly, 87*(1), 155–184.

Yancey, A. K., Ortega, A. N., & Kumanyika, S. K. (2006). Effective recruitment and retention of minority research participants. *Annual Review of Public Health, 27*, 1–28.

Yancey, A. K., Ory, M. G., & Davis, S. M. (2006). Dissemination of physical activity promotion interventions in underserved populations. *American Journal of Preventive Medicine, 31*(4 Suppl), S82–S91.

Yancey, A. K., Siegel, J., & McDaniel, K. (2002). Ethnic identity, role models, risk and health behaviors in urban adolescents. *Archives of Pediatrics and Adolescent Medicine, 156,* 55–61.

Yancey, A. K., Simon, P. A., McCarthy, W. J., Lightstone, A. S, Wold, C., & Fielding, J. E. (2006). Ethnic and gender differences in overweight self-perception and their relationship to sedentariness. *Obesity Research, 14,* 980–988.

CHAPTER FOUR

RACIAL AND ETHNIC DISPARITIES IN HEALTH CARE

Arturo Vargas Bustamante
Leo S. Morales
Alexander N. Ortega

Learning Objectives

- Understand the definition of disparity in health care
- Learn how patient-, provider-, and system-level factors contribute to disparities
- Understand the role of historical context causing disparities in health care
- Learn about efforts to reduce and eliminate disparities
- Understand how the ACA addresses disparities

Racial and ethnic disparities in health care pervade the American health care system. In 1999, the U.S. Congress commissioned a report on the health care quality and experiences of racial and ethnic minorities in the United States, which resulted in the Institute of Medicine's (IOM's) seminal report *Unequal Treatment: Confronting Racial and Ethnic Disparities in Health Care* (IOM, 2003). An earlier report on the quality of health care in the United States identified six aims for improving performance of the health care system: safety, effectiveness, patient-centeredness, timeliness, efficiency, and equity (IOM, 2001). *Equity,* as defined by the IOM, is the delivery of health services of equal quality to all individuals, regardless of such personal characteristics as gender, socioeconomic status, geographic location, and race or ethnicity. Despite the increasing awareness of health care disparities facing various racial and ethnic groups in the United States, several reviews of the scientific literature document the existence of racial and ethnic disparities in the processes and outcomes of care for a variety of diseases and clinical conditions, including cancer, HIV/AIDS, and chronic conditions such as cardiovascular disease and diabetes, as well as in the delivery of preventive care services (Department of Health and Human Services [DHHS], 2010). For example, the National Healthcare Disparities report published by the AHRQ since 2003 has consistently found that blacks, Latinos/Hispanics, Asians, and American Indians and Native Alaskans were more likely than whites to receive lower-quality care across a range of quality-of-care indicators (DHHS, 2010). Thus, the existence of disparities in health care represents a failure of the American health care system and signals the need for attention and reform.

Addressing racial and ethnic disparities in health care is of growing importance because the population of the United States is more diverse than ever. Between 2010 and 2050, the Latino population is expected to increase from 16 to 30 percent as a percentage of the U.S. population, the Asian and Pacific Islander population is expected to grow from 4 to 9 percent, while the black population is expected to remain at 12 percent of the U.S. population (U.S. Census Bureau, 2009; Ortman & Guarneri, 2009). Over the same period, the non-Latino white population is expected to decrease from 65 percent to 46 percent as a percentage of the U.S. population. If racial and ethnic minorities continue to receive lower-quality care, then in the coming years a substantial portion of the U.S. population will have suboptimal health status, which will in turn lower labor market productivity and increase national health care spending (Bound, Waidmann, Schoenbaum, & Bingenheimer, 2003).

We begin this chapter by defining our view of disparities in care. Next, we review some of the historical factors specific to racial and ethnic groups that have contributed to the patterns of disparities we observe today. In the following sections, we summarize some of the evidence documenting health care disparities by racial and ethnic groups. In the final sections of the chapter, we summarize a number of ongoing initiatives to reduce disparities in care.

Definition of Disparity in Health Care

A distinction can be made between disparity in health and *disparity in health care*. The former refers to racial and ethnic differences in morbidity and mortality and is influenced by a variety of factors (social, environmental, behavioral, and biological), only one of which is health care. With recent advances in human genomics, much more attention is being given to the genetic basis for racial and ethnic disparities in health (Fine, Ibrahim, & Thomas, 2005). Disparities in health are discussed in Chapter Three. In this chapter, we focus on disparities in health care.

Researchers have adopted various perspectives on disparities in health care over time (Carter-Pokras & Baquet, 2002; Braveman, 2006; Adler & Rehkopf, 2008; Vargas Bustamante, & Chen, 2011). Some have viewed all the differences in health care between racial and ethnic groups as constituting disparities. From this point of view, differences in the use of services are viewed as disparities regardless of coexistent differences in access to care, insurance coverage, personal preferences, clinical need, or clinical appropriateness. It has been suggested that in some cases lower use of services may constitute an advantage, in particular where overuse is thought to lead to excess morbidity or mortality.

Others have taken a narrower perspective, defining disparity as a difference in care that is not accounted for by a difference in access to care, personal preference, clinical need, or clinical appropriateness (see Figure 4.1). In this narrower view, two groups of factors are identified as being responsible for disparities in care. The first is the group of system-level factors such as the structure of health care systems and the legal and regulatory environment in which those systems operate. These may also include structural factors such as underfunding of hospitals that predominantly serve minority patients or organizational characteristics such as inadequate workforce diversity or the absence of policy and procedures that promote culturally competent care. The second group of factors is discrimination at the patient-provider level, whether it takes the form of prejudice or unconscious stereotyping.

Few datasets include information on quality of care, race and ethnicity, and patient needs. Moreover, few of these sources differentiate between the effects of structural or legal and regulatory factors on the one hand and discrimination on the other. Hence, most of the existing literature tends to support the view that disparities in health care are a result of a myriad of factors including patient preferences and behaviors, provider constraints and practices, and system or institutional policies (see Figure 4.2).

Patient Factors

Many patient-related factors are associated with access to and utilization of health care. Some of these factors are more salient to minority patients. Patient perception of health status, views of specific diseases and the patient's ability to accept and cope with illness are all associated with health care use. These points of view on health may be shaped by

FIGURE 4.1. INSTITUTE OF MEDICINE MODEL OF DISPARITIES IN HEALTH CARE

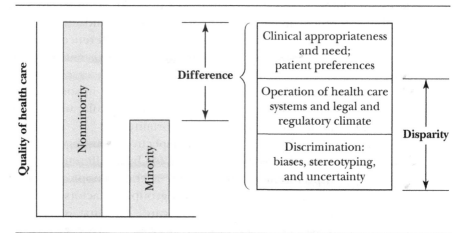

Source: Institute of Medicine, 2003.

FIGURE 4.2. FACTORS RELATED TO HEALTH CARE USE AND THEIR SYNERGIES

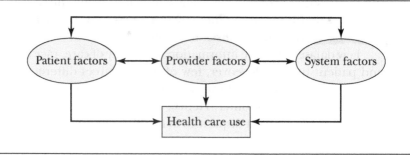

individual's cultural or traditional beliefs and practices. In addition, psychosocial constructs such as readiness for change, perceived self-efficacy, self-reliance, and fatalism are all related to individual decision making (Ortega & Alegría, 2002; Lorig & Holman, 2003; Wolff et al., 2003; Green et al., 2008). These attitudes in turn determine whether a patient will seek care, adhere to providers' recommendations, and successfully achieve desired outcomes. Patient trust, level of comfort with medical providers, and satisfaction with care are important factors for entry into the health care system as well for its continued use (Sheppard, Zambrana, & O'Malley, 2004; Shi & Stevens, 2005). Individuals' previous experiences with care providers as well as the broader minority communities' history with the health care system also influence patients' attitudes toward providers and the health care system.

Provider Factors

A number of racial and ethnic minorities in the United States come from socioeconomically disadvantaged communities and households with lower education and income levels. On the other hand, White males from affluent socioeconomic backgrounds are overrepresented in the medical establishment. Accordingly, discordance between patient and provider demographics prevails (Vargas Bustamante & Chen, 2011). It is reasonable to believe that most providers feel more comfortable communicating with patients who share similar socioeconomic backgrounds. Researchers have asserted that how providers communicate and understand their patients is likely to influence the effectiveness and continuity of care. Stereotyping or misunderstanding patients due to such differences may lead to inaccurate or inappropriate clinical decision making. For instance, Schulman and colleagues—using a sample survey of more than seven hundred physicians in videotaped, scripted interviews on their recommendations for chest pain management—found that black women were less likely to be referred for cardiac catheterization than white men (Schulman et al., 1999). They also suggest that race and gender play significant and synergistic roles in how providers manage their patients.

Recently, researchers have explored the role of unconscious bias among physicians. Social psychologists posit a dual process theory in which individuals hold attitudes and beliefs on two levels of consciousness: explicit attitudes and beliefs, which are readily available for recall and can be reported, and implicit or unconscious, automatic attitudes and beliefs that exist outside of conscious awareness (Greenwald, Poehlman, et al.,

2009). Unconscious bias refers to social attitudes and stereotypes about certain demographics or groups of people that are formed outside of their own conscious awareness and are thus "hidden" attitudes and beliefs (Dovidio, Kawakami, & Gaertner, 2002). An individual can hold egalitarian beliefs and unconscious biases simultaneously. Implicit or unconscious preferences and stereotypes are pervasive across populations and topics (Nosek et al., 2007). Implicit race attitudes are related to perceptions of a persons' trustworthiness (Stanley, Sokol-Hessner, Banaji, & Phelps, 2011). In sensitive areas such as interracial attitudes and beliefs, implicit attitudes are better predictors of the behaviors of discrimination than self-reported attitudes (Greenwald, Poehlman, Uhlman, & Banaji, 2009). In response to racial and ethnic disparities in health care, researchers have been studying implicit and explicit racial bias among physicians and have found that physicians hold implicit racial biases similar to others in society. One exploratory study found that African American physicians showed no unconscious racial bias for either white or African Americans, while physicians of other races and ethnicities showed a strong implicit pro-white preference (Sabin, Nosek, Greenwald, & Rivara, 2009).

Provider communication is associated with patient satisfaction, adherence to recommendations, and health outcomes, which may have consequential effects on the type of service sought (emergency versus primary care) (Murray-García, Selby, Schmittdiel, Grumbach, & Quesenberry, 2000; Betancourt & Maina, 2004; Johnson, Roter, Powe, & Cooper, 2004; Betancourt, Green, Carrillo, & Park, 2005). Providers who communicate effectively with their patients and are sensitive to the process tend to have patients who are satisfied and informed of their health issues; more important, such patients are more likely to follow through with treatment and continue to seek primary care services (Johnson et al., 2004; Saha, Komaromy, Koepsell, & Bindman, 1999). Hence, it is important to examine the role of providers in the process, particularly as patient-provider communications become more diverse, with the increasing participation of nonphysician medical providers such as nurses, physician assistants, pharmacists, community health workers, and office staff.

Finally, some argue that racial disparities in medical treatment are rooted in discrimination on the part of providers and health care systems, while others disagree and posit that there is insufficient empirical evidence to show that the disparities are due to conscious or subconscious discrimination (Epstein & Ayanian, 2001). Nonetheless, abundant evidence shows that disparities in health care are persistent, are deep-seated, and exist across many medical disciplines, practices, and populations, including children, adults, and the elderly.

System Factors

System factors have also been implicated in health care disparities. Lack of health insurance coverage among Latinos has been associated with uncertainty over family health care expenditures, potentially ruinous out-of-pocket payments, and lower health care access and utilization (Monheit & Vistnes, 2000; Waidmann & Rajan, 2000; Hadley, 2003; Hargraves & Hadley, 2003; Zuvekas & Taliaferro, 2003). Difficulties in navigating through a complex health care system and understanding bureaucratic procedures have been cited as major barriers to receiving quality health care for both low-income and racial and ethnic minorities (Betancourt, 2006). For example, patients who are without knowledge or tools required to access primary health care may delay seeking care or may resort to using urgent care or emergency room services. This problem is exacerbated in individuals with more serious conditions requiring secondary or tertiary care, where they would have to access complex systems of specialty care and follow-up (Scheppers, van Dongen, Dekker, Geertzen, & Dekker, 2006).

Structural and environmental conditions within clinical care settings and health care sites that serve racial and ethnic minorities may also contribute to health care disparities. The decline in funding for public clinics and community hospitals that predominantly serve racial and ethnic minorities leads to increased wait times for appointments, crowded facilities, and understaffing and negatively affects the quality of care (Hsiao, Knight, Kappel, & Done, 2011; Vargas Bustamante & Chen, 2011).

Historical Overview of Disparities in Medical Care

The historical and contemporary causes of health care disparities differ for each racial and ethnic group, given their unique experiences in the United States. While there may be overlapping reasons or commonalities among the groups, the histories of African Americans, Latinos, Asian and Pacific Islanders, and Native Americans have distinct paths and trajectories leading to the health care disparities they face. Defining and distinguishing the major forces that have influenced the emergence of health care disparities for these groups would allow health professionals and policymakers to identify appropriate policy and practice solutions specific to these groups.

Factors Related to Disparities among African Americans

The Tuskegee Syphilis Study, a forty-year study of untreated syphilis in black men from Alabama conducted by the U.S. Public Health Service, is typically cited as the central reason for nonparticipation of many African Americans in medical studies and for their reluctance to seek needed health care. However, the legacy of distrust of and mistreatment by the medical establishment among minorities predates the Tuskegee study (Gamble, 1997). Minorities, particularly African Americans, have a long history of segregation in medical care and of receiving poor-quality care (Smith, 1999). Inequity in medical care began with racial segregation and slavery in American history. Slaves were able to obtain care only in slave hospitals, which were typically staffed by other slaves, slave owners, and their family members (Gamble, 1997; Smith, 1999). After emancipation, the federal government set up more than ninety hospitals for the emancipated slaves, but only one (Howard University Medical Center) remained open until the end of the 1800s (Smith, 1999). In segregated America, no one took responsibility for the delivery of care for African Americans. In the late 1800s, African American physicians led efforts to establish black hospitals, starting with the Provident Medical Center in Chicago (Gamble, 1991).

However, in the early 1900s African Americans were excluded from mainstream professional medical societies as well as from most medical schools. In fact, in 1900 only seven medical schools were training physicians of color. Moreover, public health departments and medical societies did not begin taking responsibility for the health of African Americans until they were deemed a threat to the health of whites; thus, the type of care delivered was generally in the form of hygiene control and treatment of infectious diseases.

In addition to these historic factors that contribute to health care disparities faced by African Americans, researchers have identified a variety of other contemporary risk factors (recall Chapter Three). For example, African Americans in the United States are disproportionately represented among the poor and people who live in inner-city neighborhoods. Socioeconomic status and race are associated with a slew of disease risk factors, among them access to primary health care, behaviors (diet, smoking, and physical activity), access to resources and social capital, and environmental and psychosocial stressors. Minority and low-income populations are also less likely to receive effective public health and prevention messages that could help increase their awareness.

Studies have found that African Americans are less likely to have private insurance and more likely than whites to be publicly insured, underinsured, or uninsured (Kaiser Commission on Medicaid and the Uninsured, 2004). This is an important risk factor, because private insurance coverage is associated with better access to primary care, continuity of care, site of care, and the type and quality of care received, whereas publicly and uninsured patients often receive inadequate and poor-quality care.

Factors Related to Disparities among Latinos

Latinos make up a diverse group of people who trace their roots to several countries of origin that have distinct histories and political ties to the United States. Much like other ethnic groups in the United States, Latinos have a range of immigration and migration patterns. For instance, many Latinos in the Southwest have a family history that can be traced in the region to the time following the Treaty of Guadalupe Hildalgo, well before the colonization of the American Southwest. Puerto Ricans have a history in the United States that dates back to the Jones Act in 1917 (almost twenty years after the Treaty of Paris ended the Spanish-American War), stipulating that Puerto Rico was a U.S. territory whose inhabitants were entitled to U.S. citizenship. Other Latino groups from the Americas and the Caribbean have immigration histories that arise from refugee status, as with the Cubans who sought refuge in the United States after the Bay of Pigs fiasco in the 1960s.

Given the changing demographics of the United States, the significance of issues related to Latinos' health care access and use can be expected to rise. According to recent census data, Latinos make up approximately 16 percent of the total population (U.S. Census Bureau, 2009). Within the Latino population, those of Mexican and Puerto Rican descent make up the two largest groups, accounting for 65.5 percent and 9.1 percent respectively of the entire U.S. Latino population (not including the 3.9 million U.S. citizens in Puerto Rico). Latinos also make up the largest minority group of children and adolescents. Census data show Latinos constituting 22 percent (or sixteen million) of the U.S. population under the age of eighteen.

Studies document that compared to non-Latino Whites, Latinos tend to have worse access to health care, worse morbidity as a result of lack of medical care or treatment, and poorer quality of care. Many factors have been implicated in disparities in access to and quality of care for Latinos. Some studies have reported that Latinos, compared to non-Latino whites, have low rates of insurance coverage, usually as a result of noncitizen status or low-wage employment that does not provide employer-based health insurance; have worse geographic access to care, usually because of migration or living on farms or in rural areas; and receive low-quality care, usually because of language discordance between them and their medical providers (Vargas Bustamante & Chen, 2012). Disparities in insurance and access differ, however, within Latino subgroups. For instance, Puerto Ricans born on the island are citizens by birth, facilitating circular migration and qualifying them for certain federal and state health programs (Medicaid, SCHIP, and Medicare).

Latinos have a high presence in public insurance programs, mainly in Medicaid (IOM, 2003). Medicaid is characterized by higher per capita resource constraints and stricter limits on covered services, which are the indicators of poor access and lower quality of care. Low Medicaid capitation payments have been linked to restricted provider networks, limiting the pool of available providers for its beneficiaries, including minorities (Tai-Seale, Freund, & LoSasso, 2001).

Spanish-speaking populations in the United States face a language barrier that can affect the quality of care through poor communication with physicians and other medical care providers. As a result, there can be deficient or inaccurate transfer of important information such as details of disease symptoms, consequences of treatment or lack of treatment, and medication regimens, all of which can lead to ineffective disease management or prevention. Many Latinos delay seeking care until their condition is severe. Such delays, coupled with the need for effective medical interpreters and culturally and linguistically competent providers, make Latinos more vulnerable, potentially more expensive to treat, and more complicated to manage than other ethnic groups who are more fluent English speakers (IOM, 2003).

Factors Related to Disparities among Asians, Pacific Islanders, and Native Hawaiians

Similar to the Latino population, the Asian, Pacific Islander, and Native Hawaiian population is a heterogeneous population from different countries with diverse cultures, histories, and health statuses. While Native Hawaiians became part of the United States through the colonization of Hawaii, Asian and Pacific Islanders have a long history of immigration to the United States dating back to the late 1800s. The first large-scale immigration occurred in 1848, during the Gold Rush in California with the migration of large groups of Chinese. Subsequently, Chinese immigrants continued to fill labor demands by working on sugarcane farms in Hawaii, in various other service occupations, and also as laborers for the transcontinental railroad. Similarly, other ethnic groups such as Japanese and Filipinos experienced their own waves of migration. The passage of the Immigration and Nationality Act of 1965 eliminated the national origins quota system and opened up immigration to previously excluded South Asian and Southeast Asian groups. More recently, the United States has seen a growth in refugee migrant populations of Laotians, Hmong, and Cambodians.

Since 2000, the Asian American and Pacific Islander (AAPI) population in the United States has increased by 45 percent, surpassing the growth rate of other racial and ethnic groups (API Health Forum, 2012). The largest subgroups within the Asian population are Chinese, Indian, Filipino, and Vietnamese. Hawaiians, Samoans, and Guamanians represent the largest subgroups of the Pacific Islander population. While many AAPI subgroups have achieved high rates of education, income, homeownership, and social capital relative to non-Latino whites, substantial disparities still exist within this community. For example, while 60 percent of Asians aged twenty-five to twenty-nine reported having a college degree, after disaggregating the data only 18 percent of Native Hawaiians and Pacific Islanders and 7 percent of Hmongs had attained a college education (National Center for Education Statistics, 2012). In addition, although Asians, Pacific Islanders, and Hawaiians have high rates of employment, Asian Americans with a college degree were more likely to be unemployed in comparison to non-Latino whites (Austin, 2010). Finally, the Hmong, Laotian, and Cambodian communities continue to face high rates of poverty, ranging from 35 to 65 percent, in comparison to the national average of 17 percent (National Commission on Asian American and Pacific Islander Research in Education, 2008).

These socioeconomic variations within the AAPI population dispel the "model minority" myth that has been popularized by mainstream American society and by many policymakers (Chen & Hawks, 1995). This myth holds that AAPI groups have successfully acculturated to the U.S. lifestyle and achieved the "American dream," which masks many AAPIs' experiences of discrimination, prejudice, and limited access to resources, which in turn affect their access to health care. The heterogeneity of the Asian, Pacific Islander, and Hawaiian population poses several complexities that influence the health care disparities experienced by this community. According to U.S. Census data, 38 percent of AAPIs do not speak English fluently, and many subgroups have lower rates of English proficiency compared to other groups (Ponce et al., 2009; U.S. Census, 2003). Language barriers, along with the lack of bilingual service providers and translated health materials, have been cited as major barriers to care

(Ngo-Metzger, Sorkin, & Phillips, 2009). Equally important is the need to provide culturally competent care to diverse groups of Asians, Pacific Islanders, and Hawaiians, who have unique beliefs regarding health behaviors, outcomes, and treatment. In addition, although rates of health care insurance are high for the overall Asian population, specific subgroups (such as the recently arrived Hmong, Laotian, and Cambodian subgroups) with lower education levels, higher rates of poverty, and unemployment rely on public insurance or remain uninsured, which negatively affects their access to and receipt of health care services (OMH, 2012).

Factors Related to Disparities among American Indians and Alaska Natives

While comprising of only 2 percent of the entire U.S. population, American Indians and Alaska Natives have the longest history in the United States of any racial and ethnic group. At the time of the arrival of European settlers, scholars estimate the population of these groups to have been approximately thirty-four million, but warfare and colonization, foreign diseases, and cultural dislocation have reduced this community to roughly five million people (U.S. Census Bureau, 2009). The American Indian and Native Alaskan population is also culturally diverse; the U.S. federal government officially recognizes 566 tribes as sovereign nations (Bureau of Indian Affairs, 2012). In addition, there is a high level of geographic dispersion, with only 22 percent living on federal reservations. The states with the largest native populations include California, Oklahoma, and Arizona.

Social disparities and economic disadvantage have long been major factors in the health care disparities facing American Indians and Alaska Natives. Lower rates of education have translated into high rates of unemployment and poverty for this community. In terms of educational attainment, 77 percent have earned a high school diploma by the age of twenty-five, compared to 99 percent of non-Latino whites, and 13 percent have earned college degrees, compared to 31 percent of non-Latino whites (OMH, 2012). Twenty-eight percent of American Indians and Alaska Natives live at or below the federal poverty line, in comparison to 9.9 percent of non-Latino whites (OMH, 2012). As has been shown with other racial and ethnic groups, living in poverty contributes to poor health behaviors and limited access to social resources that promote health. Loss of cultural traditions, language, and native lands has also been attributed to the decline in health and escalation in health care disparities.

The Indian Health Service, the only federal health care system specifically established for a racial or ethnic group, has faced challenges in providing quality and accessible health care (Families USA, 2010). As a part of the treaties established in 1787, members of federally recognized tribes were guaranteed health care by the U.S. government, and the Indian Health Service (IHS) was established in 1955 to fulfill this commitment. However, only 57 percent of American Indians and Alaska Natives are serviced directly by the IHS, and members face significant restrictions on where they can access services and the extent of care they can receive (U.S. Commission on Civil Rights, 2004). Moreover, direct services from IHS are mostly provided on or near reservations, leaving the 66 percent of natives who do not live on reservations to access care through limited Urban Indian Health programs. However, due to underfunding and structural barriers, 37 percent of all Native Americans receive no services from the IHS (Urban Indian Health Institute, 2004).

Traditional insurance access is also a major barrier for American Indians and Alaska Natives. According to a report by the Kaiser Commission on Medicaid and the Uninsured, 43 percent of American Indians have employer-sponsored health insurance, in comparison to 73 percent of non-Latino whites, while 27 percent rely on public insurance programs such as Medicaid and Medicare, with nearly a quarter of the American Indian population remaining uninsured. As discussed previously, the IHS provides care for all qualified American Indians, but barriers to access place these uninsured individuals at risk of delaying care and not receiving services. Moreover, the complexity of both IHS and public insurance programs and lack of awareness are major barriers to receiving requisite care, even for qualified American Indians and Native Alaskans (U.S. Commission on Civil Rights, 2004).

Scientific Evidence of Disparities in Health Care

In this section we review some of the evidence supporting the existence of disparities in health care. Because the literature on disparities in care is extensive, spanning several decades, we have selected several condition-specific areas of research for our review: cardiovascular disease, cancer, renal disease and transplantation, HIV/AIDS, obesity, diabetes, asthma, and mental health. These areas were selected for a variety of reasons. Cardiovascular disease, cancer, renal disease and transplantation, and HIV/AIDS were selected because they are among the most studied areas of racial and ethnic disparities in care. Asthma, obesity, and diabetes were selected because various racial and ethnic subgroups are disproportionately affected by these conditions. Finally, because the other areas included in this review focus on physical domains of health status, we elected to include mental health.

Cardiovascular Disease

Coronary artery disease (CAD) and acute myocardial infarction (AMI) are the most analyzed topics among studies of racial and ethnic disparities in care. Due to data limitations and elevated risk, the most frequently studied groups are African Americans, Latinos, and whites. Although blood pressure and cholesterol screening are common among both African Americans and whites, one study using seven federal datasets found that hospitalization rates for hypertension, angina, and congestive heart failure were higher for African Americans compared to whites across almost all age groups, suggesting that screening and preventive care are insufficient to prevent heart disease in African Americans (Holmes, Arispe, & Moy, 2005). Similar findings in congestive heart failure hospitalization rates have also been found for Latinos and Native Americans in comparison to non-Latino whites (Mensah, Mokdad, Ford, Greenlund, & Croft, 2005). In addition, from 1999 to 2006 blood pressure control and cholesterol levels have improved in the United States; however, disparities persist among African Americans and Latinos compared to non-Latino whites (McWilliams, Meara, Zaslavsky, & Ayanian, 2009).

Studies of racial and ethnic disparities in cardiovascular disease have become increasingly sophisticated in their control and adjustment for confounders (Geiger, 2003). African Americans are less likely than whites to be catheterized; when it is done, they are 20 to 50 percent less likely to undergo a revascularization procedure. They are also less likely to receive beta-blockers, thrombolytic drugs, or aspirin when these interventions are indicated. There are similar findings for Latinos, as studies have found that they receive less blood pressure control, aspirin, beta-blockers, and assessments of left ventricular function (Correa-de-Araujo et al., 2006; Hicks et al., 2004).

In addition, racial and ethnic minorities are less likely to receive advanced and expensive treatments and therapies for cardiovascular disease conditions. African Americans are less likely than whites to undergo cardiac catheterization and revascularization, less likely to be given newer antiplatelet agents during hospitalization, and less likely to receive lipid-lowering agents and smoking cessation counseling at time of hospital discharge (Sonel et al., 2005). In addition, African Americans and Latinos were less likely to receive cardiac resynchronization therapy with defibrillation, even when they met clinical guidelines for receiving that treatment (Farmer et al., 2009).

The role of race in clinical decision making regarding cardiovascular disease has also been investigated. In one study where a committee of cardiologists and cardiothoracic surgeons made decisions about coronary artery bypass grafting (CABG) versus angioplasty for 938 patients after catheterization—decisions based only on a presentation by a cardiology fellow, and thus effectively blinded to the patient's race—the rate of revascularization was similar for African Americans and whites, though African Americans were more likely to receive angioplasty and whites more likely to receive CABG (Okelo et al., 2001). A study that included Medicare patients treated for myocardial infarction in 4,609 hospitals found that on average African Americans were treated at "hospitals with lower-quality medical treatment but higher-quality surgical treatment." Nevertheless, "African Americans received fewer surgical treatments than whites admitted to the same hospital" (Barnato, Lucas, Staiger, Wennberg, & Chandra, 2005). In a similar study conducted in New York state, African Americans and AAPIs who underwent CABG received treatment from lower-quality hospitals and surgeons compared to whites (Rothenberg, Pearson, Zwanziger, & Mukamel, 2004).

Cancer

Studies of racial and ethnic disparities in cancer incidence and prevalence, screening, stage at diagnosis, as well as treatment and survival have been attributed to a range of factors, among them differences in tumor biology, genetics, cultural differences and folk beliefs, socioeconomic status, problems of access to continuity of care, physician practice style and communication with patients, and interaction among all of these factors (Geiger, 2003).

For several types of cancers, racial and ethnic minorities are less likely to receive screenings and early diagnosis, which is essential for effective treatment and survivorship. One study that analyzed national cancer data found that only 52 percent of Native American women, 57 percent of Asian women, 62.6 percent of Latina women, and 68.2 percent of African American women had received a mammogram in the past two years, compared to 72 percent among non-Latino white women (Ward et al., 2004). The same study found that rates of Pap smears were similar among African American women (83.9 percent) and non-Latino white women (85.5 percent); however, rates were lower for Latinas (77.9 percent),

American Indians and Alaska Natives (78.4 percent), and Asians (68.2 percent). As a result, non-Latino white women are more likely to receive a breast cancer diagnosis when the cancer is in the localized stage as opposed to African American, Latina, and American Indian women, who have high rates of diagnoses in the regional stage. The same is true for cervical cancer, where Asian women are more likely to be diagnosed with invasive cervical cancer, followed by African American and Latina women.

Variation in cancer treatment has also been found in several reports and studies. Shavers and Brown found that, after controlling for clinical factors, African American women are less likely than white women to receive breast-conserving surgery (BCS) and radiation. After undergoing BCS, African American women and women from other racial and ethnic minority groups are less likely than whites to have radiation therapy (Shavers & Brown, 2002). In addition, Latina women were less likely to receive reconstructive surgery, and they report being less satisfied with their breast cancer treatment in comparison to African American and non-Latino white women (Katz et al., 2005). Similar patterns according to race and ethnicity were found for men and women with colorectal cancer. Both Latinos and African Americans have been shown to be treated less aggressively than non-Latino whites with similar disease, even after adjusting for insurance coverage, hospital type, and comorbidities (Elston Lafata, Cole Johnson, Ben-Menachem, & Morlock, 2001; Roetzheim et al., 2000).

Diabetes

Diabetes disproportionately affects racial ethnic minorities, including Latinos, African Americans, and Native Americans; however, the literature highlights several gaps in care facing these groups. Successful treatment and management of diabetes includes healthy eating and nutrition education, eye exams, foot inspections, prescription drug and/or insulin therapies, cholesterol and blood pressure monitoring, and glucose control.

In one review of seventy-eight articles relating to diabetes treatment and management, findings suggested that glycemic and blood pressure control was worse for racial and ethnic minorities in comparison to non-Latino whites (Kirk et al., 2006). Patient adherence and behaviors, provider practices, and health care systems all contribute to disparities in diabetes treatment faced by minority patients. For example, African American patients were found to be less adherent to medication and in turn to have less metabolic control, although the effect of race was still independent of adherence (Schectman, Nadkarni, & Voss, 2002). Similarly, a meta-analysis of several articles found that A1C levels were found to be higher among Latinos in comparison to non-Latino whites, but the causes of elevated levels were unknown (Kirk et al., 2008).

In addition, racial and ethnic minorities face more complications from diabetes when compared to non-Latino whites, which highlights failures in treatment and management. Common complications cited in the literature include glaucoma, cataract, neuropathy, cardiovascular disease, kidney disease, and mental health disease. One study examining insured patients found that Latinos, Asians, and African Americans had a higher likelihood of end-stage renal disease in comparison to non-Latino whites in the sample (Karter et al., 2002). In addition, diabetic African Americans have experienced higher rates of blindness, amputations, and amputation-related mortality, while Latinos have higher prevalence of retinopathy. Finally, Latinos, African Americans, and Native Americans have higher risks of diabetes-associated mortality compared to non-Latino whites (Peek, Cargill, & Huang, 2007).

Renal Disease and Transplantation

African Americans and Native Americans have the highest incidence of risk of illness and death from end-stage renal disease (ESRD) among racial and ethnic minorities. Among Native Americans, for example, the rate is four times that for whites. This is due to more hypertension, diabetes, and sickle cell disease among African Americans, diabetes among Native Americans, and less access to or use of early primary care interventions among both groups. The two main treatments for ESRD are dialysis and renal transplantation. Although Medicare specifically supports ESRD treatment, kidney transplantation rates vary by race (Eggers, 1995). Studies have shown that Asians, Latinos, and women initiate dialysis treatment later.

Reasons for differences in transplant rates involve numerous factors, including race. One study found that Latinos and Asians on a transplant list were less likely to receive a kidney in comparison to non-Latino whites and African Americans, after controlling for severity of the disease (Mathur, Schaubel, Gong, Guidinger, & Merion, 2010). In addition, many studies show that patient preferences, including refusal of and disinterest in transplantation, is an important contributing factor (Geiger, 2003). A study that examined physicians' beliefs about racial differences in referral for renal transplantation related that whereas physicians did not view patient-physician communication and trust as important reasons for racial differences in care, African American patients were less likely than white patients to report receiving some or a lot of information about transplantation (55 percent versus 74 percent; Ayanian et al., 2004).

HIV/AIDS

Over the past two decades, infections with HIV and progression to AIDS have disproportionately affected African Americans and Latinos. For example, in 2002 HIV/AIDS was the sixth leading cause of death among African Americans and tenth leading cause of death among Latino males, whereas it was not among the ten leading causes of death for non-Latino white males (Hoyert & Xu, 2012). Evidence from various studies indicate that racial and ethnic minorities are less likely than whites to receive various medications or to undergo some diagnostic procedures, though they vary by source of care (Geiger, 2003).

African American and Latina women have been shown to receive highly active antiretroviral therapy (HAART) less often than non-Latino white women after controlling for potential confounders (Lillie-Blanton et al., 2010). Similarly, a review of the literature found mixed effects in relation to the influence of race on the use of antiretrovirals and prophylaxis for opportunistic infection (Palacio, Kahn, Richards, & Morin, 2002). Possible reasons for the differences include misconceptions about HIV/AIDS among racial and ethnic minorities, distrust of health authorities, and "prescribing habits" of providers.

Additionally, many studies have found difficulties in physician-patient communication in HIV/AIDS cases, particularly in discussing decisions about end-of-life care and resuscitation (Haas et al. 1993) and when there was racial or ethnic discordance between patient and physician. One study found that African Americans with white physicians were less likely to receive protease inhibitors when compared to racially concordant physician-patient pairs (King, Wong, Shapiro, Landon, & Cunningham, 2004).

Finally, patient practices and beliefs are important factors in explaining disparities in HIV treatment. Appointment nonadherence was found to be an important factor in virologic failure, and it partially explained disparities in virologic failure between African American and white patients (Mugavero et al., 2009). Patient mistrust and conspiracy beliefs are also a factor. A study found that 27 percent of 520 African American adults in ten randomly selected census tracts agreed with the statement "HIV/AIDS is a man-made virus that the federal government made to kill and wipe out black people," and an additional 23 percent were undecided (Klonoff & Landrine, 1999).

Asthma

Asthma is a major health problem across many socioeconomic and racial and ethnic categories. However, African Americans and Latinos, especially Puerto Ricans, share a disproportionate burden. Asthma is the most common chronic condition afflicting children in the United States Among children, African Americans and Latinos have worse morbidity and African Americans have higher mortality due to asthma than all other racial or ethnic groups of children (Akinbami, Moorman, & Liu, 2011). The asthma death rate among African Americans is approximately three times more compared to whites (Akinbami, Moorman, & Liu, 2011). Between the ages of five and thirty-four (when asthma is easier to distinguish from other causes of ventilatory impairment), African Americans experience an asthma mortality rate approximately three to five times higher than that of whites (Akinbami, Moorman, & Liu, 2011). Multiple risk factors have been implicated for asthma morbidity and mortality for racial and ethnic minorities: tobacco smoke exposure, obesity, air pollution, house dust mite allergens, cockroaches, and cat hair (Luder, Melnik, & DiMaio, 1998; Gilliland, et al., 2000).

An elevated level of severe asthma and related hospitalization among inner-city minority children is associated with features of health care and treatment, such as inadequate use of long-term controller steroid medications and overuse of quick-acting reliever drugs such as albuterol (Ortega & Calderon, 2000). Researchers have observed that poor asthma management and control among racial and ethnic minorities is associated with a variety of factors, including poor provider-patient communication, deficient access to and use of high-quality and effective primary care, poor perceived patient and family efficacy to manage asthma, and perceived inadequate treatment efficacy by patients and their families (Ortega & Calderon, 2000).

Mental Health

Improving the access and utilization of mental health services has been a top health policy priority in the United States. The attention to mental health care comes from increasing awareness that many people who meet diagnostic criteria for mental illness do not seek or obtain needed care. Several studies have demonstrated that minorities, particularly African Americans and Latinos, are less likely to use mental health services than whites. In the U.S. Surgeon General's (2001) supplement "Mental Health: Culture, Race, and Ethnicity," it is noted that ethnic and racial minorities have less access to mental health care than whites, and that they are less likely to receive needed care and stay in care. The reasons for minorities' underuse of mental health services are multifactorial. Considerable attention in mental health services research has focused on the role of payment and insurance. Many people in the United States lack sufficient insurance coverage to cover mental health; many health plans also limit the number of visits people may have over a period of time. Further, some plans require costly copayments or do not allow people to go out of plan networks to find suitable providers. Other barriers include lack of access to providers who speak the same language, especially for low-acculturated Latinos. There are also accessibility factors, such as location and awareness of available services.

A growing body of literature indicates that other factors in addition to payment mechanisms for mental health disparity may also be in play. For example, researchers are focusing on factors such as health beliefs, knowledge of mental health problems, and coping mechanisms such as self-reliance and social networks (Ortega & Alegría, 2002). For example, two reports of island Puerto Ricans demonstrated a high level of psychiatric disorder but also high denial and self-reliance (Ortega & Alegría, 2002; Ortega & Alegría, 2005). Denial can be a maladaptive coping strategy, especially if it results in little or no usage of needed mental health care. The extent to which denial is more or less prevalent in minority populations relative to nonminority populations is unknown. For Latinos, some researchers have focused on the role of families and social networks in protecting members from morbidity (Pescosolido, Wright, Alegría, & Vera, 1998). Other factors that have been examined as potential determinants of mental health care disparities for all minorities include stigma, discrimination, and racism.

Due to these factors, racial and ethnic minorities face multiple disparities in mental health treatment, including limited access to care and lower quality of care. Among both nondepressed and depressed individuals, Asians, Latinos, and African Americans were less likely to access mental health services in comparison to non-Latino whites (Alegría et al., 2008). In addition, Asians and African Americans received lower-quality care when compared to non-Latino whites.

Future Directions

In response to the ever-growing body of literature documenting the existence of racial and ethnic disparities in care, there have been and continue to be numerous efforts to address those disparities. Examples of these efforts exist in the public and private sectors of U.S. society.

For the past thirty years, Healthy People, an initiative developed by the U.S. Department of Health and Human Services, has been outlining the national priorities for improving Americans' health. Healthy People 2000 included "reducing health disparities" as one of its major goals. Ten years later, Healthy People 2010 went one step further, with a goal of "eliminating health disparities" (DHHS, 2000). More specifically, the objectives target improving access to care and increasing immunizations as major objectives. Despite the declaration of these public efforts, studies that reviewed the progress toward Healthy People 2010 goals found mixed results in terms of improving health care access and immunizations for racial and ethnic minorities (Sonik, Stein-Wexler, Rogers, Coulter, & Wootton-Gorges, 2010). With the recognition that health care disparities continue to be a major issue, Healthy People 2020 has expanded this goal to "achieve health equity, eliminate disparities, and improve the health of all groups" according to the Office of Minority Health (OMH, 2012).

The Department of Health and Human Services has similarly called for the reduction in health disparities facing racial and ethnic minority groups and has integrated Offices of Minority Health in federal agencies under its leadership. In addition, the department organizes the Federal Interagency Health Equity Team that assembles leaders across DHHS and eleven other federal agencies to coordinate and maximize the effectiveness of the many federal efforts to eliminate disparities and to identify and evaluate new opportunities for eliminating disparities. Finally, the DHHS Disparities Action Plan, developed in 2011, provides strategic objectives over the next five years aimed at guiding agencies under DHHS to reduce health care disparities for racial and ethnic minorities (minority-health.hhs.gov/npa/files/Plans/HHS/HHS_Plan_complete.pdf).

Also, directed by Congress, the Agency for Healthcare Quality and Research has produced a yearly National Healthcare Disparities Report since 2003 documenting variations in quality of care by racial and ethnic groups. This report draws on data from numerous national surveys, including the Medical Expenditure Panel Survey, the National Health Interview Survey, the National Immunization Survey, the National Ambulatory Care Survey, and many others. The purpose of this report is to highlight areas of greatest need and track reduction in disparities over time.

In addition to monitoring efforts and goal-setting strategies, various government and private agencies have attempted to address health and health care disparities through expansion of health access and provision of care to racial and ethnic minorities. The Health Resources and Services Administration (HRSA)-supported health centers provide infrastructure support and often funding to various safety-net providers such as community clinics that provide care to the uninsured, low-income, and disadvantaged individuals. In 2010, these health centers served 19.5 million patients across the United States, where 92 percent were below 200 percent of the federal poverty guideline and 62.3 percent were racial and ethnic minorities (OMH, 2012).

Diversifying the health care workforce and promoting cultural competency have also been major initiatives of the last twenty years. Established in 1972, the National Health Service Corps places physicians, nurses, dentists, and health personnel in Health Professional Shortage Areas in exchange for scholarship and loan repayment programs (DHHS, n.d.). Also, various public and private efforts have aimed to provide more opportunities for minority students to pursue careers in medicine, nursing, dentistry, and public health. For example, Title VII of the Public Health Services Act supports the training of over ten thousand underrepresented graduates, residents, and faculty in various health professional fields (American Public Health Association, 2009). In addition, the Office of Minority Health has established national standards on Culturally and Linguistically Appropriate Services (CLAS), which guide health care organizations and providers in offering care to racial and ethnic minorities and other underserved communities (OMH, n.d.).

Finally, the Patient Protection and Affordable Healthcare Act (ACA), which passed in 2010, includes several provisions directly and indirectly intended to improve racial and ethnic disparities in health care through data collection and reporting, insurance coverage, cultural competence, access to health care, quality improvement, and research (Andrulis, Siddiqui, Purtle, & Duchon, 2010). While the full impact of these efforts is still unclear as health care reform is still being implemented, various initiatives already set into motion are projected to significantly reduce racial and ethnic health disparities.

First, the expansion of insurance and health care coverage will address significant barriers to care faced by racial and ethnic minorities. As previously discussed, compared to non-Latino whites, African Americans, Latinos, some subgroups of Asian and Pacific Islanders, and Native Americans are more likely to be uninsured. Through Medicaid expansion included in ACA, the creation of state-based health insurance exchanges, and employer-based health insurance reforms, an estimated thirty-two million individuals will gain access to health insurance (Kaiser Family Foundation, 2011). The ACA also sets out to improve access to care by providing funding and improving the infrastructure of health care systems that serve racial and ethnic minorities. For example, community health centers, which predominantly serve racial and ethnic minority and low-income patients, will receive $11 billion starting in 2011 to support expansion of operational capacity and capital improvements (National Association of Community Health Centers, 2010).

Strengthening and establishing centers to coordinate efforts to improve health and care for racial and ethnic minorities is also a priority of the ACA. In 2010, the National Center for Minority Health and Health Disparities (NCMHD) was transitioned to the National Institute on Minority Health and Health Disparities (NIMHD), which gives the institute discretion to develop research priorities and funding allocations for research focused on minorities and health disparities. In addition, federal agencies under the Department of Health and Human Services; the Agency for Healthcare Research and Quality (AHRQ); the Centers for Disease Control and Prevention (CDC); the Centers for Medicare and Medicaid Services (CMS); the Food and Drug Administration (FDA); the Health Resources and Services Administration (HRSA); and the Substance Abuse and Mental Health Services Administration (SAMHSA), in the Department of Health and Human Services, are mandated to create Offices of Minority Health to coordinate their efforts and initiatives regarding racial and ethnic minorities (OMH, n.d.).

Finally, much is still not understood about the nature and causes of health care disparities facing racial and ethnic minorities and effective solutions, therefore the ACA includes several provisions to improve research and develop effective interventions. One of the major efforts implemented in the law is the requirement to collect and utilize race, ethnicity, language, sex, and disability data in research studies and in monitoring efforts so that policymakers, practitioners, and researchers have a more holistic picture of the needs of various populations and subgroups (DHHS, 2010). To improve the quality of care for racial ethnic minorities, the law also establishes a Patient-Centered Outcomes Research Institute (PCORI) to independently investigate clinical effectiveness of medical interventions and programs for diseases, disorders, and health conditions, with a focus on what works for racial and ethnic minorities (Washington & Lipstein, 2011).

SUMMARY

According to the medical and public health literature, disparities in health care system are prevalent, with racial and ethnic minorities receiving lower-quality care in a variety of health care settings and across a range of medical conditions. A number of factors account for disparities in care, ranging from legal and structural factors to patient and provider factors. From a historical perspective, these findings are not surprising; racial and ethnic minorities have experienced discrimination and segregation in health care settings since the founding of the United States. Although efforts to address racial and ethnic disparities in care are multiple and ongoing, minority patients continue to have suboptimal health status, which will in turn affect labor market productivity and national health care spending. With the growing size of minority populations in the United States, addressing disparities in care is a paramount health policy issue.

KEY TERMS

Disparity in health care According to the Institute of Medicine (IOM), "disparity is any difference not due to clinical need or preferences for health care services" (IOM, 2003).

Equity According to the IOM, equity or equal treatment can be defined as the "delivery of health services of equal quality to all individuals regardless of personal characteristics as gender, socioeconomic status, geographic location, race or ethnicity" (IOM, 2003).

DISCUSSION QUESTIONS

1. Discuss what is meant by disparities in health care, both in terms of the relationship of disparities in health care and disparities in health, and in terms of what constitutes a disparity in health care.
2. Discuss the role that personal preference and medical appropriateness play in causing disparities in health care.
3. Discuss the role of patient provider communications in causing and also in alleviating disparities in health care.
4. Discuss the history of segregation in medical care of African American patients, physicians, and nurses and how this history might affect current racial and ethnic disparities in the delivery and receipt of medical care.
5. Discuss some of the efforts currently underway to address disparities in care, including the ACA.

6. Discuss what might be done in your community to address disparities in health care.

FURTHER READING

Aguirre-Molina, M., Molina, C. W., & Zambrana, R. E. (2001). *Health issues in the Latino community*. San Francisco: Jossey-Bass.

This book summarizes health issues among Latino populations in the United States. It includes causes of and statistics on health care disparities affecting Latinos.

Fadiman, A. (1997). *The spirit catches you and you fall down*. New York: Farrar, Straus & Giroux.

Well-written book by a journalist that describes the interactions between a Hmong family with an epileptic daughter and the health care system. This book illustrates how poor doctor-patient communication due to divergent cultural beliefs can result in poor health outcomes.

Gamble, V. N. (1995). *Making a place for ourselves: The black hospital movement*. New York: Oxford University Press.

This book examines the roles of black physicians and nurses, black community organizations, local and federal governments, and major health care organizations in the creation and demise of black hospitals from 1920 to 1945.

Institute of Medicine. (2003). *Unequal treatment: Confronting racial and ethnic disparities in health care*. Washington, DC: National Academies Press.

This report summarizes the literature on health care disparities and makes recommendations for addressing them. This is a landmark report issued by the National Research Council.

Institute of Medicine. (2012). *How far have we come in reducing health disparities? Progress since 2000: Workshop summary*. Washington, DC: National Academies Press.

Building upon previous IOM reports on health care quality and unequal treatment, the IOM held a workshop on April 8, 2010, that discussed progress toward addressing health disparities and focused on the success of various federal initiatives to reduce health disparities. This report summarizes the IOM workshop and explains the progress in the field since 2000.

LaVeist, T. A. (2005). *Minority populations and health: An introduction to health disparities in the United States*. San Francisco: Jossey-Bass.

This book describes racial and ethnic disparities in health and its causes, including disparities in health care. This book's main strength is that it includes a lot of descriptive statistics on minority health drawn from various sources.

Smith, D. B. (1999). *Health care divided: Race and healing a nation*. Ann Arbor: University of Michigan Press.

This book is a chronicle from 1920 to the present of racial segregation and discrimination in health care in the United States.

U.S. Department of Health and Human Services. (2012). *2011 National healthcare disparities report*. Rockville, MD: U.S. Department of Health and Human Services, Agency for Healthcare Research and Quality.

National report of health care disparities issued yearly by the Agency for Healthcare Research and Quality. This report uses indicators of quality of care drawn from various sources and reported by race and ethnicity.

White, A. A., III, & Chanoff, D. (2011). *Seeing patients: Unconscious bias in health care*. Boston: Harvard University Press.

This book uses the story of one of the authors, Gus White, as a way to talk about unconscious biases and their consequences in the medical profession and beyond. White is an orthopedic surgeon who grew up in Tennessee under Jim Crow, went to Ivy League schools, and was the only and first black medical student in most of those places. He was the first black chief resident at Yale, the only black surgeon in Vietnam, and the first black chief of service in a Harvard teaching hospital. The authors use an autobiographical approach, showing how Dr. White's life spans an enormous change in American race relations. They also show how great the disparities still are and make the case for "culturally competent" medical training.

Williams, R. A. (Ed.). (2011). *Healthcare disparities at the crossroads with the healthcare reform*. New York: Springer Science + Business Media.

This volume addresses how the Affordable Care Act addresses the problem of health care disparity and analyzes the benefits and shortcomings of the law as it relates to disparities.

REFERENCES

Adler, N. E., & Rehkopf, D. H. (2008). U.S. disparities in health: Descriptions, causes, and mechanisms. *Annual Review of Public Health, 29*, 235–252.

Akinbami, L. J., Moorman, J. E., & Liu, X, (2011). *Asthma prevalence, health care use, and mortality: United States, 2005–2009*. National health statistics reports; no 32. Hyattsville, MD: National Center for Health Statistics.

Alegría, M., Chatterji, P., Wells, K., Cao, Z., Chen, C. N., Takeuchi, D., . . . Meng, X. L. (2008). Disparity in depression treatment among racial and ethnic minority populations in the United States. *Psychiatric Services, 59*(11), 1264–1272.

American Public Health Association. (2009). *Public Health Services Act Title VII and VIII: Why are these programs so important?* Retrieved from http://www.apha.org /NR/rdonlyres/13E647B5-E51B-4A47-91A8-652EE973A2DB/0/TitleVIIand TitleVIII.pdf

Andrulis, D. P., Siddiqui, N. J., Purtle, J. P., & Duchon, L. (2010). *Patient Protection and Affordable Care Act of 2010: Advancing health equity for racially and ethnically diverse populations*. Washington, DC: Joint Center for Political and Economic Studies.

Austin, A. (2010). *Hidden disadvantage: Asian American unemployment and the Great Recession*. Washington, DC: Economic Policy Institute. Retrieved from http://http://www.epi.org/publication/hidden_disadvantage

Ayanian, J. Z., Cleary, P. D., Keogh, J. H., Noonan, S. J., David-Kasdan, J. A., & Epstein, A. M. (2004). Physicians' beliefs about racial differences in referral for renal transplantation. *American Journal of Kidney Diseases, 43*(2), 350–357.

Barnato, A. E., Lucas, F. L., Staiger, D., Wennberg, D. E., & Chandra, A. (2005). Hospital-level racial disparities in acute myocardial infarction treatment and outcomes. *Medical Care, 43*(4), 308–319.

Betancourt, J. R. (2006). Cultural competency: Providing quality care to diverse populations. *Consultant Pharmacist, 21*(12), 988–995.

Betancourt, J. R., Green, A. R., Carrillo, J. E., & Park, E. R. (2005). Cultural competence and health care disparities: Key perspectives and trends. *Health Affairs, 24*(2), 499–505.

Betancourt, J. R., & Maina, A. W. (2004). The Institute of Medicine Report "unequal treatment": Implications for academic health centers. *Mount Sinai Journal of Medicine, 71*, 314–321.

Bound, J., T. Waidmann, T., Schoenbaum, M., & Bingenheimer, J. B. (2003). The labor market consequences of race differences in health. *Milbank Quarterly, 81*(3), 441–473.

Braveman, P. (2006). Health disparities and health equity: Concepts and measurement. *Annual Review of Public Health, 27*(1), 167–194.

Bureau of Indian Affairs. (2012). Retrieved from http://www.bia.gov/FAQs/index.htm

Carter-Pokras, O., & Baquet, C. (2002). What is a "health disparity"? *Public Health Reports, 117*(5), 426–434.

Chen, M. S., & Hawks, B. l., (1995). A debunking of the myth of healthy Asian Americans and Pacific Islanders. *American Journal of Health Promotion, 9*(4), 261–268.

Correa-de-Araujo, R., Stevens, B., Moy, E., Nilasena, D., Chesley, F., & McDermott, K. (2006). Gender differences across racial and ethnic groups in the quality of care for acute myocardial infarction and heart failure associated with comorbidities. *Women's Health Issues, 16*(2), 44–55.

Dovidio, J. F., Kawakami, K., & Gaertner, S. L. (2002). Implicit and explicit prejudice and interracial interaction. *Journal of Personality and Social Psychology, 82*(1), 62–68.

Eggers, P. W. (1995). Racial differences in access to kidney transplantation. *Health Care Financial Review, 17*(2), 89–103.

Elston Lafata, J., Cole Johnson, C., Ben-Menachem, T., & Morlock, R. J. (2001). Sociodemographic differences in the receipt of colorectal cancer surveillance care following treatment with curative intent. *Medical Care, 39*(4), 361–372.

Epstein, A. M., & Ayanian, J. Z. (2001). Racial disparities in medical care. *New England Journal of Medicine, 344*(19), 1471–1473.

Families USA. (2010). Health reform: Help for American Indians. and Alaska Natives *(Issue Brief)*. Washington, DC: Author.

Farmer, S. A., Kirkpatrick, J. N., Heidenreich, P. A., Curtis, J. P., Wang, Y., & Groeneveld, P. W. (2009). Ethinic and racial disparities in cardiac resynchronization therapy. *Heart Rhythm, 6*(3), 325–331.

Fine, M. J., Ibrahim, S. A., & Thomas, S. B. (2005). The role of race and genetics in health disparities research. *American Journal of Public Health, 95*(12), 2125–2128.

Gamble, V. N. (1991). The Provident Hospital project: An experiment in race relations and medical education. *Bulletin of the History of Medicine, 65*(4), 457–475.

Gamble, V. N. (1997). Under the shadow of Tuskegee: African Americans and health care. *American Journal of Public Health, 87*(11), 1773–1778.

Geiger, H. J. (2003). Racial and ethnic disparities in diagnosis and treatment: A review of the evidence and a consideration of causes. In B. D. Smedley, A. Y. Stith, & A. R. Nelson (Eds.), *Unequal treatment: Confronting racial and ethnic disparities in health care.* Washington DC: National Academies Press.

Gilliland, F. D., Berhane, K., McConnell, R., Gauderman, W. J., Vora, H. Rappaport, E. B., . . . Peters, J. M. (2000). Maternal smoking during pregnancy, environmental tobacco smoke exposure and childhood lung function. *Thorax, 55*(4), 271–276.

Green, A., Peters-Lewis, A., Percac-Lima, S., Betancourt, J. R., Richter, J. M., Janairo, M. P., . . . Atlas, S. J. (2008). Barriers to screening colonoscopy for low-income Latino and white patients in an urban community health center. *Journal of General Internal Medicine, 23*(6), 834–840.

Greenwald, A. G., Poehlman, T. A., Uhlman, T. A., & Banaji, M. R. (2009). Understanding and using the Implicit Association Test: III. *Meta-analysis of predictive validity. Journal of Personality and Social Psychology, 97*(1), 17–41.

Haas, J. S., Weissman, J. S., Cleary, P. D., Goldberg, J., Gatsonis, C., Seage, G. R., III,, . . . Epstein, A. M. (1993). Discussion of preferences for life-sustaining care by persons with AIDS: Predictors of failure in patient-physician communication. *Archives of Internal Medicine, 153*(10), 1241–1248.

Hadley, J. (2003). Sicker and poorer: The consequences of being uninsured—a review of the research on the relationship between health insurance, medical care use, health, work, and income. *Medical Care Research Review, 60*(2 Suppl), 3S–112S.

Hargraves, J. L., & Hadley, J. (2003). The contribution of insurance coverage and community resources to reducing racial/ethnic disparities in access to care. *Health Services Research, 38*(3), 809–829.

Hicks, L. S., Fairchild, D. G., Horng, M. S., Orav, E. J., Bates, D. W., & Ayanian, J. Z. (2004). Determinants of JNC VI guideline adherence, intensity of drug therapy, and blood pressure control by race and ethnicity. *Hypertension, 44*(4), 429–434.

Holmes, J. S., Arispe, I. E., & Moy, E. (2005). Heart disease and prevention: Race and age differences in heart disease prevention, treatment, and mortality. *Medical Care, 43*(3 Suppl), I33–I41.

Hoyert, D. L., Xu, J. Q. (2012). *Deaths: Preliminary data for 2011.* National vital statistics reports; vol 61 no 6. Hyattsville, MD: National Center for Health Statistics.

Hsiao, W. C., Knight, A. G., Kappel, S., & Done, N. (2011). What other states can learn from Vermont's bold experiment: Embracing a single-payer health care financing system. *Health Affairs, 30*(7), 1232–1241.

Institute of Medicine (IOM). (2001). *Crossing the quality chasm.* Washington, DC: National Academies Press.

Institute of Medicine (IOM). (2003). *Unequal treatment: Confronting racial and ethnic disparities in health care.* Washington, DC: National Academies Press.

Johnson, R. L., Roter, D., Powe, N. R., & Cooper, L. A. (2004). Patient race/ethnicity and quality of patient–physician communication during medical visits. *American Journal of Public Health, 94*(12), 2084–2090.

Kaiser Commission on Medicaid and the Uninsured. (2004). *Health insurance coverage in America.* Washington, DC: Kaiser Family Foundation.

Kaiser Family Foundation. (2011). *Summary of the Affordable Care Act*. Menlo Park: Author.

Karter, A. J., Ferrara, A., Liu, J. Y., Moffet, H. H., Ackerson, L. M., & Selby, J. V. (2002). Ethnic disparities in diabetic complications in an insured population. *Journal of the American Medical Association, 287*(19), 2519–2527.

Katz, S. J., Lantz, P. M., Paredes, Y., Janz, N. K., Fagerlin, A., Liu, L., & Deapen, D. (2005). Breast cancer treatment experiences of Latinas in Los Angeles County. *American Journal of Public Health, 95*(12), 2225–2230.

King, W. D., Wong, M. D., Shapiro, M. F., Landon, B. E., & Cunningham, W. E. (2004). Does racial concordance between HIV-positive patients and their physicians affect the time to receipt of protease inhibitors? *Journal of General Internal Medicine, 19*(11), 1146–1153.

Kirk, J. K., Bell, R. A., Bertoni, A. G., Arcury, T. A., Quandt, S. A. & Goff, D. C., Jr., (2006). Ethnic disparities: Control of glycemia, blood pressure, and LDL cholesterol among U.S. adults with type 2 diabetes. *Annals of Pharmacotherapy, 39*(9), 1489–1501.

Kirk, J. K., Passmore, L. V., Bell, R. A., Narayan, K. M., D'Agostino, R. B., Jr., Arcury, T. A., & Quandt, S. A. (2008). Disparities in A1C levels between Hispanic and non-Hispanic white adults with diabetes: A meta-analysis. *Diabetes Care, 31*(2), 240–246.

Klonoff, E. A., & Landrine, H. (1999). Do blacks believe that HIV/AIDS is a government conspiracy against them? *Preventive Medicine, 28*(5), 451–457.

Lillie-Blanton, M., Stone, V. E., Snow Jones, A., Levi, J., Golub, E. T., Cohen, M. H., . . . Wilson, T. E. (2010). Association of race, substance abuse, and health insurance coverage with use of highly active antiretroviral therapy among HIV-infected women, 2005. *American Journal of Public Health, 100*(8), 1493–1499.

Lorig, K., & Holman, H. (2003). Self-management education: History, definition, outcomes, and mechanisms. *Annals of Behavioral Medicine, 26*(1), 1–7.

Luder, E., Melnik, T. A., & DiMaio, M. (1998). Association of being overweight with greater asthma symptoms in inner city black and Hispanic children. *Journal of Pediatrics, 132*(4), 699–703.

Mathur, A. K., Schaubel, D. E., Gong, Q., Guidinger, M. K., & Merion, R. M. (2010). Racial and ethnic disparities in access to liver transplantation. *Liver Transplantation, 16*(9), 1033–1040.

McWilliams, J. M., Meara, E., Zaslavsky, A. M., & Ayanian, J. Z. (2009). Differences in control of cardiovascular disease and diabetes by race, ethnicity, and education: U.S. trends from 1999 to 2006 and effects of Medicare coverage. *Annals of Internal Medicine, 150*(8), 505–515.

Mensah, G. A., Mokdad, A. H., Ford, E. S., Greenlund, K. J., & Croft, J. B. (2005). State of disparities in cardiovascular health in the United States. *Circulation, 111*(10), 1233–1241.

Monheit, A. C., & Vistnes, J. P. (2000). Race/ethnicity and health insurance status: 1987 and 1996. *Medical Care Research and Review, 57*(Suppl 1), 11–35.

Mugavero, M. J., Lin, H. Y., Allison, J. J., Giordano, T. P., Willig, J. H., Raper, J. L., . . . Saag, M. S. (2009). Racial disparities in HIV virologic failure: Do missed visits matter? *Journal of Acquired Immune Deficiency Syndrome, 50*(1), 100–108.

Murray-García, J. L., Selby, J. V., Schmittdiel, J., Grumbach, K., & Quesenberry, C. P., Jr., (2000). Racial and ethnic differences in a patient survey: Patients' values, ratings, and reports regarding physician primary care performance in a large health maintenance organization. *Medical Care, 38*(3), 300–310.

National Association of Community Health Centers. (2010). *Community health centers and health reform: Summary of key health center provisions.* Bethesda, MD: Author.

National Center for Education Statistics. (2012). *Higher education: Gaps in access and persistence study,* U.S. Department of Education, Washington, D.C.

National Commission on Asian American and Pacific Islander Research in Education. (2008). *Asian Americans and Pacific Islanders—Facts, not fiction: Setting the record straight.* Steinhardt Institute for Higher Education Policy, Asian/Pacific/American Institute at NYU, and College Board.

Ngo-Metzger, Q., Sorkin, D. H., & Phillips, R. S. (2009). Healthcare experiences of limited English-proficient Asian American patients: A cross-sectional mail survey. *Patient, 2*(2), 113–120.

Nosek, B. A., Smyth, F. L., Hansen, J. J., Devos, T., Lindner, N. M., Ranganath, K. A., . . . Greenwald, A. G. (2007). Pervasiveness and correlates of implicit attitudes and stereotypes. *European Review of Social Psychology, 18,* 36–88.

Office of Minority Health. (2012). *HHS action plan to reduce racial and ethnic health disparities,* U.S. Department of Health and Human Services, Washington D.C.

Office of Minority Health. (n.d.-b). *The National CLAS Standards.* Retrieved from http://minorityhealth.hhs.gov/templates/browse.aspx?lvl=2&lvlID=15

Okelo, S., Taylor, A. L., Wright, J. T., Jr., Gordon, N., Mohan, G., & Lesnefsky, E. (2001). Race and the decision to refer for coronary revascularization: The effect of physician awareness of patient ethnicity. *Journal of the American College of Cardiology, 38*(3), 698–704.

Ortega, A. N., & Alegría, M. (2002). Self-reliance, mental health need, and the use of mental healthcare among island Puerto Ricans. *Mental Health Services Research, 4*(3), 131–140.

Ortega, A. N., & Alegría, M. (2005). Denial and its association with mental health care use: A study of island Puerto Ricans. *Journal of Behavioral Health Services Research, 32*(3), 320–331.

Ortega, A. N., & Calderon, J. G. (2000). Pediatric asthma among minority populations. *Current Opinion in Pediatrics, 12*(6), 579–583.

Ortman, J. M., & Guarneri, C.E. (2009). *United States population projections: 2000 to 2050.* Washington DC: U.S. Census Bureau.

Palacio, H., Kahn, J. G., Richards, T. A., & Morin, S. F. (2002). Effect of race and/or ethnicity in use of antiretrovirals and prophylaxis for opportunistic infection: A review of the literature. *Public Health Reports, 117*(3), 233–232.

Peek, M. E., Cargill, A., & Huang, E. S. (2007). Diabetes health disparities: a systematic review of health care interventions. *Medical Care Research and Review, 64*(5 Suppl), 101S–156S.

Pescosolido, B. A., Wright, E. R., Alegría, M., & Vera, M. (1998). Social networks and patterns of use among the poor with mental health problems in Puerto Rico. *Medical Care, 36*(7), 1057–1072.

Ponce, N. A., Tseng, W., Ong, P., Shek, Y. L., Ortiz, S., & Gatchell, M. (2009). *The state of Asian American, Native Hawaiian and Pacific Islander health in California report.* Los Angeles: UCLA Center for Health Policy Research.

Roetzheim, R. G., Pal, N., Gonzalez, E. C., Ferrante, J. M., Van Durme, D. J., & Krischer, J. P. (2000). *American Journal of Public Health, 90*(11), 1746–1754.

Rothenberg, B. M., Pearson, T., Zwanziger, J., & Mukamel, D. (2004). Explaining disparities in access to high-quality cardiac surgeons. *Annals of Thoracic Surgery, 78*(1), 18–24.

Sabin, J., Nosek, B. A., Greenwald, A., & Rivara, F. P. (2009). Physicians' implicit and explicit attitudes about race by MD race, ethnicity, and gender. *Journal of Health Care for the Poor and Underserved, 20*(3), 896–913.

Saha, S., Komaromy, M., Koepsell, T. D., & Bindman, A. B. (1999). Patient-physician racial concordance and the perceived quality and use of health care. *Archives of Internal Medicine, 159*(9), 997–1004.

Schectman, J. M., Nadkarni, M. M., & Voss, J. D. (2002). The association between diabetes metabolic control and drug adherence in an indigent population. *Diabetes Care, 25*(6), 1015–1021.

Scheppers, E., van Dongen, E., Dekker, J., Geertzen, J., & Dekker, J. (2006). Potential barriers to the use of health services among ethnic minorities: A review. *Family Practice, 23*(3), 325–348.

Schulman, K. A., Berlin, J. A., Harless, W., Kerner, J. F., Sistrunk, S., Gersh, B. J., . . . Escarce, J. J. (1999). The effect of race and sex on physicians' recommendations for cardiac catheterization. *New England Journal of Medicine, 340*(8), 618–626.

Shavers, V. L., & Brown, M. L. (2002). Racial and ethnic disparities in the receipt of cancer treatment. *Journal of the National Cancer Institute, 94*(5), 334–357.

Sheppard, V. B., Zambrana, R. E., & O'Malley, A. S. (2004). Providing health care to low-income women: A matter of trust. *Family Practice, 21*(5), 484–491.

Shi, L., & Stevens, G. D. (2005). Disparities in access to care and satisfaction among U.S. children: The roles of race/ethnicity and poverty status. *Public Health Reports, 120*(4), 431–441.

Smith, M. B. (1999). Primary care: Choices and opportunities for racial/ethnic minority populations in the USA and UK—a comparative analysis. *Ethnicity and Health, 4*(3), 165–188.

Sonel, A. F., Good, C. B., Mulgund, J., Roe, M. T., Gibler, W. B., Smith, S. C., Jr., . . . Peterson, E. D. (2005). Racial variations in treatment and outcomes of black and white patients with high-risk non-ST-elevation acute coronary syndromes: Insights from CRUSADE (Can Rapid Risk Stratification of Unstable Angina Patients Suppress Adverse Outcomes with Early Implementation of the ACC/AHA Guidelines?). *Circulation, 111*(10), 1225–1232.

Sonik, A., Stein-Wexler, R., Rogers, K. K., Coulter, K. P., & Wootton-Gorges, S. L. (2010). Follow-up skeletal surveys for suspected non-accidental trauma: Can a more limited survey be performed without compromising diagnostic information? *Child Abuse & Neglect, 34*(10), 804–806. doi: http://dx.doi.org/10.1016/j.chiabu.2010.03.002

Stanley, D. A., Sokol-Hessner, P., Banaji, M. R., & Phelps, E. A. (2011). Implicit race attitudes predict trustworthiness judgments and economic trust decisions. *Proceedings of the National Academy of Sciences of the USA, 108*(19), 7710–7715.

Tai-Seale, M., Freund, D., & LoSasso, A. (2001). Racial disparities in service use among Medicaid beneficiaries after mandatory enrollment in managed care: A difference-in-differences approach. *Inquiry, 38*(1), 49–59.

Urban Indian Health Institute. (2004). *The health status of urban American Indians and Alaska Natives*. Retrieved from http://www.uihi.org/wp-content/uploads/2007/07/2004healthstatusreport.pdf

U.S. Census Bureau. (2009). *2009 National population projections*. Washington, DC: Author.

U.S. Commission on Civil Rights. (2004). Evaluating the Native American Health Care System, Washington D.C. Retrieved from: http://www.usccr.gov/pubs/nahealth/nabroken.pdf

U.S. Department of Health and Human Services. (2000). *Healthy People 2010: What are its goals?* Retrieved from http://www.healthypeople.gov/2010/About/goals.htm

U.S. Department of Health and Human Services. (2010). *2010 National healthcare disparities report*. Rockville, MD: Agency for Healthcare Research and Quality.

U.S. Department of Health and Human Services. (n.d.). *Key facts about the National Health Service Corps*. http://www.hhs.gov/recovery/programs/nhsc/nhscfactsheet.html

U.S. Surgeon General. (2001). *Mental health: Culture, race, and ethnicity*. Rockville, MD: Substance Abuse and Mental Health Services Administration.

Vargas Bustamante, A., & Chen, J. (2011). Physicians cite hurdles ranging from lack of coverage to poor communication in providing high-quality care to Latinos. *Health Affairs (Millwood), 30*(10), 1921–1929.

Vargas Bustamante, A., & Chen, J. (2012). Health expenditure dynamics and years of U.S. residence: Analyzing spending disparities among Latinos by citizenship/nativity status. *Health Services Research, 47*(2), 794–818.

Waidmann, T. A., & Rajan, S. (2000). Race and ethnic disparities in health care access and utilization: An examination of state variation. *Medical Care Research and Review, 57*(Suppl 1), 55–84.

Ward, E., Jemal, A., Cokkinides, V., Singh, G., Cardinez, C., Ghafoor, A., & Thun, M. (2004). Cancer disparities by race/ethnicity and socioeconomic status. *CA: A Cancer Journal for Clinicians, 54*(2), 78–93.

Washington, A. E., & Lipstein, S. H. (2011). The Patient-Centered Outcomes Research Institute: Promoting better information, decisions, and health. *New England Journal of Medicine, 365*(15), e31.

Wolff, M., Bates, T., Beck, B., Young, S., Ahmed, S. M., & Maurana, C. (2003). Cancer prevention in underserved African American communities: Barriers and effective strategies—a review of the literature. *Wisconsin Medical Journal, 102*(5), 36–40.

Zuvekas, S. H., & Taliaferro, G. S. (2003). Pathways to access: Health insurance, the health care delivery system, and racial/ethnic disparities, 1996–1999. *Health Affairs (Millwood), 22*(2), 139–153.

CHAPTER FIVE

MULTILEVEL SOCIAL DETERMINANTS OF HEALTH

Ninez A. Ponce
Michelle Ko

Learning Objectives

- Identify social determinants of health at the individual level and community level
- Understand the contribution of social determinants on population health outcomes and health inequities
- Elucidate the linkage and interactions of individual-level and community-level social determinants with the health system
- Formulate ways that information on the multiple levels of social determinants of health can guide policy action

In the United States, there are nearly three decades worth of evidence implicating social factors in the production of health and health inequities. Examining forty-seven studies in the United States from 1980 to 2007, the death toll attributed to specific social factors has been recently quantified by Galea and colleagues as comparable to the number of deaths caused by acute myocardial infarction, cerebrovascular disease, or lung cancer—the leading causes of death in the United States today (Galea, Tracy, Hoggatt, Dimaggio, & Karpati, 2011). This quantification supports a call for action to consider the *social determinants of health* (SDOH) in tandem with medical factors in formulating public policies and public health programs in the United States; globally, this has been steadfastly championed by the World Health Organization (WHO) since the establishment of the Commission on Social Determinants of Health (CSDH) in March 2005 (CSDH, 2008).

Beyond medical care, the social, economic, political, cultural, and environmental contexts contribute to population health. Over a decade ago, in their review article on the social environment and health, Yen and Syme (1999) provided optimism (though guarded) in the possible explanatory power of social context on health. At that time, they found that a majority of studies showed a significant association between community-level socioeconomic status (SES) with mortality risk and health behaviors, but a weaker association with morbidity. Most of the studies reviewed by Yen and Syme examined all causes of mortality (seventeen studies), and cardiovascular mortality (four studies). Galea and his colleagues put numbers with the associations: "approximately 245,000 deaths in the United States in 2000 were attributable to low education, 176,000 to racial segregation, 162,000 to low social support, 133,000 to individual-level poverty, 119,000 to income inequality, and 39,000 to area-level poverty" (Galea et al., 2011). Building on these findings, some of the more recent literature examines the relationship, or interaction, that each individual has with his or her environment that may mitigate these structural inequities (Ahnquist, Wamala, & Lindstrom, 2012; Poortinga, 2006, 2012; Prentice, 2006). Thus, a social determinants approach also advances the notions of "social capital" and "social cohesion" (Kawachi, Kennedy, Lochner, & Prothrow-Stith, 1997; Macinko & Starfield, 2001; Meijer, Rohl, Bloomfield, & Grittner, 2012).

As articulated by the WHO CSDH, the most consequential social determinants of health generate divisions, chasms, and stratifications in social position that advantage some individuals in income, social status, political power, favorable environmental exposures and assets in their neighborhoods, but disadvantage others. Moreover, these cumulative disadvantages may prevail over generations, and are therefore intractable without explicit policy solutions. All told, structural inequities may undermine the productivity of medical care inputs, but are also implicated in directly influencing the allocation of who gets quality health care and who does not.

In this chapter, we discuss the mechanisms of how social determinants affect health and health inequities with a specific application to the U.S. health system. The perspective of *multilevel social determinants of health* acknowledges that individual health and health behaviors occur within a larger social context. Chapter Four's discussion of disparities in health enumerated several individual-level social determinants, notably race or ethnicity, income, and education, that significantly predict population differences in mortality and self-rated health. Chapter Four also discussed medical care factors beyond need and patient preferences that lead to unequal access and unequal treatment. Here, we focus on the role of the area-level or "upstream" social determinants of health and health care outcomes, above and beyond the influences of individual and health care system characteristics. Notwithstanding the individual's and health system's role in producing good health, our goals are to demonstrate that socially produced health inequities are a crucial component of discussions on U.S. health system change, and to rouse policy action addressing the structural inequities that shape the allocation of U.S. health resources and that ultimately affect the level and distribution of health in the U.S. population.

Policy Frameworks for Social Determinants of Health

We draw on two theoretical and conceptual frameworks to elucidate why and how social determinants affect population health: (1) the WHO CSDH conceptual framework on the social determinants of health and (2) the Robert Wood Johnson Foundation Commission to Build a Healthier America. Both frameworks hold that social determinants operate at a number of levels—from individuals to households and communities, and to multiple levels of political jurisdictions—and underscore the need for shared governance by individuals and different policy actors and sectors beyond the health care delivery system.

WHO CSDH Conceptual Framework

The WHO CSDH conceptual framework on SDOH (Figure 5.1), presented by Solar and Irwin in 2007 and updated in 2010, offers an organizing lens that differentiates "structural determinants" from "the intermediary determinants of health."

The WHO's conceptual framework categorizes structural determinants of health inequities as

1. Governance: participation and accountability of policy actors in shaping health and health inequities

2. Macroeconomic policies: labor market, tax policies, and regulation of markets that may have consequences in generating inequities in allocation of socioeconomic and political resources and opportunities

3 & 4. Social and public policies that directly govern the distribution of resources and opportunities in health, education, housing, employment, and social welfare

5. Culture and societal values that reflect both preferences in how goods and services should be allocated and how much a society prioritizes good health and well-being (CSDH, 2011)

In turn, the socioeconomic and political context create the social processes—income inequality, residential segregation, and varying potencies of social capital—that we see in a society, thereby leading to inequities in socioeconomic class and social position and in differential exposures to positive community-level assets and opportunities. How these vulnerabilities and differential exposures affect health and well-being are conceptually explained in the box in Figure 5.1 labeled "intermediary determinants

FIGURE 5.1. WHO CSDH CONCEPTUAL FRAMEWORK

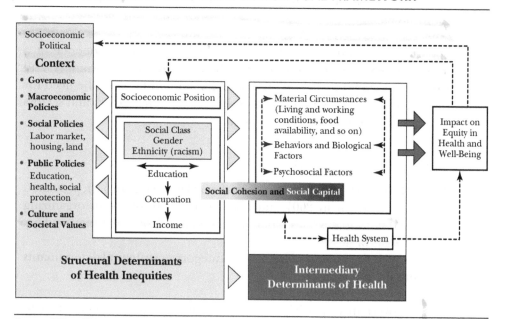

Source: CSDH, 2011.

of health." We note that in this box the health system simultaneously determines and is also determined by an individual's material circumstances, behaviors, biological factors, and psychosocial factors.

Much of the discussion of WHO's CSDH has focused on advancing the implementation of an SDOH approach through good governance and policies outside the health care system. Although the health system is identified as an intermediary determinant, the structural determinants are the centerpiece of the discussions, since the pathway of structural inequities explain inequities in health much more than inequities in health care. We posit that this perspective manifests for two reasons. First, globally, among lower-income nations, investing in social inputs can bring bigger returns than health system factors to overall population well-being (including health). Second, among wealthier nations, with the exception of the United States prior to the Affordable Care Act (ACA), health insurance coverage rates are much higher and presumed to minimize inequities associated with access to health care. For the United States, where the health sector looms large—health care spending in fiscal year 2012 was 17 percent of GNP—a framework that incorporates how social determinants influence health care is needed.

The Robert Wood Johnson Foundation Commission to Build a Healthier America

The Robert Wood Johnson Foundation (RWJF) Commission to Build a Healthier America (Braveman, Egerter, & Williams, 2011) expands upon the model developed by the WHO by explicitly recognizing that medical care is also inherently embedded in a larger social context (Figure 5.2). In other words, the way in which health care is distributed and the quality of care that is delivered do not occur independently of community context, but are also affected by these conditions. For example, a community's socioeconomic status influences an individual's access to resources such as education and employment opportunities, as well as the number of health care providers in the area. In this framework, social determinants of health also operate through the effects on the health care system.

Broadly, the social factors in Figure 5.2 are depicted as all nonmedical care and personal behavior factors. But, akin to the WHO nomenclature of "structural determinants," the outer arch in Figure 5.2 represents this upstream concept of economic and social opportunities and resources that may directly affect health but may also operate via differential effects on living and working conditions, which in turn could shape the health-related

FIGURE 5.2. RWJ COMMISSION TO BUILD A HEALTHIER AMERICA FRAMEWORK

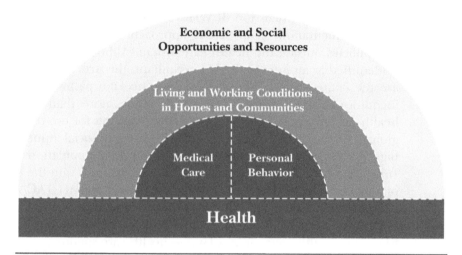

Source: Robert Wood Johnson Foundation (RWJF), 2008. Copyright 2008 Robert Wood Johnson Foundation/Overcoming Obstacles to Health.

choices and behaviors of individuals that then influence their health (Braveman et al., 2011). Social gradients in income, education, and living and working conditions in homes and communities are linked with the health divide in the United States. For example, living a few miles apart in the Washington, DC, area separates life expectancy by up to twenty years; and on average a college degree extends life expectancy by five years compared to not completing high school (RWJF, 2010). As another example, in Figure 5.3 we see that within racial and ethnic groups, lower income is associated with poorer health (RWJF, 2008; RWJF, 2010).

These gradients in education, income, race, and ethnicity signal that social determinants beyond medical care are linked to health by way of a financial enabler or as a marker of socioeconomic position and agency. For example, education is a key social indicator, and low education was the top indicator that Galea and colleagues attributed to higher mortality rates (Galea et al., 2011). Education is a financial enabler, as education leads to gains in human capital and thus employment, increased earnings capacity, and a higher likelihood of access to employment-based insurance. Lower educational attainment tends to limit these enabling factors to accessing

FIGURE 5.3. POOR OR FAIR HEALTH BY FAMILY INCOME AND RACE OR ETHNICITY

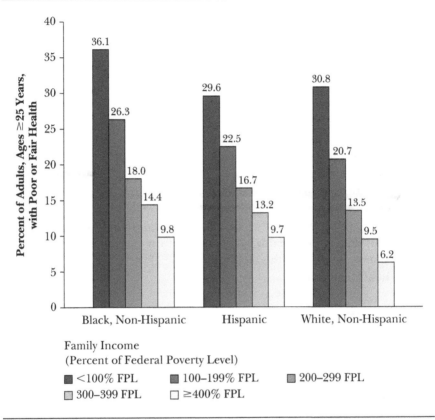

Family Income
(Percent of Federal Poverty Level)

■ <100% FPL   ■ 100–199% FPL   ▨ 200–299 FPL
▨ 300–399 FPL   ▢ ≥400% FPL

Source: Robert Wood Johnson Foundation (RWJF), 2008. Copyright 2008 Robert Wood Johnson Foundation/Overcoming Obstacles to Health.

health care. Lower educational attainment, however, may also abrade health in a different way—through perceived lower social status and self-perceived lack of control or through exposure to degrading attitudes and treatment by others with more years of schooling.

Yet the precise contribution of these SDOH linkages to health is still not clearly understood for several reasons:

1. The sources of SDOH occur over time and space, so that tracking experiences and exposures over a lifetime across different places where the individual lives and works presents a major data challenge; in many

cases, the source of disparities have been constructed from social, economic, and political inequities faced by past generations

2. Some factors are difficult to observe—such as how well an individual copes with social stressors or how well an individual harnesses assets like safe walkable public spaces in his or her neighborhood—that modify the extent to which SDOH affects health

3. Importantly, from a health services perspective, mediating factors such as the availability and quality of health care may link the relationship between SDOH and health, which needs to be better understood to inform the formulation of health policies

Although both the WHO CSDH and RWJF frameworks include the health system (WHO) or medical care (RWJF), their focus is on how structural inequities directly affect health via its interaction with individual characteristics and health behaviors. We submit an alternative approach by elaborating on how structural determinants affect the organization and delivery of health services based on our assumption that the health system mediates the linkage of social determinants with health and health inequities.

Mechanisms by Which Social Context Affects Health Care

We focus on five contextual-level social determinants that have been conceptualized as generating the social processes that lead to health and health inequities: area-based income, income inequality, racial or ethnic composition, residential segregation, and social capital. All are measured at an area or community level, and all have been conceptualized as directly affecting health and to a lesser extent as affecting health via the organization, distribution, and delivery of health services.

Area-Based Income

The income level of a community can affect health services through multiple pathways. First, higher-income areas attract a greater supply of health care providers, offering a higher quality of care, thus improving access to care, even for more disadvantaged populations. Second, higher-income areas with lower unemployment rates may also offer more options for health insurance. Third, areas with greater household incomes may be able to better support safety net services and other types of policies that can alleviate disparities in care. Alternatively, high-poverty areas can qualify for medically underserved area or population designation and be eligible for support to establish federally qualified health centers (Ko & Ponce, 2012). Low-income children in metropolitan areas with higher household incomes have higher odds of seeing a physician; the same association is found for low-income adults in areas with lower unemployment rates, above and beyond individual characteristics (Andersen et al., 2002).

Income Inequality

In addition to overall area-level income, the distribution of income and wealth within an area can also influence the delivery of health services. *Income inequality*, typically measured as the Gini index, where 0 indicates the most equal income distribution and 1 the most unequal, is at an all-time high in the United States and is one of the highest among similar economies (DeBacker, Heim, Panousi, Ramnath, & Vidangos, 2013; OECD, 2011). Although evidence from other countries is mixed on whether or not the gap between the rich and poor erodes the health of populations (Deaton & Lubotsky, 2009; Kahn, Wise, Kennedy, & Kawachi, 2000; McGrail, van Doorslaer, Ross, & Sanmartin, 2009; Subramanian & Kawachi, 2004; Wilkinson & Pickett, 2006), the findings on income inequality's negative effect on health, typically measured as mortality or as self-rated health, is most robust for the United States. And among studies that do find an effect between income inequality and health, across all nations income inequality appears to be most detrimental to the poor (Diez-Roux, Link, & Northridge, 2000; Subramanian & Kawachi, 2003; Wagstaff & van Doorslaer, 2000).

We know less as to whether income inequality affects equity in health care delivery and whether a reformed U.S. health system with near-universal access may attenuate the effects of area-based social disparities. Indeed, a study comparing pre-ACA United States and Canada suggests that the null finding on income inequality on health in Canada may be due to Canada's lower income inequality and universal coverage (Ross et al., 2000). A few studies to date have implicated high income-related inequalities as impinging primary care access (Chen & Escare, 2004; Macinko, Shi, Starfield, & Wulu, 2003).

In contrast, areas with high income inequality appear to favor the use and diffusion of expensive specialty care (van Doorslaer, Koolman, & Jones, 2004). This may be because high income inequality areas may attract specialists who are more likely to be located near academic centers. This framework embraces a market forces perspective, or a neomaterialist view, advanced by Lynch and others that income inequality promotes availability of health services, spurred by the demands of the wealthy (Lynch, 2000). The competing psychosocial view, advanced by Wilkinson and Pickett (Wilkinson & Pickett, 2006), postulates a more patient-centered and patient-provider interaction lens—that is, in our stylistic interpretation, income inequality stigmatizes patients, lessens patient agency to seek resources or information to better navigate health services and to make the best choices to improve their quality of their care. In high inequality areas, clinicians may also differentially value patients owing to the provider's perceived hierarchies by class, gender, and race in the places where they practice. Access to health services would be higher in more egalitarian, socially cohesive areas, as patients are not stigmatized and clinicians may not be discriminating based on the patient's socioeconomic position. Supporting this view, Clarkwest found that higher state-level income inequality was associated with poorer health care quality (average adherence rate for twenty-two Center for Medicare and Medicaid Services [CMS] quality-of-care measures) and also found that health care quality does indeed mediate the negative association between the Gini index and life expectancy (Clarkwest, 2008). However, another study in the United States found that income inequality is only weakly associated with maldistribution of doctors and not associated with hospital bed distribution (Horev, Pesis-Katz, & Mukamel, 2004). In sum, there is still no clear understanding of the direction of income inequality's effect on health. In health care, the evidence base on income inequality's effect on health care is still new, but the direction appears to follow a plausible pattern in which income inequality is negatively associated with primary care and safety net services, but positively associated with more expensive specialty services.

Racial and Ethnic Minority Composition

Even after controlling for socioeconomic factors, there continue to be persistent disparities in care based on community, racial, and ethnic composition. Areas with a higher percentage of black and Hispanic residents have fewer physicians per capita (Komaromy et al., 1996). Emergency departments and trauma centers are more likely to close in communities with a higher concentration of black residents, irrespective of area-level income (Hsia & Shen, 2011; Shen, Hsia, & Kuzma, 2009). Some studies have found hospitals are more likely to close in black neighborhoods, whereas others have found no association. Whereas studies of individual-level health racial and ethnic disparities have focused on mechanisms such as experiences of discrimination, cultural competency, and race concordance, studies of area-level disparities have not delineated a specific mechanism for community-level racial and ethnic-based inequities. More recent literature has argued that compositional measures at larger areal units (counties and states) may not capture the effects of community context because it is the distribution of resources within an area, not the average level, that drives disparities in access to care (Gaskin, Dinwiddie, Chan, & McCleary, 2011). Residential segregation refers to "the degree to which two or more groups live separately from one another in different parts of the urban environment" (Massey & Denton, 1989). Isolation of disadvantaged groups into concentrated neighborhoods is associated with poorer education systems, employment opportunities, access to transportation, and public safety (Wilson, 1987).

Racial and Ethnic Residential Segregation

Racial *residential segregation* may reflect cultural preferences to live in ethnic enclaves, or a constraint based on discrimination that perpetuates social divisions and blocked opportunities for racial and ethnic minorities. Segregated low-income and minority communities may experience greater difficulty in attracting health care providers and have fewer neighborhood resources such as nonprofit and governmental organizations that promote health and access care (White, Haas, & Williams, 2012). Prior research has shown that residential segregation is associated with fewer physician visits, higher odds of primary care physician shortage, fewer ambulatory surgical facilities, lower supply of general surgeons and colorectal subspecialists, lower odds of receipt of appropriate breast cancer care, and delayed time to renal transplantation (Gaskin, Dinwiddie, Chan, & McCleary, 2012; Gaskin, Price, Brandon, & LaVeist, 2009; Haas et al., 2008; Hayanga et al., 2009; Rodriguez et al., 2007). Furthermore, studies of integrated communities have found either a reduction or elimination of disparities in access to care for black residents (Gaskin et al., 2009; LaVeist, Pollack, Thorpe, Fesahazion, & Gaskin, 2011; Skinner, Weinstein, Sporer, & Wennberg, 2003).

However, the majority of earlier work focused on black racial residential segregation. New studies have identified differences for Hispanics and Asian residential segregation, showing that residents of these communities have lower odds of experiencing physician shortage (Gaskin et al., 2012). As seen with some health outcomes, the formation of Hispanic and Asian "ethnic enclaves" may offer benefits of social networks, with improved access to information and providers.

Racial residential segregation is associated with worse health outcomes, including poorer birth outcomes, higher infant mortality, lower self-rated health, lower health-related quality of life, higher mortality, higher allostatic load, and higher rates of obesity (Bellatorre, Finch, Phuong Do, Bird, & Beck, 2011; Chang, 2006; Corral et al., 2012; Hao et al., 2011; LaVeist, Gaskin, & Trujillo, 2011). The evidence is mixed or not explicitly tested whether health services mediate the relationship of racial residential segregation with health outcomes.

Social Capital

Community social capital refers to "all features of social life—networks, norms, and trust—that enable participants to act together more effectively to pursue shared objectives" (Putnam, 1993). A number of studies have found that greater community social capital at many levels—nation, state, and neighborhood—is associated with improved health outcomes, including self-rated health, health-related quality of life, and lower rates of all-cause and disease-specific mortality (Elgar et al., 2011; Engström, Mattsson, Järleborg, & Hallqvist, 2008; Islam et al., 2006; Kawachi et al., 1997; Kim, Subramanian, & Kawachi, 2006; Mansyur, Amick, Harrist, & Franzini, 2008; Poortinga, 2006).

Social capital has the potential to improve health outcomes via multiple pathways. First, social norms and information flows may encourage positive health behaviors. For example, community social capital is associated with increased consumption of fruits and vegetables, exercise, and reduced cigarette consumption and binge drinking (Brown, Scheffler, Seo, & Reed, 2006; Carpiano, 2007). Second, social networks can increase available psychosocial support. Lower-income residents of urban areas with higher social capital report lower levels of psychological distress, controlling for individual characteristics (Scheffler, Brown, & Rice, 2007). Lastly, social capital may facilitate access to a variety of resources, including health services.

Community social capital is thought to facilitate access to care, both through information flows and improved relationships between residents and health care providers. Area-level social capital is associated with increased trust in health care providers, and neighborhood cohesion is associated with a higher likelihood of children's access to a patient-centered medical home (Ahern, 2003; Aysola, Orav, & Ayanian, 2011). However, the evidence for the effects of community social capital on measures of access to care has been mixed. Some studies have shown that community-level social capital was associated with fewer reported problems in access to care, greater odds of having a regular source of care, and increased use of mental health services (Drukker, Driessen, Krabbendam, & van Os, 2004; Greenberg & Rosenheck, 2003; Hendryx, Ahern, Lovrich, & McCurdy, 2002; Lee, Chen, & Weiner, 2004; Prentice, 2006). Other studies have found that community social capital is associated with fewer visits to a general practitioner and a higher number of preventable hospitalizations (Derose, 2008; Laporte, Nauenberg, & Shen, 2008). Social capital was found to have mixed associations with provision of community services on the part of private hospitals (Lee et al., 2004). The lack of consistent findings on the relationships between community social capital and health services is likely related to different measures used across studies, the need for further research on different types of social capital, and a greater understanding of how community factors interacts with individual characteristics (Derose & Varda, 2009).

At worst, social capital could worsen inequities in health. One study has found that the associations between community social capital and self-rated health are weakened for black individuals; another has shown that the benefits of social capital accrue primarily to those who already have a high level of individual social trust (Kim et al., 2006; Poortinga, 2006).

Future Directions

To advance understanding of the impact of social context on health and health care, parallel advances in available data will be required. Ideally, longitudinal survey data spanning at least a generation and across several diverse geographic, socioeconomic, and racial and ethnic communities in the United States are needed to identify the contribution of social determinants on health and investigate the mediating effects of the U.S. health care system. Moreover, promoting linkage of individual-level data with administrative data on the supply and location of providers, community health centers and hospitals, and other data systems on U.S. health care would facilitate multilevel examinations of how social determinants interact with the health system. The impact of contextual-level social determinants, to be meaningfully measured, may require more granular definitions of communities than counties, cities, and zip codes—areas used in many of the studies reviewed. Data sources thus need to be adequately geocoded and provide a sufficient sample to conduct multilevel analysis.

Despite the data challenges, the research that informs policy on SDOH vis-à-vis the U.S. health system change is promising. More researchers are delving into conceptual frameworks and empirical studies explicitly examining structural determinants of both health and health care. In the context of the ACA, there is an implicit assumption that as coverage barriers are alleviated, the income-based inequities will diminish. But as resources are directed to spread coverage for nearly all the U.S. population, more expensive health services may be rationed on the basis of social determinants. A key question to be answered is whether income inequality and residential segregation matter more or less in accessing expensive care, tests, and procedures, especially for the poorest and for vulnerable racial and ethnic minorities. Identifying which social determinants matter more or less on specific health and health care inequities post-ACA will be instructive in formulating macroeconomic and social policies in health and other sectors to fulfill the policy goals of the ACA.

SUMMARY

Health is a product of multiple levels of social factors, and one of the intermediary factors is medical care. Because U.S. society is inherently unequal, contextual social determinants lead to structural inequities in health and in health care. Many agree globally and in the United States that the most consequential social determinants of health are the ones that generate stratifications in social position that advantage some individuals in income, social status, political power, and favorable environmental exposures and assets in their communities, but disadvantage others. For this reason, we have focused on the effects of area-based income, income inequality, racial and ethnic composition, and residential segregation on health care to determine whether these social processes that lead to structural inequities undermine the productivity or distribution of medical care and ultimately erode population health.

Our review suggests that several of these factors—income, income inequality, racial and ethnic composition, and residential segregation— likewise produce inequities in health care and may ultimately undermine population health. Income inequality appears to have a differential effect by type of health services—where a more egalitarian space is associated with more primary care and safety net services, but fewer specialty services. Residential segregation, on the other hand, is resoundingly negatively associated with a host of health services: physician visits, primary care physician supply, ambulatory surgical facilities, and supply of general surgeons and colorectal subspecialists. Further, we examined whether a community's social capital might mitigate the potential health penalties of these structural inequities, but we have found that this may not be the case. Social capital has the potential to facilitate access to care, by building connections between disadvantaged populations and health care resources; however, it may also serve to augment the advantages more privileged groups already possess. Thus, as Pearce and Davey Smith entreat, since social factors determine which groups have potent social capital and which groups have not, shifting the policy space from interventions that form and develop community-level social capital to government-level macroeconomic and social policies that reduce structural inequities may be more appropriate (Pearce & Davey Smith, 2003). In sum, social processes do generate inequities in health care and can be addressed by policies put forth by the WHO CSDH framework. The evidence favorably supports the health care returns to labor market and tax policies that curtail rising income inequality and social and public policies that equalize opportunities in education, housing, employment, and social welfare to address both racial or ethnic residential segregation and income inequality.

KEY TERMS

Area-based income An ecological measure depicting the income level of a geographically defined community, for example, a census tract, a city, or a county. This measure could be the median household income in an area or the percent of residents in an area with incomes below poverty. This is a measure of a group of individuals living in an area, not an individual-level measure. *Adults living in high-income cities compared to low-income cities are more likely to have seen a physician in the past year.*

Community social capital The resources derived from social relationships and networks within a community. *Elderly residents of communities with greater social capital are thought to experience better outcomes following natural disasters, because interconnected social networks may facilitate care and assistance of vulnerable members.*

Income inequality The degree to which income is unevenly distributed within an area. *The increasing concentration of income in the* *top 1 percent of the U.S. population in the past three decades reflects growing income inequality.*

Multilevel social determinants of health Refers to the concept that social determinants at multiple "levels"—such as the levels of the individual, neighborhood, community, health care system, state, and so on—may affect health. Low-income individuals may face barriers to care due to a lack of health insurance; residents of low-income communities may further be disadvantaged by a shortage of health care providers.

Racial and ethnic minority composition An ecological measure depicting the racial or ethnic makeup of a geographically defined community, for example, a census tract, a city, or a county. For example, this measure could be the percent of non-Hispanic whites in an area. This is a measure of a group of individuals living in an area, and not an individual-level measure. *Areas with a higher percentage of black and Hispanic residents have fewer physicians per capita.*

Residential segregation The degree to which various subpopulations, often defined by race, ethnicity, and/or socioeconomic status, live separately from one another. *The formation of urban Chinatown neighborhoods contributes to residential segregation of ethnic Chinese from other groups in urban areas.*

Social determinants of health The WHO defines social determinants of health as "the circumstances in which people are born, grow up, live, work, and age, as well as the systems put in place to deal with illness." These are shaped by the social, economic, political, cultural, and environmental factors that contribute to population health. *A considerable number of deaths in the United States are attributable to social determinants of health.*

DISCUSSION QUESTIONS

1. Why doesn't medical care alone explain the dramatic differences in the health of the U.S. population?
2. How should we intervene to improve health and reduce health inequities? At which levels?
3. What are the two frameworks presented in this chapter, and how have they advanced our understanding of the structural constructs of social determinants of health?

4. What social processes or mechanisms link the structural or upstream social determinants to differences in health care and ultimately the health of the U.S. population?
5. Reflect on whether the body of evidence shows that there are likely health care returns to public policies that directly address social determinants of health, for example, efforts to curtail the rising income inequality and policies that equalize the opportunities in education, housing, employment, and social welfare.

FURTHER READING

Braveman, P., Egerter, S., & Williams, D. R. (2011). The social determinants of health: Coming of age. *Annual Review of Public Health, 32*(1), 381–398. Additional information available at the Robert Wood Johnson Foundation Commission to Build a Healthier America: http://rwjf.org/en/topics/search-topics/S/social-determinants-of-health.html

Commission on Social Determinants of Health (CSDH). (2011). *Closing the gap: Policy into practice on social determinants of health.* Final report of the World Conference on Social Determinants of Health. Rio de Janeiro: World Health Organization. Additional information on the WHO implementation, tools, and resources: http://www.who.int/social_determinants/en

Derose, K. P., & Varda, D. M. (2009). Social capital and health care access. *Medical Care Research and Review, 66*(3), 272–306.

White, K., Haas, J. S., & Williams, D. R. (2012). Elucidating the role of place in health care disparities: The example of racial/ethnic residential segregation. *Health Services Research, 47*(3 Pt 2), 1278–1299.

REFERENCES

Ahern, M. M. (2003). Social capital and trust in providers. *Social Science and Medicine, 57*, 1195–1203.

Ahnquist, J., Wamala, S. P., & Lindstrom, M. (2012). Social determinants of health: A question of social or economic capital? Interaction effects of socioeconomic factors on health outcomes. *Social Science and Medicine, 74*(6), 930–939.

Andersen, R. M., Yu, H., Wyn, R., Davidson, P. L., Brown, E. R., & Teleki, S. (2002). Access to medical care for low-income persons: How do communities make a difference? *Medical Care Research Review, 59*(4), 384–411.

Aysola, J., Orav, E. J., & Ayanian, J. Z. (2011). Neighborhood characteristics associated with access to patient-centered medical homes for children. *Health Affairs (Millwood), 30*(11), 2080–2089.

Bellatorre, A., Finch, B. K., Phuong Do, D., Bird, C. E., & Beck, A. N. (2011). Contextual predictors of cumulative biological risk: Segregation and allostatic load. *Social Science Quarterly, 92*(5), 1338–1362.

Braveman, P., Egerter, S., & Williams, D. R. (2011). The social determinants of health: Coming of age. *Annual Review of Public Health, 32*(1), 381–398.

Brown, T. T., Scheffler, R. M., Seo, S., & Reed, M. (2006). The empirical relationship between community social capital and the demand for cigarettes. *Health Economics, 15*(11), 1159–1172.

Carpiano, R. M. (2007). Neighborhood social capital and adult health: An empirical test of a Bourdieu-based model. *Health and Place, 13*(3), 639–655.

Chang, V. W. (2006). Racial residential segregation and weight status among US adults. *Social Science and Medicine, 63*(5), 1289–1303.

Chen, A., & Escare, J. (2004). Quantifying income-related inequality in healthcare delivery in the United States. *Medical Care, 42*(1), 38–47.

Clarkwest, A. (2008). Neo-materialist theory and the temporal relationship between income inequality and longevity change. *Social Science and Medicine, 66*(9), 1871–1881.

Commission on Social Determinants of Health (CSDH). (2008). *Closing the gap in a generation: Health equity through action on the social determinants of health.* Final report of the Commission on Social Determinants of Health. Geneva: World Health Organization.

Commission on Social Determinants of Health (CSDH). (2011). *Closing the gap: Policy into practice on social determinants of health.* Final Report of the World Conference on Social Determinants of Health. Rio de Janeiro: World Health Organization.

Corral, I., Landrine, H., Hao, Y., Zhao, L., Mellerson, J. L., & Cooper, D. L. (2012). Residential segregation, health behavior and overweight/obesity among a national sample of African American adults. *Journal of Health Psychology, 17*(3), 371–378.

Deaton, A., & Lubotsky, D. (2009). Income inequality and mortality in U.S. cities: Weighing the evidence. A response to Ash [Comment]. *Social Science and Medicine, 68*(11), 1914–1917.

DeBacker, J., Heim, B., Panousi, V., Ramnath, S., & Vidangos, I. (2013). Rising inequality: Transitory or permanent? New evidence from a panel of U.S. tax returns. Washington, DC: Brookings Institution.

Derose, K. P. (2008). Do bonding, bridging, and linking social capital affect preventable hospitalizations? *Health Services Research, 43*(5p1), 1520–1541.

Derose, K. P., & Varda, D. M. (2009). Social capital and health care access. *Medical Care Research and Review, 66*(3), 272–306.

Diez-Roux, A. V., Link, B. G., & Northridge, M. E. (2000). A multilevel analysis of income inequality and cardiovascular disease risk factors. *Social Science and Medicine, 50*(5), 673–687.

Drukker, M., Driessen, G., Krabbendam, L., & van Os, J. (2004). The wider social environment and mental health service use. *Acta Psychiatrica Scandinavica, 110*(2), 119–129.

Elgar, F. J., Davis, C. G., Wohl, M. J., Trites, S. J., Zelenski, J. M., & Martin, M. S. (2011). Social capital, health and life satisfaction in 50 countries. *Health and Place, 17*(5), 1044–1053.

Engström, K., Mattsson, F., Järleborg, A., & Hallqvist, J. (2008). Contextual social capital as a risk factor for poor self-rated health: A multilevel analysis. *Social Science and Medicine, 66*(11), 2268–2280.

Galea, S., Tracy, M., Hoggatt, K. J., Dimaggio, C., & Karpati, A. (2011). Estimated deaths attributable to social factors in the United States. *American Journal of Public Health, 101*(8), 1456–1465.

Gaskin, D. J., Dinwiddie, G. Y., Chan, K. S., & McCleary, R. (2011). Residential segregation and disparities in health care services utilization. *Medical Care Research and Review, 69*(2),158–175.

Gaskin, D. J., Dinwiddie, G. Y., Chan, K. S., & McCleary, R. R. (2012). Residential segregation and the availability of primary care physicians. *Health Services Research, 47*(6), 2353–2376.

Gaskin, D. J., Price, A., Brandon, D. T., & LaVeist, T. A. (2009). Segregation and disparities in health services use. *Medical Care Research and Review, 66*(5), 578–589.

Greenberg, G. A., & Rosenheck, R. A. (2003). Managerial and environmental factors in the continuity of mental health care across institutions. *Psychiatric Services, 54*(4), 529–534.

Haas, J. S., Earle, C. C., Orav, J. E., Brawarsky, P., Keohane, M., Neville, B. A., & Williams, D. R. (2008). Racial segregation and disparities in breast cancer care and mortality. *Cancer, 113*(8), 2166–2172.

Hao, Y., Landrine, H., Smith, T., Kaw, C., Corral, I., & Stein, K. (2011). Residential segregation and disparities in health-related quality of life among Black and White cancer survivors. *Health Psychology, 30*(2), 137–144.

Hayanga, A. J., Kaiser, H. E., Sinha, R., Berenholtz, S. M., Makary, M., & Chang, D. (2009). Residential segregation and access to surgical care by minority populations in US counties. *Journal of the American College of Surgeons, 208*(6), 1017–1022.

Hendryx, M. S., Ahern, M. M., Lovrich, N. P., & McCurdy, A. H. (2002). Access to health care and community social capital. *Health Services Research, 37*(1), 87–103.

Horev, T., Pesis-Katz, I., & Mukamel, D. B. (2004). Trends in geographic disparities in allocation of health care resources in the US. *Health Policy, 68*(2), 223–232.

Hsia, R., & Shen, Y. C. (2011). Possible geographical barriers to trauma center access for vulnerable patients in the United States: An analysis of urban and rural communities. *Archives of Surgery, 146*(1), 46–52.

Islam, M. K., Merlo, J., Kawachi, I., Lindström, M., Burström, K., & Gerdtham, U.-G. (2006). Does it really matter where you live? A panel data multilevel analysis of Swedish municipality-level social capital on individual health-related quality of life. *Health Economics, Policy and Law, 1*(03), 209–235.

Kahn, R. S., Wise, P. H., Kennedy, B. P., & Kawachi, I. (2000). State income inequality, household income, and maternal mental and physical health: Cross-sectional national survey. *British Medical Journal, 321*(7272), 1311–1315.

Kawachi, I., Kennedy, B. P., Lochner, K., & Prothrow-Stith, D. (1997). Social capital, income inequality, and mortality. *American Journal of Public Health, 87*(9), 1491–1498.

Kim, D., Subramanian, S. V., & Kawachi, I. (2006). Bonding versus bridging social capital and their associations with self-rated health: a multilevel analysis of 40 US communities. *Journal of Epidemiology and Community Health, 60*(2), 116–122.

Ko, M., & Ponce, N. A. (2012). Community residential segregation and the local supply of Federally Qualified Health Centers. *Health Services Research, 48*(1), 253–270.

Komaromy, M., Grumbach, K., Drake, M., Vranizan, K., Lurie, N., Keane, D., & Bindman, A. B. (1996). The role of black and Hispanic physicians in providing health care for underserved populations. *New England Journal of Medicine, 334*(20), 1305–1310.

Laporte, A., Nauenberg, E., & Shen, L. (2008). Aging, social capital, and health care utilization in Canada. *Health Economics, Policy and Law, 3*(04), 393–411.

LaVeist, T., Gaskin, D., & Trujillo, A. J. (2011). Segregated spaces, risky places: The effects of racial segregation on health inequalities. Washington, DC: Joint Center for Political and Economic Studies.

LaVeist, T., Pollack, K., Thorpe, R., Fesahazion, R., & Gaskin, D. (2011). Place, not race: Disparities dissipate in southwest Baltimore when blacks and whites live under similar conditions. *Health Affairs, 30*(10), 1880–1887.

Lee, S. Y., Chen, W. L., & Weiner, B. J. (2004). Communities and hospitals: Social capital, community accountability, and service provision in U.S. community hospitals. *Health Services Research, 39*(5), 1487–1508.

Lynch, J. (2000). Income inequality and health: expanding the debate. *Social Science and Medicine, 51*(7), 1001–1005.

Macinko, J., & Starfield, B. (2001). The utility of social capital in research on health determinants. *Milbank Quarterly, 79*(3), 387–427, IV.

Macinko, J., Shi, L., Starfield, B., & Wulu, J. (2003). Income inequality and health: A critical review of the literature. *Medical Care Research and Review, 60*(4), 407–542.

Mansyur, C., Amick, B. C., Harrist, R. B., & Franzini, L. (2008). Social capital, income inequality, and self-rated health in 45 countries. *Social Science and Medicine, 66*(1), 43–56.

Massey, D. S., & Denton, N. A. (1989). Hypersegregation in U.S. metropolitan areas: Black and Hispanic segregation along five dimensions. *Demography, 26*(3), 373–391.

McGrail, K. M., van Doorslaer, E., Ross, N. A., & Sanmartin, C. (2009). Income-related health inequalities in Canada and the United States: A decomposition analysis. *American Journal of Public Health, 99*(10), 1856–1863.

Meijer, M., Rohl, J., Bloomfield, K., & Grittner, U. (2012). Do neighborhoods affect individual mortality? A systematic review and meta-analysis of multilevel studies. *Social Science and Medicine, 74*(8), 1204–1212.

Organisation for Economic Cooperation and Development (OECD). (2011). *Divided we stand: Why inequality keeps rising*. Retrieved from www.oecd.org/els/social/inequality

Pearce, N., & Davey Smith, G. (2003). Is social capital the key to inequalities in health? *American Journal of Public Health, 93*(1), 122–129.

Poortinga, W. (2006). Social relations or social capital? Individual and community health effects of bonding social capital. *Social Science and Medicine, 63*(1), 255–270.

Poortinga, W. (2012). Community resilience and health: The role of bonding, bridging, and linking aspects of social capital. *Health and Place, 18*(2), 286–295.

Prentice, J. C. (2006). Neighborhood effects on primary care access in Los Angeles. *Social Science and Medicine, 62*(5), 1291–1303.

Putnam, R. D. (1993). The prosperous community: Social capital and public life. *American Prospect, 13*, 35–42.

Robert Wood Johnson Foundation. (2008). *Overcoming obstacles to health: Stories, facts, and findings*. Princeton, NJ: Commission to Build a Healthier America. Retrieved from http://www.commissiononhealth.org/PDF/ObstaclesToHealth-Report.pdf

Robert Wood Johnson Foundation. (2010). *Social determinants of health factsheet*. Princeton, NJ: Commission to Build a Healthier America.

Rodriguez, R. A., Sen, S., Metha, K., Moody-Ayers, S., Bacchetti, P., & O'Hare, A. M. (2007). Geography matters: Relationships among urban residential segregation, dialysis facilities, and patient outcomes. *Annals of Internal Medicine, 146*(7), 493–501.

Ross, N. A., Wolfson, M. C., Dunn, J. R., Berthelot, J., Kaplan, G. A., & Lynch, J. W. (2000). Relation between income inequality and mortality in Canada and in the United States: Cross-sectional assessment using census data and vital statistics. *British Medical Journal, 320*, 898–902.

Scheffler, R. M., Brown, T. T., & Rice, J. K. (2007). The role of social capital in reducing non-specific psychological distress: The importance of controlling for omitted variable bias. *Social Science and Medicine, 65*(4), 842–854.

Shen, Y. C., Hsia, R. Y., & Kuzma, K. (2009). Understanding the risk factors of trauma center closures: Do financial pressure and community characteristics matter? *Medical Care, 47*(9), 968–978.

Skinner, J., Weinstein, J. N., Sporer, S. M., & Wennberg, J. E. (2003). Racial, ethnic, and geographic disparities in rates of knee arthroplasty among Medicare patients. *New England Journal of Medicine, 349*(14), 1350–1359.

Solar, O., & Irwin, A. (2007). A conceptual framework for action on the social determinants of health: Discussion paper for the Commission on Social Determinants of Health (Draft). Geneva: WHO Secretariat Commission on Social Determinants of Health.

Solar, O., & Irwin, A. (2010). A conceptual framework for action on the social determinants of health (Social Determinants of Health Discussion, Paper 2: Policy and Practice). Geneva: WHO Secretariat Commission on Social Determinants of Health.

Subramanian, S. V., & Kawachi, I. (2003). The association between state income inequality and worse health is not confounded by race. *International Journal of Epidemiology, 32*(6), 1022–1028.

Subramanian, S. V., & Kawachi, I. (2004). Income inequality and health: What have we learned so far? *Epidemiology Review, 26*, 78–91.

van Doorslaer, E., Koolman, X., & Jones, A. M. (2004) Explaining income-related inequalities in doctor utilisation in Europe. *Health Economics, 13*(7), 629–647.

Wagstaff, A., & van Doorslaer, E. (2000). Income inequality and health: what does the literature tell us? *Annual Review of Public Health, 21*, 543–567.

White, K., Haas, J. S., & Williams, D. R. (2012). Elucidating the role of place in health care disparities: The example of racial/ethnic residential segregation. *Health Services Research, 47*(3 Pt 2), 1278–1299.

Wilkinson, R. G., & Pickett, K. E. (2006). Income inequality and population health: A review and explanation of the evidence. *Social Science and Medicine, 62*, 1768–1784.

Wilson, W. J. (1987). *The truly disadvantaged: The inner city, the underclass, and public policy*. Chicago: University of Chicago Press.

Yen, I. H., & Syme, S. L. (1999). The social environment and health: A discussion of the epidemiologic literature. *Annual Review of Public Health, 20*, 287–308.

CHAPTER SIX

PUBLIC HEALTH INSURANCE

Shana Alex Lavarreda
E. Richard Brown

Learning Objectives

- Learn about the history and nature of public health insurance programs in the United States
- Understand the political process that historically has shaped and continues to influence public health insurance
- Analyze the differences among the major public health insurance programs (Medicare, Medicaid, and CHIP) in terms of eligibility and benefits
- Understand the extraordinary political process that led to the enactment of the Patient Protection and Affordable Care Act of 2010 (ACA)

The United States remains alone among the economically developed countries in not providing health care coverage to its entire population. In 2010, nearly fifty million Americans were uninsured; they have no private or public health insurance of any kind (Current Population Survey, 2011).

This chapter examines the origins and status of the American system of public health care coverage and the options that have been attempted to extend coverage to the uninsured. First, it describes the current state of public health insurance programs, with an examination of historical trends and the policies that have shaped the current system. The chapter concludes with a review of the political factors that influenced these policies, including a detailed examination of the enactment of the Patient Protection and Affordable Care Act of 2010 (ACA).

Why is health insurance coverage important? It is the principal financial means by which people can obtain health care services. The importance of health insurance coverage has been shown in cross-sectional surveys that compare the access of insured and uninsured people, and in panel or longitudinal studies that examine over time the effects of losing or gaining health insurance on access and health status (Aday, Andersen, & Fleming, 1980; Aday, Begley, Lairson, & Slater, 1998; Lurie, Ward, Shapiro, & Brook, 1984; Marquis & Long, 1996; Finkelstein et al., 2011).

The United States has repeatedly attempted to enact major reforms to establish a universal social insurance program to extend health care coverage to the entire population. Until the enactment of the ACA, each time it had failed to come to grips with this issue or has adopted partial reforms. After these repeated failures to enact comprehensive reform, and despite the partial solutions that have been adopted, the problems of lack of coverage remained a continuing challenge. Even in 2019, when the expansion provisions in the ACA have been fully implemented, the U.S. Congressional Budget Office estimates that twenty-two million people will still remain uninsured (U.S. Congressional Budget Office, 2010).

Private health insurance has not served all sectors of American society. The elderly and the poor were effectively priced out of the market for private coverage, even in its period of rapid growth during the 1950s and early 1960s. In 1958, although 86 percent of the upper-income third of all American families had some type of private health insurance, only 42 percent of the lower-income third had any coverage at all. Like the lower working class and the poor, the elderly were unable to obtain adequate private hospitalization coverage at a price they could afford. In 1958, only 43 percent of those age sixty-five and over had insurance for hospital care, compared to at least two-thirds of the nonelderly population (Somers & Somers, 1961). Although private health insurance dramatically reduced disparities in the use of health services related to income for the population with coverage, it remained for Medicare and Medicaid to significantly improve access for the elderly and the poor.

Medicare, Medicaid, and CHIP

By 1960, political pressures to enact public programs to provide for the poor, especially the low-income elderly, had become irresistible. The Kerr-Mills Act, enacted in that year, offered generous matching federal grants to states to encourage them to develop medical care programs for the elderly poor and the nonelderly disabled and blind. But the program was implemented unevenly by the states, with the bulk of the federal funds going to a handful of states that developed comprehensive programs. Senior citizen groups and the nation's major labor unions were not assuaged by this public assistance program; they continued to demand health insurance under Social Security, not a welfare program (Marmor, 2000).

The November 1964 election gave the Democrats a landslide victory (the most lopsided popular vote in the twentieth century) and President Lyndon B. Johnson both a clear mandate for his Great Society reforms and a Democratic Congress (two-thirds in both houses) to enact them. The next year, Congress established Medicare, a social insurance program for hospital care and voluntary insurance for physician services for the elderly, and Medicaid, a public assistance program for poor people who meet "categorical" requirements. Medicare was a landmark in American health care reform because, as a contributory program that afforded entitlement to health benefits without a means test, it was the first successful enactment of social insurance for health services. Medicaid was also important because of its broad potential scope of benefits and population coverage, despite its public assistance (or welfare) character resting on means testing.

Medicare: Improving Access for the Elderly

Medicare has extended coverage to virtually all the elderly and to many blind and long-term-disabled nonelderly persons for a significant portion of their medical expenses. It is the largest source of public financing for health care services in the United States. People age sixty-five and over with social security benefits are automatically entitled to receive Medicare Part A (coverage for hospital services) and to enroll in Medicare Part B (coverage for physician and other services). Part A is a mandatory program financed by a special social security tax paid by all workers and deposited in the

Medicare Trust Fund, while Part B is a voluntary plan funded by beneficiary premium payments and contributions from the U.S. Treasury. In 2009, Medicare covered forty-six million beneficiaries (thirty-eight million aged and eight million disabled enrollees), at a cost of $471 billion (Centers for Medicare &Medicaid Services, 2011).

Medicare Part A is a social insurance program. This is a very important characteristic. Like Social Security, Medicare Part A is a contributory program, which means that everyone who works contributes to it through a tax on earnings. Medicare is also an entitlement program, which means that everyone is eligible for Medicare on reaching age sixty-five or, if younger, meeting a stringent disability test. It is not a means-tested welfare program; this distinction will become clear as we discuss Medicaid.

Medicare quickly improved access to medical services, especially hospital care, for the elderly and disabled. But even under Medicare—an entitlement program with uniform benefits and standards—beneficiary access problems remain. In the program's first few years, more affluent elderly beneficiaries received more physician and hospital services than did the lower-income elderly. Similarly, non-Hispanic white beneficiaries received more health services than did African American beneficiaries. Over time, however, both income and racial differentials were reduced. Recent studies have found that the vast majority of Medicare beneficiaries report no access problems, but some groups do encounter serious barriers. About one in seven Medicare beneficiaries do not have a usual source of care or have not seen a physician for a medical problem that warranted medical attention. Studies that examine access to specific procedures consistently find differences by race in the rate of selected diagnostic and treatment procedures performed. For example, African American beneficiaries are less likely than non-Hispanic white beneficiaries to receive a variety of high-technology procedures (Davis, 1975; Gaskin, Briesacher, Limcangco, & Brigantti, 2006; Link, Long, & Settle, 1982; Long & Settle, 1984; McBean & Gornick, 1994; Mitchell & Khandker, 1995; Physician Payment Review Commission, 1994; Wenneker & Epstein, 1989; Wheeler et al., 2012).

Despite Medicare's impact in improving access to care for elderly and disabled beneficiaries, the program's cost-sharing provisions for covered services posed financial barriers for many. Premium costs for Medicare Part B, deductibles, and coinsurance impose out-of-pocket expenses on the beneficiary. In addition, physicians can bill beneficiaries for more than Medicare's allowed fee (called "balance billing"), although the Omnibus Budget Reconciliation Act of 1989 limited these extra fees to no more than

15 percent of the Medicare payment rate. Nearly nine in ten beneficiaries purchase supplemental "Medigap" coverage to offset deductibles and coinsurance as well as cover some additional services; many individually purchase private supplemental insurance or receive it through a current or former employer. An estimated 20 percent of Medicare beneficiaries also qualify for financial assistance and supplemental benefits under their state Medicaid programs because their income is very low (Kaiser Commission on Medicaid, 2012).

Many Medicare beneficiaries obtained their supplemental coverage through managed care plans (HMOs) called "Medicare+Choice" originally, but now called "Medicare Advantage." Medicare managed care plans were especially attractive because they covered services (in particular prescription drugs) that the basic Medicare program did not. They also covered preventive health services such as screening mammograms and Pap tests, which were not covered by Medicare until 1991.

By 2005, only 13 percent of Medicare beneficiaries were enrolled in a managed care plan, ranging from less than 1 percent in seventeen states to more than 20 percent in six states. Many private plans, unhappy with the amount of money they were getting per enrollee, withdrew from the program, reducing the number of Medicare managed care plans from a high of 346 in 1998 to 179 in 2005. Payments to Medicare HMOs were raised by the Congress and President Bush to attract such plans back into serving Medicare beneficiaries. As a result of increased payment to Medicare HMOs, they received more on average than the program would have spent if those enrollees had remained in the fee-for-service Medicare program—$11 billion more in 2009, according to a study by the Commonwealth Fund (Biles, Pozen, & Guterman, 2009). This issue was addressed by payment reforms in the ACA that tie financing for Medicare Advantage plans to quality health outcomes indicators.

During its first four decades, Medicare's lack of coverage for several key benefits limited its effectiveness for many types of health service, particularly for lower-income beneficiaries. One notable absence of coverage is for long-term care services. Medicare restricts coverage for nursing home stays and home health visits to posthospital use of limited duration, imposing hardship on the elderly who must use extensive personal resources to pay for care. If they become poor or impoverished because of medical expenses, they may apply to Medicaid, which has become the nation's largest payer for long-term care.

Perhaps foremost among Medicare's gaps was the lack of coverage for prescription drugs. This problem grew over time for the elderly and others who on average use more medication than younger groups do. Out-of-pocket costs for prescription drugs took an ever-increasing share of seniors' income, as a growing number of drugs were prescribed for more conditions and as the high prices charged by pharmaceutical manufacturers pushed up prescription drug expenditures. A growing demand to cover prescription drugs under Medicare eventually generated enough political support to push the Congress to enact a coverage program. The Medicare Prescription Drug, Improvement, and Modernization Act of 2003 (MMA) established a new and complex prescription drug benefit (Part D) beginning in 2006, bringing expected relief to many elderly persons with high expenses. President George W. Bush and the Republican majority in Congress created the Part D benefit as a private program, except in areas where private plans were very limited, overcoming objections by Democratic congressional leaders who argued for having the program run by the federal Medicare program. The MMA requires beneficiaries to choose among private drug plans, with a complex set of rules and options that may well test the viability of such privatization strategies in the Medicare program. As of February 2010, 38 percent of Medicare enrollees had also obtained a stand-alone drug plan, with another 21 percent gaining drug coverage through a managed care plan (Kaiser Family Foundation, 2012a). For more on Part D implementation, and on proposals to reform Medicare, see Chapter Twenty-One.

Medicaid: Improving Access for the Poor

Medicaid was enacted in 1965 to offer coverage to poor persons who were eligible for federally supported, state-run welfare programs. These welfare programs give cash assistance to families with dependent children (formerly Aid to Families with Dependent Children, or AFDC) and to the disabled, the blind, and the elderly (those receiving Supplemental Security Income or State Supplemental Payment program income). Through this latter component, Medicaid assists elderly Medicare beneficiaries who cannot afford the required cost sharing for Medicare or supplemental insurance. Medicaid is administered by the states under federal guidelines that require minimum standards for eligibility, benefits, and (in some cases) provider payments. Funding is shared between the federal government and the states, with the federal share (called the federal medical assistance percentage, or FMAP) ranging from 50 percent to 77 percent.

In 2009, Medicaid covered nearly sixty-three million persons, at a cost of $389 billion. Half of Medicaid beneficiaries are low-income children, about a quarter are low-income women, and the remaining quarter are low-income disabled and elderly persons. Medicaid spending is tilted toward the elderly (who in 2009 accounted for 10 percent of all recipients and 23 percent of the total spending) and toward the disabled (who made up 15 percent of recipients and accounted for 43 percent of total spending; Kaiser Family Foundation, 2012a).

There is substantial evidence that Medicaid is responsible for a significant increase in use of health services among low-income persons. In 1964, two years before the Medicaid program launched, poor people averaged 4.3 doctor visits per year, compared to 4.6 visits for the nonpoor. By the mid-1970s, when nearly all states were operating Medicaid programs, poor adults averaged more physician visits than nonpoor adults, and the gap between poor and nonpoor children had been reduced (though not eliminated). However, use of a greater volume of services by the poor may not necessarily indicate complete equity in access, because of the poorer health status of many low-income people (Aday & Andersen, 1983; Health Resources Administration, 1980).

Medicaid's positive effect on the utilization rate of low-income people is, of course, limited to those who are eligible for the program. Numerous studies have found that Medicaid beneficiaries, in contrast to uninsured low-income persons, use health services at a rate comparable to that of higher-income people, after adjusting for differences in health status. Among the poor and near-poor who are sick or in poor health, those uninsured during the entire year use far fewer medical services than those who have Medicaid for even part of the year (Almeida, Dubay, & Ko, 2001; Berk, Schur, & Cantor, 1995; Freeman & Corey, 1993; Davidoff, Kenney, & Dubay, 2005; Finkelstein et al., 2011; Kasper, 1986; Millman, 1993; Newacheck, 1988; Wilensky & Berk, 1982).

Studies have found that loss of Medicaid coverage has an adverse impact on the health status of low-income people, especially among persons with chronic illness. Loss of Medicaid has a serious adverse impact on access to health services and on the health status of anyone with a chronic illness such as diabetes or high blood pressure (Finkelstein et al., 2011; Lurie, Ward, Shapiro, & Brook, 1984).

Despite its important contributions, Medicaid's ability to improve access to medical care for the nation's low-income population has been hampered by several factors. State-level discretion in the Medicaid program has resulted in great variation across states in the population covered and the benefits provided. Federal guidelines define mandatory eligible populations and covered benefits, but they allow states considerable latitude beyond this floor. States vary markedly in their Medicaid income eligibility level for a family, which ranges from one state with income eligibility below 50 percent of the federal poverty level for parents of eligible Medicaid children to eleven states with income eligibility at or above 200 percent. States also differ in the benefits covered in the Medicaid program. Each state defines its own package of benefits beyond the mandatory services defined by federal Medicaid law. For example, coverage for such essential services as prescription drugs, physical therapy, occupational therapy, respiratory care services, and corrective eyeglasses are all optional. The reimbursement level for Medicaid also varies considerably across states, contributing to differences by state in the rate of physician participation (Centers for Medicaid and Medicare Services, 2011; Kaiser Commission on Medicaid and the Uninsured, 2005a; NGA Center for Best Practices, 2003).

Medicaid's limitations in covering the poor were exacerbated by budget cuts during the Reagan administration and ratcheting down by states of income limits for AFDC eligibility. As a result, Medicaid enrollees as a proportion of all poor persons declined from 51 percent in 1981 to 45 percent in 1982. Beginning in the mid-1980s, however, Congress enacted a series of expansions in Medicaid income eligibility in order to extend Medicaid's beneficial effects to more low-income pregnant women and their children. Although only 51 percent of poor children were on Medicaid in 1985, 60 percent were covered by Medicaid in 1994, an important reversal of the trend of a decade earlier (NGA Center for Best Practices, 2003).

Most of this increase was aimed at ensuring financial access to pregnant women to enable them to obtain prenatal care early in pregnancy in order to improve birth outcomes and the health of infants of Medicaid-eligible pregnant women. Congress required states to cover pregnant women up to 133 percent of the poverty level and encouraged states to voluntarily expand coverage up to 185 percent of poverty. This extension of Medicaid to a population well above the income eligibility for cash public assistance programs partially severed the historic link between Medicaid and welfare. In addition, Congress required states to increase fees for obstetric care to attract an adequate number of providers, and it appropriated other funds for enhanced perinatal care. By 2002, thirty-four states had expanded coverage of pregnant women beyond the federally mandated level, all fifty states had streamlined the eligibility process at least to some extent, and forty-four states offered Medicaid reimbursement for enhanced prenatal services. More than one-third of all births in the United States (37 percent) now are paid for by Medicaid, while other programs fund improvement in the supply and accessibility of prenatal care services and nutritional and other supports for mothers and young children (Kaiser Family Foundation, 2012a).

The Medicaid program's improvement in eligibility for pregnant women to meet specific public health goals is a valuable example of how public policy may be used directly to improve access. The findings regarding the effects of Medicaid expansion on use of prenatal care and birth outcomes vary. Some studies show improvement in access to care and birth outcomes, while others do not. These findings suggest that there are multiple components to providing prenatal care that include, but go beyond, improving financial access: outreach and educational programs, case management, and supply of providers (Hessol, Vittinghoff, & Fuentes-Afflick, 2004; Kaestner, Dubay, & Kenney, 2005; Loranger & Lipson, 1995; Ray, Mitchel, & Piper, 1997).

The expansion of Medicaid coverage appeared to come to a halt with enactment and implementation of the Personal Responsibility and Work Opportunity Reconciliation Act of 1996, better known as welfare reform. Nationally, Medicaid coverage fell from 12.5 percent of the nonelderly population overall in 1994 to 10.4 percent in 1998, but it fell even more sharply among nonworking families, from 52.8 percent in 1994 to 40.8 percent in 1998 (Holl, Slack, & Stevens, 2005; Krebs-Carter & Holahan, 2000). As the economy continued to improve, some families and individuals who formerly relied on Medicaid might have obtained low-wage jobs that permitted some access to health benefits, or earned more money that enabled them to pay the employee's share of premiums. However, many of these newly employed workers and their families found themselves in low-wage jobs without health benefits and joined the ranks of the uninsured. Although welfare reform promises public assistance recipients that they will receive transitional Medicaid coverage for at least a year when they leave public assistance, both advocates and analysts argue that this policy is inadequately implemented (Perry, Stark & Valdez, 1998).

Finally, many noncitizen families refrained from applying for Medicaid. Welfare reform legislation together with the Illegal Immigration Reform and Immigrant Responsibility Act of 1996 restricted all noncitizens' eligibility for Medicaid and greatly broadened application of a "public charge" classification for those who used any public benefits. Noncitizen parents feared being labeled a public charge if they enrolled themselves or their children (even children who were born in the United States and thus are citizens) in a means-tested program. They were concerned that the classification would be used against them if they tried to renew their visas, return to the United States from abroad, or apply for citizenship. This problem was ameliorated by policies issued in May 1999 by the Immigration and Naturalization Service (now called the U.S. Citizenship and Immigration Services), specifying that noncitizens will not be classified as a public charge if they or their children enroll in Medicaid, unless they receive long-term care under Medicaid.

One important characteristic of the Medicaid program is its origin as a public assistance program. Welfare programs, even federally supported ones such as Medicaid, tend to be administered by the states, albeit under some federal regulation. Unlike Medicare, which is administered as a social insurance program by the federal government and includes the same eligibility and benefits throughout the country, the Medicaid program is administered by the states. Medicaid is in reality fifty-one programs, with variations in eligibility and benefits across all fifty states and the District of Columbia.

Many of the problems associated with Medicaid are the legacy of its welfare-based origin. Welfare programs tend to rely on stigmatizing means tests, usually conducted in welfare offices (Perry et al., 1998). It is noteworthy that there is no stigma attached to Medicare, which is viewed as a universal entitlement, a social contract between the nation's young and old generations. Nor is there stigma associated with the tax exemption of employer-paid health insurance for largely middle- and upper-income workers, which cost the federal government over $200 billion in 2006—a health insurance subsidy program that no one calls welfare (Selden & Gray, 2006). Despite Medicaid's welfare origins, expansion of eligibility in the 1980s to low-income pregnant women and children at a higher income level—nearly twice the poverty level for pregnant women and infants—loosened the connection with welfare and created the logic for 1990s policies that went further.

A second important characteristic of Medicaid is that it is an entitlement program. Anyone who meets Medicaid's eligibility requirements is entitled to receive its benefits. Expenditures for these benefits generate a cost to the state and draw the specified federal matching payment. In this way, Medicaid differs from block grant programs, in which the federal government gives the states a maximum allocation, such that once a state has expended its allocation, any additional services for eligible persons become the fiscal responsibility of the state alone. This characteristic has been the nub of major conflict between liberals and conservatives, with liberals defending Medicaid as an entitlement and conservatives often proposing to turn it into a block grant—as they tried unsuccessfully to do in 1996, when welfare reform ended entitlement of poor children and families to cash assistance. President Bush has also proposed turning Medicaid at least partly into a block grant program, indicating that this issue remains alive and may yet alter the fundamental character of Medicaid.

With the failure to enact national health care reform prior to the Patient Protection and Affordable Care Act of 2010 (ACA), many states looked to Medicaid, among other approaches, to extend coverage to their uninsured residents. Numerous states have expanded or otherwise modified their Medicaid programs with the aid of a waiver under sections 1115 and 1915(b) and (c) of the Social Security Act. These waivers, which must be granted by the federal Health Care Financing Administration, permit states to modify eligibility, payment methods, and other characteristics in their Medicaid programs. These waivers permit states to require Medicaid beneficiaries to enroll in a managed care plan, on the expectation that managed care enables the state to slow the growth of its Medicaid expenditures and, in some cases, improve access to health services. Most of the recent waivers also extend coverage to the working poor and their families, who were not previously eligible for Medicaid, promising to use at least some of the expected savings from managed care to expand coverage to low-income uninsured persons. By 2010, 71.4 percent of all Medicaid beneficiaries were enrolled in managed care, up from 9.5 percent in 1991 (Centers for Medicare and Medicaid Services, 2011).

Medicaid managed care has a mixed record. On some measures, such as having a regular provider and receiving preventive health care services, Medicaid managed care beneficiaries appear to be doing better than their fee-for-service counterparts, but managed care enrollees are more likely to report not getting needed care and more dissatisfaction with some aspects of their care. There is, however, a growing body of evidence that, overall, managed care plans offer Medicaid beneficiaries access to health services that is at least as good as in the fee-for-service Medicaid program and quality of care that is equal to or better than care in the fee-for-service program (Coughlin & Long, 2000; Garrett, Davidoff, & Yemane, 2003; Kaiser Commission on the Future of Medicaid, 1995). Nevertheless, there is little evidence that managed care reduces Medicaid costs, in part because most Medicaid managed care enrollees have not been the higher-cost disabled or elderly for whom substantial savings might be realized, and in part because Medicaid expenditures per beneficiary were already ratcheted down to an extremely low level in many states.

The Children's Health Insurance Program (CHIP)

With the collapse in 1994 of efforts to cover the entire population, many health care reform advocates joined with children's advocacy groups to expand coverage for children. They focused a great deal of attention on the fact that there were then more than eleven million uninsured children age eighteen or younger in the United States, many of whom had low family incomes that were nonetheless above their state's often less-than-generous Medicaid income eligibility level. Children are an appealing group to cover, both because there is wide political support for public programs that benefit children and because insuring children costs much less than insuring adults.

In 1997, Congress enacted what was then called the State Children's Health Insurance Program (SCHIP), offering funds to states to expand health insurance coverage to uninsured, low-income, and moderate-income children. Although liberals and conservatives fought over whether to make SCHIP an entitlement that expanded Medicaid or a block grant that established a separate program that relies on private insurance, in the end Congress compromised on a generous block grant that could be used by the states to do either or both.

SCHIP was generous in two ways. First, it enabled states to set the income eligibility level up to 200 percent of the federal poverty level (in 2003, up to $24,240 for a family of two or $30,520 for a family of three) or even higher. Second, it gave states more generous matching funds than under Medicaid—30 percent higher than the state's federal Medicaid match, up to 85 percent of a state's expenditures. This was an incentive to induce states to implement the program quickly and vigorously. SCHIP implementation began slowly, falling short of early enrollment goals, but it has picked up speed since 2000 and significantly helped slow the growth in the uninsured population. By 2003, four million children nationwide were enrolled in SCHIP (Kaiser Commission on Medicaid and the Uninsured, 2005b).

Early examinations indicated that most of the program's enrollment came from children who were previously insured through private coverage, not uninsured children as intended. However, as states' SCHIP programs matured and outreach efforts intensified, more and more children who previously had no insurance enrolled in the program (Cunningham, Hadley, & Reschovsky, 2002; Lo Sasso & Buchmueller, 2004). Among children with chronic health conditions (such as asthma), SCHIP has achieved significant success in reducing the uninsured rate. Early research showed that access to quality health care received by SCHIP enrollees was dramatically higher than when they were uninsured (Davidoff et al., 2005; Kempe et al., 2005).

As SCHIP enrollments expanded, these state programs faced the same budgetary pressures as did Medicaid. Although some states were able to continue expanding their SCHIP programs throughout the recession from 2000 to 2003, twenty-three restricted enrollment and retention. Eight states imposed an explicit enrollment freeze, while the rest rolled back application simplifications to reduce enrollment indirectly. By July 2004, twenty-two states had imposed additional copayments on SCHIP enrollees to decrease state expenditures (Kaiser Commission on Medicaid and the Uninsured, 2005b).

SCHIP was not intended as an indefinite program, and contained a "sunset provision" that required Congressional action to maintain the program after ten years. The reauthorization of SCHIP in 2007 had broad bipartisan support in Congress, but was vetoed twice by President George W. Bush (in 2007 and again in 2008), who refused to allow the expansion of eligibility that was embedded in the bill (now called the Children's Health Insurance Program Reauthorization Act, or CHIPRA). President Bush negotiated with Congress for a limited reauthorization that would keep the program at current levels until February 2009, when a new administration could address the issue. President Obama quickly signed the CHIPRA bill, expanding eligibility to up to six million additional children nationwide. As of 2011, nearly eight million children had CHIP coverage nationwide (Kaiser Family Foundation, 2012a).

In spite of the setbacks, the SCHIP program was a successful model for modern expansion of public coverage. Together with Medicaid, CHIP expanded eligibility for and enrollment in public health insurance programs for children whose low- and moderate-income families did not have access to affordable employment-based insurance. Between the Medicaid and CHIP public programs and private employment-based coverage, the United States was clearly moving—albeit haltingly and with some steps backward—toward a policy of offering affordable health care coverage to all children.

Who is Left Out of Public Coverage?

The large and growing number of Americans who have no health care coverage continues to be one of the most compelling policy and political issues in the United States, and it spurred the push for national health care

TABLE 6.1. PERCENTAGE OF NONELDERLY POPULATION WHO ARE UNINSURED, AGES 0–64, UNITED STATES, SELECTED YEARS

Year	Percentage of Persons Age 0–64
1994	15.5
1997	17.4
2000	16.5
2003	16.0
2006	16.8
2009	17.8
2010	18.0

Source: Author's analysis of Current Population Survey Annual Social and Economic Supplement, 1995–2011.

reform for both President Clinton and President Obama. When President Clinton proposed his health care reform in 1994, 15.5 percent of the nonelderly U.S. population (ages 0–64) were uninsured, or 35.7 million Americans (see Table 6.1). The uninsured rate dipped slightly by 2000, due to the economic expansion in the late 1990s. With the recession beginning in 2001, however, the uninsurance rate again began to climb. In late 2008, the United States entered a period of extended, severe economic recession, and the uninsured rate jumped even higher.

By 2009, when President Obama argued for the need for overall health care reform, the number of the uninsured had climbed to 17.8 percent, or 47.4 million nonelderly people, ages 0 through 64. About 770,000 persons age sixty-five or over (just 2.0 percent of all persons in this age group) were completely uninsured in 2010 because nearly all the elderly receive at least Medicare coverage, and most have some other coverage that reduces Medicare's cost sharing (deductibles and coinsurance) and covers some services that are not Medicare benefits. Because the uninsured population includes so few elderly persons, most analysts of this problem focus on the nonelderly population.

About eight in ten (77 percent) of the nonelderly uninsured are working adults and their children. Three-fifths (60 percent) of the uninsured are in families headed by at least one employee who works full-time all year, and another 17 percent are in a families of part-time employees (see Figure 6.1). Nonworking families comprised nearly one-quarter of the uninsured in 2010.

FIGURE 6.1. FAMILY WORK STATUS OF UNINSURED NONELDERLY PERSONS, UNITED STATES, 2010

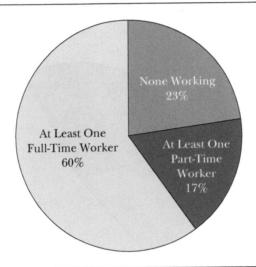

Note: Counts are presented in thousands.
Source: Author's analysis of Current Population Survey Annual Social and Economic Supplement, 2011.

Three-fourths of the uninsured have low or moderate family incomes. Over two-thirds (70 percent) have incomes below 200 percent of the federal poverty level (that is, less than about $44,100 for a family of four in 2010), and another fifth (21 percent) have moderate family incomes (between 201 percent and 400 percent of the poverty level; see Figure 6.2). The low and moderate incomes of the uninsured mean that efforts to extend coverage to them require considerable financial assistance to make it affordable, assistance that can come only from employers or government. Although 60 percent of the entire nonelderly population have a family income at least two times the poverty level, only about one in three (29 percent) of the uninsured have a family income that high. It is unlikely that any of the uninsured below this level could afford a significant share of the costs of family coverage, although those with incomes above 400 percent of poverty could help pay for their health insurance.

Because of their predominance in the population, nearly half of the uninsured are non-Latino whites (45 percent), but ethnic minorities have disproportionately high uninsured rates. One out of three nonelderly Latinos (33 percent), one in five African Americans (22 percent), and one

FIGURE 6.2. FAMILY INCOME OF UNINSURED NONELDERLY PERSONS, UNITED STATES, 2010

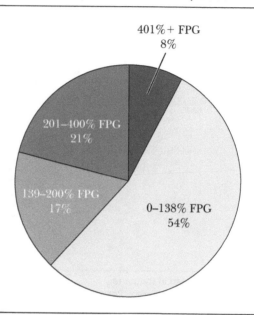

Note: Counts are presented in thousands.
Source: Author's analysis of Current Population Survey Annual Social and Economic Supplement, 2011.

in five Asian Americans and Pacific Islanders (19 percent) are uninsured, compared to 13 percent of non-Latino whites (see Figure 6.3).

Fourteen states have uninsured rates of 20 percent or more of their nonelderly population, while eight states have rates below 12 percent (Current Population Survey, 2011). Differences in uninsured rates across states are driven mainly by state variation in employment-based health insurance, which itself is explained by differences in labor market characteristics (such as firm size, industry, and unionization). But state differences in uninsured rates are also influenced by the generosity of each state's eligibility policy policies for Medicaid and other public health care insurance programs.

There is also substantial evidence that a large number of Americans are *under*insured. An estimated two-thirds (62.1 percent) of personal bankruptcies in the United States in 2007 were due to medical care costs. Three-fourths of all these individuals had health insurance at the time they incurred their expenses. The proportion of bankruptcies due to medical debt increased by 50 percent from 2001 to 2007 (Himmelstein, Thorne, Warren, & Woolhandler, 2009).

FIGURE 6.3. FAMILY INCOME OF UNINSURED NONELDERLY PERSONS, UNITED STATES, 2010

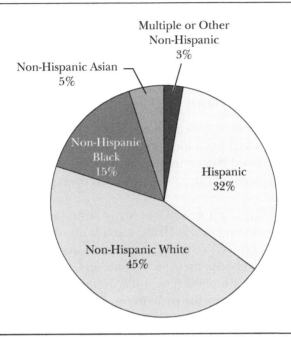

Source: Author's analysis of Current Population Survey Annual Social and Economic Supplement, 2011.

In 2010, 22 percent of all nonelderly insured adults (or 29 million people) either had out-of-pocket health care expenses greater than 10 percent of their income or deductibles that were greater than 5 percent of their income. As household income decreases, the risk of being underinsured or uninsured increases dramatically. Nearly 80 percent of adults with household incomes below $20,000 and 55 percent of those with incomes between $20,000 and $39,999 were either underinsured or uninsured (Schoen, Doty, Robertson, & Collins, 2011).

Frustrations on the Road to Universal Coverage

For at least the last half century, many Americans have found the concept of government health insurance an appealing way to cover the population. Funded by taxes and administered as a universal national program by the federal government, or by a combination of federal and state governments, such a social insurance program would pay physicians, hospitals, and other health care providers, eliminating the need for private health insurance. Since 1965, Medicare has provided virtually universal coverage for the elderly, but throughout much of the twentieth century repeated efforts to enact a universal system for the entire population have consistently foundered.

Social Insurance: The Elusive Option

Social insurance systems have many advantages. Canada's single-payer system, a social insurance program that received a great deal of attention in the United States in the late 1980s and early 1990s, has been an efficient means of extending universal coverage with comprehensive health benefits.

The Canadian system has many advantages that attracted Americans at the beginning of the 1990s. Canada's provincial-run national program features universal coverage, very good access to primary care, patients' freedom to choose their own physicians, a superior record of controlling expenditures for physicians and hospitals, lower administrative costs, lower out-of-pocket costs for patients, and less restricted clinical autonomy for physicians (Fuchs & Hahn, 1990; Hayes, Hayes, & Dykstra, 1993). However, steady reductions in federal support for the provincial programs, from 50 percent in 1971 to just 23 percent in 1997, exacerbated by the ever-rising costs of providing new medical technologies, has led to lower per capita spending, a shortage of medical personnel and facilities, and increased waiting time for specialty care and surgery. The decline in federal support and its sequelae yielded a dramatic decline in popular satisfaction with the system, with the proportion of the public saying "On the whole the system works pretty well, and only minor changes are needed to make it work better" falling from 56 percent in 1988 to just 20 percent in 1998. Growing dissatisfaction, while rooted in funding constraints, has created fertile ground for arguments by market-oriented policymakers that Canada should allow employers and individuals to supplement government-funded health care with private insurance and services, which is otherwise restricted. Nevertheless, Canada's public system retains strong popular support, even as conservative and liberal political leaders ramp up a national debate (Iglehart, 2000).

Despite their advantages and at least nominal support among the American public, social insurance proposals have not fared well in the United States since the enactment of Medicare. Although the single-payer proposals introduced into Congress in the health care reform effort of the early 1990s received substantial support from some unions and consumer-based organizations, they could not overcome the powerful opposition of an array of interest groups representing health care providers, insurers, and business. In November 1994, California voters rejected (by a 73-to-27 margin) a Canadian-style single-payer ballot initiative that was opposed by a very well-funded campaign.

A growing number of states have taken it upon themselves to expand public programs, such as the Medicaid and SCHIP expansions discussed earlier in this chapter. Along with those programs, states (and in some cases counties) have developed their own insurance programs to fill in the gaps left between Medicaid and those who earn enough to either get coverage through their employer or buy it on their own. Maine launched Dirigo Health in June 2003 as a broad strategy to improve the state's health care system, which included universal access to health coverage. California also enacted an employer mandate in 2003, which was repealed a year later. Other efforts to expand coverage at the state level range from proposals for mandates on individuals to buy coverage to proposals for universal coverage of children, building on the relatively successful expansions of Medicaid and SCHIP. In 2005 Illinois enacted a program to offer some form of coverage, private or public, to all children. Massachusetts enacted health care reform in 2006 that became a model for the ACA, including an individual mandate, an exchange (called the Connector), and expansions of public coverage to achieve universal health insurance.

Overcoming Political Barriers to Universal Health Insurance

There are many barriers to adopting policy options that would lead to universal coverage, and these have been played out on the national stage for multiple different iterations of health care reform efforts. President Theodore Roosevelt first proposed the idea of national health insurance in 1912 during his presidential campaign. President Franklin Delano Roosevelt initially intended to include universal health insurance as part of the New Deal, but dropped that proposal in order to win support for Social Security. Although President Lyndon B. Johnson successfully enacted Medicaid and Medicare in 1965, he was unable to win support for a universal plan that would include all Americans. In 1972, President Richard M. Nixon also proposed a universal health insurance plan based on requiring employers to offer affordable coverage to all. This effort was thwarted by Senator Ted Kennedy, who thought that he could gain support instead for his single-payer health insurance plan. Both plans failed to win majorities in Congress.

The effort for health care reform in the early 1990s started out with massive public support, but many forces combined to sap the political momentum for change. As we entered the 1990s, nine out of ten Americans, driven by fear of losing health insurance coverage and being unable to afford the rising cost of care, told pollsters that they believed the nation's health care system needed fundamental change or complete rebuilding (Blendon & Taylor, 1989). The same proportion of chief executive officers of Fortune 500 corporations, whose attention was focused on their rising health benefits costs, supported fundamental change or complete rebuilding of the nation's health care system (Cantor, Barand, Desonia, Cohen, & Merrill, 1991). Three-fourths of these corporate executives said the problems could not be solved by companies working on their own and that government must play a bigger role. The leaders of four major national business organizations jointly appealed to the Congress to "do something" about health care costs (Rosenblatt, 1989).

This impressive support for comprehensive reform dissipated rapidly as opposition interest groups eroded public support and threw their impressive weight against congressional efforts to find a consensus (West, Heith, & Goodwin, 1996). The Clinton administration created a cumbersome policy process to develop and promote its health care proposal, and (unlike reform opponents) the administration waged a feckless public campaign that did not mobilize grassroots support. Popular support for any specific proposal began to decline. Waning prospects for health care reform encouraged major employers to turn from policy change to other options to lower their own costs, including encouraging or forcing their employees into managed care and limiting their own costs by providing employees with a fixed contribution for health benefits.

As managed care plans tightly controlled utilization, they created a backlash in the late 1990s that, combined with extraordinary economic growth and a tight labor market, encouraged employers to seek looser arrangements for care (Marquis, Rogowski, & Escarce, 2004–2005; Mechanic, 2004). Many employers and their employees turned increasingly to preferred provider organizations (PPOs), but these PPOs in part fueled a rapid increase in health care spending, sending health insurance premiums up by double digits every year from 2001 to 2004, with no signs of relief on the horizon (Kaiser Family Foundation, 2004). Increasingly, conservative political and business leaders became advocates for "consumer-directed health plans," which are designed to make patients and families more conscious of each dollar spent on health care by making them more directly responsible for the financial consequences of their health care utilization.

President Bush and many business groups soon went further, making high-deductible health plans into their primary cost-control strategy (Robinson, 2004). These plans replace comprehensive health insurance with catastrophic coverage plans, often paired with "health savings accounts." In a high-deductible health plan, the average annual deductible for an individual is $3,365, and the average share-of-cost for covered benefits is $3,681—a total of more than $7,000 in financial exposure—even after paying annual premiums that average $1,326 for a twenty-year-old to $4,408 for a fifty-five-year-old. Family coverage imposes even more potential liability, totaling $6,366 in deductibles and out-of-pocket costs, plus annual premiums averaging $3,375 for a family with a twenty-year-old primary subscriber to $7,483 for a family with a fifty-five-year-old primary subscriber. High-deductible health plans have experienced rapid growth, as the number of covered lives increased tenfold to ten million persons between March 2005 and January 2010, according to America's Health Insurance Plans, the industry's trade association (AHIP Center for Policy and Research, 2010).

Underlying this successful frustration of health care reform efforts is the nation's political system itself. Compared to all parliamentary democracies that have developed national health insurance systems, the U.S. political system, institutions, and culture pose significant challenges to enacting major reforms.

In parliamentary democracies, the government represents a majority party or coalition in the parliament, creating a greater concentration of political power and fewer opportunities for blocking legislation that the government supports. In the United States, political power is dispersed—divided between the executive (the government), the legislative body, and the judiciary—rather than concentrated, making it more difficult for the government to push through controversial reforms. The government (headed by the president or a governor) gains office through a winner-take-all election that reduces the opportunity for third parties to influence policy; this is quite a different situation from parliamentary systems. The winner-take-all provision encourages parties to "market" themselves to the broadest part of the electorate and discourages formation of political parties with a coherent policy or political commitments that are considered binding on candidates elected in the party's name.

These systemic conditions make U.S. political parties weak institutions. They are organized as a loose coalition and more focused on fundraising than on policy guidance. The weakness of political parties opens a door widely to interest group influence in the policy process. The influence of interest groups has been greatly enhanced by the growing dominance of expensive television advertising in political campaigns and the dependence of parties and candidates on large donations from interest groups, corporations, and individuals with resources to give (Navarro, 1989; Rothman, 1993). Thus, a political party that "controls" the White House and the Congress—as the Democrats did in 1993 and 1994—lacks coherence and a means of enforcing its policy platform. In parliamentary democracies, parties have more political coherence and more leverage over legislators elected on the party slate.

Compounding the weakness of parties, labor unions in the United States historically have played a more modest political role than they do in other industrial democracies. In most parliamentary democracies, the power of the labor-controlled party, clearly generally representing working families and individuals, was a critical factor in enacting national health insurance. In the United States, throughout the twentieth century and at the beginning of the current century, labor tied itself to the Democratic Party, which it influences but does not control. In contrast to labor's relatively weak role, business-oriented interest groups in the United States assert a broad and powerful influence and have repeatedly undermined or vetoed efforts to enact national health insurance.

Finally, the United States has an ingrained political culture that supports weak government, a tradition that goes back to the very founding of the country. The United States has never developed either a strong civil service or a tradition of people looking to government to solve social problems—a different set of popular expectations than prevail in a number of other industrial democracies.

There are additional political and economic barriers for states that try to tackle these problems outside a national framework. ERISA limits states' ability to regulate employer health and welfare benefit programs. Limited state fiscal resources create competition among constituencies and interest groups, especially when the state's fiscal condition is tight—and state residents who lack health insurance coverage tend not to be among the more influential political groups. Elected officials fear raising taxes, which would be needed to fund a health insurance subsidy, because higher taxes may encourage some businesses to move to other states or countries, and a vote for higher taxes certainly would be a weapon in a challenger's hands at the next election. Finally, many elected officials worry that generous public subsidies for health insurance coverage will attract a lot of low-income people to move to the state.

Enactment of the Affordable Care Act of 2010: A Political Success Story

During the midterm election of 2006, the public's mood began moving toward pragmatic, government-based solutions to intractable economic problems. The Bush administration policies of market-based reforms were leading to expansions of health insurance that were either unaffordable or did not protect adequately against financial risk. With the passage of comprehensive health care reform in Massachusetts, a Democratic state with a Republican governor, a successful blueprint for how reform could be accomplished in a bipartisan fashion emerged (McDonough, Rosman, Phelps, & Shannon, 2006). Democrats won a majority of seats in both chambers of Congress in 2006 and began implementing a more progressive legislative agenda. In 2007, California nearly enacted a Massachusetts-style health care reform effort, but it was killed in the state legislature due to concerns about costs and a preference for single-payer reforms (Zelman, 2009). In the presidential primary debates in 2007 and 2008, candidates Barack Obama and Hillary Rodham Clinton focused on disagreements about aspects of the Massachusetts model of health care reform, but both agreed that reform was necessary and would be a strong focus of their first term in office, if elected.

President Barack Obama, elected in fall of 2008, was determined to enact health care reform as one of his first major policy changes. However, he faced the worst economic conditions in the United States since the Great Depression, as the unemployment rate soared from 5.8 percent in July 2008 to 9.5 percent by July 2009 (U.S. Department of Labor, 2012). Even with that crisis crowding out much of the policy agenda, Speaker of the House Nancy Pelosi (D-CA) and Senate Majority Leader Harry Reid (D-NV) kept the even more acute need for health insurance firmly in the forefront. In February 2009, the Children's Health Insurance Program Reauthorization Act (CHIPRA), vetoed twice previously by President Bush, was signed into law by President Obama. A further temporary health insurance expansion was included in a relief bill intended to help those who had lost their jobs and could not afford the health insurance then offered to them through COBRA. Under this new law, the federal government would pay for two-thirds of the COBRA coverage premium for up to eighteen months.

These victories set the stage for President Obama's strategy for successfully maneuvering his health care plan through Congress. The health care reform efforts of the early 1990s and the marketplace reforms under the Bush Administration both played large roles in this strategy. Eschewing the secret meetings to create a new government-run plan as in the Clinton reforms, and somewhat embracing the private market that emerged under the Bush administration, the Obama administration proposed a framework based on the Massachusetts model (privately funded insurance made available through an exchange with subsidized affordable insurance, coupled with public program expansion and an individual mandate requiring all to obtain coverage) and left the hard work of the policy process to congressional leaders.

While Congress worked on the particulars of the bill, President Obama focused on targeting key stakeholders for support. He convened a health care summit in the White House that engaged both major associations (including the Association of Health Insurance Plans and the American Medical Association) and legislators to discuss reform issues. During the course of the year, the Obama administration announced that medical trade groups such as the pharmaceutical industry had agreed to support the bill. These efforts greatly reduced the outside special interest pressures on Congress to scrap reform entirely, unlike the infamous "Harry and Louise" television ad campaign during the Clinton reform effort.

In the House of Representatives, Speaker Nancy Pelosi had personally been engaged in the Clinton reform debacle and was determined to avoid a similar fate for President Obama's reform bill. The wide consensus among Democrats as to the overall parameters of the bill helped this process, as it minimized the internal disagreements between different committee chairpersons within the House and their versions of health care reform (Oberlander, 2010). She knew that she would be unable to secure any Republican votes and so focused instead on keeping the Democratic caucus united in support of the bill. Speaker Pelosi successfully negotiated with both the liberal wing of the party, who would have preferred a more expansive single-payer bill, and the conservative wing, the so-called Blue Dog Democrats, who were insisting on more private market involvement and less government regulation. Three committees moved the same version of the bill to the House floor (the so-called Tri-Committee Bill), and on November 7, 2009, the House of Representatives passed their version of the health care reform bill, with a party-line vote of 220 to 215.

In the Senate, a more diffuse process occurred, with more power concentrated in the hands of individual committee chairpersons. Senator

Christopher Dodd (D-CT) of the Health, Education, Labor and Pensions Committee steered a health care reform bill swiftly through, with little negotiation. A straight party-line vote in July 2009 moved the bill to the floor. However, Senator Max Baucus (D-MT) of the Senate Finance Committee had released his own policy white paper on health care reform immediately following the 2008 election and was determined to engage the Republicans on his committee who had proven in the past to be supportive of public health insurance efforts. Both Senators Olympia Snowe (R-MN) and Orrin Hatch (R-UT) agreed to negotiate over the details of the bill. These negotiations dragged on through the summer, until Senator Baucus decided to end them and the bill was voted out of his committee with the sole Republican support of Senator Snowe (who later voted against the final bill) in October 2009. At this point, the Republicans in the Senate employed the filibuster rule to prevent the bill from even coming to a vote on the floor. After a grueling fight, on December 24, 2009, the Senate passed its version of the Patient Protection and Affordable Care Act, on a vote of 60 to 39 (with 60 votes needed to override the filibuster).

The conference committee to merge the two versions of the bill to send for the president's signature, however, proved to be an insurmountable hurdle for congressional leaders. They simply would not have the votes in the Senate if any of the House differences were included in the final bill. When Senator Scott Brown (R-MA) won the special election in January 2010 to fill the late Ted Kennedy's seat in the Senate, it seemed as if a Republican tide was about to sweep through Congress and that the health care reform momentum had shifted again. Speaker Pelosi and Majority Leader Reid were building support for an alternative legislative process called "reconciliation," but it would need full, unified support from the Democrats in the House and trust between the House and Senate (a difficult prospect) in order to work.

In this climate in early February 2010, the private health insurer Anthem decided to raise its rates on its individual plan members by as much as 30 percent in California, which drew the attention of the *Los Angeles Times* (Helfand, 2010). The story appeared in the newspaper and swiftly sparked a statewide, and then national, outcry over the abuses of consumers by the health insurance industry. By the end of the month, President Obama had convened a meeting of health insurance company leaders to publicly chastise them for consumer practices, and Congressman Henry Waxman had subpoenaed them in front of a congressional hearing on rate increases. Both Republican and Democratic state officeholders nationwide began to investigate rate increases, and their efforts continually made national headlines. With the political climate again in their favor, Democrats were able to implement the reconciliation process to pass the same version of the bill in both chambers, and the Patient Protection and Affordable Care Act was signed into law on March 23, 2010.

This process provides a historic example of a dedicated united majority party marshaling both legislative and public opinion forces to enact major legislation. Within a relatively short time frame in his first term in office (fourteen months), President Obama accomplished a major policy goal, which many other presidents over the preceding hundred years had attempted and failed. The scope of this accomplishment is historic. However, the lack of minority party support has hurt public opinion of the ACA, and the Republicans immediately announced that their major goal was the repeal or dismantling of what they termed "Obamacare." Just minutes after the ACA's enactment, the first major lawsuit against it was filed, with twenty-six state attorneys general and governors as the plaintiffs. They argued that the individual mandate impinged upon the freedom of their states' citizens. Numerous other lawsuits were also filed, but most were dismissed by the lower courts for lack of standing.

The United States Supreme Court decided in 2012 to review two judgments by the 11th Circuit Court of Appeals (including the multistate case), and review the constitutionality of both the individual mandate and the Medicaid expansion. They also included a review of whether the court had any standing to rule at this time (given that the "tax" in the individual mandate would not be assessed until 2015). The court ordered six hours of argument, which is more time given to any case since *Brown v. Board of Education* in 1954.

On June 28, 2012, the Supreme Court issued their decision. By a 9-to-0 vote, they upheld their right to issue an opinion at the current time. In a 5-to-4 vote, with Chief Justice John Roberts authoring the majority opinion, the court upheld the individual mandate as a tax that the IRS may administer, and therefore the law would stand. However, in a 7-to-2 vote, the court struck down the provision that mandated states had to expand their Medicaid programs in order to retain any federal Medicaid funding for the existing program (Kaiser Family Foundation, 2012b). States now had the option to reject the Medicaid expansion, giving more autonomy and power to governors, many of whom decided not to pursue the expansion after all, regardless of the increased federal funding. For more on this topic, see Chapter One.

Future Directions

With the Supreme Court decision and the reelection of President Obama in 2012, the full implementation of the ACA will occur in 2014 and beyond. However, even when it is fully in effect, the Congressional Budget Office (CBO) estimates that thirty million residents of the United States will remain uninsured (CBO, 2012). This residual uninsured population will be comprised mainly of (1) low-income families who waive out of the individual mandate, (2) higher-income families who either pay or perhaps refuse to pay the penalty, (3) American Indians with Indian Health Service access, and (4) undocumented immigrants. They will still need health care, and the concern is that the safety net will be starved for resources as funding moves elsewhere, on the assumption that the uninsured have now all gained coverage. Additionally, the exchanges might offer coverage that is still functionally unaffordable for many families.

With a large remaining group of uninsured residents, the United States might finally move in the one direction that has not yet been tried on a nationwide scale, that of establishing a government-funded default system of health insurance for everyone within our borders. The delivery system would remain largely privately owned and operated and would negotiate directly with this public payer through the insurance companies. Additionally, families could purchase private health insurance supplements, in much the same way as Medicare and Medigap policies exist today. This type of "Medicare for All" system would align our country with the insurance systems of much of the industrialized world, and would finally relieve our families and businesses of the burdens of either paying for or worrying about paying for health care. However, the United States will only move in this direction if the ACA fails to deliver on its promise of providing affordable health insurance to both the uninsured and the underinsured.

As the great experiment of the ACA unfolds, its successes and failures will define the next challenges facing the health care system.

SUMMARY

This chapter focused on the uninsured and public programs in the United States that expand health care coverage for targeted populations. It is designed to provide a basic understanding of the historical trends and current picture of Medicare, Medicaid, and the State Children's Health Insurance Program (SCHIP). Additionally, this chapter provided insights into the political barriers that blocked comprehensive health insurance expansions prior to the enactment of the Patient Protection and Affordable Care Act of 2010 (ACA) and the historic political process that coalesced to facilitate the ACA. Chapter Six covered the following topics:

- Demographics of the growing uninsured population
- Trends in Medicare, Medicaid, and SCHIP
- Previous failed attempts to extend health insurance coverage to the entire U.S. population
- The enactment of the ACA and implications of the Supreme Court decision of June 2012

KEY TERMS

Affordable Care Act (ACA) The Patient Protection and Affordable Care Act of 2010, also known as "Obamacare." This law reallocated funds in the health care system to provide new options for health insurance to the uninsured, namely the *exchanges* and the *Medicaid expansion* (discussed later in this list). An *exchange* is a state-based web portal that acts as a marketplace in which individuals or small groups can purchase health insurance. Individuals with household incomes between 139 percent and 400 percent of the federal poverty level (FPL) will be eligible to receive federal subsidies to purchase the insurance if they have no "affordable" offer of coverage through an employer.

Children's Health Insurance Program (CHIP) A federal-state partnership health insurance program designed to cover the children of the "working poor," namely those with incomes slightly above the Medicaid eligibility limit. Enrollees are not entitled to this coverage, but can only obtain it if funding is available.

Medicaid A federal-state partnership entitlement health insurance program launched in 1965 that provides comprehensive coverage (until 2014) to low-income children, their parents, and the aged, blind, and disabled. In January 2014, states will have the option of implementing the *Medicaid expansion* and providing coverage for all adults (including those without children) with household incomes up to 138 percent FPL.

Medicare A federal entitlement health insurance program launched in 1965 that provides coverage for citizens and legal permanent residents of the United States who have paid Medicare taxes through work for ten quarters and are age sixty-five or older or who are disabled. *Part A* covers hospital and other facility-based care, *Part B* covers doctor visits and other ambulatory care services, and *Part D* covers prescription drugs. Enrollees may also choose a comprehensive managed care plan through *Medicare Advantage (Part C)*.

Uninsured People who do not have medical insurance coverage through any source, including their employment, an individually purchased plan, or a public plan.

DISCUSSION QUESTIONS

1. What are the major groups that comprise the uninsured population? What factors seem most important in putting people at risk of becoming uninsured?
2. What are the different parts of Medicare, and what do they cover? What are the major differences between Medicare and Medicaid in terms of their target populations, services covered, and financing systems?
3. Medicare enjoys widespread support among the general population, while Medicaid is often targeted for program cuts, which suggests that it has less public support. What characteristics distinguish Medicare and Medicaid that might contribute to differences in political support?
4. How did the enactment process of the ACA differ from the previously failed attempts to provide comprehensive health insurance on a nationwide scale?

FURTHER READING

Altman, S., & Schactman, D. (2011). *Power, politics, and universal health care.* New York: Prometheus Books.

REFERENCES

Aday, L., & Andersen, R. (1983). Equity of access to medical care: A conceptual and empirical overview. In *Securing access to health care: The ethical implications of differences in the availability of health services.* Washington, DC: President's Commission for the Study of Ethical Problems in Medicine and Biomedical and Behavioral Research.

Aday, L., Andersen, R., & Fleming, G. V. (1980). *Health care in the U.S.: Equitable for whom?* Thousand Oaks, CA: Sage.

Aday, L., Begley, C. E., Lairson, D. R., & Slater, C. H. (1998). *Evaluating the health care system: Effectiveness, efficiency, and equity* (2nd ed.). Chicago: Health Administration Press.

AHIP Center for Policy and Research. (2010). *January 2010 Census shows 10 million people covered by HSA/high-deductible health plans.* Washington, DC: AHIP Center for Policy and Research.

Almeida, R. A., Dubay, L. C., & Ko, G. (2001). Access to care and use of health services by low-income women. *Health Care Finance Review, 22*(4), 27–47.

Berk, M. L., Schur, C. L., & Cantor, J. C. (1995). Ability to obtain health care: Recent estimates from the Robert Wood Johnson Foundation National Access to Care Survey. *Health Affairs, 14*(3), 139–146.

Biles, B., Pozen, J., & Guterman, S. (2009). Paying Medicare Advantage plans by competitive bidding: How much competition is there? *Issue brief (Commonwealth Fund), 65,* 1–12.

Blendon, R. J., & Taylor, H. (1989). Views on health care: Public opinion in three nations. *Health Affairs, 8,* 149–157.

Cantor, J. C., Barand, N. L., Desonia, R. A., Cohen, A. B., & Merrill, J. C. (1991). Business leaders' views on American health care. *Health Affairs, 10,* 98–105.

Centers for Medicare and Medicaid Services. (2011). Health expenditures by state of residence. Retrieved from www.cms.gov/nationalhealthexpenddata/downloads/resident-state-estimates.zip

Congressional Budget Office. (2012, July). Estimates for the insurance coverage provisions of the Affordable Care Act updated for the recent Supreme Court decision. Washington, DC: Author.

Coughlin, T. A., & Long, S. K. (2000). Effects of Medicaid managed care on adults. *Medical Care, 38*(4), 433–446.

Cunningham, P. J., Hadley, J., & Reschovsky, J. (2002). The effects of SCHIP on children's health insurance coverage: Early evidence from the Community Tracking Survey. *Medical Care Research and Review, 59*(4), 359–383.

Current Population Survey. (2011). *Author's analysis of data accessed from the SHADAC Data Access Center.* Retrieved from www.shadac.org/datacenter

Davidoff, A., Kenney, G., & Dubay, L. (2005). Effects of the State Children's Health Insurance Program expansions on children with chronic health conditions. *Pediatrics, 116,* 34–42.

Davis, K. (1975). Equal treatment and unequal benefits: The Medicare program. *Milbank Memorial Fund Quarterly/Health and Society, 53,* 449–488.

Finkelstein, A., Taubman, S., Wright, B., Bernstein, M., Gruber, J., Newhouse, J. P., . . . Baicker, K. (2011). *The Oregon health insurance experiment: Evidence from the first year* (NBER Working Paper No. 17190).

Freeman, H. E., & Corey, C. R. (1993). Insurance status and access to health services among poor persons. *Health Services Research, 28*(5), 531–541.

Fuchs, V. R., & Hahn, J. S. (1990). How does Canada do it? A comparison of expenditures for physicians' services in the United States and Canada. *New England Journal of Medicine, 323,* 884–890.

Garrett, B., Davidoff, A. J., & Yemane, A. (2003). Effects of Medicaid managed care programs on health services access and use. *Health Services Research, 38(2)*, 575–594.

Gaskin, D. J., Briesacher, B. A., Limcangco, R., & Brigantti, B. L. (2006). Exploring racial and ethnic disparities in prescription drug spending and use among Medicare beneficiaries. *American Journal of Geriatric Pharmacotherapy, 4(2)*, 96–111.

Hayes, G. J., Hayes, C., & Dykstra, T. (1993). Physicians who have practiced in both the U.S. and Canada compare systems. *American Journal of Public Health, 83*, 1544–1548.

Health Resources Administration. (1980). *Health of the disadvantaged: Chart book II* (DHHS Pub. No. [HRA] 80–633). Washington, DC: U.S. Government Printing Office.

Helfand, D. (2010, February 4). Anthem Blue Cross dramatically raising rates for Californians with individual health policies. Los Angeles Times.

Hessol, N. A., Vittinghoff, E., & Fuentes-Afflick, E. (2004). Reduced risk of inadequate prenatal care in the era after Medicaid expansions in California. *Medical Care, 42(5)*, 416–422.

Himmelstein, D. U., Thorne, D., Warren, E., & Woolhandler, S. (2009). Medical bankruptcy in the United States, 2007: Results of a national study. *American Journal of Medicine, 122*(8), 741–746.

Holl, J. L, Slack, K. S., & Stevens, A. B. (2005). Welfare reform and health insurance: Consequences for parents. *American Journal of Public Health, 95*(2), 279–285.

Iglehart, J. K. (2000). Revisiting the Canadian health care system. *New England Journal of Medicine, 342*, 2007–2012.

Kaestner, R., Dubay, L., & Kenney, G. (2005). Managed care and infant health: An evaluation of Medicaid in the U.S. *Social Science and Medicine, 60*, 1815–1833.

Kaiser Commission on the Future of Medicaid. (1995). *Medicaid and managed care: Lessons from the literature.* Menlo Park, CA: Henry J. Kaiser Family Foundation.

Kaiser Commission on Medicaid and the Uninsured. (2005a). *Medicaid: An overview of spending on "mandatory" vs. "optional" populations and services.* Menlo Park: Henry J. Kaiser Family Foundation.

Kaiser Commission on Medicaid and the Uninsured. (2005b). *Enrolling uninsured low-income children in Medicaid and SCHIP.* Menlo Park, CA: Henry J. Kaiser Family Foundation.

Kaiser Commission on Medicaid and the Uninsured & Urban Institute. (2012). *Estimates based on data from FY2008 MSIS.* Retrieved from www.kff.org/medicare/upload/8138–02.pdf

Kaiser Family Foundation. (2004, September). Employer health benefits 2004 annual survey. Chicago: Health Research and Educational Trust.

Kaiser Family Foundation. (2012a). State health facts. Retrieved from www.statehealthfacts.org

Kaiser Family Foundation. (2012b). A guide to the Supreme Court's Affordable Care Act decision. Retrieved from http://www.kff.org/healthreform

Kasper, J. D. (1986). Health status and utilization: Differences by Medicaid coverage and income. *Health Care Financing Review, 7*, 1–17.

Kempe, A., Beaty, B. L., Crane, L. A., Stokstad, J., Barrow, J., Belman, S., & Steiner, J. F. (2005). Changes in access, utilization, and quality of care after enrollment into a State Child Health Insurance Plan. *Pediatrics, 115*(2), 494–494.

Krebs-Carter, M., & Holahan, J. (2000). *State strategies for covering uninsured adults.* Washington, DC: Urban Institute.

Link, C. R., Long, S. H., & Settle, R. F. (1982). Equity and the utilization of health services by the Medicare elderly. *Journal of Human Resources, 17,* 195–212.

Long, S. H., & Settle, R. F. (1984). Medicare and the disadvantaged elderly: Objectives and outcomes. *Milbank Memorial Fund Quarterly/Health and Society, 62,* 609–656.

Loranger, L., & Lipson, D. (1995). *The Medicaid expansions for pregnant women and children.* Washington, DC: Alpha Center.

Lo Sasso, A. T., & Buchmueller, T. C. (2004). The effect of the State Children's Health Insurance Program on health insurance coverage. *Journal of Health Economics, 23,* 1059–1082.

Lurie, N., Ward, N. B., Shapiro, M. F., & Brook, R. H. (1984). Termination from Medi-Cal: Does it affect health? *New England Journal of Medicine, 311,* 480–484.

Marmor, T. R. (2000). *The politics of Medicare* (2nd ed.). Chicago: Aldine.

Marquis, M. S., & Long, S. H. (1996). Reconsidering the effect of Medicaid on health care services use. *Health Services Research, 30,* 791–808.

Marquis, M. S., Rogowski, J. A., & Escarce, J. J. (2004–2005). The managed care backlash: Did consumers vote with their feet? *Inquiry, 41*(4), 376–390.

McBean, A. M., & Gornick, M. (1994). Differences by race in the rates of procedures performed in hospitals for Medicare beneficiaries. *Health Care Financing Review, 15,* 77–90.

McDonough, J. E., Rosman, B., Phelps F., & Shannon, M. (2006). The third wave of Massachusetts health care reform. *Health Affairs, 25*(6), 420–431.

Mechanic, D. (2004). The rise and fall of managed care. *Journal of Health and Social Behavior, 45*(Suppl), 76–86.

Millman, M. (Ed.) (1993). *Access to health care in America.* Washington, DC: National Academy Press, Institute of Medicine.

Mitchell, J. B., & Khandker, R. K. (1995). Black-white treatment differences in acute myocardial infarction. *Health Care Financing Review, 17,* 61–70.

Navarro, V. (1989). Why some countries have national health insurance, others have national health services, and the U.S. has neither. *Social Science and Medicine, 28,* 887–898.

Newacheck, P. (1988). Access to ambulatory care for poor persons. *Health Services Research, 23,* 401–419.

NGA Center for Best Practices. (2003). *MCH update 2002: State health coverage for low-income pregnant women, children, and parents.* Washington, DC: NGA Center for Best Practices.

Oberlander, J. (2010). Long time coming: Why health reform finally passed. *Health Affairs, 29*(6), 1112–1116.

Perry, M. J., Stark, E., & Valdez, R. B. (1998). *Barriers to Medi-Cal enrollment and ideas for improving enrollment: Findings from eight focus groups in California with parents of potentially eligible children.* Menlo Park, CA: Henry J. Kaiser Family Foundation.

Physician Payment Review Commission (PPRC). (1994). *Annual report to Congress, 1994.* Washington, DC: Physician Payment Review Commission.

Ray, W.A., Mitchel, E. F., Jr., & Piper, J. M. (1997). Effect of Medicaid expansions on preterm birth. *American Journal of Preventive Medicine, 13*(4), 292–297.

Robinson, J. C. (2004). Reinvention of health insurance in the consumer era. *Journal of the American Medical Association, 291*(15), 1886–1886.

Rothman, D. J. (1993). A century of failure: Health care reform in America. *Journal of Health Politics, Policy and Law, 18*, 271–286.

Rosenblatt, R. A. (1989, November 16). Business groups plead for health-care support. *Los Angeles Times, p. A20.*

Schoen, C., Doty, M. M., Robertson, R. H., & Collins, S. R. (2011). Affordable Care Act reforms could reduce the number of underinsured U.S. adults by 70 percent. *Health Affairs, 30*(9), 1762–1771.

Selden, T. M. & Gray, B. M. (2006). Tax subsidies for employment-related health insurance: Estimates for 2006. *Health Affairs, 25*(6), 1568–1579.

Somers, H. W., & Somers, A. R. (1961). *Doctors, patients and health insurance.* Washington, DC: Brookings Institution.

U.S. Congressional Budget Office. (2010, March 18). *Letter to Speaker Nancy Pelosi.*

U.S. Department of Labor, Bureau of Labor Statistics. (2012). Retrieved from www.bls.gov

Wenneker, M. B., & Epstein, A. M. (1989). Racial inequalities in the use of procedures for patients with ischemic heart disease in Massachusetts. *Journal of the American Medical Association, 261*, 253–257.

West, M. W., Heith, D., & Goodwin, C. (1996). Harry and Louise go to Washington: Political advertising and health care reform. *Journal of Health Politics, Policy and Law, 21*, 35–68.

Wheeler, S. B., Carpenter, W. R., Peppercorn, J., Schenck, A. P., Weinberger, M., & Biddle, A. K. (2012). Structural/organizational characteristics of health services partly explain racial variation in timeliness of radiation therapy among elderly breast cancer patients. *Breast Cancer Research and Treatment, 133*(1), 333–345.

Wilensky, G. R., & Berk, M. L. (1982). Health care, the poor, and the role of Medicaid. *Health Affairs, 1*, 93–100.

Zelman, W. (2009). *Swimming upstream: The hard politics of health care reform in California.* Los Angeles: UCLA Center for Health Policy Research.

CHAPTER SEVEN

PRIVATE HEALTH INSURANCE

Nadereh Pourat
Gerald F. Kominski

Learning Objectives

- Identify key concepts in private (and public) insurance
- Understand the various markets for private health insurance in the United States, including both employment-based and individually purchased insurance
- Learn about significant trends in private insurance
- Understand the ongoing evolution of managed care

Private insurance has been the predominant source of insurance coverage in the United States since the first Blue Cross plan was established in 1929. After the enactment of Medicare and Medicaid in 1965, public insurance has grown steadily and was the primary source of coverage for 31 percent of the U.S. population as of 2010, while private insurance was the sole source of insurance for 52.7 percent of the population (DeNavas-Walt, Proctor, & Smith, 2011). The private insurance market also includes a substantial number of Medicare beneficiaries, who obtain additional coverage to supplement their Medicare benefits. Private coverage after retirement may be provided through a previous employer as part of retirement benefits, purchased through unions or other groups, or purchased in the private market.

Since 1994, the rate of employment-based insurance for the population ages 0 to 64 has declined in United States from 60.9 percent in 1994 to 55.3 percent in 2010 (see Figure 7.1) (Fronstin, 2011). However, the rate of coverage increased from 1994 to 2000, peaking at 69.3 percent with a steady decline since that year. During the same time frame, the rate of individually purchased coverage has declined slightly from 7.5 percent in 1994 to 7.1 percent in 2010.

Employment-based and individually purchased coverage vary in several respects, including premiums, comprehensiveness of benefits, cost sharing required, and predominance of types of plans available in each market. The benefits offered under private insurance range from basic medical services to additional benefits such as behavioral, dental, and vision. These additional benefits are frequently optional services or riders offered by plans that specialize in such benefits and have differential levels of cost sharing, benefits, and annual limits. The trends in choice of various plans offered and enrollment in those plans have also changed over time. These trends also vary by employment-based and individually purchased insurance.

Evolution of Private Health Insurance

The dominance of private health insurance, specifically employment-based insurance, in the United States is commonly attributed to events following WWII. Postwar economic growth led to a tight labor market and inclusion of health insurance as a noncash benefit to be used in competition for workers. Changes in federal tax laws allowing exemptions of premiums added additional incentives for employers to provide health benefits.

Between 1945 and 1964, coverage for private hospitalization insurance increased from 24 percent to 79 percent of the population, with nearly two-thirds of the insured receiving their coverage from group policies. In 1964, 71 percent also had coverage for surgical insurance, which paid fees for physicians' surgical fees (U.S. Public Health Service, n.d.). Despite these seemingly high rates of coverage in 1964, insurance benefits were at 20 percent of total national health expenditures, and national health expenditures accounted for 5.9 percent of the gross national product (U.S. Public Health Service, n.d.). Private insurance was beneficial to both the insured and providers of health care because it protected individuals from catastrophic medical expenses and insured payment to providers. The financial burden on employers was also limited, given the scope of coverage and federal tax exemptions.

FIGURE 7.1. TRENDS IN PRIVATE INSURANCE COVERAGE IN THE UNITED STATES, 1994–2010, AGES 0–64

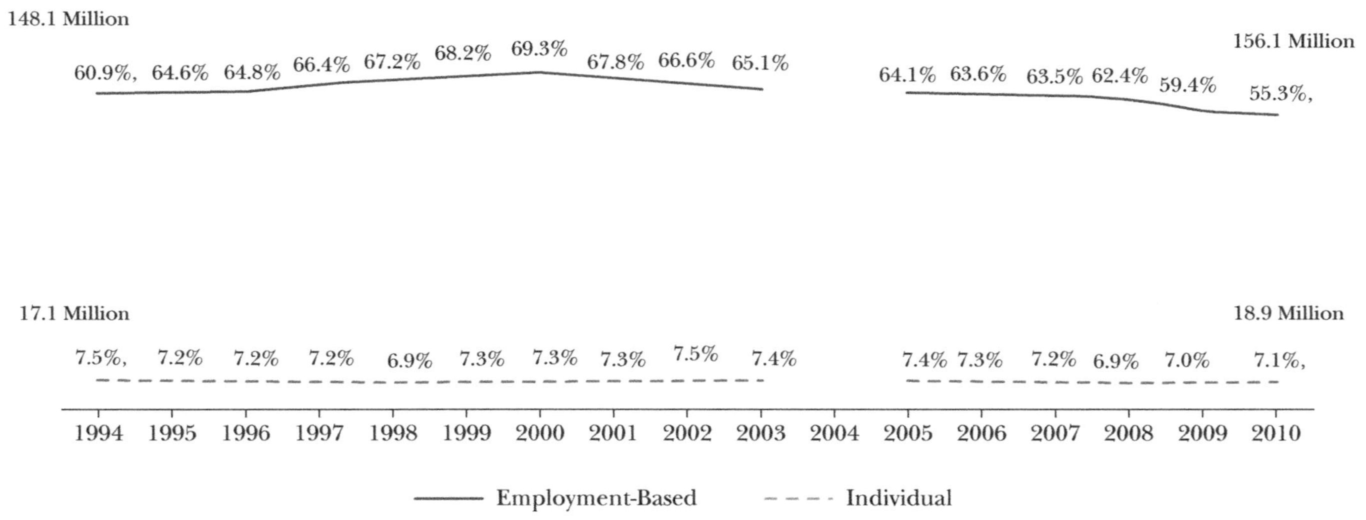

148.1 Million   156.1 Million

60.9%, 64.6% 64.8% 66.4% 67.2% 68.2% 69.3% 67.8% 66.6% 65.1%   64.1% 63.6% 63.5% 62.4% 59.4% 55.3%,

17.1 Million   18.9 Million

7.5%, 7.2% 7.2% 7.2% 6.9% 7.3% 7.3% 7.5% 7.4%   7.4% 7.3% 7.2% 6.9% 7.0% 7.1%

1994 1995 1996 1997 1998 1999 2000 2001 2002 2003 2004 2005 2006 2007 2008 2009 2010

———— Employment-Based   – – – – Individual

Note: 2004 data not available.
Source: Fronstin, 2011.

Concepts in Private Health Insurance

The meaning and implications of some concepts, such as moral hazard and premiums, are nearly universal in the field of private health insurance. However, other concepts such as those in managed care and payment methods continue to evolve or exist in multiple variations. Yet other concepts are frequently used interchangeably in various contexts. Thus, a basic description of the most common concepts in private health insurance is necessary prior to the discussion of the dominant issues in this field.

Premiums

Premiums are the monthly or annual amount paid by employers and individuals who purchase health insurance. In employment-based insurance, employers may pay the entire amount of premium, share the premium with employees who participate in that coverage, or require the participating employees to pay the entire amount. Frequently, the employee share of premium is inversely related to the employee participation rate in employment-based insurance. Nationwide trends in premiums are often used as an indication of inflation in health care prices, since premium increases are closely tied to provider payments and health care utilization levels.

Community Rating versus Experience Rating

Community rating is the practice of setting health insurance premiums based on the average health care use and expenditures of a community, frequently defined as a geographic area. Under this method, the premiums are the same for individuals regardless of their characteristics. Thus, older adults, smokers, and young athletes will all pay the same premium. In contrast, *experience rating* is the practice of setting health insurance premiums based on the health care use and expenditures of a particular group to be insured. Under this method, groups with a higher proportion of older, sicker, or at-risk individuals will have higher premiums than groups with a higher proportion of young adults and healthy children. The differences between the two methods are at times blurred, with elements of each method blended. For example, the community rating method can be "adjusted" to allow for differences in age, gender, or smoking status of the population to be insured. From the insurer's perspective, experience rating is a more representative method of setting premiums and poses a lower level of financial risk than community rating. Regulation is frequently used to modify experience rating to protect individuals or small groups who may be otherwise unable to purchase private insurance due to past illness or high-risk jobs.

Comprehensive versus Single Specialty Plans

The basic medical services or benefits covered under comprehensive health insurance policies include hospitalizations, emergency services, physician visits, laboratory, imaging, and pharmaceuticals. Other benefits such as behavioral health, dental, vision, and long-term care may be included in the package of benefits and are called riders. These benefits are often carved out or provided by plans that specialize in coverage and delivery of those services. The terms of coverage by these specialty plans differ from the major medical plans, with variations in share of premiums paid by employees, scope of services covered, deductibles and cost-sharing requirements, and annual out-of-pocket and lifetime limits.

Parity

Significant restrictions and variations in coverage by mental health specialty plans have caused concerns over unequal benefit levels, cost sharing, and annual and lifetime limits and their impact on those most in need of services. These concerns led to legislation requiring parity of mental health benefits with medical and surgical benefits. Currently, other specially plans such as dental or vision are not subject to parity.

Retrospective versus Prospective Provider Payment

As in purchase of other goods and services, providers of health care were traditionally paid for services after rendering care. This retrospective payment method was replaced by HMOs and Medicare, which employed various prospective payment systems including capitation. The prospective payment method provides a set payment for a patient or for specific services with the intention of incentivizing providers to contain costs.

Health Maintenance Organizations (HMOs)

HMOs are the traditional form of managed care. Group-model HMOs contract with a single medical group to provide care to plan members, while staff-model HMOs employ physicians directly. In group-model HMOs, the medical group usually contracts exclusively with the HMO, which is known as a closed panel; that is, providers do not treat patients outside the HMO. Staff-model HMOs are by definition closed panels. Group- and staff-model HMOs represent a traditional model of managed care that many physicians view as excessively intrusive and many consumers see as too restrictive because of their closed panels. Therefore, alternative models have evolved that allow physicians greater autonomy in how their practices are organized and permit greater choice for plan members. Network-model HMOs contract with multiple medical groups, rather than a single group, while HMOs on the independent practice association (IPA) model contract with individual physicians in solo practice. Network- and IPA-model HMOs are typically open panel; physicians do not contract exclusively with a single HMO and may continue to treat non-HMO patients.

All forms of HMOs employ some form of gatekeeper, a primary care physician who serves as the initial point of contact for receiving care and who must authorize referrals for specialty care. However, in response to competitive pressures during the 1990s, HMOs have begun offering multiple managed care products. For example, some HMOs offer an open-access product that allows self-referral within the network but imposes increased cost sharing on members who choose this option. These hybrid arrangements are likely to continue growing in response to changing perceptions of what best serves the interests of the health plans, providers, and members.

Preferred Provider Organizations (PPOs)

PPOs represent a less restrictive form of managed care than the HMO, mainly because they do not require primary care physicians to serve as gatekeepers and thus permit self-referral to specialists. They are generally formed by employers or insurers who contract with physicians and other providers to create a network of participating or preferred providers. These preferred providers generally agree to follow utilization management guidelines and to accept discounted fee-for-service payments as conditions for participating in the PPO. Health plan members are encouraged to use the preferred provider network through reduced cost sharing, although they are generally covered for care provided by nonparticipating physicians. The mechanism that allows the creation of PPOs is known as selective contracting.

A variation of PPO insurance is an exclusive provider organization (EPO). EPOs are similar to PPOs in organization and benefit structure but do not reimburse services obtained from nonparticipating physicians.

Point-of-Service (POS) Plans

POS plans are essentially the same as the open-access HMOs already described, but they also offer limited coverage for self-referral outside the network. Members may choose the level of managed care they desire at the point of service, with the degree of cost sharing increasing along with freedom of choice. Members in these three-tier plans who use a gatekeeper (HMO tier) have the lowest copayments, while those self-referring to network providers (PPO tier) have higher copayments, and those seeking care outside the network (POS tier) have the highest copayments.

Indemnity and Fee-for-Service Insurance

Indemnity refers to reimbursing or indemnifying the insured person who has already paid the provider for services rendered. Fee for service (FFS) specifically refers to the retrospective method of payment for services rendered by a provider. Frequently, the two terms are used interchangeably to refer to a form of insurance that directly reimburses the provider for services provided. The payment amount may be based on a predetermined fee schedule or a "reasonable, usual, and customary" amount, rather than providers' charges. The incentive under the FFS payment method is to provide more services per patient with no financial risk to providers.

Capitation

Under *capitation*, providers receive a fixed per-member, per-month payment for an individual who enrolls in the provider's patient panel. Thus, the provider is responsible for delivering all the care required for that enrollee regardless of the enrollee's health status. The incentive under capitation is to provide fewer services per patient. Clauses in insurer and provider contracts can modify the level of financial risk assumed by the provider or impose performance measures to change provider behavior in certain ways. For example, including share of profits to capitation in provider reimbursement can incentivize better management of chronic conditions to avoid hospitalizations and high-cost services.

Deductible

Deductible refers to a specific predetermined annual amount to be paid by the insured before the insurer pays for health care services. The main purpose of the deductible is to protect the insurer from moral hazard and reduce the liability of the insurer by sharing some of the risk and expenditures with the insured. Thus, the deductible amount varies inversely with the premium amount. Deductibles are infrequently applied in HMO policies because of more utilization oversight and restrictions in choice of providers. Some policies may apply differential amounts of deductibles per category of service such as hospitalization or emergency room visits, to further discourage use of specific services and share the risk with the insured.

Cost Sharing

Insurance policies infrequently cover the entire costs of health care used by the insured and require some level of *cost sharing*. While deductibles are also designed to share the costs of health care with the insured, cost sharing refers specifically to the amount the insured must pay for each service used. In HMO policies, cost sharing is typically a fixed dollar amount, also called a *copayment*. In PPO policies, cost sharing is typically a percentage of the total cost of the service, and is called a *coinsurance rate*.

Annual Out-of-Pocket and Lifetime Maximums

Annual out-of-pocket maximum is the total amount the insured person is expected to pay toward deductibles and cost sharing in a given year. This provision is designed to limit the undue financial burden on the insured person, but does not include the share of premiums paid by the insured with employment-based or group policies. Lifetime maximum is the amount an insurer will pay toward the costs of care incurred by an insured person in his or her lifetime and is a mechanism to protect the insurer from the high costs of catastrophic illness by the insured.

Moral Hazard

The concept of *moral hazard* in health insurance refers to the higher likelihood of use of health care in the absence of responsibility to pay for that care. For example, the insured may be more likely to use discretionary or elective health care in the absence of any cost sharing. Tools such as deductibles and cost sharing are used by insurers to address moral hazard.

Adverse Selection

Adverse selection, also referred to as cream skimming and cherry picking, occurs when health plans enroll healthier individuals and avoid enrolling those who are sicker or at higher risk. The exclusion of preexisting conditions is a manifestation of adverse selection, though other practices such as higher premiums for smokers and older individuals and targeted marketing of HMO policies to healthy Medicare beneficiaries can have the same outcomes. When individuals choose to enroll in specific plans, the process is called *self-selection*.

Rescission

An insurer has the right to rescind or cancel a policy if the insured has withheld or misrepresented information related to his or her health or committed fraud. Rescissions most frequently occur if the insured withholds or misrepresents information on the existence of preexisting conditions. The preexisting condition clauses and rescissions are most frequently applied to individual insurance policies. These practices are infrequently applied to group policies, as risk of financial loss to the insurer is spread over a larger population and is therefore considerably smaller. Regulation can be used to limit rescissions by requiring the insurer to provide proof of "intent to deceive" by the insured or disallow the insurers to apply the preexisting condition clauses. Such regulations are intended to avoid rescissions of policies for patients diagnosed with costly illnesses or enable individuals to purchase health insurance.

Guaranteed Issue

Guaranteed issue refers to a requirement that insurers will issue a policy to individuals, self-employed persons, or small groups regardless of preexisting conditions, health status, or claims history. Guaranteed issue has been required by law for all small-group employers and is now required by law under the 2010 Patient Protection and Affordable Care Act for individual insurance as well.

Underwriting

Underwriting refers to the process of evaluating the health status and past health care utilization of an applicant for insurance. Insurers use health status and past health care use of individuals to determine whether to offer coverage and at what premium.

Self-Insurance

Typically insurers accept financial risk for paying all the claims incurred by the insured population. However, an employer or other organization has the option to take on that financial risk for its employees or members and self-insure. An organization has the option to self-insure fully or partially.

Managed Competition

First proposed by Alain Enthoven in the late 1970s (Enthoven, 1978, 1993), *managed competition* is designed to build on the strengths of private insurance markets by addressing their weaknesses through regulated competition. Enthoven proposed to standardize insurance policies so that price comparison among similar products was possible, and to address inefficiencies in the demand side of the market by pooling small companies and individual purchasers into larger groups known as health insurance purchasing cooperatives (HIPCs). Enthoven's model of managed competition was based on the Federal Employees Health Benefits Program (FEHBP). It is the conceptual foundation for health insurance exchanges that are central to both the Massachusetts health reform legislation enacted in 2006 and the federal Affordable Care Act enacted in 2010, as well as international health reform efforts in the Netherlands, Switzerland, and Israel.

Employment-Based Health Insurance

Not all employers offer health insurance benefits to their employees. An estimated 60 percent of firms nationwide offered health insurance benefits to their workers in 2010, a decline from 66 percent in 1999 (Claxton et al., 2012). The decision to offer insurance is influenced primarily by the behavior of similar firms in the market, the firm's financial reserves, and the competition for qualified workers. Offer rates are highest (99 percent in 2010) among large firms with two hundred or more employees and lowest (48 percent in 2010) among smallest firms with three to nine employees. Also, firms with large proportions of young, part-time, low-wage, and nonunionized workers less often offer coverage.

The small-employer health insurance market, for firms with fewer than fifty employees, is characterized by higher premiums and fewer choice of products than the large-group market (America's Health Insurance Plans, 2010). Despite previous attempts at market reform to regulate premium levels and guaranteed issuing of policies to firms with historical high claims expenditures, the offer rates for small firms remains lower than large firms.

Not all workers are eligible for coverage offered by their employers or willing to participate. Historically, employers have excluded seasonal or part-time employees and imposed waiting times before employees can enroll. Employers who exclude coverage for dependents, do not pay any share of the employee's premium, offer high premiums policies, or offer a limited choice of plans are more likely to have lower participation levels. Among firms with health insurance benefits, participation or take-up rate among eligible employees was 81 percent in 2011 (Claxton et al., 2012).

The factors associated with offer rates and eligibility restrictions have led to higher rates of employment-based insurance coverage among certain employers. In 2010, employment-based coverage was higher for public sector (85 percent) and manufacturing (77 percent) industries than agriculture, forestry, and fishing (50 percent); higher for private sector firms with one thousand or more employees (77 percent) than private sector firms with fewer than ten employees (46 percent); and higher for managerial and professional jobs (82 percent) than construction and maintenance jobs (35 percent) (Fronstin, 2011).

Dependent coverage is a significant source of coverage for many Americans. About half of the population with employment-based insurance are dependents (Fronstin, 2011). Thus, the increasing costs of dependent coverage and the affordability of these policies are major policy concerns. Single coverage premiums are lower than premiums for family coverage, and the gap between these premiums has expanded threefold in 2012 (see Figure 7.2) (Claxton et al., 2012).

The rapid rise in premiums has led to a comparable increase in employees' share of premiums, as the increasing costs are passed on directly to employees. An increase of 160 percent in health insurance premiums from 1999 to 2011 coincides with a 168 percent increase in the employees' share of the premium during the same time period (Claxton et al., 2012). The share of premiums paid by employers is considered a business expense and is not taxed. Exemption of premiums from payroll tax is designed to encourage offering of health benefits by employers.

ERISA and Self-Insurance

Firms with sufficient financial reserves and positive outlook have the choice to self-insure rather than purchase insurance for their employees. The passage of the Employee Retirement and Income Security Act (ERISA) of

FIGURE 7.2. AVERAGE ANNUAL PREMIUMS FOR SINGLE AND FAMILY COVERAGE, 1999–2012

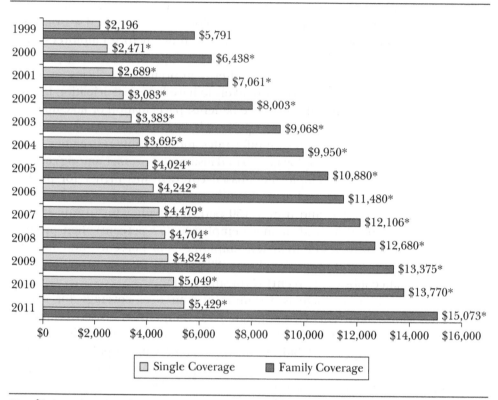

Note: *Estimate is statistically different from estimate for the previous year shown (p<.05).
Source: Claxton et al., 2012.

1974 set minimum requirements for self-insured plans, but also provided additional benefits and incentives to self-insure. The law exempted self-insured firms from state benefit mandates, making it possible for national firms to offer the benefits regardless of state mandates. The law also exempted self-insured employers from any taxes on premiums, allowing availability of high-premium plans for executives or certain employees if desired. The law also allowed employers significant flexibility in the benefits offered. Most significantly, the control of reserves needed to pay for claims remains with the self-insured firm rather than the insurer, allowing interest earnings to accrue to the employer.

Amendments to ERISA in subsequent legislation further regulated self-funded plans to prohibit unfavorable practices. The Consolidated Omnibus Budget Reconciliation Act of 1985 gave employees the right to continue their coverage after loss of their jobs for a limited time. The Health Insurance Portability and Accountability Act (HIPAA) of 1996 restricted exclusion of employees from plans due to preexisting conditions and did not allow variations in premiums among employees in the same plan. The Mental Health Parity Act of 1996 also prohibited self-insured plans who offer mental health benefits from imposing differential limits on benefits and annual and lifetime dollar limits, with some exceptions for firms with fifty or fewer employees (Purcell & Staman, 2009).

Trends in Dominant Types of Employment-Based Coverage

The dominant types of employment-based coverage have changed dramatically over the past two decades. In 1988, conventional fee-for-service plans covered 73 percent of workers in the United States with HMOs (16 percent) and PPOs (11 percent) in distant second and third places (see Figure 7.3). In 2012, conventional FFS plans covered less than 1 percent, HMOs covered 16 percent, and PPOs covered 56 percent of workers nationally (Claxton et al., 2012). These changes were primarily due to the escalating costs of health care, which translated to increasing premiums paid by employers and employees. Employers turned away from conventional FFS plans that did not include any cost-control mechanisms in favor of managed care plans to control utilization and costs. Enrollment in HMOs and POS plans increased to over half of the workers in 1999, but the backlash against the strict gatekeeping practices of these plans, particularly restricted self-referral to specialists, led to increased enrollment in PPO plans. The advent of consumer-directed ideology in health care use and the promise of reduced employer expenditures were followed by an increasing rate of covered workers in high-deductible health plans, from 4 percent in 2006 to 19 percent in 2012.

High-Deductible Health Plans

High-deductible health plans (HDHPs) are promoted as vehicles for reducing health care costs by incentivizing the insured to use less health care and seek high-quality services. HDHPs are paired with optional health savings accounts (HSAs) or health reimbursement accounts (HRAs) to encourage policyholders to save the funds that would otherwise be spent on health care and to shelter those savings from taxation.

HSAs are optional savings accounts established by the individual to pay for medical expenditures, are not affected by changes in jobs, and can roll over each year and into retirement (Reed et al., 2012). HSAs were first authorized by the Medicare Modernization Act of 2003 as a nontaxable

FIGURE 7.3. DISTRIBUTION OF HEALTH PLAN ENROLLMENT FOR COVERED WORKERS, BY PLAN TYPE, 1988–2012

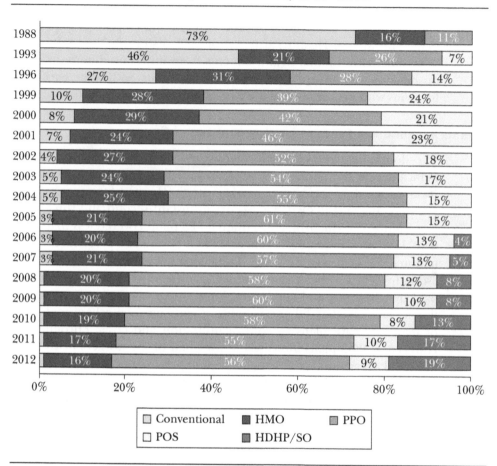

Note: A portion of the change in plan type enrollment for 2005 is likely attributable to incorporating more recent Census Bureau estimates of the number of state and local government workers and removing federal workers from the weights. Information was not obtained for POS plans in 1988.
Source: Claxton et al., 2012.

savings account established and used by the individual, to be used solely in conjunction with a high-deductible health policy. Both employers and employees can contribute to an HSA. Employer contributions are optional and not taxable to the employee. HSAs can be carried over to future years and can be retained after retirement and with any change of plans. Funds can be used for medical expenses covered by the plan and for those not covered, such as eyeglasses. Funds used for nonmedical expenses are subject to a tax penalty. Employers may contribute to employee HSAs in the amounts generally equitable to individual and family deductibles for an average PPO plan (Claxton et al., 2012). HSA annual maximum contributions are set by law annually and have been limited by ACA.

HRAs are savings accounts that were first authorized by the Internal Revenue Service in 2002 as employer-sponsored nontaxable accounts for reimbursement of medical care expenditures by the employee. HRAs are solely established and funded by the employer. The employer can decide if the unspent funds can be carried over to the next year or will remain available to the employee once he or she leaves the job. The employer contributions to HRAs are over $5,000 for single coverage and over $12,000 for family coverage, on average (Claxton et al., 2012). There are no limits on HRA contributions.

HDHPs and associated HSAs and HRAs are designed to increase patient awareness of medical costs and reduce overall expenditures. However, there is evidence of adverse selection of higher-income individuals into HSAs and healthier families and individuals into HDHPs (Galbraith et al., 2009; Naessens et al., 2008; U.S. Government Accountability Office, 2006).

Preventive services are not subject to the deductible, to make sure they get used. Despite these measures, HDHPs are shown to negatively affect health care use among chronically ill and low-income populations (Galbraith et al., 2012) and show savings in costs, but with reductions in preventive care (Beeuwkes Buntin, Haviland, McDevitt, & Sood, 2011). The short-term reduction of nonurgent emergency room visits and hospitalizations among HDHP enrollees raises concerns over deferred utilization (Wharam, Landon, Zhang, Soumerai, & Ross-Degnan, 2011). Evidence on impact of HDHP coverage on prescription drugs is inconsistent. For example, one study found discontinued use of certain classes of drugs and a reduction in brand-name drugs use (Greene, Hibbard, Murray, Teutsch, & Berger, 2008), and another study found no differences in prescription use for specific classes of drugs for three common chronic conditions (Reiss et al., 2011). HDHPs also have a significant financial burden of medical costs for covered individuals (Galbraith et al., 2011).

Erosion of Employment-Based Benefits

Employers' efforts to reduce their liability and curtail health expenditures of employees have led to availability of fewer plans in general and selection of plans with greater cost savings potential. Thus, employers have reduced the types of plans offered. The great majority of firms with fewer than two hundred employees (85 percent) offered only one plan in 2011, while fewer large firms (58 percent) offered only one plan (Claxton et al., 2012). More plan choice is associated with a higher number of employees who participate in employment-based coverage.

Employment-based insurance frequently has separate cost sharing for different services to prevent overuse of services such as emergency room and hospitalizations. Tiered cost sharing in prescription drugs following evidence-based guidelines, step therapy (first-order, second-order, or higher-order medications), and mail order drugs are also employed to reduce costs. Only about 3 percent of covered employees have no deductibles for prescription drugs most commonly in HDHP plans. Three-tier cost sharing is most common (63 percent) in 2011 with generics, preferred, and nonpreferred drugs in the first, second, and third tiers, respectively. However, four or more tiers are increasingly applied, mostly in PPO plans and for 14 percent of covered workers in 2011 (Claxton et al., 2012).

Employment-Based Retirement Benefits

Employment-based retirement benefits are traditionally offered in tandem with active employment benefits and are thus more common among large employers and certain industries. However, changes to Financial Accounting Statement No. 106 (FAS 106) in 1990 was introduced to close loopholes in accounting rules and required more accurate reporting of reserves. The employers' response to this rule change has been to reduce offer rates, restrict eligibility, increase premiums, increase cost sharing, and switch to more restrictive policies (Fronstin, 2010). The magnitude of this erosion is significant. For example, offer rates have declined among firms with five hundred or more employees, from 40 percent in 1993 to 21 percent in 2009 for Medicare eligible retirees and from 46 percent in 1993 to 28 percent in 2009 for early retirees. Also, employers have introduced requirements such as ten to fifteen years of service for eligibility for retiree benefits among employees aged fifty or more. In 1996, 2 percent of firms with one thousand or more employees had this requirement; in 2009, 6 percent of such firms had it (Fronstin, 2010).

The erosion of benefits among Medicare-age retirees can lead to reduced rates of supplemental Medicare coverage, but may also push more patients into HMOs to compensate for loss of retirement benefits with little or no additional premiums. The impact on early retirees is greater, since most do not qualify for Medicare yet and can face very large premiums in the individual market.

Weaknesses of Employment-Based Coverage

Several weaknesses of employment-based coverage can be gleaned from the trends and issues described earlier. First, employment-based coverage is expensive to employers and employees. Despite efforts to reduce costs with strategies such as increasing enrollment in HDHPs, the ability of employers to control the rapid rise in premiums has been limited. Various strategies to reduce employer expenditures, including increased cost sharing, have led to erosion of benefits.

The negotiating power of employers to purchase better and cheaper benefit packages increases significantly by employer size. Large firms have a better ability to "shop" and customize benefits, and small employers have to purchase benefits from existing "menus" of plan options at fixed costs. The low negotiating power of small employers is partly because of their vulnerability to a single catastrophic illness for an employee and the negative impact of that experience on their subsequent premiums. The Health Insurance Portability and Accountability Act of 1996 has required all health insurers to offer health insurance to small employers with two to fifty employees, regardless of the employer's past experience. Early studies of similar state-based legislation from 1993 to 1997 did not show any significant or consistent changes in a number of outcomes, including offer and participation rates or premiums (Marquis & Long, 2001).

A notable weakness of employment-based insurance has been "job lock," or restricting the ability of employees to pursue various job opportunities because other jobs may not offer benefits, offer less generous benefits, offer more costly benefits, or a combination of these. The weakness of employment-based insurance with the biggest systemwide impact is arguably leaving out the self-employed or those not in the labor force, either by choice or due to disability. The only recourse for these individuals is purchasing high-cost policies in the individual market or obtaining government-sponsored coverage if eligible.

Individually Purchased Health Insurance

Unlike employer-based insurance, where the cost of coverage is shared between the employer and the employee, the premiums for individual coverage are paid solely by the individual. The average annual premiums of over $2,900 for single coverage and $6,300 for family coverage vary significantly depending on age and type of policy. For example, average annual premiums for single policies for those ages sixty to sixty-four can be over $5,700 (America's Health Insurance Plans, 2009). These premium amounts keep this coverage out of reach of most low-income individuals, but another significant barrier in obtaining this form of coverage is whether an individual will be offered a policy given preexisting conditions. Of all the medically underwritten or evaluated applications in 2009, 12.7 percent were denied, with most denials among those fifty-five to sixty-four years of age (America's Health Insurance Plans, 2009).

The products offered in the individual market are similar to those offered in the employment-based market and include PPO, POS, HMO, EPO, and indemnity products. The majority of the individual policies sold nationally were PPO or POS products (83 percent of single and 73 percent of family policies). Most of these policies had deductibles of $2,500 or higher for a single (59 percent) or family (74 percent) policy, but were not associated with HSAs. About 11 percent of single and 24 percent of family policies sold were associated with an HSA with high deductibles starting at $1,000 for single and $2,000 for family policies (American's Health Insurance Plans, 2009).

Individually purchased health insurance is fraught with weaknesses, due to high premiums, restrictions in choice, underwriting, lack of guarantee issue, and rescissions. The United States health insurance market is segmented into employment-based health insurance, Medicare, and Medicaid. The residual category of individuals who are not eligible for these other forms of coverage face individually purchased insurance as their only option for obtaining coverage. High premiums, underwriting, and preexisting condition exclusions restrict the ability of individuals to successfully obtain coverage. Even with purchase of a policy, rescissions and lack of guarantee issue can significantly limit the scope of coverage in the event of a catastrophic illness. The recent dominance of HDHPs in this market and the potential cost burden of such plans also restrict choice of plans for individuals.

Significant Trends in Private Health Insurance

Two specific trends in private health insurance are the growth of managed care and price competition. These trends have had a significant and overreaching impact on private insurance and are discussed in detail next.

Growth of Managed Care

Managed care has existed in the United States for more than seventy years. As early as 1932, the Committee on the Costs of Medical Care called for the practice of medicine in the United States to be reorganized into prepaid group practice (Committee on the Costs of Medical Care, 1932). This recommendation acknowledged that the incentives of fee-for-service, solo-practitioner medical practice were inefficient compared to a system where physicians coordinated their care and received a fixed payment in advance for their services. Despite these conceptual advantages, the only prominent prepaid group practice for many years was the nonprofit Kaiser Permanente health plan. During the past two decades, managed care has evolved into a broad concept encompassing a variety of managed care organizations (MCOs) or managed care plans (MCPs), some of which barely resemble prepaid group practice.

Without question, managed care has grown substantially since the early 1970s, when Paul Ellwood's advocacy of health maintenance organizations was translated into national policy as the HMO Act of 1973 (Ellwood et al., 1971). This legislation gave federal grants and loans to federally qualified HMOs to promote their expansion. More important, it required employers with twenty-five or more employees already offering health insurance coverage to offer at least two HMO options, thus promoting the growth of managed care. By the time Harold Luft published his seminal book on HMO performance in 1981, slightly more than seven million U.S. residents were enrolled in HMOs (Luft, 1981), and almost half of all HMO members were concentrated in California in a single network, the Kaiser Foundation Health Plans (Gruber, Shadle, & Polich, 1988). By 1990, enrollment in HMOs increased fivefold to about thirty-five million in almost seven hundred HMOs across the United States. As the 1990s came to an end, HMO enrollment (including enrollment in POS plans) had more than doubled again, to an estimated eighty-one million, or about 29 percent of the U.S. population. Since then, HMO and POS enrollment has declined to an estimated seventy million as of 2011, or about 23 percent of the U.S. population (Kaiser Family Foundation, 2013). This decline is largely due to the growth of PPOs and has been attributed by many analysts to a managed care "backlash," discussed next.

A number of factors explain the rapid proliferation of managed care since the early 1980s. A primary driving force clearly has been employers seeking lower-cost alternatives to indemnity insurance for their employee health benefit plans. At the start of this period of growth, the cost advantages of HMOs were most thoroughly documented by Luft, who found that the long-term cost savings of HMOs were primarily attributable to a lower rate of hospitalization, rather than improved productivity or lower input costs (Luft, 1981). Thus, although the empirical evidence did not suggest that HMOs would produce substantial savings, they nevertheless gave employers an alternative to the inflationary incentives of indemnity-based, fee-for-service health benefits.

In the early years of managed care, employees faced a complex decision in choosing whether to enroll in an HMO. One major advantage was the reduction in out-of-pocket expenditures associated with most HMOs. Prior to the mid-1980s, however, this financial advantage was offset by having a limited choice of providers and by having to obtain gatekeeper approval before seeking specialty care. These disadvantages of the traditional HMO spurred development of less restrictive forms of managed care such as PPO and POS plans. Advocates of managed care cite this ability of the industry to innovate and create new products that vary across markets in response to consumer demand as a major advantage of market-driven reform. In addition to these cost considerations on the part of employers and employees, managed care also has the potential to improve quality of care, at least in part because of the financial incentives facing providers. In theory, managed care has the potential to improve coordination of care through clinical management of entire episodes of care, develop information systems to assist in care coordination, identify and eliminate wasteful or ineffective practices, and identify and manage care for the costliest conditions (such as those involving chronic illness).

In summary, HMOs as the primary form of managed care grew rapidly until the end of the 1990s and are now experiencing declining enrollment nationally in favor of less restrictive forms of managed care.

The Managed Care Backlash

At the beginning of the 1990s, HMOs were the centerpiece of President Clinton's proposal for health care reform in the United States. By the end of the decade, HMO enrollment had peaked and analysts were discussing the emergence of a managed care backlash (Enthoven & Singer, 1998). Although the causes of this backlash were complex, a major factor was dissatisfaction on the part of HMO members, with an increasing sense of restriction regarding their choice of providers and treatments, fueled by several highly visible lawsuits filed against HMOs alleging unlawful denial of care (Peterson, 1999).The policy response to this popular backlash resulted in various proposals for legislation that would have created a "patients' bill of rights" during the period from 1998 to 2001. Although none of these bills were enacted at the national level, the threat of such legislation during this period led to voluntary changes in HMO products that resulted in "open access" HMOs permitting self-referral to specialty care with prior approval from the patient's primary care provider.

These changes in the fundamental functions of HMOs, combined with the decline in HMO enrollment that began in 2000, led one health economist to conclude in 2001 that the United States was witnessing the end of managed care (Robinson, 2001). According to Robinson, despite the economic success of managed care, it has become a cultural and political failure and is being abandoned in favor of an emerging model of consumer-centered or patient-directed health care, in which individuals are empowered with both information and sufficient competing choices to make cost-effective decisions about their care. Of course, not all health economists agree that managed care has been an economic success (Miller & Luft, 2002). In contrast to declining managed care enrollment HDHPs, either alone or combined with HRAs or HSAs, are expected to grow rapidly during the remainder of this decade. Whether this trend represents the end of managed care or simply a reformulation of the role of managed care in the U.S. health care system remains to be seen. In any event, since the last edition of this book managed care is no longer being viewed as the central component of market-based health care reform. But what does the evidence show about how managed care and competition have actually changed the health care system?

Price Competition among Insurers

Selective contracting and managed care change the economic incentives faced by both insurers and providers. The ability to assemble preferred provider networks endows insurers with the potential power to channel patients away from more expensive providers. Insurers, competing with one another for subscribers, have both a financial incentive and the benefit of economies of scale to search the market for an optimal mix of high-quality and low-price providers. Under such conditions, insurers can leverage excess capacity and competitive hospital market conditions to negotiate lower prices with health care providers.

In theory, effective use of the selective contracting mechanism can generate savings for insurers, thereby leading to price advantages over other insurers who pay "too much." Such price advantages could be important in building or maintaining a subscriber base in a competitive insurance market. However, selective contracting plans operate under constraints that in all likelihood prevent them from choosing providers solely by price. If payers use only a price criterion in choosing providers, they may assemble too limited a network, thereby putting themselves at risk of diminishing their subscriber base because of unacceptable quality or access. Thus, payers must assess the relative consumer attractiveness of individual hospitals before choosing which hospitals to exclude for reasons of high price.

Faced with the pressure to reduce prices or risk being excluded from an insurer's network, providers must also balance trade-offs in negotiating with selective contracting plans. They must assess their importance to the insurer's network, which determines the likelihood of being excluded should they refuse to grant requested price concessions. Their ability to retain patients should the contract not be offered, influences their bargaining position.

Insurers may also face competitive pressure on their premiums, depending on how price-sensitive purchasers are in selecting health insurance. Managed competition and other market-oriented reforms are founded on the assumption that, in markets with a sufficient amount of choice among competing health insurers, competition on the basis of price (that is, premiums) will constrain growth in health expenditures. Of course, this assumption itself presumes that purchasers are sufficiently price-sensitive to seek lower-cost insurers, all things being equal.

Previous research on the early effects of selective contracting in California indicates that restructuring the health care market can lead to increased price competition and lower cost growth in the hospital industry. One group found that increasing price sensitivity on the part of buyers has resulted in improved price competition among hospitals, leading them to offer price discounts to secure contracts with managed care plans (Melnick, Zwanziger, Bamezai, & Pattison, 1992). In other studies, hospitals lowered their costs when faced with competitive pressure on their prices exerted by managed care plans (Robinson, 1996; Robinson, 1991; Melnick & Zwanziger, 1988).

Previous published studies showing that competition can lead to smaller increases in hospital costs and prices have been limited in several ways. Because they were done soon after the introduction of price competition, they do not address the question of whether cost-containment effects can be sustained over a long period of time, or if they are simply a one-time reduction followed by increases at previous rates.

Other work has addressed the question of whether price competition in California resulted in a long-term and sustained reduction in hospital expenditures (Zwanziger, Melnick, & Bamezai, 1994, 2000). These analyses were designed to isolate and compare the effects of competition on hospital revenues prior to and following the growth of managed care plans and selective contracting. They found that in the period from 1983 to 1997, hospital expenses in the most competitive markets were 18.4 percent lower than in the least competitive markets, while revenue in the least competitive markets was 19.4 percent lower than in the most competitive ones. They conclude that competition resulting from selective contracting has had a sustained effect, although the potential impact of reduced expenses and revenue on hospital quality is unclear.

The RAND Health Insurance Experiment (HIE) yielded the first scientifically valid estimates of individual price sensitivity to level of copayment and deductible for individual health services. But the HIE did not specifically look at price sensitivity to premiums, since individuals in that study were randomly assigned to a number of insurance plans. Of course, determining the price elasticity of demand for health insurance is a difficult task. Most studies cannot adequately control for unobserved differences among insurance plans and unobserved characteristics among those selecting the plans, and thus they are subject to selection bias. Nevertheless, several studies have examined price sensitivity to premiums.

Buchmueller (2006) found a significant price elasticity of demand for health insurance using data on retirees from a single large employer. He found that a $5 increase in out-of-pocket premiums was associated with a 0.4 percentage point decline, on average, in market share. The price sensitivity of single retirees was greater than for married retirees, with a $5 increase in out-of-pocket premiums resulting in a 1.5 percentage point decline in market share. Strombom, Buchmueller, and Feldstein (2002) found greater price sensitivity among employees in the University of California system, with a $5 increase in out-of-pocket premiums associated with a 3.2 percentage point decline among all health insurers, and a 7.6 percentage point decline among managed care plans.

Future Directions

The Affordable Care Act (ACA) is intended to address several major shortcomings of the private insurance coverage in the United States These include addressing erosion of offer and take-up rates, erosion of and variations in benefits, job lock, rescissions and exclusions, and the basic affordability of private health insurance without employer subsidies.

Preventing Erosion of Offer and Take-up Rates

The two major provisions of the ACA aimed at preventing erosion of offer and take-up rates are the employer and individual mandates. With some exceptions, the employer mandate requires employers to offer health insurance benefits to their employees or pay a penalty for not doing so. Employers with fewer than fifty employees are exempt from the mandate, and those with fewer than twenty-five employees receive premium subsidies if their employees on average earn less than $50,000 per year. However, employers with fifty or more employees will have to pay a fee if they do not offer insurance or they have employees that receive premium subsidies in the exchange.

The employer mandate is designed to prevent further erosion of offer rates or a rapid decline of offer rates due to the ACA. The response of employers to the mandate to offer coverage remains to be seen once the ACA fully takes effect. An early assessment of employers' responses to the ACA and this mandate indicated a major concern over rapidly rising insurance premiums and the potential for increases in employer costs (Darling, 2010).

The individual mandate requires proof of insurance coverage by all individuals in their income tax returns filed with the Internal Revenue Service (IRS) and penalties in the absence of proof of coverage. However, the IRS is prohibited from prosecuting individuals without coverage. Individuals are exempted from this provision of the law most notably because of financial hardship and lack of documentation. Low-income individuals will either receive Medicaid coverage or receive subsidies to purchase insurance in the exchange, depending on their income.

The individual mandate is designed to prevent erosion of take-up rates for individuals whose employers offer health insurance. Much controversy and debate surrounded this provision of the law, despite the significant amount of subsidies provided to low-income individuals. Yet the individual mandate is considered by many to be a pivotal provision, because it increases the pool of the insured populations and has the potential to keep premiums at affordable levels. A significant level of effort is spent on estimating take-up rates, since participation levels have direct implications for premium costs after full implementation of the ACA.

Reducing Erosion of and Variations in Benefits

Several provisions of the ACA will affect benefits and cost sharing of employment-based and individually purchased policies. The ACA standardizes the package of benefit provided in both markets, with some exemptions. All offered policies must include basic inpatient, emergency, and outpatient services in addition to prescription drugs and pediatric oral and vision care. The benefit levels must conform to one of the four tiers of actuarial value (bronze, silver, gold, and platinum) with a prespecified fixed ratio of premium to out-of-pocket costs. A separate maximum is set for annual out-of-pocket spending for individuals and families. Exemptions to these rules apply to "grandfather" plans and self-insured policies. Other provisions of the ACA limit the amount of medical loss ratio—the percentage of the premiums to be spent on administrative activities and lifetime limits on coverage.

The ACA also mandates guaranteed issue of policies, establishment of the exchange market to purchase subsidized policies if the employer does not offer coverage or the policy is unaffordable, and establishment of high-risk insurance pools. These provisions can prevent job lock and allow individuals to pursue other employment opportunities without concerns over the ability to purchase coverage. Also, preexisting exclusions and rescissions are no longer allowed under the ACA, leading to more stable coverage of individuals with individually purchased policies. In addition, the ACA creates a temporary reinsurance program coverage of early retirees over age fifty-five who are not eligible for Medicare by reimbursing employers or insurers for 80 percent of retiree claims between $15,000 and $90,000.

Understanding the Price Elasticity of Demand for Health Insurance

With regard to the price elasticity (or sensitivity) of individuals to the cost of insurance, specifically out-of-pocket premiums, the ACA should provide a tremendous amount of data on who takes up insurance given the availability of subsidies to purchase insurance in exchanges. Economic theory predicts that take-up will be highest among those with the largest subsidies or among those with the poorest health status, all else being equal. Previous research suggests that individuals are fairly sensitive to changes in premiums. The availability of significant subsidies for purchase of insurance through exchanges will provide a once-in-a-lifetime opportunity to measure the sensitivity of individuals to premium price changes. Moving forward after 2014, premium price information from the exchanges should also provide a unique opportunity to study consumer sensitivity to price changes over time.

SUMMARY

Employment-based insurance has been the foundation of private health insurance in the United States since the end of World War II and is still the primary source of health insurance for the majority of Americans. Ongoing increases in the costs of private insurance, however, have led to erosion of employment-based insurance in recent decades, and the private market has historically left major portions of the population without affordable options. Rather than replace the private market entirely, the United States has pursued policies since the 1960s to create public insurance programs to provide coverage to those left without affordable options in the private market. The ACA is the latest effort to provide nearly universal access to health insurance among those without affordable employment-based insurance. A major question regarding the impact of the ACA is how will it affect the private insurance market generally and employment-based insurance specifically. Will the ACA stabilize current employment-based insurance, or will it lead employers to shift away from offering health insurance directly toward offering financial support to employees for purchasing insurance in state-based exchanges? In either case, the private insurance market is likely to continue experiencing substantial change for the foreseeable future.

KEY TERMS

Adverse selection also referred to as cream skimming and cherry picking, it occurs when health plans enroll healthier individuals and avoid enrolling those who are sicker or at higher risk.

Capitation method of payment in which providers receive a fixed per-member, per-month payment for each individual who enrolls in the provider's patient panel.

Community rating the practice of setting health insurance premiums based on the average health care use and expenditures of a community, frequently defined by a geographic area.

Cost-sharing Insurance policies infrequently cover the entire costs of health care used by the insured and require some level of cost sharing, which refers to the amount the insured must pay for each service used. In HMO policies, cost sharing is typically a fixed dollar amount called a *copayment*. In PPO policies, cost sharing is typically a percentage of the total cost of the service and is called a *coinsurance rate.*

Deductible refers to a specific predetermined annual amount to be paid by the insured before the insurer pays for health care services. The main purpose of the deductible is to protect the insurer from moral hazard and reduce the liability of the insurer by sharing some of the risk and expenditures with the insured.

Experience rating the practice of setting health insurance premiums based on the health care use and expenditures of a particular group to be insured.

Health maintenance organizations (HMOs) HMOs are the traditional form of managed care. *Group-model* HMOs contract with a single medical group to provide care to plan members, while *staff-model* HMOs employ physicians directly. *Network-model* HMOs contract with multiple medical groups, while *independent practice association (IPA) model* HMOs contract with individual physicians in solo practice. Network- and IPA-model HMOs are typically open panel; physicians do not contract exclusively with a single HMO and may continue to treat non-HMO patients.

Health reimbursement accounts (HRAs) savings accounts that were first authorized by the Internal Revenue Service in 2002 as employer-sponsored nontaxable accounts for reimbursement of medical care expenditures by the employee. HRAs are solely established and funded by the employer.

Health savings accounts (HSAs) optional savings accounts paired with HDHPs to pay for out-of-pocket costs of the policyholder. Contributions can be made by individuals or by employers, or both.

High-deductible health plans (HDHPs) health insurance plans or policies with high deductibles (minimum of $1,250 for single coverage and $2,500 for family coverage in 2013) to encourage policyholders to use less health care.

Managed competition a model for health care reform proposed by Alain Enthoven in the late 1970s based on the Federal Employees Health Benefits Program (FEHBP). Its key elements are (1) price competition in regulated insurance markets between insurers based on standard insurance policies and (2) pooling of small companies and individual purchasers into larger groups known as health insurance purchasing cooperatives (HIPCs).

Moral hazard refers to the higher likelihood of use of health care services when the out-of-pocket expense is reduced due to insurance. Tools such as deductibles and cost sharing are used by insurers to address moral hazard.

Point-of-service plans (POS) POS plans are essentially the same as the open-access HMOs, but they also offer limited coverage for self-referral outside the network.

Preferred provider organizations (PPOs) these represent a less restrictive form of managed care than HMOs, mainly because they do not require primary care physicians to serve as gatekeepers and thus permit self-referral to specialists.

Premiums the monthly or annual amount paid by employers and individuals who purchase health insurance.

DISCUSSION QUESTIONS

1. What is the basis for the managed care "backlash" in the United States, and why has enrollment in PPOs grown while enrollment in HMOs has declined?

2. What are some of the major barriers to making price competition work more effectively in health care markets? Are health care markets different in some fundamental way from other markets, so that price competition is more difficult to put into effect? Or, can free markets really produce better "products" at lower cost in health care, just as they do in many other sectors of the economy? Why or why not?

3. Enthoven's theory of managed competition includes having health plans compete for enrollment within a market by bidding against each other on the basis of premiums (i.e., price). Competition among health insurers within regulated markets known as exchanges is a central component of the Affordable Care Act. Is price competition likely to be effective in controlling health care expenditures in the future under the ACA?

FURTHER READING

Claxton, G., Rae, M., Panchal, N., Damico, A., & Lundy, J. (2012). 2012 Employer Health Benefits Survey. Menlo Park, CA, and Chicago: Kaiser Family Foundation,

Health Research & Educational Trust, NORC at the University of Chicago. Retrieved from http://ehbs.kff.org/pdf/2011/8225.pdf

Excellent summary of the current state of employment-based health insurance.

Enthoven, A. C., & Kronick, R. (1989). A consumer-choice health plan for the 1990s. *New England Journal of Medicine, 320*, 29–37, 94–101.

This seminal article lays out the framework for managed competition and was the basis for much of the Clinton proposal for health reform, despite several important departures from the original model described here.

Pacific Business Group on Health (PBGH): http://www.pbgh.org/programs/value_based_purchasing.asp

This coalition of large purchasers in California is actively involved in implementing the concept of value-based purchasing through the development of quality and performance measures that can be used by individuals, employers, and government purchasers of health care to evaluate both the cost and quality of care.

Galbraith, A. A., Ross-Degnan, D., Soumerai, S. B., Rosenthal, M. B., Gay, C., & Lieu, T. A. (2011). Nearly half of families in high-deductible health plans whose members have chronic conditions face substantial financial burden. *Health Affairs, 30*(2), 322–331.

This article examines the impact of high-deductible health plans on health care for specific populations.

REFERENCES

America's Health Insurance Plans. (2009). *Individual health insurance 2009: A comprehensive survey of premiums, availability, and benefits.* Washington DC: America's Health Insurance Plans, Center for Policy and Research.

America's Health Insurance Plans. (2010). *Small-group health insurance in 2010: A comprehensive survey of premiums, product choices, and benefits.* Washington DC: America's Health Insurance Plans, Center for Policy and Research.

Beeuwkes Buntin, M., Haviland, A. M., McDevitt, R., & Sood, N. (2011). Healthcare spending and preventive care in high-deductible and consumer-directed health plans. *American Journal of Managed Care, 17*(3), 222–230.

Buchmueller, T. (2006). Price and health plan choices of retirees. *Journal of Health Economics, 25*, 81–100.

Claxton, G., Rae, M., Panchal, N., Damico, A., Lundy, J., Bostick, N., . . . Whitmore, H. (2012). *Employer health benefits 2012 annual survey.* Chicago: Kaiser Family Foundation, Health Research & Educational Trust, NORC at the University of Chicago. Retrieved from http://ehbs.kff.org/pdf/2012/8345.pdf

Committee on the Costs of Medical Care. (1932). *Medical care for the American people: The final report.* Chicago: University of Chicago Press.

Darling, H. (2010). Health care reform: Perspectives from large employers. *Health Affairs, 29*(6), 1220–1224.

DeNavas-Walt, C., Proctor, D. B., & Smith, J. C. (2011). *Income, poverty, and health insurance in the United States, 2010* (Document No. P60–239). Washington, DC: U.S. Census Bureau).

Ellwood, P. M., Anderson, N. N., Billings, J. E., Carlson, R. J., Hoagberg, E. J., & McClure, W. (1971). Health maintenance strategy. *Medical Care, 9*, 291–298.

Enthoven, A. C. (1978). Consumer choice health plan: A national health insurance proposal based on regulated competition in the private sector. *New England Journal of Medicine, 298*, 709–720.

Enthoven, A. C. (1993). The history and principles of managed competition. *Health Affairs, 12*(Suppl), 24–48.

Enthoven, A. C., & Singer, S. J. (1998). The managed care backlash and the task force in California. *Health Affairs, 17*, 95–110.

Fronstin, P. (2010). *Implications of health reform for retiree health benefits.* Washington, DC: Employee Benefit Research Institute.

Fronstin, P. (2011). *Sources of health insurance and characteristics of the uninsured: Analysis of the March 2011 Current Population Survey.* Washington, DC: Employee Benefit Research Institute.

Galbraith, A. A., Soumerai, S., Ross-Degnan, D., Rosenthal, M., Gay, C., & Lieu, T. (2012). Delayed and forgone care for families with chronic conditions in high-deductible health plans. *Journal of General Internal Medicine*, 1–7.

Galbraith, A. A., Ross-Degnan, D., Soumerai, S. B., Miroshnik, I., Wharam, J. F., Kleinman, K., & Lieu, T. A. (2009). High-deductible health plans: Are vulnerable families enrolled? *Pediatrics, 123*(4), e589–e594.

Galbraith, A. A., Ross-Degnan, D., Soumerai, S. B., Rosenthal, M. B., Gay, C., & Lieu, T. A. (2011). Nearly half of families in high-deductible health plans whose members have chronic conditions face substantial financial burden. *Health Affairs, 30*(2), 322–331.

Greene, J., Hibbard, J., Murray, J. F., Teutsch, S. M., & Berger, M. L. (2008). The impact of consumer-directed health plans on prescription drug use. *Health Affairs, 27*(4), 1111–1119.

Gruber, L., Shadle, M., & Polich, C. (1988). From movement to industry: The growth of HMOs. *Health Affairs, 7*, 197–208.

Kaiser Family Foundation. (2013). *State health facts.* Retrieved from http://www.state healthfacts.org/comparemaptable.jsp?ind=348&cat=7

Luft, H. S. (1981). *Health maintenance organizations: Dimensions of performance.* New York: Wiley.

Marquis, M. S., & Long, S. H. (2001). Effects of "second generation" small group health insurance market reforms, 1993 to 1997. *Inquiry, 38*(4), 365–380.

Melnick, G. A., & Zwanziger, J. (1988). Hospital behavior under competition and cost containment policies: The California experience. *Journal of the American Medical Association, 260*, 2669–2675.

Melnick, G. A., Zwanziger, J., Bamezai, A., & Pattison, R. (1992). The effects of market structure and hospital bargaining position on hospital prices. *Journal of Health Economics, 11*, 217–233.

Miller, R. H., & Luft, H. S. (2002). HMO plan performance update: An analysis of the literature, 1997–2001. *Health Affairs, 21*, 63–86.

Naessens, J. M., Khan, M., Shah, N. D., Wagie, A., Pautz, R. A., & Campbell, C. R. (2008). Effect of premium, copayments, and health status on the choice of health plans. *Medical Care, 46*(10), 1033–1040.

Peterson, M. A. (1999). Introduction: Politics, misperception, or apropos? *Journal of Politics, Policy, and Law, 25*, 873–886.

Purcell, P., & Staman, J. (2009). *Summary of the Employee Retirement Income Security Act (ERISA)*. Washington, DC: Congressional Research Service.

Reed, M., Graetz, I., Wang, H., Fung, V., Newhouse, J. P., & Hsu, J. (2012). Consumer-directed health plans with health savings accounts: Whose skin is in the game and how do costs affect care seeking? *Medical Care, 50*, 585–590.

Reiss, S. K., Ross-Degnan, D., Zhang, F., Soumerai, S. B., Zaslavsky, A. M., & Wharam, J. F. (2011). Effect of switching to a high-deductible health plan on use of chronic medications. *Health Services Research, 46*(5), 1382–1401.

Robinson, J. C. (1991). HMO market penetration and hospital cost inflation in California. *Journal of the American Medical Association, 266*, 2719–2723.

Robinson, J. C. (1996). Decline in hospital utilization and cost inflation under managed care in California. *Journal of the American Medical Association, 276*, 1060–1064.

Robinson, J. C. (2001). The end of managed care. *Journal of the American Medical Association, 285*, 2622–2628.

Strombom, B. A., Buchmueller, T. C., & Feldstein, P. J. (2002). Switching costs, price sensitivity, and health plan choice. *Journal of Health Economics, 21*, 89–116.

U.S. Government Accountability Office. (2006). *Health savings accounts: Early enrollee experiences with accounts and eligible health plans* (No. GAO-06-1133T). Washington, DC: Author.

U.S. Public Health Service. (n.d.) Series B 1-220: Vital statistics and health and medical care. Retrieved from http://www2.census.gov/prod2/statcomp/documents/CT1970p1–03.pdf

Wharam, J. F., Landon, B. E., Zhang, F., Soumerai, S. B., & Ross-Degnan, D. (2011). High-deductible insurance: Two-year emergency department and hospital use. *American Journal of Managed Care, 17*(10), e410–e418.

Zwanziger, J., Melnick, G. A., & Bamezai, A. (1994). Cost and price competition in California hospitals, 1980–1990. *Health Affairs, 13*, 118–126.

Zwanziger, J., Melnick, G. A., & Bamezai, A. (2000). The effect of selective contracting on hospital costs and revenues. *Health Services Research, 35*, 849–867.

PART TWO

COST OF HEALTH CARE

CHAPTER EIGHT

MEASURING HEALTH CARE EXPENDITURES AND TRENDS

Thomas H. Rice

Learning Objectives

- Distinguish between the terms *costs* and *expenditures*
- Explain how unit prices and health care expenditures are defined for purposes of measurement, as well as limitations of particular measures and the data sources used
- Provide data on health care costs and their growth, within the United States and compared to other countries
- Explain problems with current data systems

In 2010, the United States spent about $2.6 trillion on health care. It is difficult to fathom such a large number. To put it in perspective, suppose you lined $2.6 trillion one-dollar bills 'end to end. They would stretch all the way to the sun—and back to Earth—and nearly back to the sun again!

This chapter focuses on how these health care expenditures are measured and then discusses the trends. It concludes with a discussion of whether health care cost control is even necessary, as a bridge to the following chapter, where particular strategies are evaluated. Although data and measurement may seem a bit pedestrian to the analyst interested in proceeding quickly to policy issues, this is an unfortunate viewpoint.

Accurate data on national health care spending are necessary for choosing the most appropriate health policy reforms. (A blunter reason for accurate data that may ring true to the policy analyst comes from computer programming: "garbage in, garbage out.") Once these tools are in hand, one can analyze alternative methods of containing health care expenditures (see Chapter Nine).

Measuring Health Care Expenditures

As just noted, understanding measurement is essential if one is to fully appreciate many issues that are currently in the forefront of health policy. To give one example, debate continues about whether the United States—a country that relies more heavily than others on markets in its health care system—has been as successful as other countries in controlling health expenditures. Resolution of this ostensibly straightforward issue would yield insight as to the potential savings or losses, if any, that might accrue if the United States adopted some aspects of other countries' organization and financing systems. But to ascertain an accurate answer to this question, it is necessary to understand how health expenditures are compiled in various countries as well as how they can be compared. This section of the chapter discusses a number of key issues concerning measurement of health care expenditures.

Expenditures versus Costs

Most policy discussions employ the term *costs* rather than *expenditures;* indeed, the next chapter also adopts this convenience. It is important to understand that the two concepts are hardly the same.

Expenditures, of course, mean how much is spent on a particular thing. As discussed in Chapter Nine, in a fee-for-service system expenditures are simply the product of unit prices and the quantity of goods or services purchased. Total expenditures can then be broken down in a number of ways, such as by type of service (for example, by hospital expenditures or physician expenditures) or by payer source (private insurers, Medicare, or out-of-pocket).

In contrast, costs apply to the production process. Specifically, the term refers to the value of resources used in producing a good or service. There are two distinct definitions of cost: accounting and economic. The accounting definition includes only the value of the resources used in production (that is, labor and capital). The difference between the sales revenue from a good or service and the accounting cost is defined as net revenue or profit.

This differs from the economic definition of cost. To an economist, the term includes not only the value of resources expended in the production process but in addition a "normal" return on investment. Using their definition, economists predict that in a competitive market profit levels are near zero—that is, a typically efficient producer garners only a normal rate of return on investment. The persistence of an economic profit level far above zero over a long period of time may indicate the existence of "market failure," which in turn might call for government policy intervention.

Accounting and economic *profits* are therefore related to each other. The latter is approximately equal to the former minus a normal rate of return on investment. There are other distinctions in how economists and accountants define cost. Specifically, economic profits equal an organization's cash flow minus a normal rate of return on investment. Further discussion of this issue can be found in textbooks on corporate finance.

Nevertheless, both definitions of cost differ from the definition of expenditure. The distinction is shown in Figure 8.1; for simplicity, we use the economic definition of cost and compare that to the definition of expenditure. In the figure, the horizontal axis shows the quantity of a

FIGURE 8.1. DISTINCTION BETWEEN ACCOUNTING AND ECONOMIC PROFITS

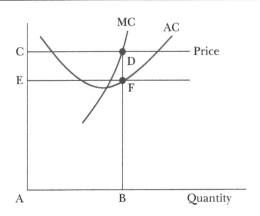

particular good or service; the vertical axis, sales prices and production costs. MC refers to marginal costs—the cost of producing the last unit of output. AC is average cost of output, and Price is the selling price. Both of the cost curves include a normal rate of return on investment.

Health care expenditures are equal to the rectangle ABCD, which is simply the selling price multiplied by the quantity sold, AB. In contrast, economic costs are shown by a smaller rectangle, ABEF: this is average costs (AE) multiplied by the quantity sold (AB). In this example, expenditure exceeds cost by the rectangle CDEF. This implies that excess profits are being obtained by firms in the industry. Other firms therefore may be stimulated to enter the market to reap these profits, which in turn may drive down price and restore profit to a normal level. If this does not occur, then some form of government intervention may be necessary to correct market failure.

With these distinctions in mind, we can address the question of whether we should spend most of our effort analyzing health care costs or expenditures. Although both are useful, it turns out to be considerably easier to conduct analyses of the entire health care system using the concept of expenditure. This is because it is extremely difficult to obtain reliable data on cost; private firms are rarely expected to report their internal cost data to any sort of governmental body. One exception is Medicare hospital costs, because such data are collected by the federal government. But for other sectors—physician care, pharmaceuticals, and the like (and for services that are covered by private insurers rather than Medicare and Medicaid)—reliable data on costs are exceedingly difficult to obtain. The remainder of this chapter, then, focuses on measurement and trends in health care expenditure rather than cost. First, however, we discuss measuring changes in unit price.

Measuring Health Care Prices

The most common measure of health care prices in the United States is the medical care component of the *Consumer Price Index (CPI)*. The CPI, which is published monthly by the Bureau of Labor Statistics (BLS), gives information on the change in prices charged to urban consumers for a variety of consumer goods and services. More information on the CPI can be found at the BLS website at http://www.bls.gov/cpi.

To obtain the index, the CPI begins with a common "market basket" of goods and services. The monthly price data are obtained from urban localities that represent about 80 percent of the United States population.

To form the index, each item in the market basket is given a weight representing its relative importance in the spending patterns of urban consumers. An index is then formed that compares the change in prices in a current time period to a base period (usually 1982 to 1984) whose index value is set to a value of 100. For example, in 2011 the medical care component of the CPI had a value of 405.6, which means that medical care prices were slightly more than four times what they were during the base period.

As shown later in this chapter when trends are presented, the medical care component of the CPI is further subdivided into several categories, making it possible to monitor inflation in various health-related markets. The two main subcategories are medical care services and medical care commodities. Within services, there are separate indices constructed for physicians' services, dental services, eye care, other medical professionals, hospital rooms, other inpatient services, and hospital outpatient services. Within commodities, separate indices exist for prescription drugs, over-the-counter drugs and medical supplies, internal and respiratory over-the-counter drugs, and medical equipment and supplies.

There are a number of limitations to the CPI (Feldstein, 2004). First, and perhaps most important, the CPI measures change in price, not in expenditure. It does not take into account change in the quantity of services provided, only the price.

Second, the CPI measures changes in prices, not price levels. The index cannot be used to compare difference in health care prices among parts of the country. Suppose, for example, that in 2011 the medical component of the CPI was 440 in New York City, and 370 in Los Angeles. All that one could say is that prices rose faster in New York than Los Angeles since the base year in which the index was set to 100. It cannot be concluded that health care prices necessarily are lower in Los Angeles than New York.

Third, the CPI measures the price charged, not the price received by a producer. This is a critical distinction because of the prevalence of discounts offered by providers and pharmaceutical companies to managed care plans. In some competitive parts of the country, such as California, providers' list or billed charges are illusory; almost no one pays them. However, these prices are exactly what are measured by the CPI. What this means is that the CPI might overstate the amount of medical care inflation in certain parts of the country because over time the true price of care has deviated further from the billed charge.

Fourth, the CPI measures changes in price for a fixed market basket of consumer goods. In fact, the entire notion of the CPI is based on the existence of such an apples-to-apples comparison. By using a standard market basket of goods, it is possible to determine how price alone has changed. But this also leads to two difficulties. First, people do change their consumption habits over time, so the market basket being measured by the CPI may become increasingly irrelevant. The Bureau of Labor Statistics (BLS), the federal agency responsible for the index, is dealing with this problem by updating the composition of the market basket more frequently than it did previously. The second difficulty is that the CPI does not take into account change in the quality of goods and services produced—although again, the BLS is currently grappling with this problem. To illustrate this issue, note that an increase in per diem hospital charges over the last twenty years is likely to be exaggerated by the CPI. Over this period, hospital rooms have become much more expensive not only from inflation but also because of enhancements in the type of services and facilities available to the hospital patient. In theory, the CPI should hold these changes constant and look only at price inflation of hospital care of a given quality. This has not been the practice, however.

Fifth, the CPI measures only changes in consumers' expenditures (premiums plus out-of-pocket payments). If, as in the case of hospital care, few expenditures are not out of pocket, then the index does not capture the vast majority of underlying inflation. This could bias the index figures because there has been a gradual movement away from out-of-pocket expenditure toward more employer and government payment, which is not included in the CPI (Feldstein, 2004). We may now be witnessing a reversal of this trend, with increased patient cost sharing as part of many job-based health insurance plans and through the expansion of high-deductible health plans and health savings accounts.

These caveats are not meant as criticism; any differently configured index would raise a host of other problems. Rather, the limitations of the CPI must simply be understood when using the index.

Measuring Expenditures

This section examines U.S. expenditures and international comparisons.

U.S. Expenditures. There are many sources of data on U.S. health expenditures; space does not permit separate discussion of each. Rather, we focus on the primary source: the national health accounts produced by the Office of the Actuary of the Centers for Medicare and Medicaid Services

(CMS), which is housed in the U.S. Department of Health and Human Services. Trends in these data are presented later in the chapter.

Data on U.S. national health expenditures are published regularly—usually annually—in the journal *Health Affairs* (Martin, Lassman, Washington, Catlin, & the National Health Expenditure Accounts Team, 2012). The data for one year can be viewed best as a matrix. Each row of the matrix represents the group that spends the money, whereas each column indicates the provider of services that receives the funds. (An example is presented later in the chapter, as Table 8.5.) A cell in the matrix therefore represents how much a particular payer (for example, a private insurer) spends on a specific service (say, hospital care). Because these same data are compiled annually, by comparing the matrices of several years one can calculate the rate of change in expenditure in various components of the health care sector.

In viewing the matrix, one might think that the data come from a single, consistent source. They do not. Literally dozens of sources are used to piece the matrices together. Some of the data are collected relatively systematically, but others are not. For example, data from the Medicare program are systemically collected by CMS through the Medicare Statistical System (MSS). One file in the MSS, the hospital insurance claims file, contains information on each beneficiary's spending for Part A (hospital) services, while the supplementary Medicare insurance file includes similar data for Part B (primarily physician) services. Although somewhat more unwieldy, Medicaid data are also collected from the states in a consistent format by HCFA.

But because there are no national data collection requirements for private insurers, other aspects of the matrices have to be pieced together from multiple data sources. Some are more systematic than others. Hospital expenditures, for example, come largely from a single source: the American Hospital Association's annual survey of hospitals. But out-of-pocket expenditures come from any number of sources: a consumer expenditures survey, conducted by the Bureau of Labor Statistics; periodic surveys of nursing homes, conducted by the National Center for Health Statistics; surveys about home health care, conducted by the Visiting Nurse Association; physician and dentist surveys, conducted by the American Medical Association and the American Dental Association; data about outpatient clinic services, collected by the Bureau of the Census; and information about Community Health Centers, collected by the Health Resources and Services Administration. As discussed at the end of the chapter, the lack of a consistent data source makes it difficult to successfully administer certain types of health care reform, particularly regulatory ones such as national expenditure targets.

Over the years, there have been various revisions to the national health accounts. There are, nevertheless, a number of problems, most of which are caused by the lack of source data:

- The accounts are unable to distinguish between some inpatient and outpatient expenditures (for example, salaried physician care counted as hospital rather than physician expenditure).
- Premium expenditures by consumers (Medicare Part B payments and private insurance premiums) are included as payment made by insurers, rather than as out-of-pocket expenditure by consumers.
- Some capital expenditures are double-counted.

International Comparisons. The primary source of data on international health care spending for more than two dozen developed (and some developing) countries is collected by the Organization for Economic Cooperation and Development (OECD), which is based in Paris. These data are published in periodic articles in the journal *Health Affairs* (and also appear in the annual government publication *Health United States*: http://www.cdc.gov/nchs/hus.htm). Much effort has gone into compiling accurate health expenditure figures across countries. For a presentation of some recent cross-national comparisons, see Anderson and Frogner (2008). Data from the OECD database are presented later in the chapter.

The previous discussion about U.S. health expenditures focused on the lack of a consistent data source. As can be imagined, the problem of lacking consistent data is even greater when one compares data from over two dozen countries. Those who compile the OECD data have attempted to make them reliable by disseminating definitions of key terms as well as common accounting principles to all member countries. Nevertheless, one must use caution in employing the data because of differences in definition, source of data, and variation in accuracy among the countries.

Among the areas of particular concern:

- *How countries distinguish between health and social services.* Some, for example, may classify certain domiciliary care to the elderly as health, while others might not.
- *How countries distinguish between hospital and long-term care.* In some countries the distinction between the two is much finer than in the United States, with more long-term care being provided in hospitals.

- *Accurate conversion of numerous currencies to a common unit.* This is typically done through purchasing power parities (PPPs), which take into account buying power in different countries. For this reason, it is probably safer to rely on figures pertaining to the proportion of a country's national income devoted to health than to an absolute monetary amount.
- *Underreporting of certain categories of expenditure by some countries,* which is due in part to data limitations.

The OECD draws on researchers and government officials from member countries to improve the quality and comparability of the data, which have improved over time.

Trends in Health Care Expenditures

This section is divided into three parts: U.S. prices, U.S. expenditures, and international expenditures.

U.S. Prices

Table 8.1 presents the values for the major components of the CPI from 1980 to 2011, while Table 8.2 shows the corresponding annual rates of change. Tables 8.3 and 8.4 present similar data for some of the items that make up the medical care component of the CPI.

Beginning with Tables 8.1 and 8.2, we see that since 1980 medical care prices have grown far faster than other prices in the U.S. economy. Between 1980 and 2011, they rose about 5.4-fold, whereas the index as a whole increased only about 2.75 times, and the other components listed grew even less. The pattern is most pronounced in the early years; between 1980 and 1990 medical prices rose by an average of 8.1 percent annually, compared to 4.7 percent for the CPI as a whole. Since then, price increases have lessened somewhat, although still usually almost double those of the other sectors of the economy.

Tables 8.3 and 8.4 show the patterns within the medical care sector. The largest growth rate was for hospital, which increased by a factor of 9.5 from 1980 to 2011. As mentioned earlier, however, one should be somewhat skeptical about this number because the CPI does not do a good job of accounting for the changing nature of the hospital product. What is most noteworthy is that after relatively low inflation in the middle to

TABLE 8.1. CONSUMER PRICE INDEX FOR SELECTED ITEMS: UNITED STATES, SELECTED YEARS, 1980–2011

Year	All Items	Medical Care	Food	Apparel	Housing	Energy
		Consumer Price Index				
1980	82.4	74.9	86.8	90.9	81.1	86.0
1990	130.7	162.8	132.4	124.1	128.5	102.1
1995	152.4	220.5	148.4	132.0	148.5	105.2
2000	172.2	260.8	167.8	129.6	169.6	124.6
2005	195.3	323.2	190.7	119.5	195.7	177.1
2010	218.1	391.9	221.3	118.1	216.1	218.0
2011	225.0	405.6	231.1	123.5	220.2	232.3

Note: 1982–1984 = 100.

Sources: (1) U.S. Department of Health and Human Services, Public Health Service. (2010). *Health United States: 2010.* Retrieved from http://www.cdc.gov/nchs/data/hus/hus10.pdf#listtables; Table 123. (2) U.S. Department of Labor, Consumer Price Index, various years. Retrieved from http://www.bls.gov/cpi.

TABLE 8.2. ANNUAL CHANGE IN CONSUMER PRICE INDEX FOR SELECTED ITEMS: UNITED STATES, SELECTED YEARS, 1980–2010

Year	All Items	Medical Care	Food	Apparel	Housing	Energy
		Average Annual Percent Change				
1980–1990	4.7	8.1	4.3	3.2	4.7	1.7
1990–1995	3.1	6.3	2.3	1.2	2.9	0.6
1995–2000	2.5	3.4	2.5	-0.4	2.7	3.4
2000–2005	2.5	4.4	2.6	-1.6	2.9	7.3
2005–2010	2.2	3.9	3.0	-0.2	2.0	4.2

Source: Calculated from data in Table 8.1.

late 1990s, there has been a resurgence in most medical price increases, although not as great as in the 1980s.

U.S. Expenditures

Table 8.5 presents 2008 data on U.S. health expenditures from the national health accounts. The rows give information on the source of funds, while

TABLE 8.3. CONSUMER PRICE INDEX FOR ALL ITEMS AND FOR MEDICAL CARE COMPONENTS: UNITED STATES, SELECTED YEARS, 1980–2011

	1980	1990	1995	2000	2005	2010	2011
	Consumer Price Index						
CPI, all items	82.4	130.7	152.4	172.2	195.3	218.1	225.0
Less medical care	82.8	128.8	148.6	167.3	188.7	210.7	216.9
CPI, all services	77.9	139.2	168.7	195.3	230.1	262.7	267.7
All medical care	74.9	162.8	220.5	260.8	323.2	391.9	405.6
Medical care services	74.8	162.7	224.2	266.0	336.7	415.1	430.0
Professional medical services	77.9	156.1	201.0	237.7	281.7	330.7	337.9
Physicians' services	76.5	160.8	208.8	244.7	287.5	334.1	343.0
Dental services	78.9	155.8	206.8	258.5	324.0	402.4	411.4
Eye care	-–-	117.3	137.0	149.7	163.2	176.9	178.2
Services by other medical professionals	-–-	120.2	143.9	161.9	186.8	215.4	218.2
Hospital and related services	69.2	178.0	257.8	317.3	439.9	621.2	653.8
Medical care commodities	75.4	163.4	204.5	238.1	276.0	317.2	327.3
Prescription drugs	72.5	181.7	235.0	285.4	349.0	412.8	429.8

Note: 1982–1984 = 100.

Sources: (1) U.S. Department of Health and Human Services, Public Health Service. (2010). *Health United States: 2010*. Retrieved from http://www.cdc.gov/nchs/data/hus/hus10.pdf#listtables; Table 123. (2) U.S. Department of Labor, Consumer Price Index, various years. Retrieved from http://www.bls.gov/cpi.

the columns indicate the provider of services receiving the funds. Some noteworthy aspects of the data are these:

- Government expenditures account for 46.5 percent of total health expenditures, most of which are federal. Government pays far more of the bill for hospital care (57 percent) than for physician services (35 percent).
- Although out-of-pocket costs make up on average 14 percent of total expenditures, this figure varies tremendously by type of service. It ranges from only 3 percent for hospital care to 27 percent for nursing home care, 34 percent for other personal care, and 21 percent for prescription drugs.
- Private insurance pays a substantial proportion (more than 30 percent) of expenditure for hospital, physician, and prescription drugs, but only 7.4 percent for nursing home care.

TABLE 8.4. AVERAGE ANNUAL CHANGE IN CONSUMER PRICE INDEX FOR ALL ITEMS AND FOR MEDICAL CARE COMPONENTS: UNITED STATES, SELECTED YEARS, 1980–2003

	1980–1990	1990–1995	1995–2000	2000–2005	2005–2010
	Average Annual Percent Change				
CPI, all items	4.7	3.1	2.5	2.5	2.2
Less medical care	4.5	2.9	2.4	2.4	2.2
CPI, all services	6.0	3.9	3.0	3.3	2.7
All medical care	8.1	6.3	3.4	4.4	3.9
Medical care services	8.1	6.6	3.5	4.8	4.3
Professional medical services	7.2	5.2	3.4	3.4	3.2
Physicians' services	7.7	5.4	3.2	3.3	3.0
Dental services	7.0	5.8	4.6	4.6	4.4
Eye care	—–—	3.2	1.8	1.7	1.6
Services by other medical professionals	—–—	3.7	2.4	2.9	2.9
Hospital and related services	9.9	7.7	4.2	6.7	7.1
Medical care commodities	8.0	4.6	3.1	3.0	2.8
Prescription drugs	9.6	5.3	4.0	4.1	3.4

Source: Calculated from Table 8.3.

TABLE 8.5. PERSONAL HEALTH CARE EXPENDITURES, BY SELECTED TYPES OF EXPENDITURE AND SOURCES OF PAYMENT, 2008

Source of Payment	Total	Hospital Care	Physician Service	Prescription Drug	Nursing Home Care	Other Personal Care
			Amount in Billions			
Personal Health Care Expenditures	1952.3	718.4	496.2	234.1	138.4	199.3
			Percentage of Total			
Out-of-pocket payments	14.2	3.2	10.1	20.7	26.7	34.1
Private health insurance	35.4	36.1	48.7	42.1	7.4	13.3
Other private funds	3.9	3.8	6.4	0	3.7	5.1
Government	46.5	56.9	34.7	37.2	62.2	47.5
Medicare	22.8	29.4	20.7	22.2	18.6	12.8
Medicaid and CHIP	16.7	17.5	7.8	9.0	40.6	27.5

Source: U.S. Department of Health and Human Services, Public Health Service. (2010). *Health United States, 2010,* Table 126. Retrieved from http://www.cdc.gov/nchs/data/hus/hus10.pdf#listtables.

TABLE 8.6. ANNUAL CHANGE IN PERSONAL HEALTH CARE EXPENDITURES, BY SELECTED TYPE OF SERVICE, UNITED STATES, 1980–2008

Year	All Expenditures	Hospital	Physician	Nursing Home	Prescription Drug	Other Personal Care
		Average Annual Percent Change				
1980–1990	11.0	96.0	12.8	11.5	12.9	11.1
1990–1995	7.2	6.2	7.0	7.2	8.6	9.6
1995–2000	5.5	3.8	4.2	4.7	14.9	5.4
2000–2008	7.0	7.0	7.0	4.8	8.6	6.0

Source: U.S. Department of Health and Human Services, Public Health Service, *Health United States 2010*, Table 126. Retrieved from http://www.cdc.gov/nchs/data/hus/hus10.pdf #listtables.

Table 8.6 shows annual rate of change in U.S. health expenditures, by type of service, between 1980 and 2008. Expenditure growth has slowed since 1990, but it is still far higher than in the rest of the economy. There has also been a resurgence of growth during the 2000s. Since 2008, expenditure growth has moderated somewhat (not shown in tables). In 2009, expenditures grew by 3.8 percent, and in 2010, by 3.9 percent (Martin et al., 2012). It is too early to know whether this lower growth rate will persist in subsequent years.

In examining types of service, note that the most important trend is the tremendous growth in spending on pharmaceuticals, which has hovered around 15 percent per year in the late 1990s and has continued to grow faster than spending for other services since then. This far exceeds all other service types, which have grown in the single digits.

Analysts have not only studied past trends in expenditures; they have also used simulation models to project what expenditures will be in future years. One recent set of projections concluded that the proportion of gross domestic project accounted for by health expenditures will increase to 19.8 percent—representing $4.6 trillion—by 2020 (Keehan et al., 2011).

In considering these figures, one should keep in mind that such projections often turn out to be quite off the mark; accurately projecting health spending is difficult at best.

Aside from a number of technical assumptions, the problem with believing these projections is that they assume, on some level at least, continuation of current expenditure trends. This is unlikely to be the case as health care further crowds out other public and private expenditures. Nevertheless, the increasing ability of new medical technologies and, increasingly, genetic therapies to improve people's health lends credence to the belief that health expenditures will continue growing rapidly in the years to come.

International Expenditures

Table 8.7 shows total health expenditures as a percentage of GDP in OECD countries over the period 1980 to 2007. The 2007 figure for the United States, 16.0 percent, is almost one-third higher than for any other country; only France reached the 11 percent threshold. Not shown in the table are per capita expenditures expressed in dollars. In 2007, the U.S. figure was about $7,290, a full 53 percent higher than the next highest country (Norway).

Future Directions

An important issue facing the United States is availability of accurate and timely data on national health care utilization rates and expenditures. The United States does not have a system in place that allows it to compute expenditures for the entire health care sector in a consistent and timely fashion. Such a dataset would be extremely beneficial, and perhaps even essential, for enacting certain types of health care reform, particularly those that are regulatory in nature.

The problem, in a nutshell, is this: the U.S. government does not require private insurers to collect and release data on expenditures. Such data, if available in a consistent format, would increase the country's flexibility in adopting various types of reform.

SUMMARY

This chapter has discussed how health care costs are measured and has shown recent levels and trends. The next chapter considers various

TABLE 8.7. HEALTH EXPENDITURES AS A PERCENTAGE OF GROSS
DOMESTIC PRODUCT: SELECTED COUNTRIES AND YEARS,
1980–2007

Country	1980	1990	1995	2000	2007
Australia	6.3%	6.9	7.4	8.3	8.9
Austria	7.4	8.3	9.5	9.9	10.1
Belgium	6.3	7.2	8.2	8.6	10.2
Canada	7.0	8.9	9.0	8.8	10.1
Denmark	8.9	8.3	8.1	8.3	9.8
Finland	6.3	7.7	7.9	7.2	8.2
France	7.0	8.4	10.4	10.1	11.0
Germany	8.4	8.3	10.1	10.3	10.4
Greece	5.9	6.6	8.6	7.9	9.6
Iceland	5.3	7.8	8.2	9.5	9.3
Ireland	8.3	6.1	6.7	6.3	7.6
Italy	6.5	6.0	6.9	7.7	8.7
Japan	6.5	6.0	6.9	7.7	8.1
Luxembourg	5.2	5.4	5.6	5.8	7.3
Netherlands	7.4	8.0	8.3	8.0	9.8
New Zealand	7.0	7.6	7.2	7.7	9.0
Norway	7.0	7.6	7.9	8.4	8.9

TABLE 8.7. HEALTH EXPENDITURES AS A PERCENTAGE OF GROSS
DOMESTIC PRODUCT: SELECTED COUNTRIES AND YEARS,
1980–2007 (Continued)

Country	1980	1990	1995	2000	2007
Portugal	5.3	5.9	7.8	8.8	9.9
Spain	5.3	6.5	7.4	7.2	8.5
Sweden	7.3	8.2	9.0	10.2	10.8
Switzerland	7.3	8.2	9.6	10.2	10.8
United Kingdom	5.6	5.9	6.8	7.0	8.4
United States	9.0	12.2	13.6	13.6	16.0

Source: U.S. Department of Health and Human Services, Public Health Service, *Health United States 2010*, Table 121. Retrieved from http://www.cdc.gov/nchs/data/hus/hus10.pdf #listtables.

methods of controlling these costs. Before doing so, one must ask a natural question: Is it even necessary to control national health expenditures?

The question is not a trivial one. If society wishes to spend more on health care, and consequently less on other things, why should it be stopped—particularly when it seems increasingly clear that certain new medical devices, products, and procedures can improve the quality and length of life?

It turns out that there are several reasons cost control is important and likely to be in the forefront of health policy for years to come. First, there are significant opportunity costs associated with additional spending. A dollar spent on health cannot be spent on such other things as education, housing, or consumer goods. Cost control continues to be a major issue simply because it is imprudent to waste money in the face of so many strong consumer desires and societal needs.

Second, there are various ways in which the health care market is imperfect, which fact may lead to more spending than is desirable. Unlike other goods and services, health care services are often well insured, which insulates consumers from facing their true cost (that is, resource value).

In addition, because consumer information is often poor, people may demand medical goods and services in part because of strong advertising or because they are "induced" to do so by providers who have a pecuniary incentive to increase demand.

Third, government now pays for almost half of U.S. health care spending. With recent government deficits, the future of social programs is worrisome. Medicare faces the prospect of more recipients and fewer contributors as the Baby Boom generation retires; problems for Medicaid are also salient, with nearly all states engaged in significant eligibility, benefit, or reimbursement cuts.

Finally, one of the major reasons that the number of uninsured persons continues to increase in the United States is rising health care costs, which make it more difficult for employers to offer coverage to employees and for individuals to pay for premiums (Kronick & Gilmer, 1999). If the Affordable Care Act is implemented as proposed, uninsurance rates will decrease by an estimated 60 percent.

In summary, there are compelling reasons to believe not only that health care costs will remain a central policy interest but also that their control is in the national interest.

KEY TERMS

Consumer Price Index (CPI) A measure published by the federal government that gauges how much the prices of a standard set of goods and services change over a specific period of time. In health care, there are separate indices for such goods and services as hospital and physician care, dental care, and prescription drugs.

Costs The value of resources used in producing a good or service. There are two distinct definitions of cost. Accounting costs include only the value of the resources used in production (that is, labor and capital). Economic costs also include a normal rate of return on investment.

Expenditures How much is spent on one or more goods or services. This is equal to the price of a good or service multiplied by the quantity used.

Profits A term that applies to a particular firm. From an accounting perspective, it is equal to how much revenue is obtained from selling its goods and services, less its cost in producing them. The economic definition of profits is slightly different, in that a normal rate of return on investment is included as a component of costs. As a result, in a competitive market economic costs are generally equal to zero.

DISCUSSION QUESTIONS

1. Economists and accountants use very different definitions of costs and profits. What definition does each employ, and how do they differ? Why has each adopted this particular definition?
2. Health care expenditures have risen far faster than medical care prices. Nevertheless, one often hears about how much the Consumer Price Index (CPI) for medical care has risen over time. What value, if any, does the medical CPI or its subindices have to health policy analysts and health care managers?
3. An article by Keehan and colleagues (2011) estimates that the proportion of national income spent on health care will rise to 19.8 percent in 2020. In the past, however, such long-range predictions have been far off target. Discuss reasons why such projections may overstate this growth.
4. Compared to other countries, what particular challenges does the United States face in compiling valid data on total health care expenditures?
5. One of the major impediments to finding accurate health care expenditure data is that the United States does not require insurers to collect or release such data, nor are these data, when collected, necessarily in a consistent format. Should the U.S. government require all private insurers to collect and turn in timely data on health care expenditures of its enrollees?
6. "It is not necessary for a country to control its health care expenditures, since they may reflect the desires of the populace. As the United States becomes wealthier, and as medical care interventions become more effective in improving health, spending more on our national wealth on medical care is good, not bad." Take a side and defend your reasons for agreeing or disagreeing with this statement.

FURTHER READING

Department of Health and Human Services, National Center for Health Statistics. (2012). *Health, United States, 2011*. Washington, DC: Government Printing Office. Retrieved from http://www.cdc.gov/nchs/hus.htm

This book provides a several hundred-page annual compendium of health statistics in the United States.

Hartman, M., Martin, A. B., Benson, J., Catlin, A., & the National Health Expenditure Accounts Team. (2013). National health spending in 2011: Overall growth remains low, but some payers and services show signs of acceleration. *Health Affairs, 32*(1), 87–98.

At time of this writing, this article offers some of the most recent statistics on U.S. health care spending. Published annually in the journal *Health Affairs.*

Keehan, S. P., Cuckler, G. A., Sisko, A. M., Madison, A. J., Smith, S. D., Lizonitz, J. M., . . . Wolfe, C. J. (2012). National health expenditure projections: Modest annual growth until coverage expands and economic growth accelerates. *Health Affairs, 31*(7), 1600–1612.

At time of this writing, this article offers some of the most recent statistics on projected U.S. health care spending.

Organisation for Economic Co-operation and Development (OECD). *Health policies and data.* Retrieved from http://www.oecd.org/health/health-systems

This website provides information on accessing OECD's data on various measures of the health care systems of developed countries (such as costs, health statistics, and supply), as well as reports from OECD researchers comparing different facets of health care systems.

U.S. Department of Labor, Bureau of Labor Statistics. Consumer Price Indices. Retrieved from http://www.bls.gov/cpi/home.htm

This website provides information on how the CPI is formed, its history and uses, as well as current and time-series data on how prices have changed over time.

REFERENCES

Anderson, G. F., & Frogner, B. K. (2008). Health spending In OECD countries: Obtaining value per dollar. *Health Affairs, 27*, 1718–1727.

Feldstein, P. (2004). *Health care economics* (6th ed.). Clifton Park, NY: Thomson Delmar Learning.

Keehan, S. P., Sisko, A. M., Truffer, C. J., Poisal, J. A., Cuckler, G. A., Madison, A. J., . . . Smith, S. D. (2011). National health spending projections through 2020: Economic recovery and reform drive faster spending growth. *Health Affairs, 30*, 1594–1605.

Kronick, R, & Gilmer, T. (1999). Explaining the decline in health insurance coverage, 1979–1995. *Health Affairs, 18*, 30–47.

Martin, A. B., Lassman, D., Washington, B., Catlin, A., & the National Health Expenditure Accounts Team. (2012). Growth in US health spending remained slow in 2010; health share of gross domestic project was unchanged from 2009. *Health Affairs 31*, 208–219.

CHAPTER NINE

CONTAINING HEALTH CARE COSTS

Thomas H. Rice
Gerald F. Kominski

Learning Objectives

- Explain and analyze the broad determinants of health care expenditures in fee-for-service and capitated systems
- Discuss methods of controlling fee-for-service costs: those focusing on price, on quantity, or directly on expenditures
- Discuss methods of controlling capitated costs
- Explore the challenges presented by alternative cost-containment methods, including the ability of providers to shift costs from one payer to another, data challenges when there is no national health care system, and unintended impacts that may compromise the quality of care

This chapter examines different ways in which a country can attempt to contain health care costs. It begins with an accounting framework to show the different components of cost increases, separately for fee-for-service and capitation systems. Using this framework, it then provides evidence on the success of various methods to control costs that have been tried either in the United States or in other developed countries.

Framework

Before embarking on an analysis of alternative cost-containment strategies, it is useful to construct a framework that groups together similar strategies. The first equation here applies to the fee-for-service system, and the second to capitated systems:

$$(1) \qquad E = \sum_{j=1}^{J} (P_j \times Q_j)$$

$$(2) \qquad E = \sum_{j=1}^{J} (C_j \times N_j)$$

where

E = total health expenditures (or costs)

P = unit price for services

Q = quantity of services in a time period

C = cost of all services per person in a time period

N = number of persons

j = index representing each payer

Equation 1 states that total expenditures are equal to the product of the price of services and the quantity of services, summed over all payers. In other words, it is the sum of P times Q for Medicare, Medicaid, Blue Cross and Blue Shield, each private insurer, and so on. In contrast, Equation 2 is oriented toward the person, not the service. In this equation, total expenditures (or costs) are simply the product of costs per person and the number of persons, again summed over all payers. Here, total expenditures would equal the number of Medicare beneficiaries multiplied by cost per beneficiary, plus the number of Blue Cross enrollees times the cost per enrollee, and so forth.

The equations employ summation signs to illustrate the potential for "*cost shifting.*" To illustrate, suppose that one payer, Medicare, successfully controls both P and Q. This clearly results in lower Medicare costs, but it does not necessarily contain systemwide health care costs. This is because hospitals and physicians might respond to Medicare's controls by trying to increase their Ps or Qs to the patients of other payers. The same thing could happen in Equation 2. A health plan with market clout might cut a particularly good deal with an HMO, and the HMO might respond by charging more to other insurers.

Our framework only defines the determinants of health expenditures; what may be hidden is the fact that the success of alternative cost-containment strategies hinges on how they affect consumer and provider behavior. In Equation 1, for example, it might appear a reasonable strategy for controlling expenditures to lower the price of services paid to physicians. This would not be successful, however, if physicians responded to these price controls by inducing their patients to obtain more services (that is, P would go down, but Q would go up).

The same is true of the capitation strategies in Equation 2. The most obvious approach for controlling expenditures seemingly is to control costs per person. However, if this is accomplished by paying HMOs less, they may in turn respond by seeking to enroll only the healthiest people, or by lowering the quality of care they provide.

In analyzing cost-containment strategies, then, we must be aware of the ability of providers (and others) to "game" the system to meet their own goals. Strategies that are difficult to game tend to be most successful. As an example, we argue that some hospital rate-setting programs were moderately successful in containing costs because it was difficult for hospitals to game the system by increasing admissions and length of stay. Instead, physicians rather than hospitals made these decisions, and physician payment rates were not affected by the rate-setting programs. In contrast, certificate-of-need programs were less successful in controlling costs because hospitals were able to respond to restrictions on growth in the number of beds by purchasing more equipment and engaging in other activities that were not regulated (or that were tolerated by the regulators). Thus, in analyzing cost-containment strategies, we focus on how they influence provider and consumer behavior, which in turn strongly influences their ultimate success or failure.

Before we proceed any further, one other caveat is necessary. This chapter focuses on ways of containing costs, but it must be remembered that cost containment is not society's only goal with regard to health services; access and quality of care also matter. Consequently, if analysts find that a particular strategy is effective in controlling costs, they must also consider any spillover effects—such as decreased quality—that result. Only by considering both benefits and costs can we make the best policy decisions for reforming our health care system.

Analysis of Cost-Containment Strategies

This section uses the framework just presented to review evidence regarding the cost-containment potential of various fee-for-service and capitated cost-containment strategies. Although it addresses more than a dozen such strategies, still others cannot be included because of space limitations.

Before embarking on this review, an explanation is in order. One cost-containment tool could just as easily be included in the fee-for-service or capitation section: increased patient cost sharing. As will be noted, patient cost sharing requirements have been increasing rapidly in order to keep utilization rates and costs down by making consumers think twice before using additional costly services. Under fee-for-service payment systems, cost sharing is designed to reduce the quantity of services (Q in the first equation); under capitation arrangements, cost sharing is designed to reduce costs per person (C in the second equation). Somewhat arbitrarily, we have included it as the last cost containment strategy in the fee-for-service section, just before capitation is discussed.

Fee-for-Service Options

Fee-for-service options can be divided into three types, each corresponding to a term in Equation 1: P, Q, and E. The discussion here is divided accordingly.

Price Options. One type of cost-containment strategy that has been attempted at various times in the United States is controlling the unit price paid to the provider. On the hospital side, examples include state hospital rate-setting programs and use of diagnosis-related groups. On the physician side, the Medicare and Medicaid programs have, at various times, attempted to control their costs by freezing (or even lowering) physician payments. There is also some experience in this regard from Canada. Since the early 1990s, Medicare and many Medicaid programs have adopted resource-based fee schedules, which are simply another form of price controls.

Before reviewing the available evidence, it is useful to outline the overall advantages and disadvantages of price-control options. There are two potential advantages. First, controlling price typically involves less administrative effort (and expense) than controlling the quantity of service. Rather than examining the appropriateness of every provider and every service, it is only necessary to ensure that payments conform to regulated amounts.

Second, and related to this, price regulation tends to be less intrusive; it does not entail the type of micromanagement often encountered in the quantity-related options discussed next.

There are some disadvantages, however. First, it addresses only one component of total expenditures. As we shall see, a price-based strategy can be circumvented if providers are able to increase the quantity of service they provide. Second, these strategies can diminish the efficiency of the market. If the wrong price is chosen, the wrong quantity or mix of services may result.

Several states adopted hospital rate-setting programs in the 1970s and 1980s. These programs varied on a number of dimensions, the most important of which were whether they were voluntary or mandatory and whether they applied to some or all payers. Most (but not all) were aimed at giving hospitals an incentive to spend less by controlling hospital charges per day.

Of the twenty-five state-level programs that were in effect by the end of the 1970s, only eight were mandatory as opposed to voluntary, and only four—in Maryland, Massachusetts, New Jersey, and New York—applied to all payers (Ashby, 1984). In most cases, these programs established uniform payments, so that public and private insurers paid the same price for the same unit of care (for example, days of care, admission, and so on). To include Medicare in their all-payer systems, these states had to apply to the Health Care Financing Administration (HCFA, now the Centers for Medicare and Medicaid Services, or CMS) for waivers exempting them from Medicare's national payment rules. In granting these waivers, HCFA limited the rate of growth in total Medicare inpatient payments, or in Medicare inpatient payments per case, under the all-payer programs (Davis, Anderson, Rowland, & Steinberg, 1990).

Since 1985, with the exception of Maryland these states have either lost their waivers or allowed them to expire. Ironically, one factor contributing to the financial pressure for these states to abandon waivers was the implementation of the Medicare diagnosis-related groups (DRG) system in 1983. Because payment rates during the first three years of DRGs were a blend of hospital-specific and national payment amounts, these states felt pressure from their hospital associations to abandon the waivers because hospitals could increase their Medicare revenue by joining the DRG system.

Most research on the subject found that these four programs were most effective, with savings on the order of 10 to 15 percent (Robinson & Luft, 1988; Thorpe, 1987). It might seem surprising that a gross strategy that limits hospital payments per day would work, but apparently it did. This is likely because of the difficulty hospitals had in "gaming" such a system. If a hospital wants to raise more revenue under an all-payer system, it has two choices: increase the number of admissions or increase length of stay. But neither option is typically available to hospitals because these decisions are made by physicians, whose fees are generally not subject to these controls. Consequently, as much as a hospital might wish to raise more revenue, it might not have the ability to do so.

Implementation of the DRG system made such gaming even more difficult (although it led to its own gaming, of course). Under the DRG system, hospitals are paid a fixed amount of money for a particular diagnosis, irrespective of how much is spent on treating a patient. Hospitals therefore cannot benefit by trying to keep patients longer. Another option for garnering more revenue is to increase the number of admissions, but this has not happened, for two reasons: the physician, rather than the hospital, makes this decision, and hospitals found it profitable to treat patients on an outpatient basis, which is paid for separately and outside the DRG system.

There remain two other avenues for increasing revenue under DRGs: earning more from treating Medicare patients on an outpatient basis and shifting costs to other payers. Although Medicare outpatient costs have risen rapidly, this increase has not been sufficient to cut deeply into Medicare savings. Since 2000, hospital outpatient care under Medicare has been paid for using an outpatient prospective payment system (PPS), thus further reducing revenue from outpatient care.

The same cannot be said about the shift to other payers. Over the years, researchers have found that hospitals do resort to shifting costs onto private payers. The magnitude of cost-shifting practice is shown in Table 9.1 (American Hospital Association, 2011). In 1990, for example, Medicare paid hospitals less than 90 percent of the costs associated with treating program patients, and Medicaid only 80 percent. In contrast, private insurers paid hospitals about 24 percent more for their patients' care than it actually cost to provide. As the table shows, trends in cost shifting have varied over the years, but overall, the amount has not changed dramatically over the past twenty years. Medicare still pays about 90 percent of the cost of its beneficiaries, Medicaid's figures have risen to almost 90 percent, and private insurers are now paying even more to hospitals for treating their enrollees.

Because of cost shifting, some analysts concluded that DRGs have done little, if anything, to control national health care spending (Chulis, 1991), evidence of substantial savings in the Medicare program notwithstanding

TABLE 9.1. HOSPITAL PAYMENT-TO-COST RATIOS, 1990–2009

Year	Medicare	Medicaid	Private
1990	89.4	80.1	124.4
1995	99.4	94.0	124.0
2000	99.1	94.5	115.7
2005	92.3	87.1	129.4
2009	90.1	89.0	134.1

Source: American Hospital Association, 2011.

(Russell & Manning, 1989). This is not necessarily an indictment of DRGs, however. If other payers were to adopt DRGs, systemwide hospital spending might be better controlled. For example, a number of state Medicaid programs have adopted payment systems based on DRGs, but most commercial insurers have not (Reinhardt, 2009).

These conclusions about the successes and failures of hospital price controls are further supported by experience with physician controls. Most studies indicate limited cost savings when physician payments are frozen or reduced, because physicians respond by providing a greater quantity of services (Gabel & Rice, 1985). In making its projections about physician payment costs under the new Medicare fee schedule that was implemented starting in 1992, the Congressional Budget Office concluded that for every 1 percent reduction in physician fees, the volume of services would rise by 0.56 percent (Christensen, 1992).

Why might these physician controls be less effective than hospital controls? It is because physicians have greater ability to game the payment system. If their payment rate drops, physicians in a fee-for-service environment can attempt to increase the volume of services (and may very well succeed). Hospitals do not generally have this ability.

Nevertheless, physicians' ability to generate additional billing is probably limited. This is illustrated by the experience of the Canadian provinces, which have tightly controlled physician fees since the early 1970s. Although the quantity of services rose faster in Canada than in the United States over this time period, it was not nearly enough to compensate for the lower fees (Barer, Evans, & Labelle, 1988). In a country like the United States, where there are multiple payers, an effective way for a payer to control physician spending is to pay so little to doctors that they do not want to treat such patients. This, of course, is what has happened in many state

Medicaid programs. Canadian provinces do not suffer from this problem because there is only one payer; the provinces are the only game in town.

Quantity Options. The next fee-for-service cost-containment strategies are those aimed at service quantity or utilization. Examples are certificate-of-need programs, technology controls, utilization management, and practice guidelines, to name just a few. Their primary advantage over price options is that they can focus on reducing waste in the system. For example, if a particular procedure is inappropriate for a patient with a given diagnosis, quantity options can focus on the problem.

There are two disadvantages. Like price options, they target only one component of expenditure. If providers can game utilization controls by increasing prices, then the savings from these programs are diminished. Second, the strategies are often cumbersome from an administrative stand-point, involving much bureaucracy, paperwork, and additional oversight over the practice of medicine.

The earliest examples of quantity controls were *certificate-of-need (CON)* programs. These programs, which became commonplace in the early 1970s, were aimed at controlling expenditures by reducing the amount of hospital resources available, both beds and equipment. Typically, hospitals needed permission for any proposed investment in excess of $100,000. A local board called the health systems agency ruled on a hospital's request for additional resources.

Many studies have been conducted on CON, and almost all reach the same conclusion: it did not succeed in saving money (Steinwald & Sloan, 1981). Although there was some effect on the number of hospital beds, capital equipment per bed rose even more quickly than before. There are a number of reasons for this failure, but the fundamental one is that the entity making the decisions on the hospital's application (the local health systems agency, and ultimately the state) was not financially accountable for the increased cost associated with approving a hospital's request. In other words, why turn down a hospital request when the cost would be borne by such payers as Medicare, Blue Cross, or commercial insurers? On the contrary, board members would have every incentive to approve requests by their local hospital, since this would be viewed as helpful to their community and constituencies.

This is not to say that technology controls can't work; they probably can. However, they need to be implemented at a broader geographic level by an entity that is at risk for additional health care spending. The Canadian provinces give us such an example.

There is no single Canadian health care system. Rather, each province has its own system, but all have to conform to various federal requirements if they are to receive federal contributions. One key point often overlooked in the literature is that provinces are 100 percent at risk for additional health care spending because annual federal contributions are fixed. Unlike the U.S. Medicaid program, where the federal government at least matches additional state spending, provinces do not receive an additional penny if they spend more on health care than anticipated.

Since provinces are also responsible for financing a host of other nonhealth programs, they must be judicious in allotting their tax revenues to health care. One way they do this is by controlling the diffusion of medical technology. If a hospital wants to expand or purchase equipment, it needs the province's permission, and provinces have not been eager to grant requests. The United States has far more of most technologies than Canada, measured per capita. For example, in 2008 the United States had 25.9 MRI units and 34.3 CT scanners per million people; Canada's figures were only 6.7 and 12.7, respectively (Squires, 2011).

Canadians often claim that they have achieved this by regionalizing their technologies, thereby making their system more efficient. Others contend, however, that the result is rationing. Indeed, evidence from 2007 and 2008 surveys of the public in seven countries (Australia, Canada, Germany, Netherlands, New Zealand, United Kingdom, and United States) found that Canadians reported the longest waits for seeing a specialist and receiving elective surgery. Regarding waiting to see a specialist, the United States reported the shortest waits, with 74 percent seeing one within four weeks; Canada ranked sixth, with a figure of only 40 percent. With respect to receiving elective surgery, the United States ranked third, with 8 percent waiting more than four months. Canada ranked last; 27 percent reported waiting more than four months (Davis, Schoen, & Stremikis, 2010).

Up to this point, the discussion of quantity has focused not on services, but on hospital beds and technologies. In the United States, however, most of the focus is aimed at particular services. This is commonly done through *utilization management (UM)*. UM programs are normally implemented by third-party payers as a way to reduce provision of unnecessary or inappropriate services. Examples are preadmission certification of hospital stays, concurrent and retrospective review of stays, management of high-cost patients, requiring a second opinion before embarking on surgery, and profiling of physicians' practices.

There is a dearth of recent literature evaluating the impact of UM in fee-for-service settings, perhaps because more attention has been paid to capitated arrangements. One review of the literature examined three types: utilization review, case management, and physician gate keeping. Prospective review of hospital stays was found to reduce admissions by about 10 percent, but concurrent review had little impact. Moreover, hospital outpatient utilization increased as a result, so the savings were even smaller. Studies show little impact of case management on cost control, in part because of the difficulty in coordinating the activities of a number of physicians. The literature on the cost-savings potential of physician gatekeeping is too sparse for making any generalization (Wickizer & Lessler, 2002). One issue for those who are concerned about controlling future health care expenditures is that UM programs are almost universal now, meaning that we may have already gained about as much in savings as can be extracted.

The wave of the future is now on developing UM for the outpatient setting, particularly through physician profiling. However, the savings potential of these programs is still largely untested. There is strong reason to believe that UM in the outpatient setting is much more difficult to implement, because of the difficulty in knowing whether a physician who is a high spender is less efficient or more profligate, or alternatively has a more severely ill group of patients than his or her peers. Normally one tries to risk-adjust a provider's case mix, but this is difficult at the level of the individual physician who experiences a relatively low caseload and therefore is more likely to have healthier or sicker patients as a result of random chance. The best we are likely to do—and this is now the emphasis—is to employ risk-adjustment formulas with physician groups.

The most recent UM efforts focus on developing *practice guidelines.* These are written protocols designed to instruct physicians on which procedures are appropriate for a patient with a particular diagnosis. The guidelines are largely being developed by researchers under the auspices of the federal Agency for Healthcare Research and Quality, although some medical specialty groups are doing so as well. One intent of the guidelines is to increase quality by reducing the amount of regional variation in health care use. It has been widely documented that parts of the country have differing surgery rates for certain procedures, and that this cannot be readily explained by variation in patient health status (Song et al., 2010).

Development of practice guidelines is still relatively new, so we cannot know the extent to which they might control costs. Moreover, because these programs aim far more at improving quality than cost containment, relatively little research has been conducted on the latter. There is reason to be skeptical, though. Just as practice guidelines could reduce resource use by physicians who overtreat patients by providing too many services, they could just as well increase spending by physicians who currently offer fewer services than are recommended by the guidelines. The issue, then, is whether the guidelines are likely to prescribe a quantity of service that is greater or less than what is currently being provided. One study that implies we are underproviding—and therefore that adherence to guidelines will result in more utilization—was conducted by McGlynn and colleagues (2003). Examining over four hundred indicators of quality for thirty medical conditions, they found that patients received only 55 percent of recommended care.

Expenditure Options. The fee-for-service options are those that directly target expenditure. Some examples are Medicare's *Sustainable Growth Rate (SGR)* system, hospital global budgets, and national and subnational health budgeting. The overriding advantage of expenditure control is somewhat tautological; it directly aims at controlling health care expenditures. The extent to which this can succeed, however, depends in large measure on whether all health care spending is targeted or just a component of total spending, such as hospital or physician expenditures. The primary disadvantage is that implementing such controls may result in a less efficient health care system, which could reduce the quality of services.

The primary example of expenditure control in the United States was implementation of Medicare Volume Performance Standards (VPS) in the early 1990s, which were replaced by the somewhat similar Sustainable Growth Rate (SGR) system. The VPS system was part of the 1989 physician payment reforms adopted by Congress that also resulted in the Medicare Fee Schedule, which is based on the *resource-based relative value scale (RBRVS)*. Congress recognized that simply redistributing physician fees to make higher payments to primary care physicians and lower payments to specialists, though more equitable, would not by itself control burgeoning program expenditures. This was left to the VPS system.

Under the system, each year Congress set a target rate of increase in Medicare Part B physician expenditures. If actual spending exceeded the target, the next year's physician fee update was normally reduced by that amount (although, of course, Congress could do whatever it chose when the time came). Conversely, if the growth in spending was less than the target, physicians would get more. Suppose, for example, that the target for a particular year was a 10 percent increase in spending. If actual spending increased by 12 percent, the target would be exceeded. Most likely, this would be extracted the next time Congress updated Medicare physician fees. If physicians were due a 5 percent cost-of-living increase, they would likely be granted only 3 percent.

The SGR system was enacted as part of the Balanced Budget Act of 1997 and implemented in 1998. The main difference between it and the VPS system was in setting the target expenditure rate of sustainable growth, which was determined by four factors: the percentage change in physician input prices, the percentage change in Part B fee-for-service enrollment, the projected change in real GDP, and the percentage change in spending for physicians' services resulting from other changes in law (Medicare Payment Advisory Commission [MedPAC], 2000).

The VPS and SGR systems have been criticized as being too blunt an instrument for affecting the individual physician's behavior. Because the systems apply nationally, individual physicians who increase their volume of services do not pay the price by experiencing a decline in fees. This happens only if all physicians behave this way. But if a physician does not increase his or her volume and other physicians do, then the first physician suffers—volume (Q) does not climb, but the fee (P) falls as a result of the behavior of other physicians. These systems therefore contain a "perverse" incentive to increase the volume of services—which is exactly what they are supposed to prevent. One way to improve the incentives is to target smaller groups of physicians, by having separate targets for each specialty, state, or state-specialty combination (Rice & Bernstein, 1990; Kominski, 1998).

The SGR system has been the subject of intense criticism. Being anchored by a formula based, in part, on growth in the economy, it does not take into account upward trends in medical technology diffusion, which is generally acknowledged as one of the leading factors in recent health care expenditure growth. This means that the payment formula has resulted in substantial annual reduction in fee updates. For nearly a decade, each year these reductions have been nullified by Congress, but this does nothing to solve the basic issue (MedPAC, 2012). The problem deepens each year. MedPAC has recommended that the SGR system be replaced by one of specific fee increases over each of the next ten years, based on growth in the number of Medicare beneficiaries as well as service usage per beneficiary. If Congress had not overridden the formula in 2011, Medicare physician payments would have been reduced by nearly 30 percent in 2012 (MedPAC, 2012).

To find an example of expenditure controls applied to the hospital level, we must again look to Canada. In each province, hospitals are paid an annual *global budget*, which is negotiated between the province and the individual hospital. If a hospital exceeds its budget, there is no guarantee that it will be compensated.

Hospital global budgets seem to work in the sense that since their inception hospital spending in Canada has risen much less quickly than in the United States. The primary way in which this has been achieved is that Canadian hospitals now have fewer nonphysician personnel than do their U.S. counterparts.(Capital expenditures have also been controlled, but for different reasons, since they are not included in the global budgets.) One perverse effect is that Canadian hospitals seem to prefer long-staying patients who might belong in nursing homes, because these patients occupy a bed but use few other resources. Another fear is that the lack of resources is diminishing the quality of care in Canadian hospitals. What little available evidence there is indicates, however, that inpatient outcomes appear to be similar in the two countries (Newhouse, Anderson, & Roos, 1988; Detsky, Stacey, & Bombardier, 1983) and that, with the exception of longer waits for elective services, quality and satisfaction indicators are comparable or favorable to Canada (Davis et al., 2010).

The two aforementioned strategies—Medicare VPS and SGR, and hospital global budgets—do not constitute a comprehensive cost-control policy because they are aimed at only one component of health care expenditures. A broader strategy might be to target all (or most) health expenditures at the same time, through a system of national or regional budgeting.

The typical way of controlling total expenditures in a fee-for-service system is through expenditure targets. Generally, under such a system unit prices are adjusted to ensure that targeted expenditures are met. This differs from the VPS and SGR systems in two primary ways: (1) it applies to all payers, not just to Medicare; and (2) it applies to most of the health care system, not just physician payment. Although the United States has the most experience with using expenditure targets for paying physicians, it could nevertheless be applied to other services, such as hospitalization. In such a case, DRG payments per admission could be tied to meeting specific growth in inpatient expenditure (Marquis & Kominski, 1994).

The advantage of such a system, of course, is that it controls expenditures directly. But there are several possible disadvantages: it might result in inefficient use of resources, it could potentially harm quality, and it requires massive amounts of timely data that currently are not being produced.

With regard to efficiency in a competitive market, in the long run price is based on the cost of producing a good or service. If the price is too high, then the incentive is to overproduce the good; if it is too low, the incentive is to underproduce. Under an expenditure target system, prices change not in response to demand and supply considerations, but rather in how closely total expenditures conform to a target. One positive aspect of this approach is that prices tend to fall when quantity is too high, so it might be argued that the system is self-correcting. Counteracting this is the fact that there is no assurance that health care inputs will be used efficiently by producers if the market mechanism is circumvented. Even more troubling is the possibility that the mix of services produced is not based on what consumers would like to buy.

This touches on the second potential problem: quality. Suppose that Congress sets an austere budget level, necessitating a subsequent decline in unit prices. This may dissuade providers from delivering necessary services for fear that they will exceed the expenditure target, which in turn can result in diminished quality. Because adequate data systems are still being developed to monitor quality, there is a strong possibility that quality will be sacrificed in favor of controlling expenditures.

Finally, there is the data problem. To make expenditure targets work in a fee-for-service system, it is necessary to have up-to-date information about the quantity of services provided to all patients. It is through this information that total expenditures are tallied and updates are made to provider prices. In the United States, however, we have no formal mechanism for obtaining timely utilization and expenditure data for privately insured patients or for publicly insured patients in managed care. It would take several years to develop such a system, but the process has not yet even started. Thus the fee-for-service method that has the greatest likelihood of controlling cost perhaps also suffers from the most shortcomings. This illustrates that there are indeed no easy answers for controlling cost under a fee-for-service system.

Patient Cost Sharing. There are many ways in which insured patients can share in the cost of the services they use. There are deductibles (amount paid out of pocket before insurance benefits kick in), copayments (fixed amount paid per covered service), and coinsurance (percentage of costs paid per service). Historically, copayment has been the most common in capitated systems, but more recently there has been a proliferation of deductibles as well, particularly of high-deductible insurance products that are included in the benefit packages of health savings accounts.

To illustrate these rapid increases, between 2006 and 2011, the percentage of workers enrolled in a health plan that contained a $1,000 or more annual deductible for single coverage tripled, from 10 percent to 31 percent. The percentage of workers in a plan with a $2,000 or higher deductible quadrupled during this time period, from 3 percent to 12 percent (Kaiser Family Foundation, 2011). In the area of prescription drugs, most employees are in so-called "three-tier" plans, which have different patient cost-sharing requirements for generic, preferred brand name, and nonpreferred brand name drugs. Between 2000 and 2011, average copayments for preferred brand name dugs nearly doubled, from $15 to $29, a period in which overall consumer prices rose just 31 percent. Copayments for nonpreferred brand name drugs rose almost 70 percent during these eleven years (Kaiser Family Foundation, 2011).

Cost sharing is designed to make consumers think twice before using additional services. Nearly all research has shown that this is the case. In the most notable research endeavor on the subject, the RAND Health Insurance Experiment (HIE), conducted between 1974 and 1982, individuals who were randomly assigned to policies with zero coinsurance used substantially more services than those who had to pay out of pocket for some of their care. Specifically, it was found that people who have to pay 95 percent of charges had annual expenditures that were 28 percent less than those who paid nothing. More relevant to policy, those paying 25 percent coinsurance had expenditures 18 percent less than those with free care (Manning, Newhouse, Duan, Keeler, & Leibowitz, 1987). Subsequent studies, none of which have had the advantage of employing a true experimental design, supported the finding that patient cost sharing requirements result in a substantially lower utilization rate (Rice & Morrison, 1994).

The impact on this lower utilization on health status, however, is less clear. In general, the HIE found few instances (notably, high blood pressure) in which free care improved health status for the general population. It did find some significant improvements for lower-income persons in poor health. One worrisome finding in the study was that those facing higher copayments did not cut back more on marginally effective services but rather cut their use across the board—reducing the use of care rated by experts as "highly effective" as much as care that is "less effective" or "rarely effective" (Lohr et al., 1986). This implies that although potentially effective, patient cost sharing is a blunt instrument that, if used injudiciously, could impair the health of the population. It is perhaps for those reasons that most other countries have relied more on strategies targeting the suppliers than the demanders of services.

The challenge, then, is to come up with a way to take advantage of the cost-saving potential of patient cost sharing, but doing so in a way that does not dissuade patients from obtaining necessary care. One promising approach, still in its infancy, is called *value-based insurance design*

(VBID). VBID tailors patient cost sharing requirements in a way that encourages patients to purchase those services that are most appropriate for their health conditions. Up until now, VBID has been applied to drugs for certain diseases. For example, a person who has diabetes pays little or nothing toward diabetes medications. This encourages him or her to refill prescriptions and can save society money by avoiding the consequences associated with more severe symptoms. Common chronic conditions for which VBID is being used include diabetes, asthma, and congestive heart failure. Early evidence indicates that its use can raise medication compliance rates (Choudhry et al., 2010).

Capitation Options

Equation 2 showed that three things are necessary to control expenditures under a capitated system: control of costs per person (C), the number of persons (N), and shifting costs between payers. This section focuses on the first component; cost shifting has already been addressed, and controlling the number of persons (say, by denying eligibility for coverage)—although clearly a cost-containment strategy—is inconsistent with the notion of equitable health care reform.

HMOs. The major way in which capitation is used in the U.S. health care system is through health maintenance organizations (HMOs). HMOs provide comprehensive care for a fixed, prepaid annual premium through a defined network of providers. The term HMO itself is attributed to Paul Ellwood in the early 1970s, but the concept goes back far earlier, to the Ross-Loos Medical Group in the late 1920s. Kaiser Permanente, the largest HMO today, has roots in the 1930s.

HMOs can be classified in different ways. One relates to whether the HMO is a single medical organization or if, alternatively, it serves more of an insurance function by contracting with numerous providers. The former are called group- or staff-model HMOs. The latter are often referred to as network-model HMOs and typically consist of several independent practice associations, or IPAs. More colloquially, these are sometimes called "HMOs without walls," because a patient does not get care from an HMO, but rather from a provider that contacts with the HMO. One other distinction is the point of service (POS) model, which is an HMO where it is possible to go outside of the network of providers—but usually at a high out-of-pocket cost to the patient.

HMOs are given an incentive to control costs by the fact that they are paid on a capitation basis. That is, they receive a fixed payment to provide an enrollee's care for a specific length of time, and this payment is unrelated to how much the HMO actually spends. Thus, if it spends less by being more efficient (say, not hospitalizing unnecessarily), then it gets to keep more money. But how much the HMO charges in premiums is kept in check by competitive pressure; if it charges too much in premiums, fewer people are likely to enroll.

Much of the early evidence on HMOs through the 1970s focused on group- and staff-model HMOs, finding that they could yield substantial savings—as much as 30 to 40 percent over fee-for-service plans. A savings rate on this order is now viewed as extremely optimistic. HMOs do save money, but it is difficult to know how much. On the one hand, comparison of HMOs and fee-for-service plans shows the savings of the former are exaggerated by the fact that historically HMOs have experienced favorable selection (healthier or less costly patients), although more recent evidence is pointing to the end of this trend (Schaefer & Reschovsky, 2002). On the other hand, HMOs probably save more than is directly attributable to them because competition between HMOs and fee-for-service plans undoubtedly results in the latter reducing their costs.

Whatever savings they generate, HMOs by themselves are probably insufficient to solve long-term problems in rising health care costs. One reason is they are subject to the same forces that raise the costs of fee-for-service medicine: overall growth in input costs and development and diffusion of expensive medical technologies. Some evidence is available on how HMOs affect the quality of care provided. One comprehensive review of the literature found equal numbers of studies reporting better and worse quality of care in HMOs than in fee-for-service plans (Miller & Luft, 2002).

In recent years, HMO enrollment has fallen as a result of the popularity of preferred provider organizations (PPOs). PPOs are not generally viewed as a form of capitation, relying more on discounted fee-for-service rates. However, PPO patients are free to go outside the organization's provider network, albeit at extra cost. Between 1999 and 2011, PPO enrollment among those with employer health plans rose from 39 percent to 55 percent. Over the same period, enrollment in standard and POS-model HMOs fell from 52 percent to 27 percent (Kaiser Family Foundation, 2011). The decline is the result largely of the flexibility that PPOs afford patients and the growth of high-deductible health plans.

Managed Competition. Analysts have recognized for years that pure competition is unlikely to work well in the health care sector. There are many reasons; two are detailed here. First, the health care market is a complicated one, with people having relatively poor information about their alternatives and the implications (for their health and their pocketbook) of making these choices. A second is biased selection; insurers may compete for the healthiest people, leaving sicker people with no source of insurance.

Advocates of *managed competition* believe that the marketplace can be trusted in the health care sector only if the players conform to certain rules (Enthoven, 1993). To facilitate consumer understanding, health plans should be required to offer specific minimum benefits or, in some proposals, conform to standardized benefits. The latter aids consumers in comparison shopping between alternative plans. Furthermore, certain practices on the part of insurers (such as cherry-picking the healthiest people, charging unaffordably high premiums to unhealthy individuals and groups, and denying coverage for preexisting conditions) are to be prohibited. To make consumers think twice before purchasing extravagant insurance policies, employers would make a defined contribution based on the lowest-cost premium in the market. As a result, those choosing more expensive health plans would have to pay more of the premiums out of pocket, given the fixed employer premium contribution. Some proposals also tax health plans that are more expensive than the cheapest approved plan in an area. All of this is to be carried out through consortia, originally called health insurance purchasing cooperatives (HIPCs) by Enthoven.

It should be obvious from the preceding description of managed competition—regulated marketplaces selling standard insurance policies to large groups pooled to maximize their purchasing power—that the ACA is based on principles originally outlined by Enthoven over thirty years ago (Enthoven, 1978). Although it can be argued that the ACA's primary objectives are to reduce the number of uninsured Americans and thus improve health status through improved access to health care, there are important elements of the ACA, described in Chapter One, dealing with cost control, or "bending the cost curve," according to current terminology. Evidence from the RAND Health Insurance Experiment suggests that it will be difficult to control total expenditures while increasing access to rather comprehensive insurance (Manning et al., 1987), at least in the short term. Clearly, the impact of the ACA on costs and total health expenditures will be a significant issue of interest to both policy analysts and policymakers during the remainder of this decade.

Future Directions

There are several reasons for ongoing research on methods to contain U.S. health care costs. First, the fact that other countries spend so much less per capita (see Table 8.7 in Chapter Eight) raises the possibility that there may be effective cost-control options available. Second, there is an opportunity cost; more spent on health care means less money available to spend on other societal needs. Third, and related to this, there are strong reasons to believe that the availability of new and effective medical technologies such as gene therapy will result in an even greater jump in spending. It would seem prudent for us to understand what options are available to control these and other costs before health care spending absorbs even more of our national income.

If continued research on cost-containment methods is appropriate, the next question is which areas of inquiry are most fruitful. One area that spans the domestic and the international is to determine the relative contribution of price versus quantity in continued health care cost inflation. In a 2003 article that received a great deal of attention from researchers and the press—"It's the Prices, Stupid: Why the United States Is So Different from Other Countries"—the authors show that whereas utilization rates are comparable between the United States and other countries, unit prices are far higher (Anderson, Reinhardt, Hussey, & Petrosyan, 2003). The issue, however, is more subtle: it may be that unit prices are higher in the United States in large part as a result of more expensive inputs (for example, more technologically advanced hospitals and better-trained doctors), which can result in better-quality care. Thus, a ripe area of cross-national research is what various countries are getting from their health care systems—an area of research that has begun (see, for example, Davis et al., 2010).

Since the late 1980s, there has been a movement toward more funded research in the areas of medical effectiveness and clinical outcomes. Infusion of more federal monies into this branch of health services research is widely viewed as a valuable investment because of the dearth of information on which medical interventions work best. We hope, however, that this recent emphasis on outcomes research does not diminish the importance of general health services research, which seeks to address some of the larger concerns discussed in this chapter.

SUMMARY

Successful containment of health care expenditures remains a critical issue not only in the United States, but internationally as well. This chapter illustrates two ways of breaking down costs, through the examination of components based on fee for service and, alternatively, capitation payment systems. A unifying theme is that economic incentives matter a great deal. However, most payment systems can be thwarted by providers or insurers, so it is essential to design such systems, as much as possible, so that the incentives facing major stakeholders will lead them to perform in a way consistent with societal goals. Otherwise, society will continue to pay an ever-increasing share of GDP for health care services at the expense of other important social investments.

KEY TERMS

Capitation A method of paying providers. In general, the capitated fee is a fixed amount per enrollee per month, irrespective of how many services are provided.

Certificate of need (CON) State regulations that require permission for hospitals or other health organizations to expand (such as by increasing the number of beds) or purchase major capital equipment. CON regulations were common in the 1970s and 1980s but are much less common now. Because of the way such programs were designed, most studies found that they were ineffective in controlling health care spending.

Cost shifting A more accurate term would be "charge shifting." The term refers to the ability of insurance companies to charge more to privately insured patients to compensate for losses from public patients and the uninsured. There is a great deal of debate on the extent to which insurers can successfully engage in this practice.

Fee for service A method of paying providers whereby a separate fee is paid every time the provider sees that patient. Separate fees are also often provided for each laboratory test.

Global budget A fixed aggregate public budget for a type of service (such as hospital care), a region, or a country.

Managed competition A model for health care reform proposed by Alain Enthoven in the late 1970s based on the Federal Employees

Health Benefits Program (FEHBP). Its key elements are (1) price competition in regulated insurance markets between insurers based on standard insurance policies and (2) pooling of small companies and individual purchasers into larger groups known as health insurance purchasing cooperatives (HIPCs).

Practice guidelines A suggested list of processes, generally aimed at physicians and based on a review of medical evidence, that should be followed to maximize the probability of obtaining desired patient outcomes.

Resource-based relative value scale (RBRVS) A kind of fee-for-service physician payment system in which payments are based on a scale that measures the complexity and cost of providing the service.

Sustainable growth rate (SGR) A method used by Medicare to control aggregate physician payments. Changes in actual expenditures are compared to a target that is based on factors such as the growth in input prices and program enrollment and change in the growth of the economy as a whole. When actual expenditures exceed the SRG, the annual increase in physician reimbursement rates is reduced. Congress, however, has overruled the formula each year for over a decade.

Utilization management Programs instituted by public and private insurers to help ensure that medically appropriate services are provided to patients. Some examples include preadmission certification of hospital stays, management of high-cost patients, requiring a second opinion before embarking on surgery, and profiling of physicians' practices.

Value-based insurance design (VBID) An insurance design system where patient cost-sharing requirements (such as coinsurance and copayments) are tailored to the medical appropriateness of a service. In such systems, cost sharing is often reduced to encourage the use of particular services or prescription drugs for conditions such as diabetes or hypertension.

DISCUSSION QUESTIONS

1. Have Medicare DRGs been a successful cost-containment strategy? How could they be modified or extended to be more effective?
2. Some researchers believe that the major reason that the United States spends more on health care than any other country is a proliferation

of "high-tech" medical interventions. By regionalizing hospitals and technologies, Canada appears to enjoy savings. What other advantages, and what disadvantages, might result from regionalized hospital and technology systems?

3. Certificate-of-need (CON) programs, according to most researchers, were not effective in controlling hospital costs. They are an example of health care regulation. But other countries rely heavily on regulation of their hospitals and appear to be more effective in controlling costs. Why do you think that these latter regulatory systems are more effective than CON?

4. What are the primary advantages and disadvantages of relying on increased patient cost sharing? Be sure to include both efficiency and equity considerations.

5. In Alain Enthoven's earlier work, he suggested that managed competition would manifest itself through competing group and staff model HMOs. What emerged, however, has been competition between PPOs and network-model HMOs, neither of which has its own set of dedicated providers. What barriers are there for effective competition among providers that contract with many HMOs and PPOs? How might these barriers be overcome to achieve effective cost control?

FURTHER READING

Anderson, G. F., Reinhardt, U. E., Hussey, P. S., & Petrosyan, V. (2003). It's the prices, stupid: Why the United States is so different from other countries. *Health Affairs, 22*, 89–105.

Cutler, D. M., & McClellan, M. (2001). Is technological change in medicine worth it? *Health Affairs, 20*, 11–29.

Enthoven, A. C. (1993). The history and principles of managed competition. *Health Affairs, 12*(Suppl), 24–48.

Manning, W. G., Newhouse, J. P., Duan, N., Keeler, E. B., & Leibowitz, A. (1987). Health insurance and the demand for medical care: Evidence from a randomized experiment. *American Economic Review, 77*, 251–277.

Miller, R. H., & Luft, H. S. (2002). HMO plan performance update: An analysis of the literature, 1997–2001. *Health Affairs, 21*, 63–86.

Squires, D. A. (2011, July). The U.S. health system in perspective: A comparison of twelve industrialized nations. Commonwealth Fund. Retrieved from http://www.commonwealthfund.org/~/media/Files/Publications/Issue%20Brief/2011/Jul/1532_Squires_US_hlt_sys_comparison_12_nations_intl_brief_v2.pdf

REFERENCES

American Hospital Association. (2011). *TrendWatch chartbook 2011.* Table 4.6. http://www.aha.org/research/reports/tw/chartbook/index.shtml

Anderson, G. F., Reinhardt, U. E., Hussey, P. S., & Petrosyan, V. (2003). It's the prices, stupid: Why the United States is so different from other countries. *Health Affairs, 22,* 89–105.

Ashby, J. L., Jr., (1984). The impact of hospital regulatory programs on per capita costs, utilization, and capital Investment. *Inquiry, 21,* 45–59.

Barer, M. L., Evans, R. G., & Labelle, R. J. (1988). Fee controls as cost controls: Tales from the frozen north. *Milbank Quarterly, 66,* 1–64.

Choudhry, N. K., Fischer, M. A., Avorn, J., Schneeweiss, S., Solomon, D. H., Berman, C., . . . Shrank, W. H. (2010). At Pitney Bowes, value-based insurance design cut copayments and increased drug adherence. *Health Affairs, 29,* 1995–2001.

Christensen, S. (1992). Volume responses to exogenous changes in Medicare's payment policies. *Health Services Research, 27,* 65–79.

Chulis, G. S. (1991). Assessing Medicare's prospective payment system for hospitals. *Medical Care Review, 48,* 167–206.

Davis, K., Anderson, G. F., Rowland, D., & Steinberg, E. P. (1990). *Health care cost containment.* Baltimore: Johns Hopkins University Press.

Davis, K., Schoen, C., & Stremikis, K. (2010, June). Mirror, mirror on the wall: How the performance of the U.S. health care system compares internationally. Commonwealth Fund. Retrieved from http://www.commonwealthfund.org/~/media /Files/Publications/Fund%20Report/2010/Jun/1400_Davis_Mirror_Mirror_on _the_wall_2010.pdf

Detsky, A. A., Stacey, S. R., & Bombardier, C. (1983). The effectiveness of a regulatory strategy in containing hospital costs: The Ontario experience, 1967–1981. *New England Journal of Medicine, 309,* 151–159.

Enthoven, A. C. (1978). Consumer choice health plan: A national health insurance proposal based on regulated competition in the private sector. *New England Journal of Medicine, 298,* 709–720.

Enthoven, A. C. (1993). The history and principles of managed competition. *Health Affairs, 12*(Suppl), 24–48.

Gabel, J., & Rice, T. (1985). Reducing public expenditures for physician services: The price of paying less. *Journal of Health Politics, Policy, and Law, 9,* 595–609.

Kaiser Family Foundation. (2011). Employer health benefits: 2011 annual survey. Retrieved from http://ehbs.kff.org/pdf/2011/8225.pdf

Kominski, G. (1998). Commentary. *Medical Care Research and Review, 55,* 479–483.

Lohr, K. N., Brook, R. H., Kamberg, C. J., Goldberg, G. A., Leibowitz, A., Keesey, J., . . . Newhouse, J. P. (1986). Effect of cost sharing on use of medically effective and less effective care. *Medical Care, 24*(Suppl), S31–S38.

Manning, W. G., Newhouse, J. P., Duan, N., Keeler, E. B., & Leibowitz, A. (1987). Health insurance and the demand for medical care: Evidence from a randomized experiment. *American Economic Review, 77,* 251–277.

Marquis, M. S., & Kominski, G. F. (1994). Alternative volume performance standards for Medicare physicians' services. *Milbank Quarterly, 72,* 329–357.

McGlynn, E. A., Asch, S. M., Adams, J., Keesey, J., Hicks, J., DeCristofara, A., & Kerr, E. A. (2003). The quality of health care delivered to adults in the United States. *New England Journal of Medicine, 348,* 2635–2645.

Medicare Payment Advisory Commission (MedPAC). (2000). *Report to Congress: Medicare payment policy.* Washington, DC: MedPAC.

Medicare Payment Advisory Commission (MedPAC). (2012). *Medicare and the health care delivery system.* Appendix A. Retrieved from http://www.medpac.gov /documents/jun11_entirereport.pdf

Miller, R. H., & Luft, H. S. (2002). HMO plan performance update: An analysis of the literature, 1997–2001. *Health Affairs, 21,* 63–86.

Newhouse, J. P., Anderson, G., & Roos, L. L. (1988). Hospital spending in the United States and Canada: A comparison. *Health Affairs, 7,* 6–24,

Reinhardt, U. E. (2009, January 23). How do hospitals get paid? A primer. Economix. *New York Times.* Retrieved from http://economix.blogs.nytimes.com/2009/01/23 /how-do-hospitals-get-paid-a-primer

Rice, T., & Bernstein, J. (1990). Volume performance standards: Can they control growth in Medicare services? *Milbank Quarterly, 68,* 295–319.

Rice, T., & Morrison, K. R. (1994). Patient cost sharing for medical services: A review of the literature and implications for health care reform. *Medical Care Review, 51,* 235–287.

Robinson, J. C., & Luft, H. S. (1988). Competition, regulation, and hospital costs: 1982–1986. *Journal of the American Medical Association, 260,* 2676–681.

Russell, L. B., & Manning, C. L. (1989). The effect of prospective payment on Medicare expenditures. *New England Journal of Medicine, 320,* 439–444.

Schaefer, E., & Reschovsky, J. D. (2002). Are HMO enrollees healthier than others? Results from the community tracking study. *Health Affairs, 21,* 249–258.

Song, Y., Skinner, J., Bynum, J., Sutherland, J., Wennberg, J. E., & Fisher, E. S. (2010). Regional variation in diagnostic practices. *New England Journal of Medicine, 363,* 45–53.

Squires, D. A. (2011, July). The U.S. health system in perspective: A comparison of twelve industrialized nations. Commonwealth Fund. Retrieved from http://www .commonwealthfund.org/~/media/Files/Publications/Issue%20Brief/2011/Jul /1532_Squires_US_hlt_sys_comparison_12_nations_intl_brief_v2.pdf

Steinwald, B., & Sloan, F. A. (1981). Regulatory approaches to hospital cost containment: A synthesis of the empirical evidence. In M. A. Olson (Ed.), *A new approach to the economics of health care.* Washington, DC: American Enterprise Institute for Public Policy Research.

Thorpe, K. E. (1987). Does all-payer rate setting work? The case of the New York prospective hospital reimbursement methodology. *Journal of Health Politics, Policy, and Law, 12,* 391–408.

Wickizer, T. M., & Lessler, D. (2002). Utilization management: Issues, effects, and future prospects. *Annual Review of Public Health, 23,* 233–254.

CHAPTER TEN

PROMOTING PHARMACEUTICAL ACCESS WHILE CONTROLLING PRICES AND EXPENDITURES

Stuart O. Schweitzer
William S. Comanor

Learning Objectives

- Understand the complex pharmaceutical market, with a network of third-party payers and price discrimination between groups of patients
- Understand how pharmaceutical prices are determined
- Understand efforts to control pharmaceutical expenditures through policies directed at patients, prescribers, and manufacturers and to stimulate thinking about other efforts that might be useful in controlling expenditures
- Understand two particularly contentious recent pharmaceutical policy issues: increased access through Part D of Medicare and the shortage of generic drugs

Despite dramatic advances in pharmaceuticals, public attitudes toward the pharmaceutical industry remain guarded. Although pleased with the technological benefits of modern drugs, which allow us all to lead longer and healthier lives, many Americans complain that pharmaceuticals are too expensive and limit their access to beneficial health care services. While the issue of drug costs is long-standing, many are unclear as to what "drug costs" actually consist of and how they are determined. People are also uncertain if there is a relationship between drug price and the supply of new innovations. The purpose of this chapter is to clarify these issues and consider some possible solutions to the problems.

Drug expenditures have grown in part because they have become a more integral part of modern medical care. Medication use is ubiquitous in all medical settings, whether it is outpatient use in the management of chronic disease or life-saving treatment in the hospital. Furthermore, drugs are often a substitute for other health care inputs, such as hospital stays and physician visits. For example, H2 antagonists such as Tagamet and Zantac have practically eliminated the need for ulcer surgery, and antipsychotic drugs have substantially reduced the need for mental hospital admissions. For both of these drug classes, pharmaceutical expenditures increased after their introduction, while at the same time total medical costs due to these illnesses declined. On the other hand, other drugs, like the so-called clot busters used in emergency rooms for heart-attack patients, are complements that make other services more efficient and improve outcomes. These drugs have led to rising pharmaceutical expenditures, but few would deny their value in improving health outcomes. Drugs can be both substitutes and complements to other health care inputs.

Concern over pharmaceutical costs is further heightened by lack of clarity about the nature of the problem. Spending on any good or service is a function of both price and quantity. Is the problem of rising drug expenditures due to rising quantities of pharmaceuticals that are consumed? Or is it due to rising prices? The answers to these questions are complicated by the role played by rapid technological innovation, which leads to frequent replacement of older products by newer ones. Newer products are often more expensive than the older ones, so that expenditures may rise due to displacement, even though prices of all drugs, new and old, and the number of prescriptions remains constant.

To understand rising drug costs, we first review trends in drug expenditures in the United States. We also discuss the difficulty of accurately measuring U.S. drug prices and how this can often inflate the perception of increasing pharmaceutical expenditures. We then look at the evidence on whether U.S. drug prices are higher than those in other countries. Next, we examine the intertemporal relationship between price increases and quality changes to determine whether pharmaceutical prices have increased after correcting for therapeutic improvements. In addition, we analyze recent governmental efforts to expand medication coverage with Part D of Medicare. We also look at drug shortages as being a potential complication to cost containment. Finally, we discuss a series of policy options for expanding access to pharmaceuticals while containing expenditures. Some are directed at consumers, some at physicians, and still others at manufacturers. Current efforts to control pharmaceutical costs are a blend of all three approaches.

The Problem of Drug Expenditures

The share of national health expenditures represented by pharmaceuticals and other components of the U.S. health care system from 1960 through 2010 is shown in Figure 10.1.

FIGURE 10.1. SHARE OF PERSONAL HEALTH EXPENDITURES, 1960–2010

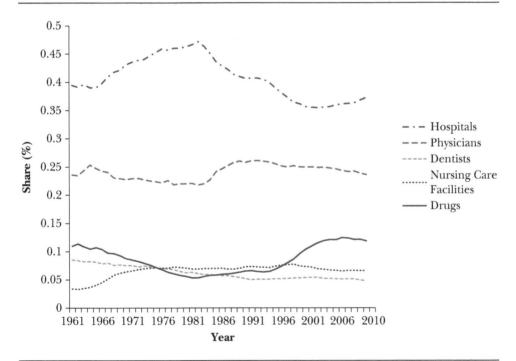

Source: Centers for Medicare and Medicaid Services, Office of the Actuary, National Health Statistics Group, 2012.

Whereas the share of health care expenditures allocated to pharmaceuticals has risen in recent years, it is still far below the proportion spent on hospitals and physician services. The pharmaceutical proportion declined from 1960 through the early 1980s and then increased, particularly since 1994, regaining its earlier position of just over 10 percent of total health care expenditures.

Of these increased outlays on pharmaceuticals, only a portion is due to higher prices charged for existing drug products. Berndt estimates that only 22 percent of the growth in drug spending since 1997 has resulted from higher prices for existing drugs (Berndt, 2001). That being said, price increases remain a minor cause of higher pharmaceutical expenditures.

To better understand this issue, we review data from the *Consumer Price Index (CPI)* and its constituent parts, including pharmaceuticals and other health care services. Figure 10.2 shows time series data on the annual change in the overall CPI and various medical care components, including pharmaceuticals, from 1960 to 2011.

FIGURE 10.2. RATE OF INCREASE OF PERSONAL HEALTH CARE COMPONENTS FROM PREVIOUS YEAR (PERCENTAGE), 1960–2011

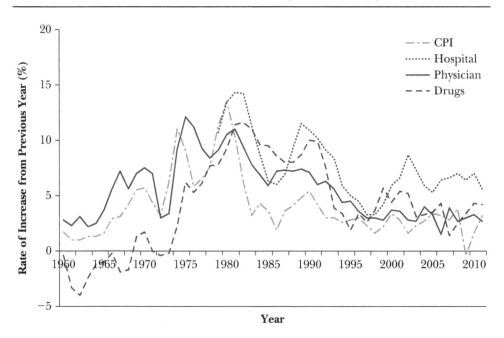

Source: U.S. Bureau of the Census, 2011.

These statistics show that the rate of price increase for health care has exceeded that of the overall CPI for the entire period; since 1980 pharmaceuticals have behaved similarly to other health care components in this matter. However, it is important to note that the rate of change of drugs has almost always been below that of hospital prices during the period for which data are available (Department of Health and Human Services [DHHS], 2010). If pharmaceuticals constitute only a small portion of overall health care expenditures, and if price increases have been similar to or below those of other health care components for many years, what explains continued public and congressional concern over drug prices and expenditures?

One answer to this query is that utilization has risen sharply, in part because of the country's aging population. Furthermore, drugs can do many more things today than in the past, so they are prescribed more frequently. Finally, *direct-to-consumer (DTC) advertising* may also lead to increased consumption. As a result of all of these factors, the number of annual prescriptions filled has risen dramatically, from 2 billion in 1993 to 3.4 billion in 2003 (Kaiser Family Foundation, 2004). Within some common therapeutic categories, the rise in quantity has been even more dramatic. From 1993 to 1997, the number of antidepressant and cholesterol-lowering drug prescriptions filled increased by 111 percent and 162 percent respectively. Oral antihistamines increased an astonishing 500 percent (National Institute for Health Care Management, 1999).

The increased quantity of filled prescriptions is the primary factor behind recent increases in pharmaceutical spending. This includes both higher spending on new drugs, accounting for about 46 percent of the total increase since 1997, and higher quantities sold of existing drugs, which accounts for 32 percent of the total (National Institute for Health Care Management, 1999; Berndt, 2001). Therefore, higher spending is mostly due to greater purchases of both new and existing drugs.

Another factor behind recent expressions of concern for these expenditures results from a fundamental difference between pharmaceuticals and other health service components: though most health care purchases are exclusively services, pharmaceuticals have both service and manufactured product components. The service role applies to knowledge of the therapeutic properties of the compound, gained from the research and development (R&D) that lies behind all pharmaceutical products, and also to professional dispensing of the drug. However, the drug itself is a manufactured product, and most drugs are produced in volumes that take advantage of economies of scale in the manufacturing process. Production costs of drugs constitute less than half of total costs (Comanor & Schweitzer, 1995).

Pharmaceutical margins must also cover the substantial research and marketing costs that accompany the introduction of new drugs. Unfortunately, due to the fact that these are mainly costs that have already been paid, consumers may not see a link with what they are charged. Further obscuring this linkage is the willingness of many pharmaceutical companies to sell the same or similar drugs at different prices through discounts to health insurers, health plans or foreign countries.

Still another reason for public concern with pharmaceutical prices lies in the fact that most insurance plans cover well under 100 percent of the total charges for drugs. At the time of the Kefauver Committee hearings in the 1950s and 1960s, there was virtually no insurance coverage for drugs. In 1960, private insurance paid little of pharmaceutical expenses, leaving consumers responsible for 96 percent of their drug costs out of pocket (Danzon & Pauly, 2002). By 1999, the situation had changed and private health insurance covered an increasing proportion of total pharmaceutical expenditures. Out-of-pocket expenditures on pharmaceuticals fell to just over 21 percent in 2009 (Centers for Disease Control and Prevention [CDC], 2011). That rate is low by historical standards, but is still higher than the out-of-pocket expenditure share for physician and clinic expenditures (9.5 percent) and that for hospital expenditures (3.2 percent). The higher share of pharmaceutical expenditures paid directly means that consumers are less sheltered from drug costs than for other health care services, making the costs more visible to consumers.

For the elderly, the problem of high drug expenditures is more complicated. The universal health insurer for the elderly is the Medicare program, but Medicare's coverage of outpatient drugs—commonly known as Part D—did not begin until 2006. It would be wrong to think that all seniors depended on Part D for coverage of drug costs. Approximately 76 percent of seniors either qualify for Medicaid coverage (which covers outpatient drugs) or have private health insurance to supplement their Medicare coverage. This leaves only 24 percent of the elderly with no extra drug coverage other than Part D, forcing them to pay a larger percentage out of pocket for their pharmaceuticals. For the rest, the "cost" of a drug consists of co-insurance and deductibles. These payments are generally linked to the type of drug used to fill a prescription and not to the drug's actual cost. For example, a prescription filled with a generic product may require only a five-dollar copayment, while the copayment for a branded product might be thirty dollars.

Interpreting Pharmaceutical Price Data

Various reports, both public and private, have disclosed rapidly rising drug prices in recent years. The 1992 report by the U.S. Government Accountability Office (U.S. GAO, 1992a), formerly the General Accounting Office, found that "during the 1980s, prescription drug prices increased by almost three times the rate of general inflation and certain drugs increased in price by over 100 percent in five years." This report reviewed price data for a sample of widely used prescription drugs, and concluded: "Prices for nearly all 29 drug products increased more than the percentage changes for all three consumer price indexes for the six year period ending December 31, 1991" (U.S. GAO, 1992a).

These conclusions are incomplete. Since adoption of the 1984 law facilitating approval of *generic drugs* upon the originator's patent expiration, the importance of generics in pharmaceutical marketplaces has expanded rapidly. By 2000, fully 47 percent of pharmaceuticals dispensed, in terms of physical units, were for generic products, up from 40 percent as recently as 1993 (Pharmaceutical Research and Manufacturers Association, 2005). Today, approximately eight of ten drug prescriptions in the United States are filled by generics (as noted previously), and there has been little suggestion that high prices for *these* products are a problem (U.S. FDA, 2012a). This is significant because average generic prices are cheaper in the United States than most foreign countries (Danzon & Furukawa, 2008).

An equally important factor is the role of large buyers who purchase pharmaceuticals on behalf of their subscribers. These buyers include health insurance companies and their pharmaceutical benefit manager affiliates, HMOs, and some large employers who supply required drugs directly to their employees. As we describe later, these purchasers typically receive a substantial discount or rebate off the price established by the drug company. Since discounts or rebates are typically not disclosed, most discussions of pharmaceutical prices simply ignore them and thereby report higher prices than those that are actually paid.

The Effect of Generic Products on Prices

Not only are generic products priced substantially below their branded counterparts; generic prices generally decline over time as the number of generic producers increases. For most products, the share of total sales for generics of a particular molecular compound expands greatly following patent expiration. Griliches and Cockburn (1994) observed that within two years of a branded drug's patent expiration, its market share of product revenues generally fell by 50 percent. Though the price of branded drugs actually *rises* after patent expiration, today's increasing role of generic products in pharmaceutical markets has surely led to a declining average price for most products (including a blend of both the branded and the generic versions) following patent expiration and the entry of generic producers. Studies showing rapid rises in drug prices must be interpreted carefully, as they typically report prices only for branded products and not those of generic substitutes.

To answer this question, one first needs to decide whether the generic version of a drug is appropriately considered the same product as its branded counterpart. How one should appraise the statistical conclusions of many of these studies depends critically on this answer. In its computations, the Bureau of Labor Statistics (BLS) assumes that branded products are inherently different from their generic versions (Griliches & Cockburn, 1994). It notes that both patients and physicians frequently react differently to the two types of product despite their bioequivalence. On this basis, it treats these products as distinct entities and reports their price changes separately. Thus the BLS data does not incorporate the increasing use of lower-priced generic drugs in its published price series (BLS, 2010).

In contrast, there is the implicit judgment of the Food and Drug Administration (FDA) that generic and branded versions of the same molecule are therapeutically identical. On this basis, one could prepare price series that include both incumbent and generic drugs that are linked according to their relative quantities. If this procedure is carried out for many individual products, average prices often decline (Griliches & Cockburn, 1994).

In their study of these issues, Griliches and Cockburn (1994) account for these views and construct adjusted price series. As might be expected, they report price series that lie between those based on the two extreme assumptions. For the most part, their price series constructed for individual drugs show some price decline after introduction of generics, although less than price series based on the assumption that branded and generic versions are the same product.

Launch Prices and Subsequent Drug Price Changes

In addition to the issue of generic substitutability, the pricing strategies employed in the years following product introduction are also important.

Two strategies are used: "skimming" and "penetration." The former involves setting a high introductory price but then reducing it over time, while the latter is the reverse, setting a low introductory price and increasing it over time. When does a manufacturer use one strategy or the other? The answer is important because with the skimming strategy one will expect to see falling prices over time, while the penetration strategy leads to a lower initial price, followed by price rises.

The skimming strategy is typically found with drugs representing a major therapeutic advance, while penetration is commonly used for imitative products (Lu & Comanor, 1998). As a result, one is more likely to find rising drug prices when imitative products are introduced but declining prices when innovative products are seen. Therefore, rising prices may be a consequence of low (penetration) launch prices, while more moderate price trends may result from high (skimming) launch prices.

Drug Prices and Quality Improvement

Branded pharmaceutical products compete not just with their generic substitutes but also among themselves. Even though a drug may be similar to others in its therapeutic category in terms of efficacy, it can differ in terms of side effects and adverse interaction profiles, and convenience; higher introductory prices can frequently be explained by such improvements (Lu & Comanor, 1998; Comanor, Schweitzer, & Carter, 2005). Indeed, a higher price for a new product generally reflects product improvement.

To investigate this issue, Berndt and his colleagues estimated a series of hedonic regression equations in which various attributes were used as proxies for the relative quality of a number of products. Through this technique, the authors were able to measure price trends while holding quality level constant. For the years between 1980 and 1996, and dealing only with antidepressant drugs, they report average price increases under three scenarios: the increase measured without accounting for generics or quality change, 7.11 percent; the increase including generics but without incorporating the improved quality of new products, 4.73 percent; and the increase incorporating both effects, 4.33 percent. Although the correction for generics was far more significant for the entire period they studied, they noted that there were particular years when the correction for quality change associated with new products was a more important factor than the increasing role of generics (Berndt, Cockburn, Griliches, Keeler, & Baily, 1996).

Comanor, Schweitzer, and Carter (2005) also employed hedonic methods to study the separate effects of generic introduction and product attributes on drug prices. Their analysis was carried out for five pharmaceutical classes. They report that generics, as expected, lead to lower drug prices but that greater efficacy, greater safety, and increased convenience in drug regimen tended to increase drug prices.

Measuring Prices When New Drugs Replace Old Ones

The BLS computes the overall CPI as well as its constituent parts as a Laspeyres index, which compares the cost of a given bundle of goods (often referred to as the "market basket") purchased at current prices to the cost of that same bundle purchased at base-year prices (Feldstein, 1993). This market basket, however, must be adjusted periodically to reflect current expenditure patterns; otherwise the index would have ever less relationship with the actual goods purchased by consumers. In health care, new treatments for old problems, such as coronary artery disease or renal failure, have totally replaced techniques in use only a few years ago. In many cases, there are new therapies available for problems that were previously untreatable. If new and improved drugs replace older ones but at a higher price, the appropriate price index should account for quality improvement as well as price increase. If price indices fail to account adequately for quality improvement, measures of price changes will be biased upward.

The method used by the BLS to measure price changes is designed to track prices for a fixed market basket, or one that changes slowly. When items in the market basket change through shifts in consumer demand, the BLS uses a "linking" technique through which the price index of a new market basket replaces the index for an older one. For example, if a new product, such as a more powerful antihypertensive drug, replaces an existing but less expensive one, price indices including the old and new products are each calculated, and the new index (with the higher-priced product) is scaled downward to equal the older one. The index including the new item then replaces the prior index in future calculations. No attempt is made to assess whether an improved drug is more or less expensive than would be justified by the quality change represented by its introduction. The price index merely tracks the prices of all items in the market basket and then recalculates the price index when a new product is included.

Failure to capture the effect of quality change is especially serious for pharmaceuticals, where turnover of products is rapid and new products frequently are an improved version of older ones, with greater efficacy, fewer side effects, or a more convenient regimen. The question of whether increases in drug prices exceed, fall behind, or accurately reflect quality changes is left unanswered.

Prices and Margins: Differences between Manufacturer and Retail Prices

There is also an important distinction between the prices set by pharmaceutical manufacturers and those ultimately paid by consumers. The difference between retail and manufacturer prices is the distribution margin, which includes the costs and profits of the dispensing pharmacy (as well as the wholesaler if one is involved in distributing the product). In many discussions of pharmaceutical costs, there is an implicit assumption that distribution margins are constant across products, such that whatever price is charged by the manufacturer is passed on to consumers, with merely a fixed amount added to cover distribution costs. However, this picture is not generally accurate. Steiner in particular has disclosed "the inverse association between the margins of manufacturers and [those of] retailers" (Steiner, 1993). His study offers empirical evidence on this relationship as well as the reasons for it. Salehi and Schweitzer (1985) also report that the relationship applies to pharmaceuticals. Branded pharmaceuticals, which typically embody a high manufacturing margin, have lower distribution margins, while generic products with lower margins at the manufacturing stage generally have much higher distribution margins. As a result, price differences between branded and generic products are greater at the manufacturing stage of production than at retail.

International Price Comparisons

Comparisons with the international community have also contributed to widespread concern that drug prices are excessive in the United States. For example, the GAO has published studies comparing U.S. drug prices with those in the United Kingdom and Canada (U.S. GAO, 1992b, 1994). These reports find that cash prices for the same branded products are generally higher in the United States than elsewhere. The GAO studies are subject to many of the same conceptual and methodological problems that were discussed earlier.

It is of particular significance that the GAO studies fail to account for generic substitution in any comprehensive way. Even though their comparison of relative prices for a particular branded drug may be correct, they do not often reflect differences in the actual prices facing consumers since generics are typically more important in the United States than elsewhere. As we have noted, the share of the market accounted for by generic drugs in the United States has grown substantially and now comprises nearly 80 percent of all drug units (doses) sold (U.S. FDA, 2012a). Simply comparing the prices of specific branded products without including the prices of generic products therefore gives a misleading picture of the relative costs to consumers of filling a doctor's prescription.

For example, suppose that half of U.S. prescriptions for cimetidine, a popular H2 blocker for gastric reflux and ulcers, are filled by the generic version, the price of which is $104 per hundred, while the price of the branded product, Tagamet, is $167. The average price is $135.50. Suppose further that the prices of both versions of the drug are lower in Canada, with Tagamet at $150 and the generic at $100. If the generic version's market share is only 20 percent in Canada, the average price there is $140, which is higher than the average U.S. price, even though the prices charged for both products are lower in Canada. Therefore, generic market shares can have important price effects.

Another important problem with the GAO approach is that it relies on established nominal prices, which do not account for the many discounts and rebates present in the United States that are generally granted to large buyers. Even if these nominal prices accurately describe charges to pharmacies, which are then applied to cash customers, they do not reflect the transaction prices used for other classes of buyers, who in fact constitute the largest segment of demand. This factor is important because these discounts appear more widespread in the United States than in Britain or Canada (Schweitzer & Comanor, 2011).

Finally, the GAO reports fail to deal with drug consumption patterns varying among the three countries studied. Not only are drugs used differently in each country, but even the same drugs are taken in a variety of forms and dosages (Payer, 1988). The GAO approach avoids the issue by asking a narrower question: Are wholesale prices higher in the United States than in Britain or Canada specifically for the highest-selling American drugs? This approach is likely to compare prices of highly popular U.S. products with those of less commonly used drugs in other countries, which is different from asking if drugs in general cost more in the United States than elsewhere.

In response to the GAO reports, Danzon and Chao (2000) carried out a more complete analysis of international drug price comparisons. They included all drugs sold in nine countries, incorporating over-the-counter drugs that substitute for prescribed drugs; they also used data on average transaction prices at the manufacturer level. The authors found that price differences between countries depend greatly on how the comparison is framed—particularly which country's quantity weights are used to construct the price index. Comparison also depends on whether one examines price per gram of active ingredient or price per "standard unit" (per capsule, per milliliter of liquid, and so on). Although by most measures average U.S. drug prices exceed those in most other countries, this result does not always apply, and it does not include the more significant role played by generic products in the United States.

Determining Drug Prices

We now turn to the causative factors that determine pharmaceutical prices. Costs are of two topes: fixed and variable. The former, including R&D and marketing, do not rise with output and, in the pharmaceutical industry, these largely occur before production and are referred to as "sunk" costs. A considerable literature points out that sunk costs do not determine price—only variable costs do.

The R&D costs required to introduce a new drug are substantial, frequently in the hundreds of millions of dollars per drug. Researchers at the Tufts Center for Drug Development report that these expenditures reached $802 million per new drug introduced in 2002 (DiMasi, Hansen, & Grabowski, 2003). Research costs include not only direct expenditures on research and testing but also the time costs incurred from the substantial differences between the dates that the outlays are made and the revenues received. This lag represents the extended time it takes for a drug to reach the stage of FDA application, as well as the time spent waiting for the FDA to evaluate a new product.

R&D, marketing, and manufacturing costs are all factors reflecting conditions on the supply side of the market. None have a major impact on pharmaceutical prices. Instead, prices depend predominantly on demand-side considerations. As we show shortly, by example, the prices charged for pharmaceuticals are determined largely by how valuable they are to consumers and what consumers are willing to pay for them. The critical factor is "willingness to pay," which in turn depends on various factors. At this point, we consider these factors: therapeutic advance, competitive forces, and buyer characteristics.

Therapeutic Advance

The most important demand-side factor in determining the price of a pharmaceutical is its therapeutic advance compared to products already on the market. Doctors, patients, and HMOs are willing to pay a larger amount for an improved product compared to one without a substantial therapeutic advance. With increased willingness to pay, sellers can set higher prices without driving customers away.

The relative importance of demand in comparison to supply factors can be explored with the help of a simple example. Suppose Drug A has been under development for many years. Costs have been high because its preclinical tests had to be redone, and clinical tests were also fraught with problems and took longer than expected. When its final (phase three) trials are completed, the manufacturer learns to its surprise that the new product is no more effective than competing drugs already on the market. In contrast, Drug B follows another path. Its development and clinical trials go smoothly and quickly; best of all, the phase three trials show it to be more effective than existing therapies.

Which product, A or B, will be priced above similar medications already on the market? Although Drug A has higher R&D costs, therapeutic equivalence to existing drugs leaves it unable to command a higher price. On the other hand, Drug B yields improved therapy, which leads physicians and patients to be willing to pay a higher price. Lower R&D costs have no affect on the price that the seller can set. What is most significant, therefore, is relative effectiveness, not relative costs.

To explore empirically the importance of therapeutic advance, Lu and Comanor (1998) examined the price premium for new products compared to their existing rivals by evaluating the ratio of median price of new drugs to existing drugs. Among drugs that demonstrate an important therapeutic advancement, the price ratio for new acute drugs relative to existing drugs was 2.97 and 2.29 for chronic drugs. Among drugs representing a modest therapeutic advance, the ratios were 1.72 and 1.19, respectively. Finally, among drugs representing little or no therapeutic advance, the ratios were 1.22 and 0.94.

This data shows that the launch prices of drugs that embody important therapeutic gain are two to three times greater than existing drugs for the same conditions. In contrast, drugs with moderate gains are priced at about one and one-half times greater, while products with little or no therapeutic advance are generally priced at or near the same level as existing products.

Competitive Forces

For any new product introduced—regardless of whether it embodies a small or large therapeutic advance—there are typically existing products used for similar indications. Physicians prescribe these alternate products in the absence of the newer one and thus can be considered competing goods. Together, this set of products, which defines a specific economic market, depends on particular therapeutic indications and is much narrower than the conventional therapeutic category. Classifications such as antibiotics or antihypertensives are so broad that they include pharmaceuticals with quite differing indications and hence products that do not actually compete with one another.

If there are alternative products available for similar indications, prescribing physicians must select among rival drugs. Physician and patient willingness to pay for specific drugs is influenced by perceived therapeutic effectiveness and price differences that exist. Sellers can hope to increase sales by cutting prices, and the more rival products that compete in the market, the more price cutting will occur.

The Lu and Comanor study (1998) found that launch prices are substantially lower when there are more branded rivals in direct competition, and subsequent price changes are lower as well. Despite frequent disdain for imitative products on the part of industry critics, they play an essential role in promoting competitive behavior and leading to lower final prices (Kessler, Rose, Temple, Schapiro, & Griffin, 1994). Imitative products are an important competitive factor in the pharmaceutical marketplace.

Generic pharmaceuticals also have an important impact on market competition and price level. Generic producers typically start production after the relevant patent has expired. They do so by gaining FDA approval of an abbreviated new drug application (ANDA), which requires simple demonstration of bioequivalence to the original product. The prices set by generic producers are much lower than those charged by the original developer of the product because they compete largely by price. It is important to note that the number of sellers also affects the prices of generic products. With more sellers, price competition becomes more vigorous, and prices decline below the level when there is only a single generic entrant.

A study of antimicrobials found that the largest price effects occurred when the fourth and fifth generic firms entered. Average prices per prescription declined from nearly $30 with two or three sellers to less than $20 with the presence of a fourth rival, and eventually approached $4 for products with forty or more sellers (Wiggins & Maness, 2004). The reported decline in average price took place despite the fact that prices charged for the original branded products typically increased rather than fell when entry occurred (Frank & Salkever, 1992). The original manufacturers do not typically compete with generic entrants on the basis of price, but find it more profitable to concentrate on the segment of the market that consists of brand-loyal customers. Such buyers are physicians and patients who know a particular brand and prefer it, so they continue to use it despite the presence of a lower-priced substitute. After generic manufacturers enter production, the price differential expands as the prices charged for the original branded products increase.

Insured and Cash Buyers

The largest market segment for pharmaceuticals, representing about two-thirds of total expenditures, is comprised of insured patients. Actual purchases are made by an intermediary, which can be a government agency, private insurance company, or HMO; this frequently involves the assistance of a pharmacy benefit manager (PBM) to help organize the complicated system of pricing and distribution. The transaction price is negotiated between the drug manufacturer and the intermediary or PBM. In most circumstances, manufacturers grant substantial (and nondisclosed) rebates and discounts to these buyers; their net prices are often significantly lower than those charged to cash buyers (Comanor et al, 2005). For this reason, the pricing studies that rely on reported prices can be misleading when applied to insured patients.

For these patients, the out-of-pocket price for a pharmaceutical product is set not by the drug manufacturer but rather by the insurance company, HMO, or government agency. Their copay is the relevant price that influences their purchasing decision (Esposito, 2003). Furthermore, in most cases the copay is not based on the amount actually paid by the intermediary for the specific product. For this reason, insured patients are largely insulated from the price manufacturers charge.

Most health plans link copays to a multitier *formulary*, which is a restrictive list of approved products. The formularies are often three-tiered, where the health plan sets a relatively low copayment for generics, a moderate copayment for the branded version of a drug whose manufacturer has agreed to a large discount in the wholesale price (this product is often called the "preferred brand"), and the largest copayment for all other branded products in the particular drug class. The expectation is that patients will pressure their physicians to select products with lower copayment, thus allowing the health plan to reduce drug costs.

While researchers have not tested this effect, two studies have shown that patients are not very willing to switch drug products when their former product is placed in the more expensive copayment category (Huskamp et al., 2003; Goldman, Joyce, & Zheng, 2004). However, it is possible that patients already familiar with a particular drug may be relatively insensitive to price changes for the drug, while patients who are newly introduced to a drug class are more willing to purchase the cheapest product available. This argument suggests that the physician-patient demand elasticity may depend on whether the patient has used the drug in the past. In this case, both physician and patient may recognize the possible costs and risks associated with switching away from a drug that "works" to a lower-priced alternative. In contrast, patients who are new to a drug class do not face the same switching costs.

Although the prices paid by intermediaries can affect health insurance premiums and thereby insured patients indirectly, the fact that pharmaceuticals account for only about 10 percent of health care expenditures suggests that these premiums are largely determined by other factors. For the larger channel of pharmaceutical distribution and expenditures, actual prices are generally lower than the prices widely reported and they are not paid directly by the patients.

In contrast, the smaller channel of distribution involves cash prices, which are borne directly by patients. Only 15 to 20 percent of written prescriptions are paid for out of pocket for branded products. While this is not an inconsequential proportion (and prices can be high for these buyers), it does not represent a dominant share of pharmaceutical sales. However, the problem surrounding high drug prices, as they have an impact on consumers, largely applies only to such purchases.

For uninsured patients who purchase pharmaceuticals, demand is often fairly price-elastic. Although the buyer is limited to a prescribed product, he or she can influence the physician's prescribing decision by calling attention to the prices of alternate products. When a generic version of the drug is available, patients can ask the pharmacist to substitute it for the branded product. The patient also has the option of not filling the prescription—which occurs in a large number of cases (Cooper, Love, & Raffoul, 1982; Clark, 1991).

In effect there are different price-setting mechanisms in place for the two distinct distribution channels. The channels need to be approached independently. Although some factors apply to both, there are many factors that affect only one or the other.

The Role of the Pharmacy Benefit Manager

The Pharmacy Benefit Manager (PBM) is the intermediary between health plans and pharmaceutical manufacturers. It purchases the pharmaceuticals from the manufacturer or wholesaler and handles reimbursement to patients and pharmacies. The insurer subcontracts most decisions pertaining to pharmaceuticals to the PBM. Thus, it is relevant for the larger, insured distribution channel. For these sales, the PBM plays an important role and has a major effect on the prices paid to drug manufacturers by HMOs, health insurance companies, and many large employers. The beneficiaries of these buyers obtain their prescribed pharmaceuticals from local pharmacies, where their payment is the copay.

The affiliated PBM has contractual relations not only with the large buyer clients but also with drug manufacturers and pharmacies. Pharmacies are reimbursed for the drugs provided to the beneficiaries. The reimbursement amount is determined by the amount paid by the pharmacy for the pharmaceutical, and also the copayment received from the consumer. Reimbursement typically includes a dispensing fee in addition to a profit margin.

To cover this outflow, the PBM receives payments from two sources. The first and primary revenues are received from the affiliated contractor: the payer who provides for the particular patient. The payment made for the drug reimburses the PBM for payment to the pharmacy, minus a share of any rebates received by the PBM from the drug company. Absent any rebate, this payment merely equals the cash price. Without rebate, the payer would pay the same amount as any cash purchaser (albeit through a circuitous route).

What sets the stage for large payers to pay lower prices than cash customers are the rebate payments made by the drug manufacturers to PBMs. In most cases, drug companies rebate a portion of the payments received from pharmacies for their products to the PBMs who support these sales. These rebates are the subject of negotiation between the PBM and the manufacturer and can differ with the product and the buyer. In effect, the manufacturer receives a net price for the product, which equals the cash price minus the rebate. Finally, depending on the contractual arrangements between the PBM and the payers, a portion of the rebates received by the PBM are remitted to the supporting payer.

There is also a third stream of revenues which is used by the largest firms in this industry. The three leading PBMs all have affiliated mail-order pharmacies with protected monopoly positions in that no independent rivals are permitted into the market. For pharmaceuticals purchased through insurance or other third party plans which use these PBMs, their unwillingness to affiliate with independent mail order pharmacies has prevented entrants from competing for mail order sales. Furthermore, these PBMs have structured copays to incentivize subscribers to use mail order pharmacies for maintenance drugs. These companies have then exploited their positions which has led these sales to become a major portion of their revenues. From the vantage point of the parties concerned, this complicated system has various advantages. For the drug manufacturer, the system permits it to separate product flows from payment flows in a way not commonly found in the American economy. Generally, a manufacturer ships products to a wholesaler who subsequently sends to a retailer; payment flows move in the reverse sequence. The presence of rebates permits manufacturers to effectively price discriminate, charge varying prices to buyers, and thereby create a complicated system of differential pricing. The system is feasible because the ultimate consumer of these products does not typically bear the predominant share of their costs. Similarly, the payers benefit by receiving a lower price for the drugs furnished to their beneficiaries compared to cash buyers. These buyers gain this advantage thanks to their greater bargaining power or more elastic demand. Finally, insured or covered patients benefit from the availability of prescribed medicines at lower prices. Their effective price is merely the copayment, although the same products are available through the same pharmacies to other buyers who must pay the higher cash price.

A major source of the rebates obtained by PBMs is their ability to switch consumers between alternate products. For pharmaceuticals, as for most other products, a manufacturer may be willing to accept a lower price in return for increased sales. As a result, PBMs who promise to expand sales for one product at the expense of another are rewarded with lower prices, which in this system take the form of higher rebates. To receive a higher rebate, a PBM seeks to switch patients from one product to another. The switching process often involves rearranging products within a therapeutic class between formulary tiers. This may also entail the pharmacy having to contact the prescribing physicians by telephone to request a change from the original prescribed product for an individual patient.

The process of switching customers among competing products allows for the generation of a large share of the rebates received by PBMs.

However, this switching process creates two sets of concerns. The first is division of rebates between the PBMs and the payers; the second is the effect of the switching process itself on the patient and the physician. Although the contractual relationships between PBMs and drug manufacturers are complex, there are commonalities running through them. Rebates are typically larger as product sales increase, relative to either some benchmark or its share of product category sales.

Since PBMs receive information on an individual physician's prescriptions for specific patients, they can influence the prescribing decision. PBM representatives commonly seek to persuade physicians to shift their patients to drugs that offer a larger rebate. The physician, of course, has the final word, but these efforts are often quite effective and account for the large sums received by PBMs.

A striking feature of the rebate process is that it is designed specifically to place one product at a more advantageous position than another. However, since one product's gain is achieved at the expense of another, producers of the latter have an incentive to respond. If there are sufficient PBMs to service competing manufacturers, then the rebate percentage should increase to a competitive level. Note that since higher rebates imply lower prices, this process can lead to competitive pricing. Alternatively, if there are only a few major PBMs, then a manufacturer's affiliation with a PBM may have a substantial effect on market shares, with some drug companies offering larger rebates and gaining increased shares. In this case, there can be a wide disparity in rebates paid between products, PBMs, and payers.

Differential Pricing

Where prices depend on demand conditions and where there are clear distinctions among types of buyer, we expect to find different prices charged to different buyers. The economist's model of price discrimination presents a clear description of this process and indicates that prices depend on the relevant price elasticity of demand. Where the elasticity differs with the class of consumer, final price differs as well. This pattern is pervasive throughout the pharmaceutical industry.

Even though pharmaceutical companies establish a list price for each drug, known as the Average Wholesale Price or AWP, most sales are made by discounting that price. These discounts can be substantial. A survey of drug prices in one area found that the average price charged for a selection of well-known products sold to hospitals was only 19 percent of that charged to a local pharmacy (Fritz, 1994). Since hospital demand for specific products is likely to be more elastic than for an individual pharmacy, which must stock a large number of products in order to fill individual prescriptions, hospital prices should be lower than those charged to pharmacies. Where prices are demand-driven, demand elasticity is reflected in price differences.

These discounts may also differ for individuals and chain store pharmacies, and between hospitals and HMOs. An important feature of the pharmaceutical industry is that there is no single price for an individual product even at a specific point in time; prices depend on the demand conditions presented by particular buyers.

Generic products entering the marketplace typically appeal more to some buyers than to others. For example, HMOs and hospital pharmacies are more likely to use generic drugs because they have the knowledge and expertise required to evaluate them, in contrast to individual physicians. Therefore, one expects that generic rivals will make greater sales to some buyers than to others. As a result,, producers of branded products will respond to generic competition more strongly in some market segments than in others. By setting much lower prices where generic competition exists but keeping original prices or higher where generic competition is less important, many sellers of branded products can maintain a large proportion of their original sales.

The evidence that major pharmaceutical firms have followed this type of strategy is that they are sometimes able to maintain a substantial market share following patent expiration and generic entry. There is little evidence of this, but one older study found that by the sixth year after patent expiration, average market shares for thirty-five products between 1984 and 1987 were fully 62 percent in physical units and 85 percent in dollar sales compared to the previous level (Office of Technology Assessment, 1993). The strategy of charging lower prices where firms face strenuous competition but higher prices where they do not is used by many drug companies to maintain sales and market share.

Approaches for Containing Pharmaceutical Costs

Pharmaceutical companies have sought to maintain or expand revenues, but health care consumers, providers, and insurers have looked for methods to limit drug expenditures. Here as elsewhere, buyers and sellers face opposing incentives. Some buyers seek to reduce the quantity of drugs consumed, but most look for means to lower the price paid for a specific product or to redirect patients toward lower-priced alternatives. These methods can be divided into those focused on consumer behavior, physician prescribing patterns, and manufacturer actions. At this point, we review some of the measures that have been used.

Patient-Focused Measures

Consumer behavior can be altered through economic incentives or education. Economic incentives typically mean cost sharing, through which patients bear more of the financial consequences of their actions. As the out-of-pocket cost of drugs increases, the quantity purchased declines, with patients either going without the prescribed drugs or shifting to less expensive alternatives such as generic products or over-the-counter options.

Cost sharing is sometimes criticized as being an overly blunt instrument, because it may discourage use of necessary as well as unnecessary therapies. The RAND Health Insurance Experiment studied the effect of cost sharing on consumption of prescribed drugs. Leibowitz, Manning, and Newhouse (1985) reported that pharmaceutical expenditures by individuals without cost sharing were as much as 60 percent higher than for those with cost sharing. These authors also found that consumers were generally more likely to reduce purchases of discretionary rather than essential drugs in response to increased cost sharing.

An alternative to economic incentives in dealing with consumer behavior is patient education. An example of this type of program is informing patients that generic drugs are equivalent to branded products. Another is explaining to patients that extensive use of certain drugs, such as antibiotics, is unnecessary and may even be harmful, thereby lowering the quantity purchased. Such programs can reduce consumer demand for specific products, but they are unlikely to limit very much the aggregate demand for pharmaceuticals. Many patients still expect a prescription at the conclusion of each physician visit, and physicians respond accordingly.

Provider-Focused Measures

Despite the presence of consumer-oriented programs, most efforts at cost containment for pharmaceuticals are directed at those who make the decision on drug therapy: the physician, hospital, or managed care provider. Because physicians, particularly those in private practice, have few incentives to limit pharmaceutical costs, physician-directed policies are not much different from those aimed at consumers. When financial constraints are removed from patients, they are also generally removed from their physicians.

However, physicians are also the subject of education programs that seek to improve the quality of prescribing and reduce overall drug expenditures. These programs are present especially in HMOs and other managed care programs; they have great potential because the pace of new-drug introduction is rapid and physicians have difficulty keeping abreast of new therapeutic options. Without such programs, the primary means the physician has for learning about new products is pharmaceutical company marketing efforts, which are designed to increase rather than reduce spending on pharmaceuticals.

Physicians have few incentives to limit costs; this is not so for the organizations that actually pay for pharmaceuticals. Generic versions of drugs are generally favored, and newer, more expensive drugs often discouraged (Harris, Stergachis, & Reid, 1990). In addition, these payers promote the shift of certain products to over-the-counter status. These drugs can be obtained without a visit to the physician's office, and such products are typically not reimbursed.

Furthermore, hospitals, HMOs, and government reimbursement plans have adopted formularies designed explicitly to restrict the drug choices available to physicians in order to reduce costs. These lists of approved drugs depend in principle on the relative cost and effectiveness of alternative products. Though nearly every formulary program permits exceptions, the burden of obtaining an exemption is often great enough to discourage a physician from doing so unless he or she feels that a nonlisted drug is absolutely necessary (Grabowski, Schweitzer, & Shiota, 1992).

Formularies, however, have the potential for increasing rather than decreasing health care costs if they are so restrictive that patients are prescribed less-effective drugs. Even expensive drugs are generally less costly than a physician visit or hospital episode, suggesting that using suboptimal drugs may be penny wise but pound foolish. The question of whether or not a formulary lowers or raises drug or overall health care costs depends on the relative prices of the drugs included and excluded from the formulary, the number of patients who use the more expensive product when it is not necessary, and the treatment ramifications for patients who are switched to a less expensive drug when they need the more expensive one. Sloan, Gordon, and Cocks (1993) found that "limiting the number of drugs [through a formulary] appears to have been a very good idea for gastrointestinal disease patients and for those with asthma, but a bad one for coronary disease patients.'' In the latter case, total medical costs actually increased with adoption of the formulary. Other studies have also shown that Medicaid formularies are not effective in lowering drug expenditures or reducing overall health care costs (Schweitzer & Shiota, 1992; Moore & Newman, 1993).

Manufacturer-Focused Measures

A more direct approach to cost containment is the exercise of a payer's *monopsony* power to limit the prices charged by pharmaceutical manufacturers. These actions are frequently adopted by governments that offer coverage for pharmaceuticals in their national programs. Increasingly, foreign governments and insurance funds have sought to reduce drug prices as a means of cost control. In most countries, the question is not whether to fix prices but how to do so, and in particular how to set prices without removing the incentive to develop new and improved pharmaceuticals. A typical response is to permit use of a product and reimburse costs in accordance with its relative therapeutic benefits. Ideally, this objective would lead to the same prices as those set in a competitive market. Regulatory objectives are thereby similar to those enforced by competitive markets.

Australia has progressed further than most other countries in attempting to calculate the cost-effectiveness of new drugs and setting reimbursement rates accordingly (Office of Technology Assessment, 1993). Canada uses this model at the national level as well. Britain, on the other hand, used to incorporate the profitability of the pharmaceutical company into its calculation of allowable prices that the National Health Service (NHS) was willing to pay for new products. More recently, however, drug prices must be analyzed by an agency within the British National Health Service, called the National Institute for Health and Clinical Excellence. This agency calculates the resulting cost per quality-adjusted life year (QALY) for the proposed price. It then sends the resulting cost-effectiveness ratio to the NHS, which decides whether to (a) accept the price, (b) reject reimbursement for the product, or (c) negotiate some lower price in order to achieve an acceptable C-E ratio (National Institute for Health and Clinical Excellence, n.d.). This brings Britain into the group of countries that are explicitly using value-based pricing as the basis for reimbursement.

Advertising is often suggested as a cause of rising pharmaceutical expenditures. With the FDA's relaxation of prohibitions against direct-to-consumer advertising in 1995, this particular marketing approach is increasingly visible to the general public. The criticism of direct-to-consumer (DTC) advertising is that it influences prescribing and consumption decisions adversely by inflating patient demand for unneeded products that can have unintended consequences, such as adverse side effects (Spence, Teleki, Cheetham, Schweitzer, & Millares, 2005). Even though the FDA monitors advertising carefully to guard against unsubstantiated claims, it has followed the guidance of the Federal Trade Commission in recognizing that advertising is inherently biased in favor of the sponsor's product (for any product or service); one should not expect different behavior on the part of pharmaceutical advertisers.

Firms are permitted to present information regarding their products that is favorable, and leave it to other producers to do the same for their own products. If there is a need for unbiased information on competing products, it should be provided separately. In the case of pharmaceuticals, there are already a number of independent newsletters, some directed to physicians and others to patients, that compare alternative therapies. The potential of the Internet to expand this sort of information is considerable but also worrisome in terms of accuracy and misinformation.

Prescribing quality would also be improved if the NIH sponsored more head-to-head clinical trials of competing drugs within a class so that competing claims could be evaluated. Drug firms, which sponsor most drug trials in connection with the drug approval process, have little incentive to conduct multiproduct trials currently, despite such trials being precisely what physicians and health plans need.

The Link Between Pharmaceutical Expenditures and Research

One of the most serious questions raised in discussion of pharmaceutical cost containment concerns whether success can be achieved without sacrificing the large investment in R&D. If cost containment is pursued too severely, many fear that diminished returns will lead to decreased spending on R&D, resulting in fewer subsequent pharmaceutical innovations.

Scherer (2001) sought to answer this question through exploring the link between pharmaceutical profitability and R&D expenditures (Scherer, 2001). Since these outlays are largely financed from internally generated funds, research levels are likely to depend on gross industry margins, which is the difference between firm revenue and costs. Finding substantial "cyclical co-movement in pharmaceutical industry gross margins and R&D outlays," Scherer concluded: "As profit opportunities expand, firms compete to exploit them by increasing R&D investments, and perhaps also promotional costs, until increases in costs dissipate most, if not all, supranormal profit returns . . . This interpretation . . . has self-evident implications for policy interventions aimed at reducing industry prices and profits" (Scherer, 2001).

Recent Events Surrounding Pharmaceutical Costs and Access

With significant advances in drug utility, rising drug costs per episode of care, and increasing life expectancy, ambulatory medication costs have become a significant aspect of health care expenditures.

Medicare Part D

Ambulatory medication costs are especially significant for the elderly, as 64 percent of individuals over the age of sixty-five use three or more medications (Gu, Dillon, & Burt, 2010). The Medicare Prescription Drug, Improvement and Modernization Act of 2003 (MMA), widely known as Part D, aimed to correct Medicare's exclusion of outpatient prescription drug coverage that brought significant financial hardship for many. This represented the largest expansion of Medicare since its inception in 1966. While the fact that Medicare did not originally cover outpatient medication may seem odd, it is important to remember that pharmaceuticals were relatively inexpensive fifty years ago and much less prominent in the provision of health care services, representing a minor expense in terms of total expenditures.

The structure of Medicare Part D is a collection of numerous private drug insurance plans; in April 2010, there were over 156 different plans available, albeit many were regional in coverage (Hoadley, Cubanski, Hargrave, Summer, & Neuman, 2009). Although this may seem peculiar given Medicare is a government run insurance program, it is nothing new. Since 1985, Medicare has adopted the private insurance sector in two alternative structures offered to its beneficiaries: Supplemental Medicare Insurance Policies and Medicare+Choice. The former policy, known publicly as Medigap, allows private insurance companies to sell supplemental plans that cover some of the Medicare cost sharing and additional services not paid by Medicare. Medicare+Choice is a program by which Medicare beneficiaries join managed care organizations (MCOs) that accept the totality of the individual's care. For most beneficiaries, the most attractive aspect of Medigap policies and Medicare+Choice options was inclusion of coverage for ambulatory pharmaceuticals. Approximately two-thirds of Medicare beneficiaries were able to obtain some pharmaceutical coverage through either of these two Medicare benefit plans, leaving approximately one-third without any coverage for outpatient drugs (Safran et al., 2005). This demonstrates that the common complaint that the elderly had no coverage for outpatient pharmaceuticals was incorrect.

Part D plans were offered as free-standing supplemental insurance programs. The plans offered for sale differed in coverage, in terms of cost-sharing and formularies. Medicare created a website to enable potential Part D purchasers to compare drug formularies, so that people could be assured that the drugs they were presently taking were covered by a particular plan they were contemplating purchasing. A Medicare beneficiary can elect to join a Part D plan at any time but there is a financial penalty for joining after one joins Medicare itself. This penalty was enacted in order to reduce the effect of asymmetric information for consumers, who would decide to buy a Part D plan only when their drug consumption was expected to become very expensive.

While the additional coverage created by Part D has made prescription medications more affordable, the program does have its shortcomings. With significant financial constraints imposed by Congress, Part D's net cost was strictly limited, leading to an unique coverage decision. Congress wanted to spread the benefits of Part D coverage to as many beneficiaries as possible, and so it wanted near first-dollar coverage. But it also wanted the plan to cover catastrophic drug costs. But offering near first-dollar coverage at the low end, along with unlimited coverage at the high end was going to be too expensive. Rather than removing coverage at either the low or high end, Congress did something else. It removed coverage in the middle! Until the 2010 reform, Part D covered annual pharmaceutical expenditures between approximately $300 and $2,700, and then those expenditures in excess of $6,154. Expenditures between $2,700 and $6,154 were not covered. This gap was nicknamed the "donut hole." It wasn't until the 2010 passage of the Affordable Care Act that Congress authorized funds to fill in that donut hole in coverage.

Drug Shortages

In recent years, another pharmaceutical access issue has appeared: pharmaceutical shortages. This situation is unusual historically and has surprised both patients and their physicians, presenting a bewildering situation that has never been encountered before. Ironically, the shortages are not where one might expect them—in new, expensive products. Rather, they are occurring in the cases of older products that are available generically. Currently, there are 103 distinct medication listed on the Food and Drug Administration's website for drug shortages (U.S. FDA, 2012b). Recent studies have implied that the problems are limited to selected therapeutic classes of drugs—especially oncology medications—and have suggested that lack of information pertaining to plant closures are the major cause (Chabner, 2011; Gatesman & Smith, 2011). However, the problem appears to be more pervasive than this and requires addressing structural shifts in the generic drug market.

The generic pharmaceutical industry has undergone important changes in recent years that have increased its prominence, which has provided consumers with more affordable drug products. However, it has also created a significant risk to the broader health care sector in the form of drug shortages. Three factors have created the "perfect storm" involving generic pharmaceuticals that has resulted in this crisis:

- A reduction in the price of generic drugs due to the consolidation of buyers and manufacturers
- An increased penetration of generic drugs in the pharmaceutical marketplace
- An increased dependence on drug products—either manufactured drugs or their active ingredients—from less regulated foreign sources

The first major trend within the generic pharmaceutical industry has been the consolidation of producers and purchasers. Manufacturers are not only merging but often creating potential conflicts of interest as some producers are now selling branded drugs alongside generic products ("branded generics"). In some cases, the mergers have enabled manufacturers to achieve economies of scale in manufacturing, which is important in a market characterized by strong downward pressure on prices. Consolidation among buyers has been the result of mergers and acquisitions of pharmaceutical purchasers—health insurers, managed care organizations, and pharmacy benefit managers. This consolidation of buyers increases their ability to negotiate substantial price reductions from manufacturers. The lower prices have decreased profit margins significantly, which results in fewer firms interested in entering the generic drug market.

The second major trend has been increased penetration of generic drugs in the pharmaceutical market. This is in large part due to three key reasons. First, generic drugs are less expensive than branded drugs because of the use of three-tiered drug formularies in managed care plans, which create a direct incentive for consumers to purchase generic drugs whenever possible. Second, the lower prices have also led to fierce price competition among retailers. Today, over three hundred popular, albeit older, drugs are offered in very low-cost programs such as Wal-Mart's and Kroger's $4 Generic Drug Plans, greatly expanding the reach of generic medications. Third, the expansion of the generic market is the result of the inexorable increase in the number of drugs that lose their patent protection. Each year several major brand name drugs lose their patent protection, which further increases the generic share of the pharmaceutical market.

The third major trend in the generic industry resulting from the strong downward price pressure has been increased reliance on pharmaceutical chemical products and finished drugs from abroad. These are often imported from low-cost, developing countries, which further increases the generic drug supply chain's vulnerability to interruptions. The failure of the FDA to enforce safe manufacturing standards in production of heparin—which led to over sixty-seven deaths in 2008 due to drug impurities at a Chinese manufacturing plant—illustrates the difficulty of maintaining standards of *good manufacturing practice (GMP)* in countries where inspections are particularly awkward to conduct (Schweitzer, 2008).

The consequence of the perfect storm is the recent rise in drug shortages. Shortages result from producers having reduced incentives to stock inventory that enables them to continue selling products in the event of an interruption of production, such as a firm's temporary closure. For branded products, the profit margin is large enough to assure that firms will maintain the supply chain; however, the generic market has markedly reduced profit margins that lessen this incentive. Furthermore, given the recent increased reliance on foreign sources for active ingredients and generic drug manufacturing—often from countries that lack stringent regulatory oversight—the possibility of production interruptions have become more likely. Furthermore, necessary increases in production from suppliers may not be feasible in the short run if demand for a certain generic grows. The result is often an unstable generic drug market that may have dire consequences for the rising number of Americans that have come to depend on the more affordable medication option (see Schweitzer, 2013, for a more comprehensive analysis of the shortage issue together with a suggestion of a policy remedy).

Future Directions

Recent trends in pharmaceutical prices can be examined from various vantage points. Although it is true that the prices of the most advanced drugs have increased over time, this statement is based largely on the increasing benefits of the new products. Prices for the same-quality products have tended to decline over time. Since "*inflation*" traditionally describes price changes for the same or similar products, one cannot conclude from recent experience that there has been much pharmaceutical price inflation. What has occurred instead is that the prices of newer products (especially their branded versions) have increased substantially, even while prices of competing products and generic alternatives have declined.

Our picture of drug price control is a mixed one. The share of health expenditures devoted to pharmaceuticals is relatively low, and there is a history of moderate price increases, albeit with some acceleration, in recent years. Furthermore, in the last few years there have been rapid changes in the market for drugs, with increasing importance for provider-driven rather than patient-driven competition. These changes have had a growing impact on both average rates of price increase and patterns of price dispersion for pharmaceuticals. The increased segmentation of pharmaceutical markets on the basis of insurance coverage also means that the average price level conveys less information about what is actually taking place. Traditional measures of price changes are inadequate and tend to inflate the actual rate of increase; international comparisons also yield inconclusive results.

A critical policy issue for the cost of pharmaceuticals is whether uniform pharmaceutical prices should be mandated for various customer classes. If this type of proposal were enacted, whether through legislation or judicial decision, pricing practices would change sharply. Berndt noted that under these conditions the vigor of competition in many pharmaceutical markets would diminish sharply, potentially resulting in *higher* overall prices (Berndt, 1994).

SUMMARY

This overview of the major factors determining the cost of pharmaceuticals illustrates three important areas where additional information would assist policy analysts. The first is the need to understand better the relationship between drug price and quality level. Preliminary data show that prices are positively affected by a drug's therapeutic advance, but the extent of this relationship is not well explored. This question is especially important because of our present inability to account for quality improvement in measures of pharmaceutical price increase. Second, we know little about how the quality level for a drug is determined. In the past, the FDA assigned a three-level quality improvement score to each drug for which marketing approval was sought. This designation was crude at best and sometimes contradicted by the marketplace. However, the FDA currently does not provide even these designations, and there is no agreed-on measure of the extent of therapeutic improvement represented by new drugs. Third, we need a better understanding of the extent of competition in pharmaceutical markets. This factor is especially critical, because we are now observing another wave of consolidation in the pharmaceutical industry. Better understanding of the appropriate breadth of pharmaceutical markets is also needed. How much rivalry is there within or across therapeutic categories? Understanding of how pharmaceutical markets are structured and interact would assist in creating appropriate public policies for this industry.

NOTE

The authors express their gratitude to Brian Raffetto for providing excellent research assistance in the preparation of this chapter.

KEY TERMS

Consumer Price Index (CPI) a measure of the overall inflation rate and its components. It is calculated monthly by the Bureau of Labor Statistics.

Direct-to-consumer (DTC) advertising Advertising directly to the general public, rather than to prescribers. As patients cannot prescribe drugs, all these ads end with the suggestion that the viewer ask the physician for the drug.

Formulary A list of all drugs covered by a health insurance plan. While formularies used to be simple lists of drugs (a product that *was* covered was on the list, and products not covered were *not* on the list), modern formularies cover far more drugs than before, but divide them into groups, or tiers, depending on patient copay.

Generic drugs Drugs manufactured that copy products that were originally patented. Patents for drugs expire twenty years after the application for a patent was originally filed with the U.S. Patent Office. Generic drug manufacturers must provide data to the FDA showing that the active ingredient of the generic product is the same molecule as was in the innovative product (chemical equivalence) and that the drug is absorbed by patients at the same rate as the innovative product (bioequivalence).

Good manufacturing practice (GMP) A designation by the Food and Drug Administration (FDA) that a drug manufacturing facility (domestic or foreign) meets minimum product safety standards.

Inflation The rise in price over time for particular goods or services. The assumption is that the goods and services are the same from one period to another; otherwise an adjustment for quality change must be made.

Monopsony A market composed of a single buyer (in contrast to a "monopoly," characterized by a single seller).

DISCUSSION QUESTIONS

1. Comment on this statement: "Drug prices are higher in the United States than in other wealthy countries."
2. Do all new drugs lower the cost of health care? Why should we continue using those drugs that do not?
3. There are three attributes of drugs that determine their price in the market. What are those three attributes?
4. What does "value-based pricing" mean?
5. "Me too" drugs are new drugs that are very similar to products that are already on the market. What value do those products have for consumers?
6. Shortages of drugs in the United States primarily occur with what kind of drugs?
7. Should the FDA have increased responsibility for regulating foreign pharmaceuticals to assure drug safety?
8. In what ways will the Patient Protection and Accountable Care Act affect pharmaceutical delivery? Will pharmaceutical manufacturers' profits increase or decrease? Why?

9. When a drug's patent expires, what incentives exist to encourage prescribers and patients to switch to generic versions of the drugs?

FURTHER READING

Comanor, W. S., & Schweitzer, S. O. (Eds.). (2013). *Readings in pharmaceutical economics and policy*. Cheltenham, U.K.: Edward Elgar.

The authors present a broad summary of pharmaceutical economics and policy and then present some of the most important literature that explains how those issues work.

Danzon, P. M., & Furukawa, M. F. (2008). International prices and availability of pharmaceuticals in 2005. *Health Affairs, 27*(1), 221–233.

Danzon and Furukawa analyze international data on pharmaceutical consumption and prices. They find that drug spending is higher in the United States than in other countries, but this is primarily because prices of branded products are higher than they are elsewhere. They note that generic drugs tend to be cheaper in the United States than in other countries and that the share of generic drug sales is increasing.

Lu, Z. J., & Comanor, W. S. (1998). Strategic pricing of new pharmaceuticals. *Review of Economics and Statistics, 80*, 108–118.

This study shows the strong influence of pharmaceutical quality (efficacy, safety, and convenience) on launch prices. The results imply that drug prices are more strongly determined by demand factors than supply factors.

Scherer, F. M. (2010). Pharmaceutical innovation. In B. Hall & N. Rosenberg (Eds.), *Handbook of the economics of technological innovation* (pp. 542–543). Amsterdam: North-Holland.

Scherer analyzes the determinants of pharmaceutical R&D and innovation. With an industry so dependent on new products and technological progress, it is critical to understand what factors make firms successful in developing new therapies.

Schweitzer, S. O. (2007). *Pharmaceutical economics and policy* (2nd ed.). New York: Oxford University Press.

The author surveys a large number of pharmaceutical industry issues in a comprehensive analysis of the entire industry. The book looks at the demand for pharmaceuticals, the characteristics of the industry that produces them, and market factors that ultimately determine both price and quantity.

Spence, M., Teleki, S., Cheetham, C. M., Schweitzer, S. O., & Millares, M. (2005). The effect of direct-to-consumer pharmaceutical advertising on prescribing. *Medical Care Review and Research, 62*(5), 544–559.

The authors present research linking different data sets in order to determine whether direct-to-consumer advertising is associated with greater sales of pharmaceuticals and whether this increased demand improves prescribing patterns or worsens them.

REFERENCES

Berndt, E. R. (1994). *Uniform pharmaceutical pricing: An economic analysis.* Washington, DC: American Enterprise Institute.

Berndt, E. R. (2001, March–April). The U.S. pharmaceutical industry: Why major growth in times of cost containment? *Health Affairs, 20,* 107.

Berndt, E. R., Cockburn, I. M., Griliches, Z., Keeler, T. E., & Baily, M. N. (1996). Pharmaceutical innovations and market dynamics: Tracking effects on price indexes for antidepressant drugs. *Brookings Papers on Economic Activity: Microeconomics,* p. 174.

Bureau of Labor Statistics. (2010). Measuring price change for medical care in the CPI. Retrieved from http://www.bls.gov/cpi/cpifact4.htm

Centers for Disease Control and Prevention. (2011). Health, United States, 2011. National Center for Health Statistics. Retrieved from http://www.cdc.gov/nchs/data/hus/hus11.pdf

Centers for Medicare and Medicaid Services, Office of the Actuary, National Health Statistics Group. (2012). National Health Expenditure Accounts (NHEA): Historical. Retrieved from http://www.cms.gov/Research-Statistics-Data-and-Systems/Statistics-Trends-and-Reports/NationalHealthExpendData/NationalHealth AccountsHistorical.html

Chabner, B. A. (2011). Drug shortages: A critical challenge for the generic-drug market. *New England Journal of Medicine, 365,* 2147–2149.

Clark, L. T. (1991). Improving compliance and increasing control of hypertension: Needs of special hypertensive populations. *American Heart Journal, 121,* 664.

Comanor, W. S., & Schweitzer, S. O. (1995). Pharmaceuticals. In W. Adams & J. W. Brock (Eds.), *Structure of American industry* (9th ed.). Upper Saddle River, NJ: Prentice-Hall.

Comanor, W. S., Schweitzer, S. O., & Carter, T. (2005). A hedonic model of pricing innovative pharmaceuticals. In M. R. DiTommaso & S. O. Schweitzer (Eds.), *Health policy and high-tech industrial development: Learning from innovation in the health industry.* Cheltenham: Edward Elgar.

Cooper, J. K., Love, D. W., & Raffoul, P. R. (1982). Intentional prescription nonadherence (noncompliance) by the elderly. *American Geriatrics Society, 30,* 329.

Danzon, P. M., & Chao, L. W. (2000). Cross-national price differences for pharmaceuticals: How large, and why? *Journal of Health Economics, 19,* 159–195.

Danzon, P. M., & Furukawa, M. F. (2008). International prices and availability of pharmaceuticals in 2005. *Health Affairs, 27*(1), 221–233.

Danzon, P. M., & Pauly, M. V. (2002). Health insurance and the growth in pharmaceutical expenditures. *Journal of Law and Economics, 45*(2, Part 2), 587–614.

Department of Health and Human Services. (2010). *Health United States, 1999.* Hyattsville, MD: National Center for Health Statistics.

DiMasi, J. A., Hansen, R. W., & Grabowski, H. G. (2003). The price of innovation: New estimates of drug development and costs. *Journal of Health Economics, 22*(2), 151–185.

Esposito, D. (2003). *You get what you co-pay for: The influence of patent co-payments on the demand for drugs.* Doctoral dissertation, Department of Economics, University of California, Santa Barbara.

Feldstein, P. J. (1993). *Health care economics* (4th ed.). Albany, NY: Delmar.

Frank, R., & Salkever, D. (1992). Pricing patent loss and the market for pharmaceuticals. *Southern Economic Journal, 50,* 165–179.

Fritz, S. (1994, Jan. 30). Prescription drug pricing hurting the poor, elderly health. *Los Angeles Times.*

Gatesman, M. L., & Smith, T. J. (2011). The shortage of essential chemotherapy drugs in the United States. *New England Journal of Medicine, 365,* 1653–1655.

Goldman, D. P., Joyce, G. F., & Zheng, Y. (2004). Pharmacy benefits and the use of drugs by the chronically ill. *Journal of the American Medical Association, 291,* 2344–2350.

Grabowski, H. G., Schweitzer, S. O., & Shiota, S. R. (1992). The Medicaid drug lag: Adoption of new drugs by state Medicaid formularies. *Pharmacoeconomics, 1*(Suppl.), 32–40.

Griliches, Z., & Cockburn, I. M. (1994). Generics and new goods in the pharmaceutical price indexes. *American Economic Review, 84*(5), 1213–1232.

Gu, Q., Dillon, C. F., & Burt, V. L. (2010). Prescription drug use continues to increase: U.S. prescription drug data for 2007–2008. *National Center for Health Statistics, 42.*

Harris, B. L., Stergachis, A., & Reid, L. D. (1990). The effect of drug co-payments on utilization and cost of pharmaceuticals in a health maintenance organization. *Medical Care, 28*(10), 907–917.

Hoadley, J., Cubanski, J., Hargrave, E., Summer, L., & Neuman, T. (2009, November). Medicare Part D spotlight: Part D plan availability in 2010 and key changes since 2009. Menlo Park, CA: Kaiser Family Foundation. Retrieved from http://www.kff.org/medicare/upload/7986.pdf

Huskamp, H. A., Deverka, P. A., Epstein, A. M., Epstein, R. S., McGuigan, K. A., & Frank, R. G. (2003). The effect of incentive-based formularies on prescription drug utilization and spending. *New England Journal of Medicine, 349,* 2224–2232.

Kaiser Family Foundation. (2004, October). *Prescription drug trends: Update* (Publication No. 3057-03). Menlo Park, CA: Kaiser Family Foundation.

Kessler, D., Rose, J. L., Temple, R. J., Schapiro, R., & Griffin, J. P. (1994). Therapeutic class wars: Drug promotion in a competitive marketplace. *New England Journal of Medicine, 331,* 1350–1353.

Leibowitz, A., Manning, W. G., & Newhouse, J. P. (1985). The demand for prescription drugs as a function of cost-sharing. *Social Science and Medicine, 21,* 1063–1069.

Lu, Z. J., & Comanor, W. S. (1998, February). Strategic pricing of new pharmaceuticals. *Review of Economics and Statistics,* p. 116.

Moore, W. J., & Newman, R. J. (1993, April). Drug formulary restrictions as a cost-containment policy in Medicaid programs. *Journal of Law and Economics, 36,* 71–97.

National Institute for Health Care Management. (1999). *Issue brief: Factors affecting growth of prescription drugs expenditures.* Washington, DC: Author.

National Institute for Health and Clinical Excellence. (n.d.). NICE quality standards. Retrieved from www.nice.org.uk

Office of Technology Assessment (OTA). (1993, February). *Pharmaceutical R&D: Costs, risks and rewards* (OTA-H-522). Washington, DC: U.S. Government Printing Office.

Payer, L. (1988). *Medicine and culture: Varieties of treatment in the United States, England, West Germany, and France.* New York: Penguin.

Pharmaceutical Research and Manufacturers Association. (2005). *Annual report 2004–05.* Washington, DC: Author.

Safran, D. G., Neuman, P., Schoen, C., Kitchman M. S., Wilson I. B., Cooper B., . . . Rogers W. H. (2005). Prescription drug coverage and seniors: Findings from a 2003 national survey. *Health Affairs, 24,* w152–w166.

Salehi, H., & Schweitzer, S. (1985). Economic aspects of drug substitution. *Health Care Financing Review, 6*(5), 59–68.

Scherer, F. M. (2001, September–October). The link between gross probability and pharmaceutical R&D spending. *Health Affairs, 20,* 216–220.

Schweitzer, S. O. (2008). Trying times at the FDA: The challenge of ensuring the safety of imported pharmaceuticals. *New England Journal of Medicine, 358*(17), 173–177.

Schweitzer, S. O. (2013). How the US Food and Drug Administration can solve the prescription drug shortage. *American Journal of Public Health, 103*(5), e10–e14.

Schweitzer, S. O., & Comanor, W. S. (2011). Prices of pharmaceuticals in poor countries are much lower than in wealthy countries. *Health Affairs, 30*(8), 1553–1561.

Schweitzer, S. O., & Shiota, S. R. (1992). Access and cost implications of state limitations on Medicaid reimbursement for pharmaceuticals. *Annual Review of Public Health, 13,* 399–410.

Sloan, F. A., Gordon, G, & Cocks, D. L. (1993). Do hospital drug formularies reduce spending on hospital services? *Medical Care, 31*(10), 851–867.

Spence, M., Teleki, S,. Cheetham, C. M., Schweitzer, S. O., & Millares, M. (2005). The effect of direct-to-consumer pharmaceutical advertising on prescribing. *Medical Care Review and Research, 62*(5), 544–559.

Steiner, R. L. (1993). Inverse association between the margins of manufacturers and retailers. *Review of Industrial Organization, 8,* 717–740.

U.S. Bureau of the Census. (2011). Statistical abstract of the United States. Section 14: Prices. Retrieved from http://www.census.gov/prod/2011pubs/12statab/prices.pdf

U.S. Congress, General Accounting Office (GAO). (1992a). *Prescription drugs: Changes in prices for selected drugs* (GAO/HRD-92–128). Washington, DC: Author.

U.S. Congress, General Accounting Office (GAO). (1992b). *Prescription drugs: Companies typically charge more in the United States than in Canada* (GAO/HRD-92–110). Washington, DC: Author.

U.S. Congress, General Accounting Office (GAO). (1994). *Prescription drugs: Companies typically charge more in the United States than in the United Kingdom* (GAO/HEHS-94–29). Washington, DC: Author.

U.S. Food and Drug Administration (FDA). (2012a). Facts about generic drugs. Retrieved from http://www.fda.gov/drugs/resourcesforyou/consumers/buying usingmedicinesafely/understandinggenericdrugs/ucm167991.htm

U.S. Food and Drug Administration (FDA). (2012b). Current drug shortages index. Retrieved from http://www.fda.gov/Drugs/DrugSafety/DrugShortages/ucm050792.htm

Wiggins, S. N., & Maness, R. (2004). Price competition in pharmaceuticals: The case of anti-infectives. *Economic Inquiry, 42*(2), 247–263.

PART THREE

QUALITY OF HEALTH CARE

CHAPTER ELEVEN

MEASURING HEALTH-RELATED QUALITY OF LIFE AND OTHER OUTCOMES

Patricia A. Ganz
Ron D. Hays
Robert M. Kaplan
Mark S. Litwin

Learning Objectives

- Understand how health-related quality of life (HRQL) is defined and conceptualized
- Learn about the history of HRQL assessment and its incorporation into health services, clinical research, and other outcome studies
- understand the role of quality-adjusted life years and cost-effectiveness applications in outcomes research
- Become familiar with different types of HRQL measures
- Appreciate the purpose of comparative effectiveness research and its relationship to the Affordable Care Act

In the first installment of a six-part series on the quality of health care that appeared in the *New England Journal of Medicine* in 1996, David Blumenthal culled several definitions to support his premise that medical outcomes are a critical component of quality (Blumenthal, 1996). One of the earliest attempts to define quality came from the American Medical Association, which in the mid-1980s stated that high-quality care was that "which consistently contributes to the improvement or maintenance of quality and/or duration of life" (Council on Medical Service, 1986). Blumenthal went on to note that the Institute of Medicine held in the 1990s that quality consists of the "degree to which health services for individuals and populations increase the likelihood of desired health outcomes" (Lohr, Donaldson, & Harris Wehling, 1992). He contended that the most important new development in our current understanding of medical outcomes was the recognition that it is patients who define which outcomes are most important and whether or not they have been achieved. "Using psychometric techniques," he argued, "researchers have developed better measures of patients' evaluations of the results of care, thus allowing patients' views to be assessed with greater scientific accuracy" (Blumenthal, 1996).

Blumenthal's emphasis on *quality of life* in the context of quality of care underscored a body of research that has grown rapidly. Figure 11.1 summarizes the number of publications under the topic of quality of life

FIGURE 11.1. QUALITY-OF-LIFE PUBLICATIONS BY YEAR

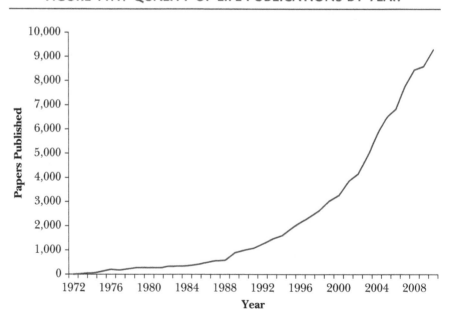

identified in PubMed between 1972 and 2010. In 1972, PubMed did not identify any publications under the quality-of-life topic heading. Over the next thirty-eight years the number of articles that use the quality-of-life key word grew dramatically. In 2010, it identified 9,291 articles. It is noteworthy that the number of publications increased 72 percent between 2005 and 2010. In these nearly four decades, the tools for quality-of-life measurement became more refined, allowing sophisticated analysis of patients' perceived outcomes in a variety of illnesses. Today, *health-related quality of life (HRQL)* is studied in a variety of subjects throughout the stages of life (Liao, McGee, Cao, & Cooper, 2000; Wolfe et al., 2000) and as a measure of community health (Centers for Disease Control and Prevention, 2000).

This work has largely been built on a stage set by Paul Ellwood in his 1988 Shattuck lecture (Ellwood, 1988) in which he advocated using a technology of patient experience, drawing on a common patient-understood language of health outcomes. He proposed that "outcomes management would draw on four already rapidly maturing techniques. First, it would place greater reliance on standards and guidelines that physicians can use in selecting appropriate interventions. Second, it would routinely and systematically measure the functioning and well-being of patients, along with disease-targeted clinical outcomes, at appropriate time intervals. Third, it would pool clinical and outcome data on a massive scale. Fourth, it would analyze and disseminate results from the segment of the data base most appropriate to the concerns of each decision maker." Later, Ellwood went on to say that "the centerpiece and unifying ingredient of outcomes management is the tracking and measurement of function and well-being or quality of life. Although this sounds like a hopelessly optimistic undertaking, I believe that we already have the ability to obtain crucial, reliable data on quality of life at minimal cost and inconvenience" (Ellwood, 1988).

Ellwood's support for active inclusion of quality-of-life data as a key component of outcomes management lends important support to advancement of the field. Now, a quarter century later, outcome assessment has gone through adolescence and has emerged as an important aspect of health care policy. For example, the Affordable Care Act created the Patient-Centered Outcomes Research Institute (PCORI) that connects studies on patient centered outcomes to reimbursement. Despite these advances, however, many challenges remain. For example, quality-of-life data must be collected prospectively and cannot be retrieved from the administrative databases that are commonly used by health services researchers.

Definition, Conceptualization, and Measurement of Quality of Life

Great energy has traditionally been expended by clinicians and other health care professionals attempting to lengthen the duration of survival in patients with chronic diseases (Tarlov, 1992). During the last few decades, dramatic advances in diagnosis, management, and overall understanding of the mechanisms of human disease have refined the treatment approaches to many medical conditions such that patients are now living longer with their disease. This is particularly true in oncology, where some patients live for years after their initial diagnosis (Ganz, 1994).

Historically, evaluation of the success of medical therapies has focused on specific clinical parameters and survival. However, the recent surge of interest in patient-centered endpoints has generated great support for the medical-outcomes movement. Not only clinicians but also payers and managers are interested in assessing outcomes to begin measuring quality of care. Indeed, some would argue that the thrust of the outcomes movement stems largely from outside the biomedical establishment, as clinicians are held ever more accountable to external authorities. To understand better how medical outcomes fit into the framework of health services research, it is necessary to focus on assessing quality of care.

In the well-known Donabedian model (Donabedian, 1980), health care quality is examined in three parts: structure, process, and outcomes of care. *Structure of care* refers to how medical and other services are organized in a particular institution or delivery system. It may include such diverse variables as specialty mix in a multi-physician medical group, access to timely radiological files in a hospital, availability of pharmacy services in a hospice program, or convenience of parking at an outpatient surgery center. It may also involve nonmedical support services such as an organized system of care, social work, home care, or clothing and housing for the socially disadvantaged.

Process of care refers to the content of the medical and psychological interactions between patient and provider. It may include variables such as whether or not a blood culture is ordered for a baby with a fever, the nature of the treatment prescribed for a patient with abdominal pain, how much compassion a doctor demonstrates when presenting a negative diagnosis with a patient, how many times a psychologist interrupts a client during a session, or whether a nurse regularly turns a bedridden patient to prevent bedsores.

Outcomes of care refer to specific indicators of what happens to the patient once care has been rendered. This may include clinical variables, such as blood sugar level in a diabetic, blood pressure in a hypertensive, abnormal chest X-ray during treatment for pneumonia, or kidney function after transplantation. It may also include complications of treatment, such as bleeding after colonoscopic biopsy, allergic reaction to an antibiotic or injection of iodinated contrast material, graft occlusion after cardiac bypass surgery, infant mortality following emergency Cesarean delivery, or hospital death rate.

Outcomes of care may also include HRQL, another variable commonly studied in the field of medical outcomes research. The general concept of quality of life encompasses a range of human experience: access to the daily necessities of life such as food and shelter, intrapersonal and interpersonal response to life events, and activities associated with professional fulfillment and personal happiness (Patrick & Erickson, 1993a). A subcomponent of overall quality of life relates to health. HRQL focuses on the patient's own perception of well-being, and the ability to function as a result of health status or disease experience. The World Health Organization (WHO) defines health as a "state of complete physical, mental, and social well-being and not merely the absence of disease" (WHO, 1948). In the Donabedian framework, HRQL is considered an important outcome variable. Figure 11.2 presents a framework described by Patrick and Bergner for the theoretical relationships among HRQL concepts, disease, the environment, and prognosis (Patrick & Bergner, 1990).

Although quantity of life is relatively easy to assess (as survival or disease-free interval, in days, months, years), measuring HRQL presents more challenges primarily because it is less familiar to most clinicians and researchers. Typically, HRQL data are collected with self-administered questionnaires, called instruments. These instruments contain questions, or items, that are organized into scales. Each scale measures an aspect, or domain, of HRQL. Some scales comprise dozens of items, while others may include only one or two items.

HRQL instruments may be general or disease-targeted. General HRQL domains address the essential or common components of functioning and well-being, while disease-targeted domains focus on the impact of particular organic dysfunctions that affect HRQL (Patrick & Deyo, 1989).

FIGURE 11.2. CONCEPTUALIZATION OF HRQL

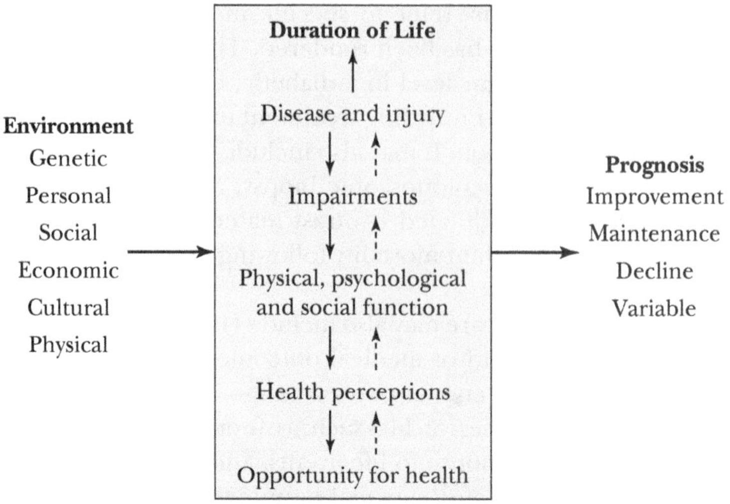

Duration of Life

↑

Environment

Genetic

Personal

Social

Economic

Cultural

Physical

Disease and injury

↓ ↑

Impairments

↓ ↑

Physical, psychological
and social function

↓ ↑

Health perceptions

↓ ↑

Opportunity for health

Prognosis

Improvement

Maintenance

Decline

Variable

Source: Adapted from Patrick & Bergner, 1990.

Generic HRQL instruments typically address general health perception; sense of well-being; and physical, emotional, and social function. Disease-targeted HRQL instruments focus on special or directly relevant domains, such as anxiety about cancer recurrence, dizziness from antihypertensive medication, or suicidal thoughts during depression therapy.

Many HRQL instruments are available. The *Quality of Life Research* journal is dedicated exclusively to presenting this research. A significant body of work has been published on HRQL in patients with various conditions (McDowell & Newell, 1996; Patrick & Erickson, 1993b; Spilker, 1990, 1996).

Evaluation of HRQL Instruments

Developing and evaluating new instruments and scales is a long and arduous process; it should not be undertaken lightly. Simply drawing up a list of questions that seem appropriate is fraught with potential traps and pitfalls. Two important characteristics to assess in new instruments are reliability and validity. Reliability is the term used to indicate the amount of measurement error in a test instrument. If a measure were applied in exactly the same situation at two points in time, the same results would be expected. For example, if you use a ruler to measure the width of this book on several occasions, you would expect the same number of inches on each application. If you get a varying width, something about the measurement process is unreliable. Assuming no changes in health, the reliability of HRQL measures is assessed by their ability to produce the same scores on repeated administration. Validity indicates the extent to which the instrument measures what it is intended to measure. Validity of HRQL instruments is evaluated by examining the extent to which the associations (correlations) of the measures with other variables are consistent with prior hypotheses (construct validity). Reliability and validity should be supported before using an instrument; therefore it is preferable to use established HRQL instruments if they are available and conceptually appropriate.

When scales and instruments are developed, they are first pilot-tested to ensure that the target population can understand and complete them with ease. Pilot testing (such as cognitive interviewing) reveals problems that might otherwise go unrecognized by researchers. For example, patients may not understand terms that are commonly used by medical professionals. This may result in missing data if patients leave questions blank or provide unreliable data if they answer questions they don't understand (Fongwa et al., 2010; Paz, Liu, Fongwa, Morales, & Hays, 2009). Furthermore, since older patients may have poor eyesight, pilot testing can identify easily corrected visual barriers such as type size and page layout. In addition, self-administered instruments with complicated skip patterns ("If you answered yes to item 16b, continue with item 16c; if you answered no to item 16b, skip to item 19a") may be confusing. This too can result in missing data and introduce difficulties in the analysis. Pilot testing is a necessary and valuable part of instrument development; it serves as a reality check for scale developers.

Caveats on Collecting HRQL Data

Once an instrument is thoroughly tested and has evidence supporting its reliability and validity, it must be administered in a manner that minimizes bias. HRQL data cannot and should not be collected from patients directly by the treating health care provider to avoid socially desirable responses (Tannock, 1990). This introduces measurement error. No matter how objective the treating clinician may claim to be, it is impossible for him or her to collect objective and unbiased outcome data through direct questioning. Variations in phrasing, inflection, eye contact, rapport, mood, and other factors are difficult or impossible to eliminate. Third parties impartial to the results should collect the data using established HRQL measures.

There is a need for basic descriptive information on the HRQL of differing patient groups, simply from an epidemiological perspective. Physical function and emotional well-being form the cornerstone of this approach, but research should also explore issues such as eating and sleeping habits, anxiety and fatigue, depression, and social interaction. Characterization of these domains often addresses not only the actual functions but also the relative importance of these issues to patients.

Beyond the descriptive analysis, HRQL outcomes need to be compared in patients undergoing various types of therapy for the same condition. From the perspective of health policy, both general and disease-targeted HRQL should be measured to facilitate comparison among common diseases or conditions. HRQL outcomes may also be correlated with clinical variables such as comorbidity, sociodemographic variables (such as age, race or ethnicity, gender, education, and income), insurance status, geographic region, and access to health care.

Quality-Adjusted Life Years

Traditional measures of health outcome include life expectancy, infant mortality, and disability days. The difficulty with these indicators is that they do not reflect most of the benefits of health care and are insensitive to minor variations in health status. Treatment of most common illnesses may have relatively little effect on life expectancy. Infant mortality does not register the effect of health services delivered to people who are older than one year (Stein, Stanton, & Starfield, 2005).

Survival analysis is an attractive generic measure of health status. It gives a unit of credit for each year of survival. Suppose, for example, that a person has a life expectancy of eighty years and dies prematurely at age fifty. In survival analysis, the person is scored as one for each of the first fifty years and zero each year thereafter. The problem is that years with disability are scored the same as years in perfect health. For example, a person with severe arthritis who is alive is scored exactly the same as someone in perfect health. Adjusted survival analysis has been proposed to address this problem. Using this method, we can summarize outcomes in terms of *quality-adjusted life years (QALYs)*. In quality-adjusted survival analysis, years of wellness are scored on a continuum ranging from 0 for dead to 1.0 for optimum function (Kaplan et al., 2001).

QALYs are a measure of life expectancy with adjustment for quality of life (Kaplan, 1993; Russell, 1999; Weinstein et al., 1996). QALYs integrate mortality and morbidity to express health status in terms of equivalents of well-years of life. If a woman dies of breast cancer at age fifty and one would have expected her to live to age seventy-five, the disease was associated with twenty-five lost life years. If one hundred women died at age fifty (and also had life expectancy of seventy-five years), 2,500 (100 × 25 years) life years would be lost. Death is not the only outcome of concern. Many adults suffer from the disease leaving them somewhat disabled over a long period of time. Although they are still alive, the quality of their lives has diminished. QALYs take into consideration the quality-of-life consequences of these illnesses.

For example, a disease that reduces quality of life by one-half takes away 0.50 QALYs over the course of one year. If it affects two people, it takes away one year (2 × 0.50) over a one-year period. A pharmaceutical treatment that improves quality of life by 0.20 for each of five individuals results in the equivalent of one QALY if the benefit is maintained over a one-year period. The basic assumption is that two years scored as 0.50 add up to the equivalent of one year of complete wellness. Similarly, four years scored as 0.25 are equivalent to one completely well year of life. A treatment that boosts a patient's health from 0.50 to 0.75 produces the equivalent of 0.25 QALYs. If applied to four individuals, and the duration of the treatment effect is one year, the effect of the treatment would be equivalent to one completely well year of life. This system has the advantage of considering both benefits and side effects of programs in terms of the common QALY units. Although QALYs are typically assessed for patients, they can also be measured for others, including caregivers who are placed at risk because they experience stressful life events. In several different reports, the Institute of Medicine (IOM) recommended that population health metrics be used to evaluate public programs and to assist the decision-making process (Field & Gold, 1998). Most recently, the IOM Committee on Public Health Strategies to Improve Health recommended that QALYs or related metrics be used to monitor the health status of all communities. In 2010 alone, more that 650 new studies applying QALYs appeared in the literature. Further, there have been significant advances in the methodologies for measuring and reporting QALYs (Adami, 2010; Adolfsson, 2010; Fowler et al., 2006; Sessions & Detsky, 2010). But there have also been significant obstacles. In particular, the Affordable Care Act specifically notes that QALYs can not be used for resource allocation decisions (Neumann & Weinstein, 2010).

Cost-Effectiveness Decisions

In addition to health benefits, programs also have costs. Resources are limited and good policy decisions require allocations that maximize life expectancy and HRQL. Methodologies for estimating costs have now become standardized (Gold, Siegel, Russell, & Weinstein, 1996). From an administrative perspective, cost estimates include all costs of treatment and costs associated with caring for any side effects of treatment. From a social perspective, costs are broader and may include costs for family members who are not working in order to provide care. Comparing programs for a given population with a given medical condition, cost-effectiveness is measured as the change in costs of care for the program compared to the existing therapy or program, relative to the change in health measured in a standardized unit such as QALYs. The difference in costs over the difference in effectiveness is the incremental cost-effectiveness, usually expressed as the cost per QALY. Since the objective of all programs is to produce QALYs, the cost per QALY can be used to show the relative efficiency of various programs (Gold, Siegel, Russell, & Weinstein, 1996).

Figure 11.3 compares programs that have been analyzed using cost per QALY. Some traditional interventions, such as mammography for women

FIGURE 11.3. COST-PER-QALY RATIOS

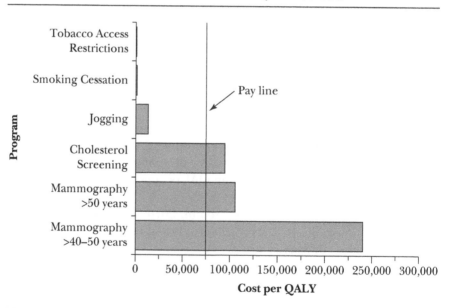

age forty to fifty, may cost as much as $240,000 to produce a QALY (Eddy, 1989). Screening programs, such as testing for high cholesterol, may also require many resources to produce a QALY (Taylor, Pass, Shepard, & Komarov, 1987). On the other hand, public health programs such as tobacco control may produce a QALY at very low cost (Kaplan et al., 2001). The figure shows a hypothetical "pay line." It might be argued that programs to the left of the pay line should be funded but those with a cost-per-QALY ratio to the right of the line be examined more carefully.

Contrary to the portrayal of cost-effectiveness analysis in the popular media, the purpose of the analysis is not to cut costs but rather attempt to identify which interventions produce the greatest amount of health using the resources that are available. Because of the confusion about cost-effectiveness analysis, the Office of Disease Prevention and Health Promotion in the Public Health Service appointed a panel to develop standards for such analysis (Gold, Siegel, Russell, & Weinstein, 1996).

The primary appeal of these approaches to summarizing the quality of various health states is their simplicity. By using QALYs, clinicians, managers, payers, and investigators can compare outcomes and health service utilization among individuals or populations with a uniform unit of measurement that is easily quantified. However, these approaches raise important ethical concerns for the physician providing care to an individual patient (Dean, 1990). Although a range of variables contribute to the physician's recommendations for treatment (or no treatment), there is nothing more relevant to decision making than the patient's own assessment of HRQL. Even if a treatment may be life-saving, ethical principles suggest that the patient's preference regarding treatment must be respected. If the patient feels that his or her quality of life is so poor that no treatment would make it better, then we should respect the patient's wishes.

The component of the Affordable Care Act (ACA) that legislates against QALYs remains controversial. Most aspects of the ACA are aimed at achieving greater efficiency. Critics believe that the restrictions against cost-effectiveness analysis were motivated by special interest groups worried about restrictions on the particular services that they provide (Neumann & Weinstein, 2010).

Feedback to Patients

To give better information to patients facing such decisions, it is important to have HRQL outcome data on individual treatments to facilitate clinical decision making. Specific examples of currently available information include the finding that HRQL is better when chemotherapy is given continuously rather than intermittently in women with advanced breast cancer (Coates et al., 1987), and that the HRQL of women receiving breast conservation treatment is no different than it is for women undergoing mastectomy (Ganz, Schag, Lee, Polinsky, & Tan, 1992). In addition, information is available to understand HRQL in men treated for localized prostate cancer (Litwin et al., 1995) and other cancers (Reeve et al., 2009). However, there are limited data of this type. We need to expand our database on HRQL outcomes to improve information for managers, payers, health care executives, and policy makers involved in the process of distributing limited health care resources, as well as to physicians and patients involved in clinical decision making (Frosch et al., 2011; Legare et al., 2011).

Contributions From the Literature

In this section, we review seminal research in health services where HRQL methods were developed or incorporated as important outcomes. Although this section is not exhaustive, we present an historical framework for research in this area.

Alameda County Human Population Laboratory Studies

More than a half century ago, Lester Breslow and colleagues recruited a probability sample of adults from Alameda County, California, to examine the health status and well-being of a community. This research program conceptualized health in broader terms than the traditional categories of disability and disease. Their work drew heavily on the World Health Organization (WHO) definition of health to guide their assessment of the population, focusing on the physical, emotional, and social dimensions of well-being (WHO, 1948; Breslow, 1972). Although they examined some social indicators (such as employment, income, and marital status) in their study sample, the focus of their work was on the self-reported evaluation of physical, mental, and social health identified in the WHO definition. They established the feasibility of asking people about their HRQL and demonstrated similar responses to personal interview, telephone, and mailed questionnaires as strategies for data collection. Further, they showed that data from the three administration strategies were nearly interchangeable.

In addition to the conceptually and methodologically pioneering work of this group, this research program made several critical observations:

- Those who were employed were healthier than those who were out of work or retired (Belloc, Breslow, & Hochstim, 1971).
- Separated persons were less physically healthy than those in other marital-status groups (Belloc et al., 1971).
- There was a positive association between physical health and mental health, independent of gender, age, or income adequacy (Berkman, 1971).
- There was a positive association between socioeconomic status and mental health (Berkman, 1971).
- Certain common health habits (hours of sleep, exercise, and abstention from alcohol and tobacco) were positively related to physical health (Belloc & Breslow, 1972) and inversely related to subsequent mortality (Belloc & Breslow, 1972) and disability (Breslow & Breslow, 1993).

The RAND Health Insurance Experiment

The RAND Health Insurance Experiment (HIE) was one of the first large health services research intervention trials. It was conceived in the early 1970s, at a time when there was considerable discussion about national health insurance reform and new approaches to limiting the rapidly expanding health care budget (Starr, 1982). The HIE randomly assigned 2,005 families (3,958 individuals between fourteen and sixty-one years of age) to health insurance plans that provided free care, varying degrees of copayment, or care through a health maintenance organization (Brook et al., 1983; Newhouse et al., 1981; Manning, Leibowitz, Goldberg, Rogers, & Newhouse, 1984). In addition to examining the cost of care and utilization of services, this comprehensively designed study looked at a number of important health outcomes, among them physiological measures (for example, blood pressure or far vision), health habits (smoking, weight, and cholesterol level), and self-reported health (physical functioning, role functioning, mental health, social contacts, and health perception). The high standards set for reliable and valid measures of self-reported health in the RAND HIE led to extensive exploration of the conceptualization of health and the methodologies required for measuring HRQL.

Although it is not possible in this chapter to examine all of the advances in measurement of HRQL that were developed as part of the RAND HIE, a few key concepts and measures should be described. Ware

(1984) noted that the "attention of society, government and health care providers has broadened beyond survival and biomedical status into the areas of behavioral and psychosocial outcomes. There also seems to be a shift in the objectives of health care toward more socially relevant health and quality-of-life outcomes and increased awareness of the interest in the psychological and economic costs of disease and disability" (Ware, 1984).

Ware (1984) noted that "quality of life encompasses personal health status and other factors such as family life, finances, housing and jobs" such aspects being the content of much of the social indicators research movement; however, not all of these factors are expected to be influenced by the health care system. Therefore, he suggests, it is more important to consider the concept of health as separate from the larger arena of quality of life, with health representing proper functioning and well-being (hearkening back to the WHO definition of health) (WHO, 1948). In this explication of a framework for measurement of HRQL, Ware identifies the dimensions seen in Figure 11.4: the disease, personal functioning, psychological distress and well-being, general health perceptions, and social and role functioning.

Using this framework, the RAND investigators developed a number of large questionnaire batteries to examine HRQL. These questionnaires were developed and evaluated specifically for the HIE. Detailed

FIGURE 11.4. FRAMEWORK FOR MEASURING HEALTH STATUS

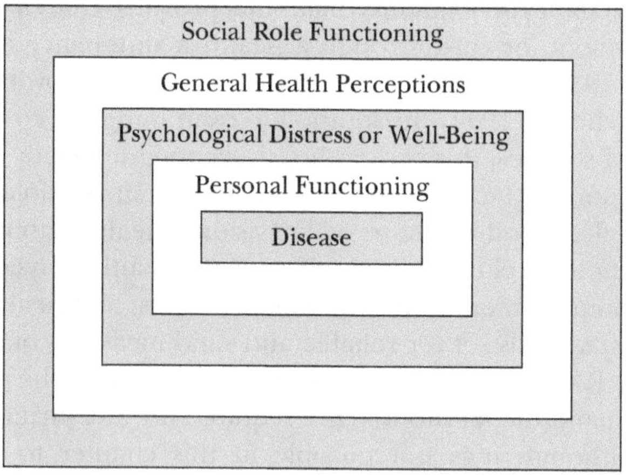

Source: Adapted from Ware, 1984.

descriptions of these measures are available as separate reports prepared through the RAND Corporation, and also through many publications.

One of the most widely used measures is the Mental Health Inventory (MHI), described by Veit and Ware in 1983 (Veit & Ware, 1983). In contrast to existing psychological measures designed to diagnose mental illness, the MHI was developed to look at psychological distress and well-being in the general population. Ware and associates drew heavily on existing measures of well-being in developing the MHI. However, they performed much additional work to conceptualize the issues of importance to this domain of HRQL and were careful to separate mental health from physical health. What resulted was a thirty-eight-item index of mental health that could be separated into two main constructs: (1) psychological distress (anxiety, depression, or loss of behavioral or emotional control) and (2) psychological well-being (general positive affect and emotional ties).

There are many important legacies from the RAND Health Insurance Experiment. From the point of view of HRQL research, conceptualizing HRQL as a key outcome of health care is critical. In addition, the HIE developed reliable and valid tools for measuring the dimensions of HRQL. However, in addition to the tools themselves, data from this study also constitute important reference points for the relative value of specific changes in scores. That is to say, what does a change in HRQL score mean? The reader is referred to a review by Testa and Nackley (1994) for an excellent discussion of this issue. Efforts to understand the meaning of differences in HRQL scores continue today, focusing on estimation of clinically important or minimally important differences (Hays, Farivar, & Liu, 2005).

The Medical Outcomes Study

The Medical Outcomes Study (MOS) is another example of a major health services research study that in its design and conceptualization included HRQL as a key outcome of care (Tarlov et al., 1989) (see Table 11.1). Many of the key investigators for this study had been involved in the RAND HIE. Again, Ware and colleagues at RAND were central figures in developing the health outcome measures for the MOS. Thus, it is not surprising that the measures drew heavily on the prior measures developed for the HIE (Stewart & Ware, 1992).

The HRQL measures used at baseline in the MOS were quite lengthy (Stewart & Ware, 1992). However, one of the major methodological advances from this project was the realization that shorter measures might

TABLE 11.1. CONCEPTUAL FRAMEWORK FOR THE MEDICAL OUTCOMES STUDY

Structure of Care	Process of Care	Outcomes
System Characteristics	*Technical Style*	*Clinical End Points*
Organization	Visits	Symptoms and signs
Specialty mix	Medications	Laboratory values
Financial incentives	Referrals	Death
Workload	Test ordering	
Access and convenience	Hospitalizations	*Functional Status*
	Expenditures	Physical
Provider Characteristics	Continuity of care	Mental
Age	Coordination	Social
Gender		Role
Specialty training	*Interpersonal Style*	
Economic incentives	Interpersonal manner	*General well-being*
Beliefs and attitudes	Patient participation	Health perceptions
Preferences	Counseling	Energy and fatigue
Job satisfaction	Communication level	Pain
		Life satisfaction
Patient Characteristics		
Age		*Satisfaction with Care*
Gender		Access
Diagnosis or condition		Convenience
Severity		Financial coverage
Comorbid conditions		Quality
Health habits		General
Beliefs and attitudes		
Preferences		

Source: Adapted from Tarlov et al., 1989.

be as effective as the lengthier measures traditionally used in this type of research. Longer measures lead to added precision, but they also increase the burden on the respondent and the likelihood of missing data. Furthermore, they are too cumbersome for most clinical settings. An additional conceptual breakthrough was developing a generic HRQL tool that could facilitate comparing common diseases across specific dimensions of HRQL. Noteworthy results from this research include development of the MOS short form, first published as a twenty-item questionnaire (Stewart, Hays, & Ware, 1988; Stewart et al., 1989) and later an expanded version known as the MOS Short Form 36 or RAND 36-Item Health Survey 1.0 (Ware & Sherbourne, 1992; Hays, Sherbourne, & Mazel, 1993). The goal of parsimony generated interest in an even shorter form of the MOS instrument, known as the SF-12 (Ware, Kosinski, & Keller, 1995). This twelve-item questionnaire summarizes HRQL in two domains: the mental component summary and the physical component summary. Although there is some sacrifice in richness of the data, the SF-12 physical and mental component summary scales are equivalent to the SF-36 counterparts. The short forms of the MOS instruments are widely used in a variety of research and clinical settings to examine health outcomes of care (Hess et al., 2012; Hsiao et al., 2012; Meyer et al., 1994). These measures were been translated for use in multinational studies as well as national studies that include diverse populations (Aaronson et al., 1992).

Because of the desirability of preference-based scores for cost utility analyses and other applications, preference scores have been estimated from the SF-36. Fryback and colleagues derived regression equations to predict the Quality of Well-Being Scale (QWB) from the SF-36 (Fryback, Lawrence, Martin, Klein, & Klein, 1997). A six-variable regression model accounted for 57 percent of the variance in QWB scores. Nichol and colleagues (Nichol, Sengupta, & Globe, 2001) used a similar method to predict HUI-2 preference scores from the SF-36 in a sample of 6,921 patients with Kaiser health insurance. Fifty percent of the variance (adjusted R-squared) in the HUI-2 was accounted for, and each of the SF-36 scales had a significant and unique positive association with the HUI-2 in the regression model.

In addition, a preference-based score was derived for the SF-36 using a six-dimensional health classification scheme and a subset of the items (Brazier et al., 1998). Multiattribute utility theory was used to derive preference weights for nine thousand health states based on ratings by a sample of 166 health professionals, health service managers and administrators, staff at the University of Sheffield medical school, undergraduates, and patients at hospital outpatient clinics. Visual analog and standard gamble estimating equations were developed to predict the preference scores. A larger study of 611 people from the U.K. general population was subsequently used to derive more definitive weights (Brazier, Roberts, & Deverill, 2002).

An inventory of HRQL instruments is available at www.proqolid.org. In addition, Staquet and colleagues proposed uniform guidelines for reporting HRQL data from clinical trials (Staquet et al., 1996).

Efficacy Studies

HRQL has long been an implied outcome of treatment for a variety of common, chronic medical conditions. For a disease such as rheumatoid arthritis, self-assessed response to anti-inflammatory agents (pain relief and increased mobility) has been critical in evaluating new treatments (Potts, Mazzuca, & Brandt, 1986). In the case of antihypertensive treatments, side effects from medication may interfere with compliance and affect successful control of this clinically silent condition (Croog et al, 1986; Testa et al., 1993). Cancer treatments are another area where quality-of-life outcomes are salient (Ganz et al., 1992; Litwin et al., 1995; Reeve, Smith, Arora, & Hays, 2008). Randomized clinical trials of treatment efficacy are the most compelling studies in which HRQL measures have been used.

Several authors have used HRQL measures to estimate the effectiveness of clinical interventions. Two excellent examples of policy analysis associated with prospective randomized clinical trials were published. In each case, the HRQL measurement was incorporated into the study protocol and the cost-effectiveness analysis was part of the study planning. These studies were the Diabetes Prevention Program (DPP) and the National Emphysema Treatment Trial (NETT).

Diabetes Clinical Trial

In the DPP, patients at risk for type 2 diabetes were randomly assigned to one of three conditions: intensive lifestyle modification, metformin, or placebo (Diabetes Primary Prevention Group, 2003). The DPP included 3,234 adults with impaired glucose tolerance. The intensive lifestyle intervention was designed to reduce the initial body weight by 7 percent through regular physical activity and diet. The metformin group took one 850 mg tablet each day. The placebo group also took one tablet per day. The patients were evaluated prior to randomization and at annual intervals over the course of three years.

HRQL was measured using the QWB. The measure was chosen because it can be used to estimate QALYs. Over the course of three years, those randomly assigned to the lifestyle intervention accrued 0.050 more QALYs than those assigned a regular dose of metformin. Among the three interventions, the lifestyle approach was the most expensive (total cost US$27,065 in year 2000 dollars). Metformin was less expensive ($25,937), while the placebo was the least expensive option ($23,525). Figure 11.5

FIGURE 11.5. COST PER QALY IN DPP

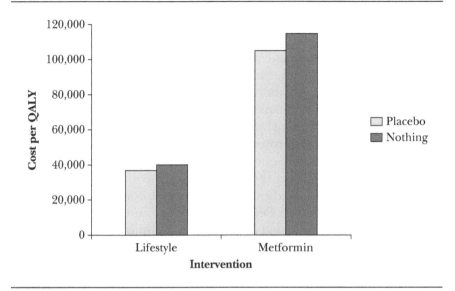

summarizes the cost per QALY for the lifestyle and metformin conditions from a health care system perspective. The figure shows the cost per QALY attributable to the interventions in comparison to placebo and to doing nothing. Although both interventions offer significant benefits over placebo or doing nothing, the cost per QALY for the lifestyle invention was significantly lower than that for metformin. A ten-year follow-up showed that the cost-effectiveness was maintained over time (Diabetes Primary Prevention Group, 2012). However, while the long-term results suggest that the health effects of metformin and lifestyle are similar, metformin is less expensive over this extended period. So, in the long run, medical management may be the most cost-effective program.

The second example is an evaluation of surgery for emphysema. Emphysema is the dominant cause of chronic obstructive pulmonary disease (COPD), which is the fourth leading cause of death and a major cause of disability in the United States (National Center for Health Statistics, 2004). COPD is caused by loss of elastic recoil of lung tissue in addition to chronic inflammation in airways. Lungs often become hyperinflated and there is an increase in the functional residual capacity. Hyperinflation may place greater strain on the muscles of respiration, increasing the effort required to breathe and reducing capacity for exercise. COPD is associated with activity limitations, premature death, and reduced HRQL (Pauwels & Rabe, 2004). Despite major advances in diagnosis and medical therapeutics, standard medical therapy often has little effect on HRQL (Sutherland & Cherniack, 2004). Thus many patients seek surgical treatments that may produce more dramatic improvements.

Lung volume reduction surgery (LVRS) is an intervention designed to reduce the volume of the hyperinflated lung. The procedure was introduced in the 1950s, but one in six patients died from the surgery. As a result, the procedure was abandoned by the late 1950s (Brantigan & Mueller, 1957; Lefrak et al., 1997). An improved procedure was reintroduced in the 1990s, and the initial results were encouraging. Shortly thereafter, patient testimonials and marketing efforts resulted in popular enthusiasm for the procedure and pressure for Medicare to pay for it (Cooper et al., 1996). A report commissioned by the Center for Medicare and Medicaid Services (CMS) cited a paper noting that more than twelve hundred LVRS procedures had been performed on Medicare beneficiaries (Huizenga, Ramsay, & Albert, 1998). Further, the rate of growth was exponential (Huizenga et al., 1998). On the other hand, the technology assessment raised significant questions about the benefits of the procedure. For example, it was noted that about one-quarter of the Medicare beneficiaries who received LVRS died within one year (Huizenga et al., 1998). In response to these concerns, Medicare decided to halt payment for the procedure until it could be studied.

The National Emphysema Treatment Trial is a multicenter randomized clinical trial designed to evaluate LVRS (Fishman et al., 2003). Subjects with moderate to severe emphysema were randomly assigned to usual medical therapy alone or to usual medical therapy plus LVRS. All patients in the trial participated in pulmonary rehabilitation prior to randomization. HRQL was one of the primary outcome measures because surgery was not expected to improve life expectancy. HRQL was measured using four methods, two generic and two disease-specific. One measure was chosen because it could be used to estimate QALYs in cost-effectiveness analysis. The study was unusual because it included a prospective plan for policy analysis.

The NETT trial randomized 1,218 patients to either maximum medical therapy or to the combination of maximal medical therapy plus LVRS (Fishman et al., 2003). Over the first twelve months of the study, LVRS patients had significantly more hospital days, ambulatory care days, and nursing home admissions. However, utilization began to change by the thirteen-to-twenty-four-month interval. During the second year, those in the maximal medical arm used more hospital days and had more emergency room visits. In the third year, utilization was equivalent between the two groups. Figure 11.6 summarizes the cumulative QALYs per person

FIGURE 11.6. MEAN CUMULATIVE QALYS, YEARS 1 THROUGH 3

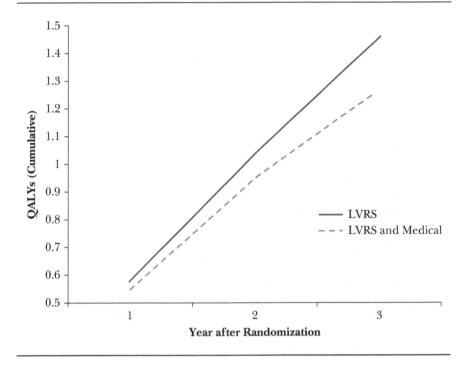

over the first three years of the project. After one year, the groups differed but the effect was nonsignificant. However, by year two the groups began separating, and this difference grew by year three.

Cost per QALY was evaluated three years following randomization (Ramsey et al., 2003). Using best estimates for cost, mortality, and HRQL, it was concluded that LVRS was more expensive than maximal medical therapy ($98,952 versus $62,560). However, QALYs were also greater in the LVRS arm (1.463 versus 1.271). Thus the incremental cost per QALY was approximately $190,000.

To capture potential long-term gains, the analysis also estimated projected benefits over an extended period of time. The analyses suggested that at five years the incremental cost per QALY was $88,000 for non-high-risk patients; at ten years it was $53,000 (Ramsey et al., 2003).

The NETT trial demonstrated that the cost-effectiveness of LVRS is comparable to several other surgical procedures. The relative cost-effectiveness of LVRS is particularly impressive if benefits of the procedure are projected into the future. The NETT was a milestone study because the cost-effectiveness analysis was planned and executed as a companion to the RCT. Further, the NETT trial allowed rapid diffusion of the findings (Ramsey et al., 2003). The trial and cost-effectiveness analysis were used as the basis of Medicare policy funding LVRS surgery. By early 2004, Medicare coverage for LVRS was approved. The trial offers an excellent example of rapid translation from research to policy.

These two examples demonstrate the importance of evaluating HRQL endpoints in efficacy studies because they provide an additional outcome that includes the patient perspective. This is most important in therapeutic situations where the toxicity of treatment is high and the benefits may be few.

HRQL assessment has been widely adopted by the pharmaceutical industry as a component of the drug approval process (McLeod, Coon, Martin, Fehnel, & Hays, 2011; Testa, 1993; Bombardier et al., 1986; Johnson & Temple, 1985). These assessments are also an expanding part of large clinical treatment trials for patients with cancer and AIDS. There has been a move toward more abbreviated HRQL outcome measures for integration into large multicenter trials (Moinpour, Hayden, Thompson, Feigl, & Metch, 1990; Wu, Hays, Kelly, Malitz, & Bozzette, 1997). In these situations, the burden on respondents and staff is an important consideration. It is hoped that these shorter forms will be equally sensitive to measuring difference in HRQL outcomes.

Comparative Effectiveness Research

Given the lack of randomized trial efficacy data on so many areas of clinical medicine and treatment decision making, other strategies are necessary to provide data for patients, clinicians, and other health care stakeholders. While comparisons of outcomes from observational data sources are potentially unreliable, these sources of data may be the only information available on which to make clinical care decisions. Thus, developing standardized approaches to the interpretation of observational data is emerging as an important area for outcomes research.

Emergence of Comparative Effectiveness Research

The field of study that concentrates on the evaluation of the benefits and risks of health care from the patient's perspective is known as *comparative effectiveness research (CER)*. Although the conceptual underpinnings of this line of scientific inquiry have been discussed for decades, CER did not exist as a formal field of study until 2009. In the early years of the Obama administration, there was extensive discussion among advisers about the costs, risks, and benefits of health care. During extensive debates about health care reform, the U.S. Congress approved legislation to develop the infrastructure for comparing the effectiveness of health care interventions. What emerged from the discussion was the basis for developing an important new infrastructure for comparing treatments and analyzing which interventions are most effective for patients. Of particular importance was the investment of $1.1 billion as part of the American Recovery and Reinvestment Act of 2009 (ARRA). The ARRA, more commonly known as the Stimulus Package, provided funding for a variety of federal agencies to begin developing the infrastructure needed for systematic and comprehensive CER studies. These agencies include the National Institutes of Health (NIH), the Agency for Healthcare Research and Quality (AHRQ), and the Centers for Disease Control (CDC).

Definition of Comparative Effectiveness Research

The purpose of comparative effectiveness research is to make informed decisions about the best alternatives for improving the health of individuals or populations. Clearly this is a worthy goal. Yet, there is significant disagreement about how this new science should proceed. To understand these controversies, it is illuminating to consider the definition of comparative effectiveness research (CER). The Institute of Medicine (IOM) defines CER as "the generation and synthesis of evidence that compares the benefits and harms of alternative methods to prevent, diagnose, treat, and monitor a clinical condition or to improve the delivery of care. The purpose of CER is to assist consumers, clinicians, purchasers, and policy makers to make informed decisions that will improve healthcare at both the individual and population levels" (Iglehart, 2009; Committee on Comparative Effectiveness Research Prioritization & Institute of Medicine, 2009).

Each phrase of this definition has engendered controversy. For example, there are disagreements about methods for synthesizing evidence, concerns about the benefits and the harms of alternative treatments, and different opinions about how these benefits and harms are optimally determined. There are also major disagreements about the meaningfulness of outcomes and from whose perspective the outcomes are best evaluated. In this chapter, we consider various facets of the debate, beginning with the philosophical background of CER.

Advocates for CER tend to look at the world of health care differently from traditional biomedical investigators. Typically, CER researchers consider the risks and benefits of treatment from a patient perspective. AHRQ favors the term "patient-centered outcomes research" instead of comparative effectiveness research. This definition emphasizes that the focus of the science is patient rather than disease or physiological system oriented (Patel, 2010).

Cost-Effectiveness Research in the Affordable Care Act

The ACA created the Patient-Centered Outcomes Research Institute (PCORI) (www.pcori.org), which is required to implement a research agenda focused on CER that is funded through the ACA legislation. A lot of controversy surrounds the use of costs in evaluating medical treatments. It is widely acknowledged that the health care crisis is really about controlling medical care costs. However, discussions of cost are conspicuously absent from many of the discussions of CER in health care reform legislation. It is not an accident that cost discussions are difficult to find. Many people believe that cost should not be part of the discussion. On the other hand, economists convincingly argue that there are opportunity costs. For example, if we spend an excessive amount of money on health care services that do not make patients better, we will have less money to spend on services known to provide benefit. Virtually all participants in the discussion acknowledge that health care costs must be controlled. Yet, the ACA specifically states that the oversight entity (PCORI) "shall not develop or employ a dollars-per-quality adjusted life year (or similar measure that discounts the value of life because of an individual's disability) as a threshold to establish what type of healthcare is cost-effective or recommended. The Secretary shall not utilize such an adjusted life year (or such similar measure) as a threshold to determine coverage, reimbursement, or incentive programs."

This provision appears to refer to the use of cost-effectiveness research in decision making (Neumann & Weinstein, 2010). The ACA specifically prohibits PCORI from developing cost- or quality-adjusted life year (QALY) thresholds.

Perhaps one reason for the aversion to QALYs in the ACA legislation was the suggestion by policy pundits that systematic methods for evaluating the benefits of treatment might lead to rationing of health care by big government—frequently cited as "death panels." Yet the ACA is about affordable care and it does make reference to using resources wisely. It is noteworthy that the World Health Organization as well as other, expert groups in many other countries, including Great Britain, Canada, and Australia, favor QALYs over other methodologies to help make rational decisions about resource allocation. Most important, these methodologies give priority to aspects of health that consumers report as most important. The decision not to use systematic models to guide choices does not avert the need to choose between competing alternatives. However, the alternatives are more subjective and less transparent. Of course, few health services analysts advocate cost or QALY as the only criterion for making difficult decisions. These methodologies provide information that can guide decision makers through a minefield of difficult choices (Neumann & Weinstein, 2010).

Future Directions

A great deal of work remains to inform health policy in the United States. Improved strategies are needed to make HRQL assessment a routine component of research, clinical care, and policy decisions. Several workshops among health services researchers (Lohr, 1989; Lohr, 1992) sponsored through the National Institutes of Health (NIH), the National Cancer Institute (NCI) (Nayfield & Hailey, 1990; Furberg & Schuttinga, 1990; Reeve et al., 2007), and the Institute of Medicine have emphasized the need for incorporating HRQL endpoints into research and clinical care settings. The technologies, though not yet perfect, are much more accessible and feasible than just a short time ago. Scannable, user-friendly instruments are available, and normative databases are being developed rapidly. Health care consumers and providers would like access to HRQL outcomes information.

As has been emphasized by several prominent health services researchers (Ellwood, 1988), it is the patient outcome that must drive our policy decisions. Prolonged survival with poor HRQL may not be desirable to patients. Consumers are anxious to have information about the HRQL impact of new treatments. If there is uncertainty about the efficacy or effectiveness of a treatment or choices among treatments, then HRQL endpoints will take on paramount importance.

All studies of efficacy and effectiveness must include patient-reported measures of HRQL whenever there is a potential HRQL question. Common core measures should be shared across studies so that relevant comparisons can be made. An example of how this is being done is the

NIH-sponsored Roadmap Initiative (now "Common Fund") Patient-Reported Outcomes Measurement Information System (PROMIS®) project (www.nih.promis.org) PROMIS was designed to establish a national resource for accurate and efficient measurement of HRQL in clinical practice and research (Cella et al., 2010; Reeve, Hays, Chang, & Perfetto, 2007). The effort has produced a plethora of item banks to assess adult and child HRQL using short-forms or computer-adaptive testing based on item response theory (DeWitt et al., 2011; Rothrock et al., 2010; Liu et al., 2010).

However, we must not fail to ask critical questions related to new therapies, to better understand their relevance to patients. For enough data to materialize, these measures of HRQL must be considered routine and not exceptional. The additional costs of data collection should be borne by funding agencies, insurers, and providers so that the value of new tests or procedures can be fully evaluated.

HRQL Endpoints and Changing Health Policy

Are HRQL endpoints sufficient to force a change in health policy? In asking this about HRQL outcomes, we must ask whether statistically significant changes in evaluating HRQL are clinically significant. To obtain more precise evaluation of the quality of our tools, it is necessary to reference or calibrate our HRQL instruments against known outcomes of clinical importance to patients, purchasers of health care, and health care providers. For this work to proceed, we must invest in collecting important clinical information along with our HRQL data. Research in HRQL needs to be supported to extrapolate effectively from the HRQL endpoint to decisions on public health policy. Short-term management applications include using HRQL endpoints and other outcomes and effectiveness research as part of quality assurance (QA).

SUMMARY

As Andersen, Davidson, and Ganz (1994) have described, "There are symbiotic relationships between Health Services Research (HSR) and HRQL studies." First, the HSR paradigm gives guidance for including structure and process in designing HRQL studies. HSR suggests what leads to HRQL improvement. It supplies ways to conceptualize, and relates the many important forces that contribute to, HRQL in addition to specific clinical interventions. Second, HRQL is an important outcome in the HSR paradigm. Early studies in HSR did not focus primarily on HRQL as an outcome indicator. Health service utilization was investigated as a means to improve access to care and change the organization and delivery of care, rather than as a direct vehicle to enhance HRQL. HRQL, however, is a key outcome in the emerging model of HSR (Andersen et al., 1994).

The expansion and development of HRQL measurement has emerged primarily from clinical research. What is needed urgently is careful and appropriate inclusion of HRQL outcomes in traditional health services research. Similarly, researchers in clinical settings who are measuring HRQL should account for the structure and process of care in designing their research and data collection. As suggested by Andersen and colleagues, ''This era of health care reform calls for a paradigm shift, away from the heroic and costly therapeutic measures that extend the quantity of life, to a patient or consumer-focused approach aimed at health promotion and disease prevention, using HRQL measures as the ultimate criteria for success'' (Andersen et al., 1994). As indicated throughout this chapter, the potential for accomplishing this goal is here today.

KEY TERMS

Comparative effectiveness research (CER) the generation and synthesis of evidence that compares the benefits and harms of alternative methods to prevent, diagnose, treat, and monitor a clinical condition or to improve the delivery of care.

Health-related quality of life (HRQL) a subcomponent of overall quality of life that relates to health and that focuses on the patient's own perception of well-being and the ability to function as a result of health status or disease experience.

Outcomes of care refers to specific indicators of what happens to the patient once care has been rendered.

Process of care refers to the content of the medical and psychological interactions between patient and provider.

Quality-adjusted life years (QALY) a measure of life expectancy with adjustment for quality of life that integrates mortality and morbidity to express health status in terms of equivalents of well-years of life.

Quality of life a range of human experience, including but not limited to access to the daily necessities of life such as food and shelter, intrapersonal and interpersonal response to life events, and activities associated with professional fulfillment and personal happiness.

Structure of care refers to how medical and other services are organized in a particular institution or delivery system.

DISCUSSION QUESTIONS

1. Discuss the potential value added from incorporation of patient-reported outcomes into health services research.
2. Describe common barriers to incorporation of patient-reported outcomes into research studies and clinical care.
3. Discuss the characteristics of a good HRQL instrument and considerations in selecting the appropriate measure for different applications.
4. How can QALYs be used to inform health policy? Should they be a requirement of new health care programs that may be costly to implement?

FURTHER READING

Barofsky, I. (2012). *Quality*. New York: Springer.

Integrating concepts from psychology, philosophy, neurocognition, and linguistics, this book attempts to answer complex questions related to quality-of-life assessment and measurement. It also breaks down the cognitive-linguistic components that comprise the judgment of quality, including description, evaluation, and valuations, and applies them to issues specific to individuals with chronic medical illness. This book is for those who want to dive deep into the conceptual aspects of quality-of-life assessment.

Detmar, S. B., Muller, M. J., Schornagel, J. H., Wever, L.D.V., & Aaronson, N. K. (2002). Health-related quality-of-life assessments and patient-physician communication: A randomized controlled trial. *Journal of the American Medical Association, 288*(23), 3027–3034.

Describes a potential application of health-related quality of life assessment in the clinical setting.

Fayers, P., & Hays, R. (Eds.). (2005). *Assessing quality of life in clinical trials: Methods and practice* (2nd ed.). Oxford, U.K.: Oxford University Press.

A rigorous, broad, comprehensive coverage of all aspects of quality-of-life measurement, methods, and practice.

Gold, M. R., Seigel, J. E., Russell, L. B., & Weinstein, M. C. (Eds.). (1996). *Cost-effectiveness in health and medicine*. New York: Oxford University Press.

This book reports recommendations of the Panel on Cost-Effectiveness in Health and Medicine regarding standards for conducting cost-effectiveness analysis. Since it was first published, the book has been consistently used to guide the design and interpretation of studies.

Guyatt, G. H., Feeny, D. H., & Patrick, D. L. (1993). Measuring health-related quality of life. *Annals of Internal Medicine, 118*(8), 622–629.

Classic article describing rationale and methods for measuring health-related quality of life.

Lenderking, W. R., & Revicki, D. A. (Eds.). (2005). *Advancing health outcomes research methods and clinical applications.* McLean, VA: Degnon Associates.

This book offers overviews of historical issues, contemporary methods, and applications of measures in clinical studies.

REFERENCES

Aaronson, N. K., Acquadro, C., Alonso, J., Apolone, G., Bucquet, D., Bullinger, M.,...Ware, J. E., Jr., (1992). International Quality of Life Assessment (IQOLA) Project. *Quality of Life Research, 1*(5), 349–351.

Adami, H. O. (2010). The prostate cancer pseudo-epidemic. *Acta Oncologica, 49*(3), 298–304.

Adolfsson, J. (2010). Screening for prostate cancer—will we ever know? *Acta Oncologica, 49*(3), 275–277.

Andersen, R. M., Davidson, P. L., & Ganz, P A. (1994). Symbiotic relationships of quality of life, health services research and other health research. *Quality of Life Research, 3*(5), 365–371.

Belloc, N. B., & Breslow, L. (1972). Relationship of physical health status and health practices. *Preventive Medicine, 1,* 409–421.

Belloc, N. B., Breslow, L., & Hochstim, J. R. (1971). Measurement of physical health in a general population survey. *American Journal of Epidemiology, 93,* 328–336.

Berkman, P. L. (1971). Measurement of mental health in a general population survey. *American Journal of Epidemiology, 94,* 105–111.

Blumenthal, D. (1996). Part 1: Quality of care—what is it? *New England Journal of Medicine, 335*(12), 891–894.

Bombardier, C., Ware, J., Russell, I. J., Larson, M., Chalmers, A., & Read, J. L. (1986). Auranofin therapy and quality of life in patients with rheumatoid arthritis: Results of a multicenter trial. *American Journal of Medicine, 81*(4), 565–578.

Brantigan, O. C., & Mueller, E. (1957). Surgical treatment of pulmonary emphysema. *American Surgeon, 23*(9), 789–804.

Brazier, J., Roberts, J., & Deverill, M. (2002). The estimation of a preference-based measure of health from the SF-36. *Journal of Health Economics, 21*(2), 271–92.

Brazier, J., Usherwood, T., Harper, R., & Thomas, K. (1998). Deriving a preference-based single index from the UK SF-36 Health Survey. *Journal of Clinical Epidemiology, 51*(11), 1115–1128.

Breslow, L. (1972). A quantitative approach to the World Health Organization definition of health: Physical, mental and social well-being. *International Journal of Epidemiology 1,* 347–355.

Breslow, L., & Breslow, N. (1993). Health practices and disability: Some evidence from Alameda County. *Preventive Medicine, 22,* 86–95.

Brook, R. H., Ware, J. E., Rogers, W. H., Keeler, E. B., Davies, A. R., Donald, C. A., . . . Newhouse, J. P. (1983). Does free care improve adults' health? *New England Journal of Medicine, 309,* 1426–1434.

Cella, D., Riley, W., Stone, A., Rothrock, N., Reeve, B., Young, S., . . . Hays, R. D. (2010). Initial item banks and first wave testing of the Patient-Reported Outcomes Measurement Information System (PROMIS) network: 2005–2008. *Journal of Clinical Epidemiology, 63*(11), 1179–1194.

Centers for Disease Control and Prevention. (2000). Community indicators of health-related quality of life, United States, 1993–1997. *Journal of the American Medical Association, 283,* 2097–2098.

Coates, A., Gebski, V., Bishop, J. F., Jeal, P. N., Woods, R. L., Snyder, R., . . . Gill, G. (1987). Improving the quality of life during chemotherapy for advanced breast cancer: A comparison of intermittent and continuous treatment strategies. *New England Journal of Medicine, 317*(24), 1490–1495.

Committee on Comparative Effectiveness Research Prioritization & Institute of Medicine. (2009). *Initial national priorities for comparative effectiveness research.* Washington, DC: Institute of Medicine of the National Academies.

Cooper, J. D., Patterson, G. A., Sundaresan, R. S., Trulock, E. P., Yusen, R. D., Pohl, M. S., & Lefrak, S. S. (1996). Results of 150 consecutive bilateral lung volume reduction procedures in patients with severe emphysema. *Journal of Thoracic and Cardiovascular Surgery, 112*(5), 1319–1329.

Council on Medical Service. (1986). Quality of care. *Journal of the American Medical Association, 256*(8), 1032–4.

Croog, S. H., Levine, S., Testa, M. A., Brown, B., Bulpitt, C. J., Jenkins, C. D., . . . Williams, G. H. (1986). The effects of antihypertensive therapy on the quality of life. *New England Journal of Medicine, 314*(26), 1657–1664.

Dean, H. E. (1990). Political and ethical implications of using quality of life as an outcome measure. *Seminars in Oncology Nursing, 6,* 303–308.

DeWitt, E. M., Stucky, B. D., Thissen, D., Irwin, D. E., Langer, M., Varni, J. W., . . . DeWalt, D. A. (2011). Construction of the eight item PROMIS Pediatric Physical Function Scales: Built using item response theory. *Journal of Clinical Epidemiology, 64*(7), 794–804.

Diabetes Primary Prevention Group. (2003). Within-trial cost-effectiveness of lifestyle intervention or metformin for the primary prevention of type 2 diabetes. *Diabetes Care, 26*(9), 2518–2523.

Diabetes Primary Prevention Group. (2012). The 10-year cost-effectiveness of lifestyle intervention or metformin for diabetes prevention: An intent-to-treat analysis of the DPP/DPPOS. *Diabetes Care, 35*(4), 723–730.

Donabedian, A. (1980). *The definition of quality and approaches to its assessment.* Ann Arbor, MI: Health Administration Press.

Eddy, D. M. (1989). Screening for breast cancer. *Annals of Internal Medicine, 111*(5), 389–399.

Ellwood, P M. (1988). Shattuck lecture—outcomes management. A technology of patient experience. *New England Journal of Medicine, 318*(23), 1549–1556.

Field, M. J., & Gold, M. R. (1998). *Summarizing population health.* Washington, DC: Institute of Medicine, National Academy Press.

Fishman, A, Martinez, F, Naunheim, K, Piantadosi, S., Wise, R., Ries, A., . . . Wood, D. E. (2003). A randomized trial comparing lung-volume-reduction surgery with medical therapy for severe emphysema. *New England Journal of Medicine, 348*(21), 2059–2073.

Fongwa, M. N., Setodji, C. M., Paz, S. H., Morales, L. S., Steers, N. W., & Hays, R. D. (2010). Readability and missing data rates in CAHPS 2.0 Medicare survey in African American and white Medicare respondents. *Health Outcomes Research in Medicine, 1*(1), e39–e49.

Fowler, F. J., Jr., Barry, M. J., Walker-Corkery, B., Caubet, J. F., Bates, D. W., Lee, J. M., . . . McNaughton-Collins, M. (2006). The impact of a suspicious prostate biopsy on patients' psychological, socio-behavioral, and medical care outcomes. *Journal of General Internal Medicine, 21*(7), 715–721.

Frosch, D. L., Moulton, B. W., Wexler, R. M., Holmes-Rovner, M., Volk, R. J., & Levin, C. A. (2011). Shared decision making in the United States: Policy and implementation activity on multiple fronts. *Zeitschrift fur Evidenz, Fortbildung und Qualitat im Gesundheitswesen, 105*(4), 305–312.

Fryback, D. G., Lawrence, W. F., Martin, P. A., Klein R., & Klein, B. E. (1997). Predicting quality of well-being scores from the SF-36: Results from the Beaver Dam Health Outcomes Study. *Medical Decision Making, 17*(1), 1–9.

Furberg, C. D., & Schuttinga, J. A. (Eds.). (1990). *Quality of life assessment: Practice, problems, promise.* Bethesda, MD: Department of Health and Human Services.

Ganz, P A. (1994). Quality of life and the patient with cancer: Individual and policy implications. *Cancer, 74*(4 Suppl), 1445–1452.

Ganz, P. A., Schag, A. C., Lee, J. J., Polinsky, M. L., & Tan, S. J. (1992). Breast conservation versus mastectomy: Is there a difference in psychological adjustment or quality of life in the year after surgery? *Cancer, 69*(7), 1729–1738.

Gold, M. R., Siegel, J. E., Russell, L. B., & Weinstein, M. C. (Eds.). (1996). *Cost-effectiveness in health and medicine.* New York: Oxford University Press.

Hays, R. D., Sherbourne, C. D., & Mazel, R. M. (1993). The RAND 36-item health survey 1.0. *Health Economics, 2*(3), 217–227.

Hays, R. D., Farivar, S. S., & Liu, H. (2005). Approaches and recommendations for estimating minimally important differences for health-related quality of life measures. *COPD: Journal of Chronic Obstructive Pulmonary Disease, 2*, 63–67.

Hess, R., Thurston, R., Hays, R. D., Chang, C.C.H., Dillon, S. N., Ness, R. B., . . . Matthews, K. A. (2012). The impact of menopause on health-related quality of life: Results from the STRIDE longitudinal study. *Quality of Life Research, 21*, 535–544.

Hsiao, A-F., York, R., Hsiao, I., Hansen, E., Hays, R. D., Ives, J., & Coulter, I. D. (2012). Farabloc efficacy for veterans with chronic phantom limb pain. *Archives of Physical Medicine and Rehabilitation, 93*, 617–622.

Huizenga, H. F., Ramsey, S. D., & Albert, R. K. (1998). Estimated growth of lung volume reduction surgery among Medicare enrollees: 1994 to 1996. *Chest, 114*(6), 1583–1587.

Iglehart, J. K. (2009). Prioritizing comparative-effectiveness research: IOM recommendations. *New England Journal of Medicine, 361*(4), 325–328.

Johnson, J. R., & Temple, R. (1985). Food and Drug Administration requirements for approval of new anticancer drugs. *Cancer Treatment Reports, 69*(10), 1155–1159.

Kaplan, R. M. (1993). Quality of life assessment for cost/utility studies in cancer. *Cancer Treatment Reviews, 19*(Suppl A), 85–96.

Kaplan, R. M., Ake, C. F., Emery, S. L., & Navarro, A. M. (2001). Simulated effect of tobacco tax variation on population health in California. *American Journal of Public Health, 91*(2), 239–244.

Lefrak, S. S., Yusen, R. D., Trulock, E. P., Pohl, M. S., Patterson, A., & Cooper, J. D. (1997). Recent advances in surgery for emphysema. *Annual Review of Medicine, 48,* 387–398.

Legare, F., Stacey, D., Gagnon, S., Dunn, S., Pluye, P., Frosch, D., . . . Graham, I. D. (2011). Validating a conceptual model for an inter-professional approach to shared decision making: A mixed methods study. *Journal of Evaluation in Clinical Practice, 17*(4), 554–564.

Liao, Y., McGee, D. L., Cao, G., & Cooper, R. S. (2000). Quality of the last year of life of older adults: 1986 vs. 1993. *Journal of the American Medical Association, 283,* 512–518.

Litwin, M. S., Hays, R. D., Fink, A., Ganz, P. A., Leake, B., Leach, G. E., & Brook, R. H. (1995). Quality-of-life outcomes in men treated for localized prostate cancer. *Journal of the American Medical Association, 273*(2), 129–135.

Liu, H. H., Cella, D., Gershon, R., Shen, J., Morales, L. S., Riley, W., & Hays, R. D. (2010). Representativeness of the PROMIS Internet panel. *Journal of Clinical Epidemiology, 63*(11), 1169–1178.

Lohr, K. N. (1989). Advances in health status assessment: Overview of the conference. *Medical Care, 27*(3 Suppl), S1–S11.

Lohr, K. N. (1992). Applications of health status assessment measures in clinical practice: Overview of the third conference on advances in health status assessment. *Medical Care, 30*(5 Suppl), MS1–MS14.

Lohr, K. N., Donaldson, M. S., & Harris Wehling, J. (1992). Medicare: A strategy for quality assurance, V: Quality of care in a changing health care environment. *Quality Review Bulletin, 18*(4), 120–126.

Manning, W. G., Leibowitz, A., Goldberg, G. A., Rogers, W. H., & Newhouse, J. P. (1984). A controlled trial of the effect of a prepaid group practice on use of services. *New England Journal of Medicine, 310,* 1505–1510.

McDowell, I., & Newell, C. (1996). *Measuring health: A guide to rating scales and questionnaires.* New York: Oxford University Press.

McLeod, L. D., Coon, C. D., Martin, S., Fehnel, S. E., & Hays, R. D. (2011). Interpreting patient-reported outcome results: FDA guidance and emerging methods. *Expert Review of Pharmacoeconomics and Outcomes Research, 11,* 163–169.

Meyer, K. B., Espindle, D. M., DeGiacomo, J. M., Jenuleson, C. S., Kurtin, P. S., & Davies, A. R. (1994). Monitoring dialysis patients' health status. *American Journal of Kidney Diseases, 24*(2), 267–279.

Moinpour, C. M., Hayden, K. A., Thompson, I. M., Feigl, P., & Metch, B. (1990). Quality of life assessment in Southwest Oncology Group trials. *Oncology, 4*(5), 79–84, 89; discussion 104.

National Center for Health Statistics. (2004). Chronic obstructive pulmonary disease (COPD) includes: Chronic bronchitis and emphysema. Retrieved from www.cdc.gov/nchs/fastats/copd.htm

Nayfield, S. G., & Hailey, B. J. (Eds.). (1990). *Quality of life assessment in cancer clinical trials*. Bethesda, MD: Department of Health and Human Services.

Neumann, P. J., & Weinstein, M. C. (2010). Legislating against use of cost-effectiveness information. *New England Journal of Medicine, 363*(16), 1495–1497.

Newhouse, J. P., Manning, W. G., Morris, C. N., Orr, L. L., Duan, N., Keeler, E. B., . . . Brook, R. H. (1981). Some interim results from a controlled trial of cost sharing in health insurance. *New England Journal of Medicine, 305*, 1501–1507.

Nichol, M. B., Sengupta, N., & Globe, D. R. (2001). Evaluating quality-adjusted life years: Estimation of the health utility index (HUI2) from the SF-36. *Medical Decision Making, 21*(2), 105–12.

Patel, K. (2010). Health reform's tortuous route to the patient-centered outcomes research institute. *Health Affairs (Millwood), 29*(10), 1777–1782.

Patrick, D. L., & Bergner, M. (1990). Measurement of health status in the 1990s. *Annual Review of Public Health, 11*, 165–183.

Patrick, D. L., & Deyo, R. A. (1989). Generic and disease-specific measures in assessing health status and quality of life. *Medical Care, 27*(3 Suppl), S217–S232.

Patrick, D. L., & Erickson, P. (1993a). Assessing health-related quality of life for clinical decision-making. In S. R. Walker & R. M. Rosser (Eds.), *Quality of life assessment: Key issues in the 1990s* (pp. 11–64). Dordrecht: Kluwer Academic.

Patrick, D. L., & Erickson, P. (1993b). *Health status and health policy: Allocating resources to health care*. New York: Oxford University Press.

Pauwels, R. A., & Rabe, K. F. (2004). Burden and clinical features of chronic obstructive pulmonary disease (COPD). *Lancet, 364*(9434), 613–620.

Paz, S. H., Liu, H., Fongwa, M. N., Morales, L. S., & Hays, R. D. (2009). Readability estimates for commonly used health-related quality of life surveys. *Quality of Life Research, 18*, 889–900.

Potts, M. K., Mazzuca, S. A., & Brandt, K. D. (1986). Views of patients and physicians regarding the importance of various aspects of arthritis treatment, correlations with health status and patient satisfaction. *Patient Education and Counseling 8*, 125–134.

Ramsey, S. D., Berry, K., Etzioni, R., Kaplan, R. M., Sullivan, S. D., Wood, D. E., & National Emphysema Treatment Trial Research Group. (2003). Cost effectiveness of lung-volume-reduction surgery for patients with severe emphysema. *New England Journal of Medicine, 348*(21), 2092–2102.

Reeve, B. B., Hays, R. D., Bjorner, J. B., Cook, K. F., Crane, P. K., Teresi, J. A., . . . Cella, D. (2007). Psychometric evaluation and calibration of health-related quality of life item banks: Plans for the Patient-Reported Outcome Measurement Information System (PROMIS). *Medical Care, 45*, S22–S31.

Reeve, B. B., Hays, R. D., Chang, C.-H., & Perfetto, E. M. (2007). Applying item response theory to enhance health outcomes assessment. *Quality of Life Research, 16*(Suppl 1), 121–132.

Reeve, B. B., Potosky, A. L., Smith, A. W., Han, P. K., Hays, R. D., Davis, W. W., . . . Clauser, S. B. (2009). Impact of cancer on health-related quality of life of older Americans. *Journal of the National Cancer Institute, 101*, 860–868.

Reeve, B. B., Smith, A. W., Arora, N. K., & Hays, R. D. (2008). Reducing bias in cancer research: Application of propensity score matching. *Health Care Financing Review, 29*(4), 69–80.

Rothrock, N. E., Hays, R. D., Spritzer, K., Yount, S. E., Riley, W., & Cella, D. (2010). Relative to the General US Population, Chronic Diseases are Associated with Poorer Health-Related Quality of Life as Measured by the Patient-Reported Outcomes Measurement Initiative (PROMIS). *Journal of Clinical Epidemiology, 63*(11), 1195–1204.

Russell, L. B., (1999). Modeling for cost-effectiveness analysis. *Statistics in Medicine, 18,* 3235–3244.

Sessions, S. Y., & Detsky, A. S. (2010). Incorporating economic reality into medical education. *Journal of the American Medical Association, 304*(11), 1229–1230.

Spilker, B. (1990). *Quality of life assessments in clinical trials.* New York: Raven Press.

Spilker, B., Ed. (1996). *Quality of life and pharmacoeconomics in clinical trials* (2nd ed.). New York: Lippincott-Raven.

Staquet, M., Berzon, R., Osoba, D., & Machin, D. (1996). Guidelines for reporting results of quality of life assessments in clinical trials. *Quality of Life Research, 5*(5), 496–502.

Starr, P. (1982). *The social transformation of American medicine.* New York: Basic Books.

Stein, R.E.K., Stanton, B., & Starfield, B. (2005). How healthy are US children? *Journal of the American Medical Association, 293,* 1781–1783.

Stewart, A. L., Greenfield, S., Hays, R. D., Wells, K., Rogers, W. H., Berry, S. D., . . . Ware, J. E., Jr., (1989). Functional status and well-being of patients with chronic conditions: Results from the Medical Outcomes Study. *Journal of the American Medical Association, 262*(7), 907–913.

Stewart, A. L., Hays, R. D., & Ware, J. E. (1988). The MOS short-form general health survey: Reliability and validity in a patient population. *Medical Care, 26*(7), 724–735.

Stewart, A. L., & Ware, J. E. (Eds.). (1992). *Measuring functioning and well-being: The medical outcomes study approach.* Durham, NC: Duke University Press.

Sutherland, E. R., & Cherniack, R. M. (2004). Management of chronic obstructive pulmonary disease. *New England Journal of Medicine, 350*(26), 2689–2697.

Tannock, I. F. (1990). Management of breast and prostate cancer: How does quality of life enter the equation? *Oncology, 4*(5), 149–156.

Tarlov, A. R. (1992). The coming influence of a social sciences perspective on medical education. *Academic Medicine, 67*(11), 724–731.

Tarlov, A. R., Ware, J. E., Greenfield, S., Nelson, E. C., Perrin, E., & Zubkoff, M. (1989). The Medical Outcomes Study: An application of methods for monitoring the results of medical care. *Journal of the American Medical Association, 262*(7), 925–930.

Taylor, W. C., Pass, T. M., Shepard, D. S., & Komaroff, A. L. (1987). Cholesterol reduction and life expectancy. *Annals of Internal Medicine, 106,* 605–614.

Testa, M. A. (1993). Parallel perspectives on quality of life during antihypertensive therapy: Impact of responder, survey environment, and questionnaire structure. *Journal of Cardiovascular Pharmacology, 21*(Suppl 2), S18–S25.

Testa, M. A., Anderson, R. B., Nackley, J. F., & Hollenberg, N. K. (1993). Quality of life and antihypertensive therapy in men: A comparison of captopril with enalapril—the Quality-of-Life Hypertension Study Group. *New England Journal of Medicine, 328*(13), 907–913.

Testa, M. A., & Nackley, J. F. (1994). Methods for quality-of-life studies. *Annual Review of Public Health, 15*, 535–559.

Veit, C. T., & Ware, J. E. (1983). The structure of psychological distress and well-being in general populations. *Journal of Consulting and Clinical Psychology, 51*(5), 730–742.

Ware, J. E. (1984). Methodology in behavioral and psychosocial cancer research: Conceptualizing disease impact and treatment outcomes. *Cancer, 53*(10 Suppl), 2316–2326.

Ware, J. E., Kosinski, M., & Keller, S. D. (1995). *SF-12: How to score the SF-12 Physical and Mental Health Summary Scales* (1st ed.). Boston: Health Institute, New England Medical Center.

Ware, J. E., & Sherbourne, C. D. (1992). The MOS 36-item short-form health survey (SF-36). I. Conceptual framework and item selection. *Medical Care, 30*(6), 473–483.

Weinstein, M. C., Siegel, J. E., Gold, M. R., Kamlet, M. S., & Russell, L. B. (1996). Recommendations of the Panel on Cost-Effectiveness in Health and Medicine. *Journal of the American Medical Association, 276*(15), 1253–1258.

Wolfe, J., Grier, H. E., Klar, N., Levin, S. B., Ellenbogen, J. M., Salem-Schatz, S., . . . Weeks, J. C. (2000). Symptoms and suffering at the end of life in children with cancer. *New England Journal of Medicine, 342*, 326–333.

World Health Organization. (1948). Constitution of the World Health Organization: Basic documents. Geneva: Author.

Wu, A. W., Hays, R. D., Kelly, S., Malitz, F., & Bozzette, S. A. (1997). Applications of the Medical Outcomes Study health-related quality of life measures in HIV/AIDS. *Quality of Life Research, 6*(6), 531–554.

CHAPTER TWELVE

EVALUATING THE QUALITY OF CARE

Elizabeth A. McGlynn

Learning Objectives

- Learn about two key conceptual frameworks for defining and evaluating quality of care
- Understand methods by which quality is measured
- Know how well the United States is performing currently on different quality dimensions
- Identify common sources of information on current performance that are routinely updated

Evaluations of health care quality are designed to assess the degree to which the U.S. health care system is successful in achieving its purpose, which is to "continually reduce the burden of illness, injury, and disability, and improve the health and functioning of the people of the United States" (Committee on Quality Health Care in America & Institute of Medicine, 2001). Quality assessment can also be used to determine whether quality improvement interventions are effective.

The main purpose of this chapter is to review a variety of methods for assessing quality of care and highlight what is known about the current level of quality in the United States. The chapter begins by describing the multiple dimensions on which quality may be evaluated and criteria for selecting assessment topics. Next, a conceptual framework is offered to organize approaches to evaluating quality. Finally, definitions, methods, and key results are presented within this conceptual framework.

The United States has made significant advances in the last decade in recognizing the importance of routinely measuring quality and developing the tools necessary to evaluate performance at all levels of the health care system. An ongoing challenge is to integrate quality measurement at the point of care delivery so that more effective and efficient progress can be made in closing the current quality chasm.

The Multiple Dimensions of Quality

Quality is a multidimensional concept reflecting the variety of perspectives held by the multiple participants in the health care system. In 2010, the Institute of Medicine (IOM) updated its widely used conceptual framework for quality (Ulmer, Bruno, & Burke, 2010). The framework includes six components of quality care:

1. *Safe:* service delivery that is free of accidental injury
2. *Effective:* services are based on scientific knowledge and provided to all who could benefit and not to those unlikely to benefit
3. *Patient- or family-centered:* services are delivered in a manner that demonstrates respect for and honors patients' individual preferences and values
4. *Timely:* services are provided free from undesirable and unnecessary delays
5. *Efficient:* producing the best set of outputs from a given set of resources or inputs
6. *Accessible:* timely use of personal health care services to achieve the best possible outcomes

The IOM framework, which is presented as a three-dimensional figure, also includes two cross-cutting dimensions (equity and value) and two foundational elements (care coordination and health systems infrastructure). The framework is used by the Department of Health and Human Services (HHS) to organize the congressionally mandated National Healthcare Quality Report (U.S. Department of Health and Human Services, 2011a) and National Healthcare Disparities Report (U.S. Department of

Health and Human Services, 2011b). Although other groups have developed their own conceptual frameworks, most contain some or all of the elements recommended by the IOM.

Criteria for Evaluating Quality Measures

It is neither feasible nor desirable to measure everything that occurs in the health care system. Quality assessment or monitoring is conducted by selectively examining specific aspects of performance across each of the six components of quality. Most groups undertaking this exercise evaluate measures on four criteria: (1) importance, (2) scientific support, (3) usability, and (4) feasibility (McGlynn, 2003). Each of these is briefly described.

A topic or measure of quality is deemed important if at least one stakeholder can use the results to inform an action. The potential uses of measures include making policy decisions (on the part of private or public groups), shaping clinical decisions (the focus for quality improvement programs), choosing where to go for health care services, or determining the structure of payment for particular providers. Importance may be defined in a variety of ways, among them how common a particular problem is (disease prevalence, utilization rate), the impact the problem has on health care or health (cost of care, major determinant of death or disability), the likelihood that improvement could affect the health and well-being of the population, whether the area is likely to affect choices made by patients, the amount of variation in the attribute across the system, and the degree to which performance is substandard. How importance is evaluated reflects the likely use of the measure as well as the group responsible for obtaining the necessary information. For example, the National Quality Forum (NQF) was asked by HHS to prioritize high-impact conditions for the Medicare population considering cost, prevalence, improvability, variability, disparities, and burden of disease. The top ten conditions (in order) from this exercise were: major depression, congestive heart failure, ischemic heart disease, diabetes, stroke or transient ischemic attack, Alzheimer's disease, breast cancer, chronic obstructive pulmonary disease, heart attack, and colorectal cancer.

Scientific support is used, sometimes indiscriminately, to refer to either the evidence that underlies a particular element of care delivery or the performance characteristics of the measure itself. For example, a group could decide to focus on heart disease because it is a leading reason for death across most age and gender groups in the population and because there are effective ways to prevent and treat the condition; these criteria are used to establish that heart disease is "important." In selecting measures related to effectiveness, the group will likely evaluate the areas in which scientifically rigorous studies have established that a particular care process (such as giving beta blockers to people who have had heart attacks) is likely to significantly improve outcomes (here, the likelihood that a patient will not have a subsequent cardiac event resulting in death or disability). Because this care process has been evaluated in randomized controlled clinical trials, the scientific support is considered to be at the highest level. However, there is an additional aspect of scientific support related to the measure itself. The question is whether it is possible to evaluate this care process in a way that is *valid* (measures the actual process of interest) and *reliable* (repeated measures would arrive at the same conclusion). Further, if the measure was intended to be used to compare performance at one hospital to that at another, additional considerations would apply, such as whether the patient populations are similar enough to permit fair comparisons or whether adequate statistical adjustments have been made to account for differences (that is, adequate methods of risk or case-mix adjustment).

Usability refers to whether the information produced by a measure can be understood and acted on by the intended audience. For a measure to be useful, it has to be a key element in decision making, subjected to analysis that determines whether the results should be used in making a decision, and presented in a way that is understandable to the user and available when a decision has to be made. Relatively little attention has been paid to the influence of data presentation on the usability of the data (and the choices made). The methods by which performance information is presented (visual cues, ordering data, trending cues, and summarizing measures) can significantly affect the choices made by consumers; the addition of cues to help consumers evaluate health plan choices results in optimal decisions being made more frequently (Hibbard, Slovic, Peters, & Finucane, 2002). Greater attention to the usability dimension will be necessary in the future for all audiences.

Feasibility refers to the ease with which a measure can be implemented for routine use (as opposed to its use in a research study). Feasibility is largely determined by the availability of necessary data elements for constructing quality measures. In general, measures that can be constructed using administrative claims data are most easily implemented. Measures that require surveys, clinical information from medical records, or onsite observation are more costly and difficult to implement. Despite recent federal investment to encourage adoption of electronic medical records by physicians and hospitals, obtaining quality measures from medical records remains challenging. Significant improvements in the information and analytic infrastructure available for managing care and evaluating quality is a necessary step to improving quality.

These criteria can be used hierarchically to evaluate potential quality measures. If a measure is not important, the remaining criteria are not particularly relevant. If a measure is not scientifically sound, then it likely is not usable. If a measure is not usable, then it does not matter if it is feasible. Criteria such as these are frequently used to winnow a large number of competing measures down to a manageable set.

A Conceptual Framework for Quality Assessment

A conceptual framework is a useful mechanism for defining which aspects of care should be evaluated in assessing quality. The most commonly used conceptual framework for quality assessment is the one proposed by Avedis Donabedian (1980). He identified three dimensions of quality: structure, process, and outcomes (see Figure 12.1). For this chapter, his

FIGURE 12.1. CONCEPTUAL FRAMEWORK FOR QUALITY ASSESSMENT

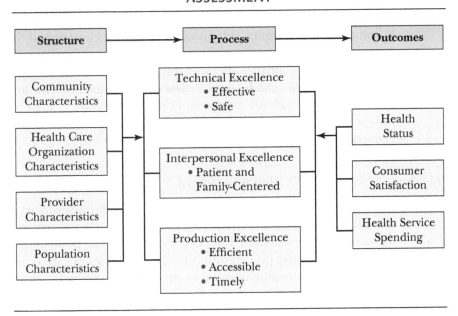

framework was modified to integrate the IOM quality components into this evaluation approach. The review of quality assessment is organized around these three dimensions. Each section includes a definition of the quality dimension, discusses methods available for assessing that dimension, and highlights empirical assessments of that aspect of quality of care in the U.S. health care system today.

Structure

Information about the structure of the health care delivery system is used to describe the context in which care is delivered and to explore potential explanations for variations in the patterns of care delivery. The IOM made this a foundational element of quality. Structural measures are most often used as proxies for other, more difficult to measure constructs such as access and care coordination.

Definition of Structural Quality

Structural quality refers to those stable elements of the health care delivery system in a community that facilitate or inhibit access to and provision of services. The elements include community characteristics (say, prevalence of disease), health care organization characteristics (such as number of hospital beds per capita, adoption of health information technology), provider characteristics (specialty mix or board certification status), and population characteristics (demographics or insurance coverage). Structural characteristics can be used to describe both the need for health care (prevalence or incidence of disease) and the capacity of the community or health care delivery system to meet those needs (availability of properly trained personnel).

Methods of Structural Quality Assessment

The elements of structure that are useful for quality assessment are those that (1) predict variations in the processes or outcomes of care and (2) can be modified. For example, the characteristics of the population residing in a community may predict differences in processes of care or outcomes. Persons without health insurance, or who are otherwise economically disadvantaged, may experience barriers to accessing the health service system; a comparatively lower rate of using necessary services among certain populations might indicate such barriers exist. In turn, lower utilization might be associated with less favorable outcomes. However, policymakers are unlikely to be able to change the characteristics of the population. The more appropriate focus for quality improvement is on reducing barriers to access, through changes in either the availability of insurance or characteristics of the health services delivery system (for example, number of public health clinics, hours of operation for other health providers). Because the relationship between the structure of the health services delivery system and the processes or outcomes of care is indirect, policymakers may find direct action on such measures more difficult than for results from measures of process quality or outcomes.

Community characteristics represent the context in which the health services delivery system operates; they offer one perspective for evaluating the adequacy of the service system to respond to community needs. The 2011 HHS national quality strategy includes population health as a key feature, with a focus on the health of communities (www.healthcare.gov /law/resources/reports/quality03212011a.html). The prevalence of disorders in the community, for instance, may be useful in estimating specific community needs. Information about the availability of health resources may be an indicator of the potential for meeting those needs. One common measure of resource availability is the physician-to-population ratio; the general tendency is to interpret a higher ratio as representing better quality (though this is not always the case) (Fisher et al., 2000). The location of the community relative to health resources is another key indicator of the ease with which residents may obtain certain services; inner-city and rural residents may have to travel farther than others to obtain services. Although an evaluation of community characteristics is not generally included in quality assessment, it may be an important precursor to understanding the particular quality challenges likely to be faced in a community. The Patient Protection and Affordable Care Act of 2010 (PPACA) requires that non-profit hospitals and health systems conduct a community needs assessment every three years as a condition of maintaining their tax-exempt status.

Health care organization characteristics have been evaluated in terms of the capacity of the organization to provide high-quality services. Various factors—notably the quality of the physical plant and equipment, ownership, accreditation, staffing patterns, organizational culture, distribution of reimbursement by source of payment, organizational structure, and governance mechanisms—have been considered markers of the likelihood that an organization provides good quality of care. Most of these factors at best can be viewed as facilitating or inhibiting the likelihood of delivering good care; because these factors always appear in combination, it is difficult to evaluate the incremental effect each has on quality. The volume of procedures performed by hospitals is used as a proxy for outcomes because it is much easier to measure and because evidence has previously established a relationship between these factors.

Organizational accreditation is a common method of assessing structural quality. Several organizations conduct accreditation programs. Generally accreditation requires that an onsite survey team inspect the facility and verify that the organization meets established standards. The Joint Commission (TJC) accredits hospitals, health care networks, clinical laboratories, and organizations that offer home care, long-term care, behavioral health care, and ambulatory care. The National Committee for Quality Assurance (NCQA) accredits managed care organizations, managed behavioral health care organizations, credentials verification organizations, physician organization certification, and preferred provider organizations. The American Accreditation Healthcare Commission (known as URAC) accredits utilization review programs, preferred provider organizations, and managed care organizations.

Provider characteristics have been included as explanatory factors in quality assessments, among them age (or years in practice), gender, race or ethnicity, medical school attended, location of residency training program, specialty, board certification status, job satisfaction, and method of compensation. Board certification is the professional indicator of quality; additional years of training and an examination are required to become board-certified. Various specialty boards are responsible for granting board certification. Overall, about 85 percent of licensed physicians receive initial board certification (Horowitz, Miller, & Miles, 2004). The American Board of Medical Specialties (ABMS), representing twenty-four specialty boards has mechanisms to evaluate professional competence throughout a physician's career. The ABMS maintenance of certification initiative includes four elements: (1) professional standing, (2) lifelong learning and periodic self-assessment, (3) cognitive expertise, and (4) performance in practice (Brennan et al., 2004). For physicians who were initially board-certified in 1990 or later (1987 for critical care medicine and 1988 for geriatric medicine), participation in the maintenance of certification program is required to continue to be board-certified. Renewal of certification occurs at least every ten years.

Population characteristics may be useful in predicting the likelihood that an individual receives high-quality care. Information may be used to identify individuals who are at risk for receiving lower-quality care; in particular, organizations that provide services to individuals at high risk should be aware of the special needs of these populations. Various population characteristics have been examined: sociodemographics, insurance coverage and type, presence of comorbid conditions, functional status, health literacy, and so on.

What Do We Know about Structural Quality?

This section offers some highlights from research on structural quality to illustrate the use of common approaches to measurement of this construct.

Community Characteristics. Although the characteristics of communities in the United States vary widely, there is little evidence of a systematic relationship between those characteristics and the processes or outcomes of care. A study of the Medicare population in the United States found substantial variation in the amount spent on health care in the last six months of life; however, higher spending was not generally associated with better quality of preventive services or care for heart attacks (Fisher, et al., 2003a). In fact, areas in the lowest quintile of spending performed best on eight of the ten measures of quality. The study also found that as spending at the end of life increased, the relative risk of death also increased; there was no relationship between the level of spending and decline in functional status or satisfaction (Fisher et al., 2003b). Similarly, a comprehensive study of the quality of care delivered in twelve diverse metropolitan areas in the United States (Boston; Cleveland; Greenville, South Carolina; Indianapolis; Lansing, Michigan; Little Rock, Arkansas; Miami; Newark, New Jersey; Orange County, California; Phoenix, Arizona; Seattle; and Syracuse, New York) found remarkably little variation. The health care markets in these metropolitan areas varied by median income ($19,672 to $32,890), the proportion of the population living below the poverty line (10 to 25 percent), the proportion of the nonelderly who did not have health insurance (8.1 to 23.0 percent), the number of hospital beds per thousand population (1.6 to 5.0), the number of physicians per thousand population (1.7 to 3.3), and the penetration of managed care (13 to 52 percent). Despite these differences in the economic and resource profile of the communities, the proportion of recommended care received overall ranged from 51 percent in Little Rock and Orange County to 59 percent in Seattle (Kerr, McGlynn, Adams, & Keesey, 2004). The absence of a relationship between the amount of money spent on health care and the quality of care received has fueled efforts to identify sources of waste or inefficiency in delivery of health services. If substantial amounts of waste were eliminated, the United States could use the savings to either reduce health care expenditures or increase access to care for underserved populations.

Health Care Organization Characteristics. The relationship between the volume of procedures performed in an institution or by a provider and the outcomes of those procedures has been studied extensively, with mixed results. One review of 135 studies published between 1980 and 2000 reported statistically significant relationships between outcomes and hospital volume (71 percent of studies) and physician volume (69 percent of studies) (Halm, Lee, & Chassin, 2002). The magnitude of the relationship varied with the type of service or procedure; AIDS treatment and surgery for pancreatic cancer, esophageal cancer, abdominal aortic aneurysm, and pediatric cardiac problems demonstrated the largest difference in outcomes related to volume. The authors of the review noted that studies using risk adjustment models based on clinical data were less likely to find significant differences than those using risk adjustment models based on administrative data. Another review of seventy-six studies published between 1990 and 2000 found a significant relationship between hospital volume and mortality in about two-thirds of the studies (twenty-two of thirty-three) and in about half of the studies (six of fifteen) of physician volume and mortality (Gandjour, Bannenberg, & Lauterbach, 2003). Consistent with the other review, the volume-outcome relationship was particularly strong for pancreatic cancer. A recent Cochrane review of studies published between 1990 and 2011 on volume and outcomes for colorectal cancer surgery found a statistically significant relationship between both hospital and surgeon volume and five-year survival (Archampong, Borowsky, Wille-Jorgensen, & Iversen, 2012). By contrast, a study of the volume-outcome relationship in coronary artery bypass surgery found mortality rates had declined in all hospitals and that hospitals with the lowest volume surgery rates had experienced the largest decrease in in-hospital mortality over the sixteen-year study period (Ricciardi et al., 2008). A study of the volume-outcome relationship for coronary artery bypass graft (CABG) surgery found that low-volume hospitals were more likely to operate on higher-risk patients and in urgent circumstances (Peterson, Coombs, DeLong, Haan, & Ferguson, 2004). Further, no relationship between volume and outcome was found for patients under age sixty-five and those at low operative risk. A study of the relationship between the volume of very low birth weight (VLBW) babies admitted to a hospital and mortality found that only 9 percent of the variation in mortality was explained by volume (Rogowski et al., 2004). Rankings based on risk-adjusted mortality were more reliable, predicting 34 percent of the variation in outcomes.

The presence of computerized physician order entry (CPOE) systems in hospitals is another structural measure that has been used as a proxy for safety. In 2010, about 22 percent of hospitals had such systems (Lewis, 2011). The American Recovery and Reinvestment Act of 2009 (also known as the stimulus bill) included incentives for hospitals and doctors to purchase and use electronic health records systems. The incentives are tied to the "meaningful use" of those systems and CPOE offers one such example of a meaningful use. To obtain incentives in stage 1, hospitals have to prescribe at least 30 percent of medications using CPOE.

A systematic review of the literature identified five randomized trials that evaluated the effect of CPOE on medication safety; two reported a significant reduction in the rate of serious medication errors (Kaushal, Shojania, & Bates, 2003). The authors concluded that most studies did not have sufficient power to detect differences in adverse drug events and had evaluated homegrown systems rather than commercial products. Nonetheless, there is considerable encouragement by large employers for hospitals to implement such systems. A study conducted at the University of Pennsylvania found that many errors persisted even after implementation of CPOE, and other problems were introduced as a result of the system (Koppel et al., 2005). Examples of problems with the system that may contribute to increased medication errors are fragmented displays, pharmacy inventory displays mistaken for dosage guidelines, orders placed in paper charts rather than in the CPOE system, separation of functions that can result in double dosing and incompatible orders, and inflexible ordering formats.

Another structural measure of safety is the patient safety culture in an organization. In 2004, the Agency for Healthcare Research and Quality (AHRQ), contracted with Westat to develop a standardized survey of hospital staff, the Hospital Survey on Patient Safety Culture (www.ahrq.gov/qual/hospsurvey12/index.html#Contents). In 2012, 1,128 hospitals reported results for the Comparative Data Base Project, with 650 hospitals reporting more than once to allow for trending. The survey results are reported in twelve composite categories. Eighty percent of respondents rated teamwork within units (extent to which staff support one another, treat one another with respect, and work together as a team) positively, and 75 percent rated supervisor or manager expectations and actions promoting patient safety positively. Areas for improvement included nonpunitive response to error (44 percent positive response), handoffs and transitions (45 percent positive response), and adequacy of staffing and workloads (56 percent positive).

Hospital, health plan, and other organizational accreditation status is a commonly used structural measure. One study found that hospitals accredited by TJC had better baseline performance on sixteen measures of process quality and four composite scores than nonaccredited hospitals, that those hospitals experienced greater gains in performance over time, and that they were more likely to perform at or above the ninetieth percentile in thirteen of sixteen measures (Schmaltz, Williams, Chassin, Loeb, & Wachter, 2011). NCQA incorporates the results of quality measures into its determination of accreditation status. In 2010, accredited commercial health maintenance organizations (HMOs) had higher absolute scores than nonaccredited HMOs on 64 of 77 quality measures and accredited commercial preferred provider organizations (PPOs) had higher absolute scores on 25 measures (National Committee on Quality Assurance, 2011). In the HMOs, differences in performance ranged from 0.2 percentage points (appropriate medications for asthma) to 8.7 percentage points (control of cholesterol among those with cardiovascular disease).

Provider Characteristics. Board certification is commonly used as a structural measure of physician quality. Relatively few studies have examined the relationship between board certification status and other indicators of quality. One study found that board certified physicians were more likely to have passed and performed well on licensing examinations (Jeffe & Andriole, 2011). Another study found that higher scores on the maintenance of certification (MOC) examination were associated with better performance on diabetes quality measures, particularly intermediate outcome measures (Hess, Weng, Holmboe, & Lipner, 2012). Physicians with higher scores on the MOC examination also demonstrated better performance on diabetes processes and mammography screening among Medicare patients, but performed no better on lipid testing for patients with cardiovascular disease (Holmboe et al., 2008). Physicians with higher MOC examination scores had higher scores on a forty-six-measure composite and performed better on the preventive care composite (Holmboe et al., 2010).

Population Characteristics. Equity is most often evaluated by comparing the experience of patients in population subgroups (race, income, insurance, education, and gender). A review of the literature on disparities in provision of health services found lower quality and intensity of services delivered to racial and ethnic minorities across a range of conditions and interventions (Smedley, Stith, & Nelson, 2003). Studies that controlled for sociodemographics, insurance status, and health status found that these disparities were smaller though rarely eliminated. A review of the literature on disparities in children's health and health care found significant differences on a range of measures of quality and health (Flores & the Committee on Pediatric Research, 2010). Considerable policy attention is currently being devoted to interventions that reduce or eliminate disparities in health care delivery.

Process

Comparison of organizations for consumer choice or accountability is dominated by process quality measures because these events occur more frequently than negative outcomes and are consistent with the structure of clinical practice guidelines.

Definition of Process Quality

Process quality refers to what occurs in the interaction between a patient and a provider. Donabedian identified two dimensions of process quality: technical excellence and interpersonal excellence (Donabedian, 1980). The former means that the intervention was effective (that is, only those services were provided that, according to scientific evidence, are likely to benefit patients) and that it was provided safely. The latter means the intervention was patient and family-centered. Production excellence was added to Donabedian's definition of technical quality to provide a category for the IOM aims of timeliness, access and efficiency. Production excellence refers to services provided without waste.

The focus of technical quality assessment is on those processes of care that are likely to produce optimal outcomes: either improvement in health or reduction in the rate of decline in functioning or effective use of resources. The best evidence of the relationship between processes and clinical outcomes is from randomized controlled trials because they can prove conclusively that an intervention is efficacious (produces desired outcomes under ideal circumstances). Evidence from other scientific methods, though not as conclusive, is often used to demonstrate the importance of a variety of interventions in medical care. Other methods are used to examine relationships between the remaining categories of process and the outcomes of interest.

Methods of Process Quality Assessment

Four methods are commonly used to evaluate the quality of medical care processes: (1) appropriateness of an intervention, (2) adherence to practice guidelines or standards of care, (3) practice profiling, and (4) consumer reports. These four methods share some features, but they are discussed separately to emphasize some methodological considerations.

Appropriateness. Appropriateness of an intervention means that, for individuals with particular clinical and personal characteristics, the expected health benefit from doing an intervention (diagnostic or therapeutic procedure) exceeds the expected health risk by a sufficient margin and that the intervention is worth doing. RAND and UCLA pioneered a method of assessing the appropriateness with which a variety of interventions are evaluated (Brook, 1994). The basic method involves five steps:

1. *Review the literature.* A detailed literature review summarizes what is known about the efficacy, utilization, complications, cost, and indications for the subject intervention. Where possible, outcome evidence tables are constructed for clinically homogeneous groups.

2. *List indications.* A preliminary list of indications (reasons for doing the procedure) categorizes patients by symptoms, past medical history, results of previous diagnostic tests, and clinically relevant personal characteristics (such as age). The indications list is designed to be detailed enough that patients within an indication are homogeneous with respect to the clinical appropriateness of performing a procedure; the indications are comprehensive enough that nearly all persons presenting for the procedure can be categorized.

3. *Convene a panel to select indications.* A nine-person multispecialty panel evaluates the preliminary indications. The panel is chosen to be diverse with respect to geographic location, practice style, and other characteristics. Both "doers" and "nondoers" of a procedure are included on the panel.

4. *Rate the indications.* The indications are rated using a modified Delphi process. In the first round, panelists individually rate the indications (the literature review prepared in step one is made available); the panelists may also recommend changes to the structure of the indications. In the second round, the panel meets face-to-face for a discussion of the results

from the first round and makes final ratings. The indications are rated from 1 to 9, where 1 means that the procedure is very inappropriate for persons within an indication and 9 means that the procedure is very appropriate for persons within an indication. The median panel rating is used to determine the appropriateness rating for each indication; a median rating of 1 to 3 is considered inappropriate, 4 to 6 is equivocal or of uncertain value, and 7 to 9 is appropriate. There is also a requirement that the panel have a reasonable and statistically determined level of agreement among themselves.

5. *Evaluate appropriateness of interventions.* The appropriateness with which interventions are used can then be evaluated. Generally, information is abstracted from the medical record (inpatient or outpatient) because of the level of clinical detail required to assign patients to indications. An alternative approach that has been applied when appropriateness is assessed prospectively is to interview both the patient and the physician.

The appropriateness method has also been used to develop valid quality indicators for evaluating adherence to evidence-based medicine. The reliability and validity of the appropriateness method has been extensively evaluated. The test-retest reliability of individual panel members' ratings and the reproducibility of overall panel ratings have been found comparable to the levels of common diagnostic tests (Shekelle, Kahan, et al., 1998b). The content and construct validity of ratings of appropriateness is supported by the studies done (Shekelle, Chassin, & Park, 1998a). For example, regression analysis performed on indications for patients with chronic stable angina undergoing coronary angiography demonstrated that the procedure was more likely to be considered appropriate (1) as severity increased, (2) among patients who had failed medical therapy, and (3) among patients who had positive findings on noninvasive tests (Kravitz et al., 1995).

The ratings of each indication are the explicit standards by which care is evaluated. The indications can be linked to the quality of scientific evidence, and ratings can be updated as knowledge changes. Sensitivity analyses can be used to evaluate the importance of certain factors in the indication structure in determining appropriateness. For example, in a study of appropriateness of hysterectomy, among women who wanted to maintain fertility, the expert panel required considerable evidence of efforts to find an alternative solution to the presenting problem before the hysterectomy was considered appropriate (Bernstein, Fiske, McGlynn, & Gifford, 1997). Because there are no standards for the expected appropriateness of care, most of the comparisons have been made among groups (hospitals, managed care organizations) participating in a study (Leape et al., 1993; Bernstein, McGlynn, et al., 1993).

Most studies of appropriateness were conducted in the 1980s and early 1990s, when overuse was the major quality issue. Although the appropriateness method can be used to evaluate both underuse and overuse, its application to the problem of overuse is more common. As initiatives to control rising health care costs were implemented (such as managed care), concern shifted to underuse of services. The pendulum is once again swinging back toward concern about overuse, which may give rise to a new generation of appropriateness studies (Lawson, Gibbons, Ingraham, Shekelle, & Ko, 2011; Dimitrow, Airaksinen, Kivela, Lyles, & Leikola, 2011; Sanmartin et al., 2008). The appropriateness method represents one method for evaluating the IOM domains of effectiveness and safety.

Adherence to Guidelines. Adherence to practice guidelines or professional standards is a method of process quality assessment that evaluates the extent to which care is consistent with professional knowledge, either by examining adherence to specific practice guidelines or by evaluating whether care meets certain professional standards. The IOM defines practice guidelines as "statements that include recommendations intended to optimize patient care that are informed by a systematic review of evidence and an assessment of the benefits and harms of alternative care options" (Graham, Mancher, Wolman, Greenfield, & Steinberg, 2011). Adherence to guidelines is one method used to evaluate the IOM domains of effectiveness and safety.

Thousands of guidelines are available today produced by groups including specialty societies, disease advocacy groups, the U.S. Preventive Services Task Force, health plans, and other types of organizations (Graham et al., 2011). A searchable data base of guidelines is maintained by AHRQ (www.guidelines.gov). The IOM reviewed the state-of-the-art in producing clinical practice guidelines as well as the quality of those guidelines. The report highlights a number of significant concerns with guidelines and proposes eight standards (transparency, conflict of interest, composition of guideline development group, quality of systematic evidence review, ratings of evidence, articulation of recommendations, external review, and updating) for trustworthy guidelines, which in turn serve as an acceptable basis for developing quality measures (Graham et al., 2011). A related IOM report recommended five sets of standards for high-quality systematic reviews that are used as the evidence base for guidelines (Eden, Levit, Berg, & Morton, 2011).

For purposes of quality assessment, it is almost always necessary to translate guidelines into review criteria by establishing operational definitions of adherence and nonadherence to the guidelines, as well as definitions for key clinical concepts employed in the guidelines. Many practice guidelines, for example, contain vague clinical terms ("mild," "moderate," and "severe") that must be explicitly defined in order to evaluate whether a particular patient qualifies for an element of the guidelines and then to assess adherence to the guideline. The performance expectation is generally 100 percent adherence to the guideline, and comparisons are made either among similar groups or compared to a benchmark.

Three data sources are used to determine the degree of adherence to practice guidelines: administrative data, medical records, and patient surveys. Administrative data are generated to pay claims for reimbursement under health insurance plans. Because claims are filed only for those services included in a benefit package, administrative data can be used to evaluate quality only where the service is covered and when the conditions for appropriate use can be ascertained from such data sources; preventive services are often evaluated using claims data. Medical record data are used when greater clinical detail is required to determine the population that should be receiving an intervention or to evaluate some types of interventions; medical records may be used to assess elements of chronic disease care, particularly if severity of disease is necessary for determining the needed interventions. Surveys are used to obtain patient reports on interventions such as immunization, mammography, and cholesterol testing that are indicators for technical process quality. The National Immunization Survey, for example, tracks the rate of immunizations for children in the first two years of life. Such reporting is particularly useful if the intervention is likely to be remembered accurately by consumers and if the intervention is difficult to identify in other data sources.

Practice Profiling. Practice profiling is a method for comparing the patterns of cost, utilization, and quality of processes among providers. The method usually compares practice patterns to an empirical norm (say, the average of other physicians in the organization). Profiles are generally constructed as a rate of occurrence of some process (such as office visit, service, surgical procedure, laboratory test) over a specified period of time for a defined population. Recently, practice profiles have been used to evaluate relative resource use (Adams, Mehrotra, Thomas, & McGlynn, 2010). Profiling is commonly distinguished from appropriateness or guideline adherence approaches by the lack of a gold standard benchmark for performance.

Profiles can be constructed at any level in the health delivery system: nationally; regionally; or by health plan, specialty, medical group, or individual physician. Profiling is most often used to examine utilization or cost of a variety of services: hospital admission, ambulatory visit, laboratory test use, referral pattern, diagnostic test use, and medication prescription. A systematic review of efficiency measures used in practice profiling found that they had not been subjected to rigorous testing of reliability and validity (Hussey, et al., 2009). Profiling methods are used to assess the IOM domain of efficiency.

Today, large employers and health plans are using profiling methods to construct tiered networks of providers on the basis of relative resource use (such as establishing lower copayment amounts for patients using providers whose practice is deemed more "efficient") and to reward providers whose profiles suggest they use resources less intensively. Most of the profiling tools in use today are proprietary and rely on claims data. An evaluation of these methods for assessing relative resource use found that 59 percent of physicians' cost profile scores did not meet common thresholds for reliability and 22 percent of physicians would, as a result, be misclassified (Adams, McGlynn, Thomas, & Mehrotra, 2010). More routine use of statistical techniques could improve the performance of some of these metrics. Similar problems with reliability have been identified for physician profiling on quality metrics (Scholle et al., 2008).

Consumer Ratings. Consumer ratings are used to evaluate the interpersonal quality of care (that is, the IOM domain of patient and family-centeredness) and production excellence (that is, the IOM domains of access and timeliness). Surveys of individuals are the most common method for eliciting information from individuals about their health care. Two types of information are generally sought: (1) reporting of events and (2) ratings of care. This section discusses reporting of events; ratings of care are discussed in the outcomes section.

Consumer reports are used to evaluate a variety of access issues, among them waiting time for an appointment or to see the doctor, distance to the nearest health facility, hours of operation, ability to see the provider one wants to see, and other similar questions regarding the consumer's experience in trying to obtain services. Consumers may also report on what the physician did during an encounter (explain options, furnish requested information, and counsel about health habits). Patients' ability to report on events varies with the time frame (a shorter time span produces more reliable information) and the type of event (invasive events, such as surgery, may be more memorable than health promotion counseling).

In an effort to standardize the survey methods used to elicit information from consumers, beginning in 1995 AHRQ awarded cooperative agreements to several academic institutions to develop the Consumer Assessment of Healthcare Providers and Systems (CAHPS) family of surveys (www.cahps.ahrq.gov). Separate CAHPS instruments are available for health plans, clinicians and groups, hospitals, nursing homes, and dialysis facilities. AHRQ maintains a benchmarking database to compare the performance of entities on these metrics (www.cahps.ahrq.gov/CAHPS-Database/About.aspx).

What Do We Know about Process Quality?

It is beyond the scope of this chapter to summarize all of the literature regarding process quality. However, this section highlights key results that have been published in each of the IOM domains. Together they illustrate application of the methods described here for measuring process quality.

Technical Excellence: Effectiveness. The most comprehensive assessment of health care quality ever undertaken reported that American adults receive just 55 percent of recommended care for the leading causes of death and disability and for the main reasons they seek health care services (McGlynn et al., 2003). The study analyzed performance on 439 indicators of effectiveness across thirty chronic and acute health problems as well as preventive care. Deficits were reported across the continuum of care from screening (52 percent) to diagnosis (56 percent), treatment (58 percent), and follow-up (59 percent). The quality of care varied substantially by health condition. For example, 68 percent of recommended care was delivered for patients with coronary artery disease, compared to 25 percent for atrial fibrillation. Among patients with a diagnosis of depression noted in the medical record, just 58 percent of recommended care was delivered. People with diabetes received 45 percent of recommended care, which is of particular concern given the increased prevalence of diabetes related to the epidemic of obesity in America. A higher rate of failure to deliver needed care (underuse) was reported compared to delivering care that was of no benefit or potentially harmful to the patient (overuse).

Beginning in December 2003, Congress required AHRQ to produce an annual report on health care quality in the United States (U.S. Department of Health and Human Services, 2011a). The section on effectiveness addresses care related to cancer, diabetes, end-stage renal disease, heart disease, HIV/AIDS, maternal and child health, mental health and substance abuse, respiratory diseases, lifestyle modifications, functional status preservation and rehabilitation, and supportive and palliative care; both process and outcome measures are reported. While two-thirds of the 179 measures tracked in the report showed improvement, the rate of change is slow—about 2 percent per year. A few specific results are highlighted here.

The 2011 report found that 56 percent of adults over the age of 50 had been screened for colorectal cancer. The proportion of patients diagnosed with colon cancer who received recommended treatment increased from 52 percent in 2003 to 77 percent in 2007. For diabetes, the report indicates that 38 percent of adults received three recommended care processes (blood sugar test, retinal examination, and foot examination). In 2008, 95 percent of patients with heart failure received recommended care. In 2008, 66 percent of children ages three to six had their vision checked by a health professional. Counseling about healthy eating and the importance of physical activity are important interventions for preventing children from becoming overweight. In 2007, 58 percent of children had been counseled about healthy eating and 39 percent about exercising. Effective management of asthma can prevent hospitalizations. In 2007, only 29 percent reported taking preventive medicine for asthma daily.

NCQA produces an annual report on the effectiveness of care delivered to people enrolled in health plans (NCQA, 2011). In 2010, NCQA collected standardized information from more than one thousand HMOs and PPOs on thirty-two effectiveness-of-care measures across preventive, chronic disease, and acute condition care. A few of the HMO results are highlighted here.

In 2010, 41 percent of commercial, 50 percent of Medicare, and 42 percent of Medicaid HMO enrollees had their body mass index (a measure of obesity) calculated by a physician. Among persons with diabetes, 86 percent of commercial, 88 percent of Medicare and 75 percent of Medicaid HMO enrollees were screened for high cholesterol. For patients with chronic lung disease, 42 percent of commercial, 34 percent of Medicare, and 31 percent of Medicaid enrollees had appropriate tests to diagnose and assess their condition. About 60 percent of commercial enrollees received a follow-up visit within seven days of being discharged from a hospital with a mental illness diagnosis compared with 37 percent of Medicare and 45 percent of Medicaid enrollees. Performance rates among PPOs in 2010 were better than HMOs for some measures and worse for others.

Results of quality measures in hospitals became publicly available for the first time through the Centers for Medicare and Medicaid Services (CMS) in late 2003 (www.hospitalcompare.hhs.gov) and TJC in July 2004. CMS reports process measures for four clinical areas: heart attack or chest pain, heart failure, children's asthma, and pneumonia. TJC publishes an annual report on quality and safety that provides trend analyses of hospital performance on both accountability measures (those that are typically in common with CMS reporting) and nonaccountability measures (required as part of accreditation) (The Joint Commission, 2011). The report documents the improvements in quality that have occurred since these measures began being publicly reported. For example, on the composite measure of hospital performance, 92 percent of hospitals achieved an overall score at or above 90 percent compared with just 20 percent of hospitals in 2002 (the first year of reporting) (The Joint Commission, 2011).

CMS also maintains web-based information on the performance of nursing homes, home health agencies, and dialysis facilities. At this writing, CMS was working on developing information on physicians but had only made public basic information about practices, such as office location and phone number, where they trained, and whether they accept Medicare assignment.

Technical Excellence: Safety. Safety is most often assessed using structure or outcome measures; however, process measures of safety are being used more frequently. NCQA reports on the proportion of elderly receiving one or more high risk medications as well as on potentially harmful drug-disease interactions. In 2010, 22 percent of Medicare HMO enrollees received at least one high risk medication and 5 percent received at least two (NCQA, 2011). The most common potentially harmful drug-disease interaction reported was among patients with dementia who were receiving tricyclic antidepressants or anticholinergic agents (NCQA, 2011). CMS reports on surgical safety in hospitals using the Surgical Care Improvement Project (SCIP) measures. Performance on these twelve measures (say, receiving an antibiotic within one hour before surgery) is high on average nationally. Beginning in 2002, TJC developed national patient safety goals for different settings (http://www.jointcommission .org/standards_information/npsgs.aspx). The 2012 measures for hospitals are grouped into seven goals: identifying patients correctly, improving staff communication, using medications safely, preventing infection, identifying patient safety risks, and preventing mistakes in surgery.

Interpersonal Excellence: Patient- and Family-Centeredness. Consumer ratings and reports are the principal means by which patient and family-centeredness is evaluated. Most of the public reports in this area are based on CAHPS measures. An important aspect of patient-centeredness is effective communications between doctors and patients. The CAHPS benchmarking database reports in 2011 that 73 percent of commercial, 70 percent of adult Medicaid, 75 percent of child Medicaid, and 76 percent of Medicare enrollees reported that their doctors always communicated well (www.cahps.ahrq.gov).

Health plans are evaluated in this area by the quality of their customer service, which includes the degree to which information and help that is needed is available and whether consumers believe they have been treated with courtesy and respect. In 2010, 59 percent of commercial, 66 percent of Medicare, and 58 percent of Medicaid HMO enrollees reported that they had always or usually had positive experiences with their plans.

Production Excellence: Efficient. Efficiency is a relatively new addition to the definition of quality, and there are few systematic studies available that rigorously document the relative use of resources to produce a specific health care service. Much of the measurement currently focuses on inappropriate use of medications and services such as hospitals and emergency departments. In 2010, the national healthcare quality report indicated that there was little improvement between 2002 and 2007 in the proportion of older persons receiving one of thirty-three potentially inappropriate drugs (U.S. DHS, 2011a). The report also indicates that in 2007 for every 100,000 hospital admissions, about 1,700 were inappropriate or avoidable; the costs associated with those admissions were about $27 billion in 2007.

NCQA reports that nearly one-quarter of commercial HMO and PPO enrollees with low back pain had an inappropriate imaging study in 2010 (NCQA, 2011). NCQA also calculates relative resource use measures for asthma, cardiovascular disease, chronic lung disease, diabetes, and hypertension. When resource use is compared to quality performance, NCQA (like other previous studies) finds little relationship between spending and quality.

Production Excellence: Accessibility. CAHPS includes an assessment of whether people are able to get needed care (such as appointments, tests, or treatments), one way of evaluating access. In the 2011 CAHPS benchmarking database, 54 percent of adult commercial, 51 percent of adult Medicaid, 55 percent of child Medicaid, and 65 percent of Medicare health plan enrollees reported that they were always able to obtained needed care (www.cahps.ahrq.gov/CAHPSIDB/Public). The group with the greatest access challenges, adult Medicaid enrollees, reported that 22 percent of the time they were never or only sometimes able to get needed care.

Production Excellence: Timely. CAHPS includes patient reports on whether they were able to get needed care quickly. The National CAHPS Database reported that in 2011, 58 percent of commercial, 66 percent of Medicare, 56 percent of adult Medicaid, and 71 percent of child Medicaid enrollees reported that they always were able to receive care and get appointments as soon as they thought care was needed (NCQA, 2011).

Timeliness can also be a factor in delivery of clinical care processes. Three of the publicly reported hospital measures evaluate the number of minutes it takes from the time a patient arrives at the hospital to the time a needed care process is delivered; timeliness is critical to good outcomes in these areas. TJC reports that the proportion of heart attack patients receiving appropriate surgical or medical intervention within ninety minutes of arriving at the hospital has improved from 68 percent in 2006 to 92 percent in 2010 (The Joint Commission, 2011).

Outcomes

Many people argue that outcomes are the best way to evaluate quality. This section highlights some of the benefits and challenges inherent in using outcomes to assess quality.

Definition of Outcomes

Outcomes can be defined as the result of efforts to prevent, diagnose, and treat various health problems encountered by the population. Outcomes are seen by many as the bottom-line measure of the degree to which the health care delivery system is achieving its purpose. A range of potential dimensions can be included in the broad category of outcomes. Figure 12.1 provides three general categories of outcomes: health status, consumer satisfaction, and health services spending.

Health status can include both clinical and functional measures. Clinical status refers to biological, physiological, and symptom-based aspects of health; examples are blood pressure, blood sugar level, cholesterol level, lung function, and mortality. These are the outcomes that are generally of interest to physicians because they are most directly amenable to treatment. Functional status captures multiple dimensions, among them physical, mental, role, and social functioning. Assessments of functional status typically ask respondents to indicate the frequency or extent to which physical or mental disorders interfere with their ability to perform their usual activities. Functional status is of interest to consumers because it represents how changes in clinical status affect their everyday life.

Consumer satisfaction assesses the extent to which experiences in the health service system were consistent with expectations and were acceptable to those receiving care.

Resource use can refer either to the total amount spent on health care or to the amount spent per capita. The increased concern over the effect of spending ever growing proportions of the nation's economic product on health care has raised this issue as a critical element of a high performing health care system.

There are two challenges in using outcome assessments for evaluating the quality of care. Both challenges reflect the fact that outcomes are produced through the interaction of a variety of factors inside and outside of the health service delivery system. First, to use outcomes to make externally valid comparisons among health plans or providers, adequate methods must be employed to control for differences in the severity of illness or the health profile of the populations being compared. A common illustration of an initial failure to do this was the release by the Health Care Financing Administration (HCFA) of hospital mortality data. Initially, the data were not adjusted for differences in the severity of illness for patients, and not surprisingly some of the hospitals that had the worst performance records were those serving the sickest patients (for example, hospices for the terminally ill) (Berwick & Wald, 1990). In response to complaints from hospitals and physicians about deficiency in the measures and lack of uptake from consumers, HCFA ceased publication of hospital mortality data in 1993 (Galvin & McGlynn, 2003). There is still considerable controversy as to whether the severity adjustments introduced by HCFA subsequent to the initial release were adequate, but the addition of severity adjustments substantially improved the discriminant validity of the model (Fleming, Hicks, & Bailey, 1995). The relative paucity of mortality measures publicly reported on today reflects the difficulty in adequately measuring this aspect of quality.

The second challenge for the use of outcomes data is the issue of attribution—that is, determining the extent to which the health plan or physician that is currently being evaluated is responsible for the observed outcomes. Health outcomes are affected by a variety of factors, not all of which can be modified by the health delivery system. One study estimated that 40 percent of mortality can be attributed to behavioral factors, 20 percent to social circumstances and environmental exposures, 30 percent to genetics, and 10 percent to inadequacies in medical care (McGinnis, Williams-Russo, & Knickman, 2002). Because these factors may be distributed differently among populations enrolled in health plans and those seeking care from primary care physicians, these external effects must be controlled for in statistical analyses in order to understand the extent to which variations in the quality of care contribute to the observed variations in outcomes. For interventions that take place over a long period of time (chronic disease care), outcomes observed in the current time period may be the result of action taken (or not taken) much earlier in the course of illness when the physicians or health plan currently responsible for treating the patient were not involved. To the extent that individuals change providers frequently, discontinuity in service may further contribute to a less-than-optimal course of treatment. Who bears the responsibility for these complex series of events remains a question open to debate.

Methods of Outcome Assessment

Three approaches to outcome assessment are commonly used to evaluate quality of care: (1) condition-specific; (2) generic; and (3) sentinel events or adverse outcomes.

Condition-Specific Approach. The condition-specific approach, sometimes referred to as a "tracer" condition approach, examines the outcomes for individuals who have a particular diagnosis (say, hypertension). The condition-specific approach is used to evaluate the IOM domain of effectiveness. The outcomes for condition-specific approaches may emphasize clinical status (blood pressure control for hypertension), although disease-specific measures of functional status should also be assessed (for prostate cancer, treatment assessments should include incontinence, impotence, and bowel function). The advantage of condition-specific outcome assessment from a quality perspective is that it may most closely reflect a link to the processes of care delivered. For example, if one health plan has a higher proportion of individuals with hypertension whose blood pressure is outside the "controlled" range, one might reasonably conclude that the plan has problems in managing the disease (medication, diet, monitoring for complications). The difficulty with condition-specific approaches to quality assessment is that they require substantial investment in developing methods across a sufficient range of diseases to produce a picture of the overall quality of care delivered in a health plan or hospital.

Research suggests that quality is not consistent from condition to condition (McGlynn et al., 2003). This implies that outcomes are likely to vary by condition; some organizations may have good outcomes for adult chronic diseases and be less successful in achieving good outcomes for chronic disease in childhood. One study of quality at the hospital level found that the relative rates of complications were similar within institutions, but there was less correlation between medical and surgical cases (Iezzoni et al., 1994). The other difficulty in the context of today's information systems is that one may not be able to easily identify individuals who have particular health problems (the denominator population) so that population-based outcomes can be estimated.

Generic Approach. The generic approach examines outcomes that can be assessed for all individuals, regardless of their health problems. The generic approach is used to evaluate the IOM domains of safety, patient-centeredness, timeliness, accessibility, and efficiency. Outcomes regarding mortality, general functional status, level of health care spending, and patient satisfaction are most commonly assessed in generic approaches. The advantage to the generic approach is that it can be applied across the entire population enrolled in a health plan, receiving care from a hospital, or seeing a particular physician. The difficulty with this approach is that research has yielded considerably less understanding of the link between what is done in the medical care system and the resulting generic outcomes for the population. There is reason to believe that other factors (education, socioeconomic status) enter into determining these outcomes. Further, the need to control for variation in severity and case mix of a population in making comparisons of generic outcomes is extremely important, and few reliable methods for doing so currently exist.

Consumer satisfaction may be the most commonly evaluated generic outcome. Consumer satisfaction measures evaluate the quality and acceptability of care. CAHPS is the standardized set of instruments most commonly used to evaluate consumer satisfaction today.

Sentinel Event Approach. The sentinel event approach identifies some occurrence, usually an adverse outcome, which is likely to be associated with poor quality of care and tracks the frequency with which the event occurs. Sentinel events are used to evaluate the IOM domains of effectiveness and safety and sometimes timeliness. Examples of adverse outcomes are mortality, early readmission to a hospital, complications of a surgical procedure (transfusion, reoperation), nosocomial infection in the hospital, suicide, adverse drug reaction (especially as a result of interactions among one or more drugs), and very low birth weight. Sentinel events can be useful for identifying potential problems, but it is almost always necessary to conduct further assessments to conclude whether an adverse event was "preventable" or not. The frequency with which adverse events occur affects their practicality for quality assessment. Events that occur rarely are less useful for quality monitoring because it is more difficult to determine whether differences are statistically meaningful. An exception to this is identification of "never events," that is, outcomes that should never occur, such as surgery on the wrong site or the development of serious pressure ulcers while an inpatient.

What Do We Know about Outcomes?

As with the literature on process quality, it is beyond the scope of this chapter to summarize everything that is known about the outcomes of care. Rather, some of the important findings from the published literature and websites reporting quality performance are highlighted.

Outcomes: Health Status. Condition-specific outcomes are used primarily to evaluate the effectiveness of care. For example, NCQA reports on the proportion of enrollees in health plans with hypertension whose blood pressure is controlled. In 2010, 63 percent of commercial enrollees, 62 percent of Medicare enrollees, and 56 percent of Medicaid enrollees with hypertension had their blood pressure controlled (NCQA, 2011). Performance on this measure has actually declined somewhat since 2005. NCQA uses three outcome measures to assess effectiveness of care for diabetes: good control of blood sugar (glycosylated hemoglobin), control of blood pressure, and control of cholesterol (lipids). In 2010, 62 percent of commercial, 66 percent of Medicare, and 47 percent of Medicaid enrollees with diabetes had a blood sugar level that was well controlled. Blood pressure control was achieved for 66 percent of commercial, 62 percent of Medicare, and 60 percent of Medicaid enrollees with diabetes. Lipid control was 48 percent for commercial, 35 percent for Medicaid, and 52 percent for Medicare enrollees with diabetes. Outcome measure thresholds can change over time as new scientific evidence is acquired or more effective therapies become available.

Mortality and changes in functional status are two commonly used generic outcomes measures. For example, one study found that veterans were more likely than Medicare Advantage enrollees to be alive with the same or better physical health and mental health outcomes scores over a two-year period (Selim et al., 2010). CMS reports outcomes for nursing home residents on the Nursing Home Compare website (www.medicare.gov/nhcompare). For example, on average nationally, 15 percent of nursing home residents have become more depressed or anxious over time; the statewide average for California is 10 percent. The proportion of patients reporting an increase in their need for help with activities of daily living is 14 percent nationally and 11 percent in California. CMS also reports risk-adjusted mortality rates for patients admitted to hospitals with heart attacks, heart failure, or pneumonia (www.hospitalcompare.hhs.gov). In 2010, about 16 percent of Medicare fee-for-service enrollees who were admitted to a hospital with a heart attack died within thirty days of that admission. For heart failure patients, 11 percent died within thirty days and among Medicare patients admitted with pneumonia, about 12 percent died within thirty days. These measures are available for individual hospitals along with an assessment of whether the hospital-specific rate is statistically significantly different from the national rate.

Mortality is also evaluated at the population level, either for the nation as a whole or at smaller geographic units. Two common measures are the infant mortality rate and life expectancy. In 2012, the United States ranked forty-ninth in the world in infant mortality with a rate of 5.98 deaths per thousand live births, considerably higher than Japan, at 2.21 (CIA, 2012). The life expectancy at birth in the United States in 2009 was 78.5 years (CDC, 2012) and ranks fiftieth in the world (CIA, 2012).

Adverse events are a common method for measuring outcomes related to safety. In 2001, the National Quality Forum (NQF) introduced the term "never event" or medical errors that should never occur, such as surgery on the wrong side of the body. Since then the list of sentinel events has expanded to include adverse events that are clearly identifiable and measurable, serious (death or disability results), and usually preventable. These events are reported by hospitals to TJC and are categorized into six groups (wrong site surgery, suicide, operative or postoperative complications, delays in treatment, medication errors, and patient falls). In 2009, hospitals reported 6,428 events to TJC, with the most common category being wrong-site surgery (www.psnet.ahrq.gov). In 2007, CMS announced that Medicare would not pay for additional costs (such as extended stay in the hospital or return to surgery) associated with these events.

Outcomes: Consumer Satisfaction. The CAHPS benchmarking data base reports that a majority of patients rated their personal doctor or specialists as 9 or 10 on a ten-point scale. Overall ratings of health care were lower with 50 percent of commercial, 49 percent of adult Medicaid and 61 percent of Medicare enrollees giving a 9 or 10 rating. Health plan ratings were lowest for commercial enrollees, with 39 percent rating their plan a 9 or 10; Medicaid and Medicare enrollees rated their plans higher, with 54 percent of adult Medicaid and 62 percent of Medicare giving a rating or 9 or 10.

Outcomes: Health Services Spending. One overall measure of health care spending is the proportion of gross domestic product (GDP) accounted for by health services. In 2010, health care accounted for 17.9 percent of GDP. Fisher and colleagues reported on the relationship between health care spending and risk of death following a hip fracture, treatment for colon cancer, and heart attack as well as over time for a general cohort of Medicare patients (Fisher et al., 2003b). For each cohort, every 10 percent increase in the expenditure index was associated with an increase in the risk of death. The study found no relationship between increased spending and changes in functional status over time. Similarly, no statistically significant relationship was found between level of health care spending and patient satisfaction with care. A test for trend suggested overall satisfaction with care was lower and satisfaction with interpersonal care was higher in higher-spending regions.

Future Directions

Health care quality assessment is likely to continue to evolve in the methods, data sources, displays, and uses. Currently, there is great interest in developing quality measures that could be routinely extracted from electronic medical records. This development has the potential to significantly increase the feasibility of using this data source which in turn might enhance the content and number of measures. A number of technical challenges must be addressed before such measures become a routine part of quality assessment.

Social media represents another potential source of information on consumer experiences and may make it easier to routinely obtain quality measures related to patient- and family-centered care. An attractive feature of this data source is the ability to acquire information more rapidly.

Across all sources of information, there are calls to improve the timeliness of measures. Today, as can be seen in many of the examples, assessments commonly reflect practice from two years prior to the report. While the slow rate of improvement nationally might suggest that older reports are reasonably accurate, delays do not appropriately acknowledge those institutions and individuals that are improving.

Much of the current discussion around payment reform includes mechanisms to incorporate quality measurement into payment methods. The general direction is to move from paying for volume to paying for value. As quality measurement becomes more widespread and robust, using measures to drive or adjust payment becomes more possible.

As the stakes for uses of measures increase, there will be continued need to improve the methods, particularly those that enable appropriate design of composite measures (likely to be necessary for payment methods), accounting for differential risk or population characteristics, accounting for differences in the measures themselves (such as how difficult it is to perform well on a measure), and to enable the use of disparate data sources.

SUMMARY

Tremendous progress has been made over the past two decades in developing methods for measuring quality, applying those methods in a variety of settings, and publicly reporting the results. In areas where quality measurement is routinely applied and reported, progress is being made. However, significant deficits exist in the structural elements of care, processes of care, and outcomes. The consequences of failure to deliver effective health services are significant in terms of preventable disability and death as well as avoidable expenditures. Large investments in the health care information infrastructure are currently under way, partly motivated by evidence that this functionality is associated with higher performance. Where such investments have been made, greater progress is evident; nevertheless, few organizations today have adequate information infrastructures in place. The infrastructure investment must include mechanisms for regularly obtaining reports and ratings from patients.

The information infrastructure is necessary but not sufficient to improve quality. Performance must be evaluated across the multiple dimensions outlined by the IOM at all levels in the health care system, from individual providers up to the nation. If performance assessment systems do not include a broad set of measures, the incentive for the health care industry will be to improve only the handful of areas measured. Further, information about performance should be made available regularly to all stakeholders in the health care system. For providers, having information available at the point of care increases the likelihood of needed services being delivered as opportunities arise; this is likely to be both more effective and more efficient than the current system.

Increasing the information about performance that is routinely available also expands opportunities to pay high performers differentially or to tailor benefit designs to incent patients to seek care from high-performing providers. Emerging evidence suggests that pay-for-performance programs in hospitals, however, have not been associated with better outcomes (Jha, Joynt, Orav, & Epstein, 2012).

Each of these policy changes will facilitate redesign of the health care delivery system from one that is reactive and inefficient to one able to proactively and efficiently manage the health service needs of the population in achieving the highest levels of health and functioning possible.

KEY TERMS

Accessible timely use of personal health care services to achieve the best possible outcomes

Effective services are based on scientific knowledge and provided to all who could benefit and not to those unlikely to benefit

Efficient producing the best set of outputs from a given set of resources or inputs

Feasibility the ease with which a measure can be implemented for routine use

Outcomes the result of efforts to prevent, diagnose, and treat various health problems encountered by the population

Patient- or family-centered services are delivered in a manner that demonstrates respect for and honors patients' individual preferences and values

Process quality what occurs in the interaction between a patient and a provider, including technical, interpersonal, and production dimensions

Reliable repeated measures would arrive at the same conclusion

Safe service delivery that is free of accidental injury

Structural quality the stable elements of the health care delivery system in a community that facilitate or inhibit access to and provision of services

Timely services are provided free from undesirable and unnecessary delays

Usability the information produced by a measure can be understood and acted on by the intended audience

Valid the measure accurately assesses the actual process of interest

DISCUSSION QUESTIONS

1. To what extent is quality of care routinely and effectively measured in the United States?
2. Which organizations play key roles in obtaining ongoing assessments of quality in the United States? To what extent are their approaches similar?
3. What sources of information are best in class for developing process quality measures?
4. What are the major challenges to using outcomes as a basis for assessing quality?
5. How good is the quality of care in the United States?

FURTHER READING

Donabedian, A. (1980). *Explorations in quality assessment and monitoring. Vol. I: The definition of quality and approaches to its assessment.* Ann Arbor, MI: Health Administration Press.

This remains the classic, foundational reference on quality of care and is worth reading for its elegant argument and historical importance.

Institute of Medicine. (2001). *Crossing the quality chasm: A new health system for the 21st century.* Washington, DC: National Academy Press.

This report from the Institute of Medicine is another classic reference about quality that established a framework for viewing quality as multidimensional. This framework, though modified by subsequent IOM reports, continues to drive how many organizations approach quality measurement.

McGlynn, E. A., Asch, S. M., Adams, J., Keesey, J., Hicks J., DeCristofaro, A., & Kerr, E. A. (2003). The quality of health care delivered to adults in the United States. *New England Journal of Medicine*, *348*(26), 2635–2645.

This article is the most comprehensive assessment of quality of care in the United States that has been done to date. It is frequently referenced both in the academic literature and by organizations who are working to improve their own quality performance.

U.S. Department of Health and Human Services. (2011). *National healthcare quality report* (AHRQ Publication No. 11-0004). Rockville, MD: Agency for Healthcare Research and Quality.

This is the most recent congressionally mandated annual report from HHS about the state of quality of care in the United States. It pulls together data collected for a variety of reasons from several federal and other sources.

U.S. Department of Health and Human Services. (2011). *National healthcare disparities report* (AHRQ Publication No. 11-0004). Rockville, MD: Agency for Healthcare Research and Quality.

This is a congressionally mandated report that serves as a companion to the report on quality, providing an assessment of disparities in health and health care.

REFERENCES

Adams, J. L., Mehrotra, A., Thomas, J. W., & McGlynn, E. A. (2010). Physician cost profiling: Reliability and risk of misclassification. *New England Journal of Medicine*, *362*(11), 1014–1021.

Adams, J. L., McGlynn, E. A., Thomas, J. W., & Mehrotra, A. (2010). Incorporating statistical uncertainty in the use of physician cost profiles. *BMC Health Services Research*, *10*(1), 57.

Archampong, D., Borowski, D., Wille-Jorgensen, P., & Iversen, L. H. (2012). Workload and surgeon's specialty for outcome after colorectal cancer surgery (review). *Cochrane Database of Systematic Reviews*, *3*.

Bernstein, S., Fiske, M. E., McGlynn, E. A., & Gifford, D. S. (1997). *Hysterectomy: A review of the literature on indications, effectiveness, and risks* (MR-592/2-AHCPR). Santa Monica, CA: RAND Corporation.

Bernstein S. J., McGlynn, E. A., Siu, A. L., Roth, C. P., Sherwood, M. J., Keesey, J. W., . . . Brook, R. H. (1993). The appropriateness of hysterectomy: A comparison of care in seven health plans. *Journal of the American Medical Association*, *269*(18), 2398–2402.

Berwick, D. M., & Wald, D. L. (1990). Hospital leaders' opinions of the HCFA mortality data. *Journal of the American Medical Association*, *263*, 247–249.

Brennan, T. A., Horwitz, R. I., Duffy, F. D., Cassel, C. K., Goode, L. D., & Lipner, R. S. (2004). The role of physician specialty board certification status in the quality movement. *Journal of the American Medical Association*, *292*, 1038–1043.

Brook, R. H. (1994). The RAND/UCLA appropriateness method. In K. A. McCormick, S. R. Moore, & R. A. Siegel (Eds.), *Clinical practice guideline development: Methodology perspectives* (AHCPR Publication No. 95–0009). Rockville, MD: Agency for Health Care Policy and Research, Public Health Service, U.S. Department of Health and Human Services.

Centers for Disease Control and Prevention. (2012). *Deaths: Final data for 2009.* Retrieved from http://www.cdc.gov/nchs/data/dvs/deaths_2009_release.pdf

Central Intelligence Agency. (2012). *World fact book.* Retrieved from https://www.cia .gov/library/publications/download/index.html

Committee on Quality Health Care in America & Institute of Medicine. (2001). *Crossing the quality chasm: A new health system for the 21st century.* Washington, DC: National Academy Press.

Dimitrow, M. S., Airaksinen, M.S.A., Kivela, S-L., Lyles, A., & Leikola, S.N.S. (2011). Comparison of prescribing criteria to evaluate the appropriateness of drug treatment in individuals aged 65 and older: A systematic review. *Journal of the American Geriatrics Society, 59,* 1521–1530.

Donabedian, A. (1980). *Explorations in quality assessment and monitoring. Vol. I: The definition of quality and approaches to its assessment.* Ann Arbor, MI: Health Administration Press.

Eden, J., Levit, L., Berg, A., & Morton, S. (Eds.) (2011). *Finding what works in health care: Standards for systematic reviews.* Washington, DC: National Academies Press.

Fisher, E. S., Wennberg, J. E., Stukel, T. A., Skinner, J. S., Sharp, S. M., Freeman, J. L., & Gittlesohn, A. M. (2000). Associations among hospital capacity, utilization, and mortality of U.S. Medicare beneficiaries, controlling for sociodemographic factors. *Health Services Research, 34,* 1351–1362.

Fisher, E. S., Wennberg, D. E., Stukel, T. A., Gottlieb, D. J., Lucas, F. L., & Pinder, E. L. (2003a). The implications of regional variations in Medicare spending. Part 1: The content, quality, and accessibility of care. *Annals of Internal Medicine, 138,* 273–287.

Fisher, E. S., Wennberg, D. E., Stukel, T. A., Gottlieb, D. J., Lucas, F. L., & Pinder, E. L. (2003b). The implications of regional variations in Medicare spending. Part 2: Health outcomes and satisfaction with care. *Annals of Internal Medicine, 138,* 288–298.

Fleming, S. T., Hicks, L. L., & Bailey, R. C. (1995). Interpreting the Health Care Financing Administration's mortality statistics. *Medical Care, 33,* 186–201.

Flores, G. F., & the Committee on Pediatric Research. (2010). Racial and ethnic disparities in the health and health care of children. *Pediatrics, 125*(4), e979–e1020.

Galvin, R. S., & McGlynn, E. A. (2003). Using performance measurement to drive improvement: A road map for change. *Medical Care, 41*(1, Suppl.), I48–I60.

Gandjour, A., Bannenberg, A., & Lauterbach, K. W. (2003). Threshold volumes associated with higher survival in health care: A systematic review. *Medical Care, 41*(10), 1129–1141.

Graham, R., Mancher, M., Wolman, D. M., Greenfield, S., & Steinberg, E. (Eds.). (2011). *Clinical practice guidelines we can trust.* Washington, DC: National Academies Press.

Halm, E. A., Lee, C., & Chassin, M. R. (2002). Is volume related to outcome in health care? A systematic review and methodologic critique of the literature. *Annals of Internal Medicine, 137,* 511–520.

Hess, B. J., Weng, W., Holmboe, E. S., & Lipner, R. S. (2012). The association between physicians' cognitive skills and quality of diabetes care. *Academic Medicine, 87*(2), 157–164.

Hibbard, J. H., Slovic, P., Peters, E., & Finucane, M. L. (2002). Strategies for reporting health plan performance information to consumers: Evidence from controlled studies. *Health Services Research, 37,* 291–313.

Holmboe, E. S., Wang, Y., Meehan, T. P., Tate, J.P., Ho, S-Y., Starkey, K. S., & Lipner, R. S. (2008). Association between maintenance of certification examination scores and quality of care for Medicare beneficiaries. *Archives of Internal Medicine, 168*(13), 1396–1403.

Holmboe, E. W., Weng, W., Arnold, G. K., Kaplan, S. H., Normand, S-L., Greenfield, S., . . . Lipner, R. S. (2010). The comprehensive care project: Measuring physician performance in ambulatory practice. *Health Services Research, 45*(6 Pt 2), 1912–1933.

Horowitz, S. D., Miller, S. H., & Miles, P. V. (2004). Board certification and physician quality. *Medical Education, 38,* 10–11.

Hussey, P. S., de Vries, H., Romley, J., Wang, M. C., Chen, S. S., Shekelle, P. G., & McGlynn, E. A. (2009). A systematic review of health care efficiency measures. *Health Services Research, 44*(3), 784–805.

Iezzoni, L. I., Daley, J., Heeren, T., Foley, S. M., Hughes, J. S., Fisher E. S., . . . Coffman, G. A. (1994). Using administrative data to screen hospitals for high complication rates. *Inquiry, 31,* 40–55.

Jeffe, D. B., & Andriole, D. A. (2011). Factors associated with American Board of Medical Specialties member board certification among U.S. medical school graduates. *Journal of the American Medical Association, 306*(9), 961–970.

Jha, A. K., Joynt, K. E., Orav, E. J., & Epstein, A. M. (2012). The long-term effect of premier pay for performance on patient outcomes. *New England Journal of Medicine, 366*(17), 1606–1615.

The Joint Commission. (2011). *Improving America's hospitals: The Joint Commission's annual report on quality and safety.* Chicago: Author. Retrieved from www.joint commission.org/2011_annual_report

Kaushal, R., Shojania, K. G., & Bates, D. W. (2003). Effects of computerized physician order entry and clinical decision support systems on medication safety: A systematic review. *Archives of Internal Medicine, 163,* 1409–1416.

Kerr, E. A., McGlynn, E. A., Adams, J., Keesey, J., & Asch, S. M. (2004). Profiling the quality of care in 12 communities: Results from the CQI study. *Health Affairs, 23,* 247–256.

Koppel, R., Metlay, J. P., Cohen, A., Abaluck, B., Localio, A. R., Kimmel, S. E., & Strom, B. L. (2005). Role of computerized physician order entry systems in facilitating medication errors. *Journal of the American Medical Association, 293,* 1197–1203.

Kravitz, R. L., Laouri, M., Kahan, J. P., Guzy, P., Sherman, T., Hilborne, L., & Brook, R. H. (1995). Validity of criteria used for detecting underuse of coronary revascularization. *Journal of the American Medical Association, 274*(8), 632–638.

Lawson, E. H., Gibbons, M. M., Ingraham, A. M., Shekelle, P. G., & Ko, C. Y. (2011). Appropriateness criteria used to assess variations in surgical procedure use in the United States. *Archives of Surgery, 146*(12), 1433–1440.

Leape, L. L., Hilborne, L. H., Park, R. E., Bernstein, S. J., Kamberg, C. J., Sherwood, M., . . . Brook, R. H. (1993). The appropriateness of use of coronary artery bypass graft surgery in New York state. *Journal of the American Medical Association, 269,* 753–760.

Lewis, N. (2011). Hospitals lag in computerized physician order entry. *Information Week.* Retrieved from http://www.informationweek.com/news/healthcare/CPOE /231500041

McGinnis, J. M., Williams-Russo, P., & Knickman, J. R. (2002). The case for more active policy attention to health promotion. *Health Affairs, 21,* 78–93.

McGlynn, E. A. (2003). Selecting common measures of quality and system performance. *Medical Care, 41*(Suppl.), I39–I47.

McGlynn, E.A., Asch, S. M., Adams, J., Keesey, J., Hicks J., DeCristofaro, A., & Kerr, E. A. (2003). The quality of health care delivered to adults in the United States. *New England Journal of Medicine, 348*(26), 2635–2645.

National Committee on Quality Assurance. (2011). *Continuous improvement and the expansion of health care quality: The state of health care quality, 2011.* Washington, DC: Author.

Peterson, E. D., Coombs, L. P., DeLong, E. R., Haan, C. K., & Ferguson, T. B. (2004). Procedural volume as a marker of quality for CABG surgery. *Journal of the American Medical Association, 291,* 195–201.

Ricciardi, R., Virnig, B. A., Ogilvie, J. W., Dahlberg, P. S., Selker, H. S., Baxter, N. N. (2008). Volume-outcome relationship for coronary artery bypass grafting in an era of decreasing volume. *Archives of Surgery, 143*(4), 338–344.

Rogowski, J. A., Horbar, J. D., Staiger, D. O., Kenny, M., Carpenter, J., & Geppert, J. (2004). Indirect vs. direct hospital quality indicators for very low-birth-weight infants. *Journal of the American Medical Association, 291,* 202–209.

Sanmartin, C., Murphy, K., Choptain, N., Conner-Spady, B., McLaren, L., Bohm, E., . . . Noseworthy, T. (2008). Appropriateness of healthcare interventions: Concepts and scoping of the published literature. *International Journal of Technology Assessment in Health Care, 24*(3), 342–349.

Schmaltz, S.P., Williams, S. C., Chassin, M. R., Loeb, J. M., & Wachter, R. M. (2011). Hospital performance trends on national quality measures and the association with Joint Commission accreditation. *Journal of Hospital Medicine, 6*(8), 454–461.

Scholle, S. H., Roski, J., Adams, J. L., Dunn, D. L., Kerr, E. A., Dugan, D. P., & Jense, R. E. (2008). Benchmarking physician performance: Reliability of individual and composite measures. *American Journal of Managed Care, 14*(12), 833–838.

Selim, A. J., Berlowitz, D., Kazis, L. E., Rogers, W., Wright, S. M., Qian, S. X., . . . Fincke, B. G. (2010). Comparison of health outcomes for male seniors in the Veterans Health Administration and Medicare Advantage plans. *Health Services Research, 45*(2), 376–396.

Shekelle, P. G., Chassin, M. R., & Park, R. E. (1998a). Assessing the predictive validity of the RAND/UCLA appropriateness method criteria for performing carotid endarterectomy. *International Journal of Technology Assessment in Health Care, 14,* 707–727.

Shekelle, P. G., Kahan, J. P., Bernstein, S. J., Leape, L. L., Kamberg, C. J., & Park, R. E. (1998b). The reproducibility of a method to identify the overuse and underuse of medical procedures. *New England Journal of Medicine, 338,* 1888–1895.

Smedley, B. D., Stith, A. Y., & Nelson, A. R. (Eds.). (2003). *Unequal treatment: Confronting racial and ethnic disparities in health.* Washington, DC: National Academies Press.

Ulmer, C., Bruno, M., & Burke, S. (Eds.). (2010). Future directions for the national healthcare quality and disparities reports. Committee on Future Directions for the National Healthcare Quality and Disparities Reports, Board on Health Care Services. Washington, DC: National Academies Press.

U.S. Department of Health and Human Services. (2011a). *National healthcare quality report* (AHRQ Publication No. 11-0004). Rockville, MD: Agency for Healthcare Research and Quality.

U.S. Department of Health and Human Services. (2011b). *National healthcare disparities report* (AHRQ Publication No. 11-0005). Rockville, MD: Agency for Healthcare Research and Quality.

CHAPTER THIRTEEN

PUBLIC RELEASE OF INFORMATION ON QUALITY

Elizabeth A. McGlynn
John L. Adams

Learning Objectives

- Identify leading sources of public information about quality across different entities and gaps in information availability
- Understand key methodological issues in constructing public reports of performance
- Understand how the design of public reports on quality affects their use
- Learn about the effects of public reporting on consumer choice of health plans and providers and the effects on quality improvement

Information about the quality of care delivered by entities in the health care system—health plans, hospitals, nursing homes, medical groups, and physicians—is becoming more routinely available. Although it remains easier to find out how well a variety of consumer products are likely to perform than it is to determine the probability that a specific physician or hospital will deliver evidence-based medicine, significant progress is being made. Publicly available information on quality (or, more broadly, performance) may be used by consumers and payers to choose among health plans, hospitals, and physicians, and by providers to improve their performance (Berwick, James, & Coye, 2003). The motivation for improvement may be professional (providers want to perform at the top of the class), financial (incentives or disincentives tied to level of performance), or regulatory (reaching a baseline level of performance required to stay in business).

Changes in the organization and financing of care have also increased concern about variation in quality. In the unrestricted-choice model characterized by fee for service, individual providers were accountable for ensuring the delivery of high-quality health care. Physicians were trusted to be effective advocates for their patients' needs. However, as third-party purchasers and their agents began to use financial incentives to control costs and restrict choices, the perception (if not the reality) was that physicians could no longer act solely in the patient's interest. High-deductible plans with catastrophic insurance (also known as consumer-directed health plans) are intended to make consumers more aware of differences among providers in the cost and quality of care.

Rising health care costs that appear to threaten the viability of the American economy have caused private and public purchasers to ask for evidence that they are getting good value for their money. These questions have been stimulated in part by evidence that serious deficits in quality exist. For example, the Institute of Medicine highlighted the problem of medical errors in hospitals and estimated that as many as ninety-eight thousand people die each year as a result of such errors (Kohn, Corrigan, & Donaldson, 1999). A national study of the quality of medical care delivered found that American adults receive only 55 percent of recommended care for the leading causes of death, disability, and utilization (McGlynn et al., 2003) and that children receive 47 percent of recommended ambulatory care (Mangione-Smith et al., 2007).

Taken together, these concerns and challenges lead to calls for more transparency about the performance of the health care system. The purpose of this chapter is to (1) describe the type of information that is currently being publicly released, (2) discuss some of the methodological issues that arise in producing information for public release, and (3) summarize what is known about the use of information on quality for selection and quality improvement.

Public Information on Quality

The Health Care Financing Administration (the predecessor agency to the Centers for Medicare and Medicaid Services) released data on mortality rates by hospital among Medicare beneficiaries in the early 1980s. Criticisms about the methodology led to the discontinuation of those reports. The next major effort in public reporting was undertaken by the National Committee for Quality Assurance (NCQA) which developed a system for reporting on health plan quality in the 1990s. Today, the breadth and depth of information about quality that is publicly available varies by type of entity. The Patient Protection and Affordable Care Act of 2010 (ACA) has both greatly accelerated the number of entities for which public quality reports are required and has formalized a progression of approaches from *voluntary reporting* to *mandatory reporting*, from *pay-for-reporting* to *pay-for-performance*, and finally *value-based purchasing*. In this section, we discuss some of the key reports available publicly for several entities.

Health Plans

NCQA is responsible for the widespread availability of information on health plan *performance*. NCQA annually collects and reports information on selected *processes* and outcomes of care, patient experiences with care, and accreditation. Most report cards on health plan performance are based primarily, or solely, on the NCQA measures.

Health plans report their performance to NCQA using standardized specifications contained in a reporting system known as the Healthcare Effectiveness Data and Information Set (HEDIS). For HEDIS 2012, plans were asked to report on their performance in calendar year 2011 on seventy-six measures in eight domains. In 2011, more than one thousand health plans reported data for public release (National Committee for Quality Assurance, 2011).

NCQA also collects and reports information on patients' experiences with care using a standardized survey known as the Consumer Assessment of Healthcare Providers and Systems (CAHPS) (Crofton, Lubalin, & Darby, 1999). The survey, initially developed by RAND, Harvard, and RTI under a cooperative agreement with the Agency for Healthcare Research and Quality (AHRQ), is fielded by independent vendors on behalf of participating health plans. Surveys are returned directly to the vendor, which prepares the results and sends the data to NCQA. The results can be reported as either single-item ratings (health plan, personal doctor or nurse, or all health care) or multiple-item composites (getting needed care, getting care quickly, courteous and helpful office staff, customer service, and claims processing). There are versions of health plan CAHPS for enrollees in commercial, Medicare, and Medicaid plans.

NCQA also accredits managed care plans using a set of standards that cover structural dimensions of the organization as well as indicators of performance based on a subset of HEDIS and CAHPS results. NCQA reports the overall accreditation outcome as excellent, commendable, accredited, provisional, or denied. *Accreditation* is also reported in consumer-oriented categories (access and service, qualified providers, staying healthy, getting better, and living with illness), using one to four stars. Both types of accreditation results are available on the NCQA website (www.ncqa.org). Users can construct their own report card for a specific geographic area using the aggregate categories. Some detail about performance on select chronic disease indicators in the living-with-illness category is also available on the website. Additional detail on other measures is available in NCQA's commercial product, Quality Compass.

NCQA partners with *Consumer Reports* to provide health plan rankings for HMOs, PPOs, and POS plans to their subscribers. In 2011, 830 plans in all fifty states and the District of Columbia were ranked. To arrive at the rankings, information was combined on multiple measures in four categories: enrollee satisfaction, prevention, treatment and accreditation. Prior to the *Consumer Reports* collaboration, NCQA and *U.S. News & World Report* annually produced "America's Best Health Plans" (2009), parallel to the annual report on hospitals. The top fifty commercial, twenty-five Medicare, and twenty-five Medicaid plans were listed in the magazine. Complete rankings on all health plans were reported on the website (www.usnews.com/healthplans), along with a listing of health plans that did not participate in HEDIS or NCQA accreditation.

The Centers for Medicare and Medicaid Services (CMS) introduced the Five-Star Quality Rating System in 2008 to help Medicare beneficiaries choose among Medicare Advantage plans. For the Medicare-eligible population enrolled in managed care, this system takes many of the CAHPS and HEDIS measures, along with other measures from NCQA, and presents them in a unified format. Plans are given ratings of one to five stars, with five being the best. Beneficiaries can use the CMS website (www.cms.gov) to compare plans in their geographic area. Beginning in 2010, CMS piloted a financial incentive program attached to performance on Medicare STAR measures. Bonuses for all Medicare Advantage plans are being phased in starting in 2012.

Hospitals

Beginning late in 2003, information on how hospitals performed on a set of clinical quality measures was released publicly by CMS (www.hospitalcompare.hhs.gov). The Joint Commission (TJC) released its first public report in July 2004 (www.qualitycheck.org). National data on ten measures of clinical quality were released by CMS in November 2004 through the efforts of a consortium called the Hospital Quality Alliance (HQA). Although public reporting among hospitals began as a voluntary effort, the Medicare Prescription Drug, Improvement, and Modernization Act of 2003 (which introduced prescription drug coverage for Medicare enrollees for the first time) added a financial incentive for hospitals to participate (the Hospital Inpatient Quality Reporting Program). Hospitals that reported the ten measures publicly in FY 2005 were eligible to receive a 0.4 percent annual reimbursement update. In FY 2006, hospitals that did not report and meet a set of data exchange and validation requirements received a reduction of 0.4 percent in their annual payment update; the reduction for nonreporting subsequently increased to two percentage points. Virtually all eligible hospitals were participating by FY 2005. Beginning in October 2012, Hospital Compare will include new surgical outcomes measures submitted on a voluntary basis by hospitals participating in the American College of Surgeon's National Surgical Quality Improvement Program database (ACS NSQIP®).

In addition to information available to consumers on the CMS and TJC websites, insurers and large employers purchase reports on hospital quality performance from a number of private vendors. The results are generally made available through an insurance company portal or employer portal and may be the information most routinely seen by employed and insured populations. Most of these report cards depend on publicly available measures and data as their source, most notably the quality indicators (QIs) from AHRQ (www.qualityindicators.ahrq.gov). The QIs cover prevention (for example, evidence of hospital admissions that could have been avoided through better outpatient management), quality of inpatient care (mortality rate by condition and procedure), and patient safety (avoidable complications and iatrogenic events).

At the state level, hospital mortality rates have been released for coronary artery bypass graft (CABG) surgery. Perhaps the leading example of this is New York State's Cardiac Reporting System, which releases risk-adjusted, in-hospital mortality rates for CABG surgery for all hospitals in New York. The Pennsylvania Health Care Cost Containment Council has also released public information on risk-adjusted, in-hospital mortality rates for the same surgery. The Pacific Business Group on Health (PBGH) led development of the California Coronary Artery Bypass Graft (CABG) Surgery Mortality Reporting Program, which released its first report in 2001 on 79 of the 118 hospitals that perform the surgery; hospitals voluntarily participated in the program (the New York and Pennsylvania efforts were mandatory). In 2001, the California state legislature mandated all hospitals to report their mortality rate following CABG surgery annually to the state Office of Statewide Health Planning and Development. The most recent report was released in 2009. PBGH has also released data on risk-adjusted mortality rates following various transplant procedures for hospitals in California.

Accreditation status represents another type of information publicly available on hospital quality. TJC is responsible for conducting hospital accreditation in the United States. Hospitals that wish to serve Medicare beneficiaries must obtain accreditation, which means most hospitals in the United States seek it. The methods used by TJC to make accreditation decisions changed in 2004 with the adoption of the Shared Visions–New Pathways initiative (http://www.medscape.com/viewarticle/482384). One innovative aspect of this new approach is the tracer methodology. On-site surveyors select a patient from the list of those currently in the hospital and follow the person's experience through the entire stay, from admission through current status. On average, about eleven patient tracers are selected during the weeklong visit. Following the patient through the hospital process gives surveyors a different view of how well the various systems and procedures are operating within a hospital. As of 2011, approximately 4,168 general, children's, long-term acute, psychiatric, rehabilitation, and specialty hospitals are accredited, and 378 critical access hospitals are accredited through a separate program. Approximately 82 percent of the nation's hospitals are currently accredited by TJC.

In the popular press, perhaps the most familiar report card on hospitals is *U.S. News & World Report's* annual issue on "America's Best Hospitals" (www.health.usnews.com/best-hospitals). Introduced in 1990, these reports have been produced since 2005 by RTI. In 2009 a patient safety dimension was incorporated. The magazine examines four major aspects of performance in developing its rankings: reputation, mortality rate, patient safety, and nursing and patient services. Annual surveys by the American Hospital Association are one of the data sources used. Rankings are calculated for all hospitals in each of sixteen specialty areas (cancer; cardiology and heart surgery; diabetes and endocrinology; ear, nose, and throat; gastroenterology; geriatrics; gynecology; nephrology; neurology and neurosurgery; ophthalmology; orthopedics; psychiatry; pulmonology; rehabilitation; rheumatology; and urology). Separate rankings of children's hospitals have been produced since 2007. An Index of Hospital Quality (IHQ) is calculated for each hospital in twelve of the specialty areas. Reputation scores are based on a survey of 4,100 board-certified physicians who are asked to rank the top five hospitals in the nation in their specialty (results are averaged for the most recent three years). Mortality scores are based on the ratio of observed to expected risk-adjusted mortality rates from Medicare data. The safety measure is based on AHRQ's patient safety indicators. The final category is composed of a variety of structural elements: whether the hospital is a member of the Council of Teaching Hospitals, availability of high-technology services, medical and surgical volume, nurse-to-patient ratio, availability of a state-certified trauma center and the level of that center, patient-community services index, availability of geriatric services, availability of obstetric care and birthing rooms, medical and surgical intensive-care beds, hospice and palliative care, National Cancer Institute designated cancer center, nurse magnet facility, and epilepsy center certification. The weights for combining these structural elements into a score for each specialty are based on factor analysis. Each of the four major components is assigned a factor analytic weight in determining the final overall ranking for each specialty. Notably, the safety component has a much lower weight than the other major components (approximately 5 percent of the combined score).

Medical Groups

As information on quality has become more systematically available, interest in having such information at the medical group level has increased. Many consumers do not understand the role health plans play in ensuring provision of high-quality care and would prefer information closer to the point of service delivery. This is particularly true in states such as California and Massachusetts where medical groups are a dominant form of physician organization and many medical groups contract with multiple health plans.

The state of California produces report cards on 212 medical groups that contract with the nine largest commercial HMOs in California. The report cards include seventeen quality measures reflecting national standards of care and five patient survey measures of care experience. The results are presented in categories (excellent, good, fair, and poor). Numeric results are also available (using bar graphs) for the individual items that make up the categorical results. Reports are available on a website (reportcard.opa.ca.gov/rc2013) that also includes reports on health plans and hospitals in California.

Minnesota initiated a statewide reporting system on medical groups in 2004. In 2010, the Minnesota legislature required providers to report on quality measures. For medical groups, performance is assessed in fourteen clinical areas. The measures are technical process and outcomes measures based on guidelines from the Institute for Clinical Systems Improvement. The results are presented graphically with the point estimate and 95 percent confidence interval; comparisons to performance across all medical groups are also provided. The website includes information for consumers about what they can do to improve their health in the target area as well as the role their provider plays (www.mnhealthscores.org).

Massachusetts Health Quality Partners has also developed a statewide medical group reporting system based on the HEDIS measure set. Data supplied by the five largest commercial plans in Massachusetts are used to calculate the scores. The results are displayed using one to four stars; one star indicates the group had a sufficient number of patients eligible for the measure to report (thirty minimum), and each additional star reflects performance that is better than each of three benchmark comparisons (the national average of health plans reporting to NCQA, the ninetieth percentile of health plans reporting to NCQA, and the statewide average of providers reporting to MHQP). Consumers can access the group scores via the web (www.mhqp.org). In addition, MHQP partnered with *Consumer Reports* in 2012 to produce rankings of physician groups on patient experience measures using the CAHPS instrument designed for medical groups. The results are published in a special issue of *Consumer Reports*. Minnesota and Wisconsin have now also produced reports on medical groups in collaboration with *Consumer Reports*.

In 2007, AHRQ created the Chartered Value Exchanges program, which brought together twenty-four communities to collaborate on quality improvement and transparency initiatives. In a related effort, the Robert Wood Johnson Foundation's Aligning Forces for Quality promoted *transparency* and public reporting as a mechanism for quality improvement. As a result of these efforts, Oregon, Washington, and Ohio have also produced reports on medical group quality.

In 2010, the Society of Thoracic Surgeons partnered with *Consumer Reports* to rate 363 cardiac surgical groups in forty-two states. The measures include risk-adjusted thirty-day mortality rates, complication rates, whether patients receive recommended medications, and whether they get at least one optimal surgical graft. The reports are available to subscribers of *Consumer Reports.* Performance is displayed on the website and in one issue of the magazine using one to three stars.

Physicians

Consumers are probably most interested in the quality of individual physicians, but little information is publicly available at this level. Most of the reports on individual physicians have been developed for internal use by health plans or medical groups as part of determining compensation. Risk-adjusted mortality rates following CABG surgery were one of the first physician-level reports produced, and these are mandated in California, Massachusetts, New York, and Pennsylvania.

NCQA has developed voluntary programs for recognizing provider performance in four areas: diabetes, heart and stroke, physician office practice, and primary care medical home. A new program recognizing specialists' participation in care coordination activities that parallels the primary care medical home recognition program is expected in March 2013. The Diabetes Physician Recognition Program requires physicians seeking recognition to complete an application and abstract data on twenty-five patients from medical records or administrative databases on eleven diabetes process and outcome measures. The Heart/Stroke Recognition Program is cosponsored by the American Heart Association and American Stroke Association and contains five clinical measures. The Physician Practice Connections Program recognizes physicians who have systems in place to offer evidence-based medicine, provide patient education and support, and manage the care of patients with complex issues. There are nine modules in which assessments are conducted; recognition is furnished for participating in any module. For all of the recognition programs, physicians who have successfully met the thresholds established by NCQA are recognized on the NCQA website with a seal. NCQA has developed collaborative arrangements with the American Boards of Internal Medicine and Family Practice to enable physicians participating in recognition programs to get some credit or to use data to meet maintenance of certification requirements.

Report Cards on Other Entities

The Centers for Medicare and Medicaid Services (CMS) have developed report cards on nursing homes, home health, and dialysis centers. The ACA established programs for several other entities including rehabilitation hospitals, cancer specialty hospitals, inpatient psychiatric facilities, hospital outpatient facilities, ambulatory surgical centers, and hospice. Because the approaches are similar, we focus here on just a few entities.

Nursing Homes

The CMS report card on nursing homes, which was introduced late in 1998, can be found at www.medicare.gov/NursingHomeCompare. Originally, the report card had mostly descriptive information; quality measures were added in 2002. The results are based on data collected on all nursing home residents at specific intervals during their stay. The website has a search tool that enables the user to identify nursing homes by state, county, city, zip code, or name. The report card gives general information about the nursing home, such as whether it participates in Medicare, how many beds are certified, whether the owner is a nonprofit or for-profit corporation, whether it is located in a hospital or part of a chain, and whether there are resident and family councils. The report card displays performance ratings overall, as well as for the three components (health inspection, staffing, and quality measures) using the Five-Star approach, which was introduced in December 2008. Performance on five quality measures for short-stay patients and thirteen measures for long-stay patients is available in both table and graphic forms; the graphs include average performance in the state and the nation. There is additional detail on deficiencies, including the date the deficiency was corrected, the level of harm (on a four-point scale), and the number of residents affected (few, some, or many).

Dialysis Facilities

CMS makes Dialysis Facility Compare available on its website (http://www .medicare.gov/dialysisfacilitycompare/). Three quality measures are available: control of anemia, adequacy of hemodialysis, and patient survival (actual versus expected). In addition, there is information about the facility (address, date of initial Medicare certification, whether evening appointments are available, number of treatment stations, types of dialysis offered, facility ownership type, and performance on the value-based purchasing initiative). The quality results are displayed on a bar graph and compare facility performance to that in the state overall and the nation. The data in the report are about two years old.

Home Health Agencies

CMS reports on the performance of home health agencies at www .medicare.gov/homehealthcompare. Agencies can be identified by state and/or zip code. The top level provides information on whether agencies offer services in each of six areas: nursing, physical therapy, occupational therapy, speech therapy, medical social services, and home health aides. Twenty-two measures in five domains of quality are included in the report: managing daily activities, managing pain and treating symptoms, treating wounds and preventing pressure sores, preventing harm, and preventing unplanned hospital care. Patient experiences in five areas are also reported. Information on state and national average performance is provided in both the tables and graphs. The data in the report are fairly current, with about a six-month lag between the reporting period (which is displayed on the website) and the current date.

Some Methodological Issues in Performance Reporting

Current report cards vary along a number of dimensions, reflecting lack of agreement on (or lack of attention to) how best to communicate information to various audiences. CMS is notable for having developed a fairly standard format for the reports it produces. However, the proliferation of report cards in different formats, along with evidence that the methodological choices made are likely to influence how the information is received and used, underscore the need to use greater rigor in developing these tools. We discuss here a number of methodological issues that are likely to be encountered (explicitly or implicitly) by report card developers and what is known about the importance of some of these issues.

Number of Measures

As the amount of information collected on quality performance expands, attention shifts to how this information can be meaningfully transmitted to consumers. Both methodological and communications issues arise and interact. Cognitive psychology affords some insight into the amount of information humans can use in making a decision. Typically, five to seven "bits" of information are the maximum that can be held in short-term memory and incorporated into a single decision. Thus, minimizing the amount of information on a report card facilitates use by the intended audience. However, a single number about performance (for example, overall hospital mortality or mortality following CABG surgery) may not be adequate to characterize all the important decision dimensions for consumers. Further, most studies of quality that examine multiple dimensions of performance find considerable heterogeneity in the results, suggesting that the user needs to be cautious in drawing inferences about the relationship between performance in the area reported and performance in an unreported area (Asch et al., 2004). This balancing act between offering enough information but not too much continues to be debated among those producing report cards. Making information available on the Internet offers an opportunity for individuals to tailor results to their decision. High-level aggregate results can be displayed on the first page of a website, and then users can seek additional detail relevant to their own circumstances on subsequent pages. CMS has taken this approach in designing its web-based report cards.

Display of Results

Report cards present results in a variety of formats, including giving results on individual performance measures versus summary scores for multiple measures. Some present both summary scores and individual results, as CMS and the California Office of the Patient Advocate do. A review of the literature on decision making suggests strongly that the scale approach is preferable because it serves the purpose of reducing the amount of information that consumers must consider in making a decision (Hibbard, Slovic, & Jewett, 1997). The authors note that there is an apparent contradiction between the amount of information people can typically use in making a decision and the desire frequently expressed by consumers for more information.

A study by one of those authors yielded an interesting insight into this conflict (Slovic, 1982). Handicappers for horse races were given the option of selecting five to forty variables from among eighty-eight possible to predict the winners of horse races. Their confidence in prediction increased with the number of variables, but their accuracy did not improve. The handicappers were as accurate in predicting results with five variables as they were with forty; as the number of variables increased, the level of consistency decreased. The authors of the review article conclude that "the approach of giving consumers the maximum amount of information is not the most effective path to informed consumer choice" (Hibbard et al., 1997). Further, they report that in focus groups consumers "commonly respond that they find the information overwhelming and confusing and that they do not know how to bring all the pieces of information together into a decision" (Hibbard et al., 1997). In these focus groups, consumers were looking at report cards with about twenty measures or pieces of information (plan characteristics) on them; in some cases, as many as thirty-eight plans were included.

Research on approaches to displaying information reveals that the type of presentation can affect both the interpretation of results and the relative weight placed on multiple dimensions (Hibbard, Slovic, Peters, & Finucane, 2002). The authors found that adding visual cues about performance (stars, stacked bar with stars, and so on) increased the weight placed on quality results compared to report cards without evaluation signals. Similarly, ordering plans according to quality performance increased the weight consumers placed on this dimension in choosing among health plans. They also found that if people were given information on time trends in performance, they weighted positive trends (improvement) more highly than the absolute level of current performance. Finally, in this experiment, the authors found that participants had difficulty consistently weighting multiple performance measures in their choices and were unaware of the influence that data display had on their decision.

Credibility of Data Source

One of the challenges for public reporting is the credibility of the data source. Users may be suspicious of information that is produced by the entity being evaluated. For example, a study of employer responses to a report card produced by a medical center found that 45 percent thought the report was hospital advertising (Longo, 2004). Among consumers seeing the report, 30 percent thought it was hospital advertising or public relations. Consumers, however, were more likely than employers to report that the information was useful in decision making.

Two approaches are commonly used to enhance the credibility of the information. In some cases, a third party collects and analyzes the data. This is true for TJC and NCQA accreditation and for the consumer surveys used by NCQA (CAHPS). The other approach is to audit the performance data. NCQA requires that HEDIS results, based on plans' analyses of their own administrative and medical record data, be audited by an outside group certified to perform this function. Auditors essentially look at both the integrity of the process used to produce the result and the reproducibility of the results in determining whether the information is accurate.

Risk Adjustment

For comparisons between entities to be fair, the data must be adequately adjusted for differences in the populations receiving services; this is known as risk or case-mix adjustment. A number of issues related to *risk adjustment* should arise when results are used to make comparison among entities. First, in this application there is often lack of clarity around the factors that should be adjusted for. For quality measurement, the key question is whether the factor inherently causes quality differences (for instance, people who have comorbid heart failure are more likely to die from a heart attack) or whether that factor is associated with quality differences but neither clinically nor biologically causes the difference (as with socioeconomic characteristics). Adjusting for the second type of factor can mask important differences in quality for subpopulations. Second, one must consider the adequacy of the data source for representing the factors of interest. For example, in New York state, a comparison of administrative versus clinical data concluded that clinical data were superior, largely due to the importance of three clinical factors in predicting cardiac surgical outcomes (ejection fraction, reoperation, and 90 percent occlusion of the left main trunk) that were available only in the clinical dataset (Hannan, Kilburn, Lindsey, & Lewis, 1992). The adequacy of data sources varies considerably by the type of measure, with no single source being adequate for all dimensions of performance. Third, one must consider whether application of risk-adjustment methods significantly changes the conclusion one is likely to draw. The methods themselves are complex and create additional challenges for communicating results; if no significant differences are found, the complexity may not be justifiable.

Outcome data are more likely to require risk adjustment than process measures because a larger number of factors that contribute to observed performance are outside the control of the organization being evaluated (McGlynn, 1998). The reports on hospital mortality have paid the greatest attention to risk-adjustment issues. Process measures may require adjustment less often because the criteria used to define eligibility for an indicator generally exclude individuals for whom the process is not indicated. However, clinical data sources are better than others at excluding inappropriate candidates on the basis of comorbid conditions or other clinical considerations. Patient-reported information may be necessary to capture preferences, including refusals. Attention has also been given to the role of case-mix adjustment with patient experience measures (Zaslavsky, Zaborski, & Cleary, 2000).

Missing Data

In our previous work on developing reporting strategies, we considered a number of potential solutions to handling missing data (McGlynn, Adams, Hicks, & Klein, 1999a). These issues are particularly important if one is developing scales (groups of measures), but some of the same issues may arise if one is reporting performance on single items. Reports based on surveys routinely face this issue because respondents may not answer all questions. One always has the option of noting nonresponse (NR) for entities that do not report on one or more measures, but it may be difficult for consumers to compare NR with an actual performance result. For this reason, we prefer some type of imputation strategy. Three are summarized here.

Mean imputation takes the average value of all entities that have reported on a measure and assigns this average to entities whose results were missing for the measure. Imputing the mean value maintains the mean of the observed values and is a conservative approach suggesting that in the absence of other information we assume an entity's performance is average.

Regression imputation is a more sophisticated approach to imputing the means because it uses more information to estimate what the entity's performance might have been, given other characteristics (for example, number of enrollees or profit status) or performance on other measures. This method is likely to estimate a missing value closer to the true performance than simple mean imputation. There are also more modern methods of imputation (for instance, multiple imputation) used in statistical analysis. Their failure to be adopted for performance reporting may be a consequence of organizations not having staffs that are accustomed to using these methods as well as the difficulty in explaining these complex methods to lay audiences.

We can also impute zero, or the lowest observed value, for entities not reporting results. Both represent a more punitive approach to dealing with missing data. In previous work, we used the lowest observed value because it represented real performance (compared with zero, which is unlikely) and because most entities that report results could likely outperform the worst entity. This approach, which may be most useful in voluntary reporting programs, is designed to encourage complete reporting by penalizing entities that fail to report.

Report cards that present summary scales must choose an imputation method. Because the method used is likely to affect the results, it would be preferable for report card developers to indicate the method they used to deal with missing data. Most report cards are not explicit about the methods used to address problems with missing data.

Aggregation Issues

A number of other analytic issues arise in constructing aggregate or composite scales. Conclusions can vary with the choices in these areas.

Choosing an Organizing Framework. There are two strategies for creating a framework. The first approach, which might be called "bottom-up," starts with the individual measures that are available and creates summary categories that maximize the number of measures used. This can be done quantitatively, using factor analysis or other methods designed to identify patterns in data, or it can be done qualitatively by obtaining expert opinion.

The second approach, which might be called "top-down," starts with the information that potential users would like to have to make decisions and identifies measures that communicate the desired information. The Institute of Medicine framework is frequently used (Committee on Quality Health Care in America, 2001; Ulmer, Bruno, & Burke, 2010). The methods for identifying what information the target audience wants may include surveys, focus groups, or semistructured interviews.

The bottom-up approach is more frequently associated with research or decision analysis. This approach has the advantage of trying to use all available information. Since the approach is empirically driven, another advantage is the opportunity to identify patterns in data that might otherwise escape notice. The disadvantage of this approach, particularly if done quantitatively (say, using factor analysis), is that it may produce results that are difficult to interpret and not valued by the intended audience. In analyzing Medicare plan performance data using factor analysis, we found some of the resulting categories impossible to interpret (McGlynn, Adams, Hicks, & Klein, 1999b).

The top-down approach is more audience-sensitive because it identifies attributes that are important to those making a decision. Because decision makers generally come to a task with some questions already in mind, an optimal top-down approach organizes information into categories that respond to the questions on the mind of the potential user. The disadvantage of this approach is that there may be categories of interest to decision makers for which few measures currently exist.

Scaling. Individual measures that are combined to create summary categories may have differing means and variances. This potentially presents a problem for scaling in that it can permit some measures to have a greater (or lesser) effect on the results because of their distributional properties.

Standardization is a simple calculation, but it is frequently misunderstood owing to its similarity to related statistical calculations. The idea is to transform item scores so that entities are ranked on a comparable scale across items. This prevents an item with a large range (say, 0 to 100) from completely dominating an item with a small range (say, 0 to 1). A common form of standardization is to divide scores by the standard deviation of the entity scores.

The benefit of standardization is that it simplifies comparing items and understanding the meaning of weights applied to those items. The standard deviation scale makes using a simple rule of thumb based on the normal distribution easy; thinking of a standard deviation increase of one in each item is often easier than comparing a 35-point increase on a 100-point scale with a .012 increase in a dichotomous variable.

Weights. A basic starting point in constructing new scales is to give each measure in a scale equal weight. This implies that every element of the scale is equally important in arriving at a summary assessment. For many performance measures, this assumption of equal importance is at odds with both consumer and expert assessments of the measures. In previous work, we considered six options for weighting measures within scales (McGlynn et al., 1999a):

1. *Equal weights.* We start with equal weights as the base case since it is the option requiring the least judgment and offers a convenient method for evaluating the effect of other weighting methods on the results. All alternative weight schemes should be compared to the results on the basis of equal weights.
2. *Consumer weights.* A second option would be to ask consumers to assign weights to measures. This could be done either by surveying consumers to establish standardized weights for printed publications or by establishing an interactive mechanism that allows each individual to assign weights reflecting his or her own preferences.

3. *Expert weights.* Under this approach, experts assign weights according to their assessment of the relative importance of the measured process. Importance may be determined relative to the effect on outcomes, or it may reflect expert assessment of what is important to consumers. This is the approach used in NCQA's Diabetes Physician Recognition Program.

4. *Population weights.* Under this approach, measures are assigned a weight that reflects the proportion of the population eligible for the service represented by the measure. Importance is established on the basis of the number of people to whom the measure might be relevant.

5. *Factor weights.* If a factor-analytic approach was used to construct the reporting framework, one could use the resulting factor weights in creating aggregate scales. This is the approach used by *U.S. News & World Report* for hospital performance on the technology scale.

6. *Clinical importance weights.* This approach would adopt a particular outcome (such as mortality or quality-adjusted life years) and develop weights that quantify the effect of the measures on the outcome. Values could be obtained from the literature or expert assessment.

Assessing the Reliability of Performance Measures

Reliability is a characterization of the suitability of a measure for profiling. It describes how well one can confidently distinguish the performance of one provider from another (Scholle et al., 2008; Hofer et al., 1999). The reliability of a performance measure can be studied for different levels of a system. For example, a performance measure can have different reliabilities at the physician, hospital, or plan level. Conceptually, it is the ratio of signal to noise. The signal in this case is the proportion of the variability in measured performance that can be explained by real differences in performance.

There are three main drivers of reliability: sample size, differences among providers, and measurement error. At any provider level, sample size can be increased by increasing the number of patients in the data as well as by increasing the number of measures.

Although sample size and power have always been important considerations, reliability has recently come into focus as a key issue. The reason this has occurred is the strong relationship between reliability and profiling providers on their performance relative to their peers. This is a logical consequence of the way that stakeholders are using profiling information.

When discrete categories are used for performance reports (such as the star ratings being used by CMS), the key question becomes the probability of misclassification. If the categories are based on relative comparisons, reliability tells you most of what you need to know about the risk of misclassification in these systems. For example, in a simple high-performance network system that flags a subset of the physicians as high performing, there are two types of errors: (1) flagging a lower-performance physician as high performance and (2) failing to flag a high-performance physician as high performance.

Whether a measure is useful for profiling providers depends on how different the providers are from one another. Measures that may be useful in one group of providers or for one level of the system may not be useful in another group or level with little provider-to-provider variation. Similarly, as the providers under study increase their performance, the reliability may decrease if the provider-to-provider variance decreases over time. This is especially true as measures hit the upper limits of their ranges.

Relatively few studies have estimated misclassification probabilities in the presence of suboptimal reliability. It is likely that the most challenging application in terms of misclassification is physician level profiling due to the small sample size. Adams, Mehrotra, Thomas, and McGlynn (2010) examined the misclassification rates for a hypothetical physician-level cost profiling system. Median reliabilities ranged from 0.05 for vascular surgery to 0.79 for gastroenterology and otolaryngology. Overall, 59 percent of physicians had cost-profile scores with reliabilities of less than 0.70, a commonly used marker of suboptimal reliability. Using these reliability results, they estimated that 22 percent of physicians would be misclassified in a simple two-tiered system. However, the misclassification rate was as high as 36 percent for vascular surgery. Approaches with more performance categories (such as the CMS Five-Star system) are likely to have even higher misclassification rates.

Statistical Evaluation of Differences

The final analytic consideration for public reporting is to evaluate whether results are statistically significantly different from one another. In general, ignoring statistical significance is likely to increase misinformation. The challenge is how to present the results in a way that is interpretable by users. Given that one is committed to using statistical significance to distinguish performance, some additional analytic issues must be addressed in terms of the reference point for comparison. Performance for any one entity could be compared to (1) the average performance of all entities nationally, state, or by market; (2) the average performance of a peer group; (3) a benchmark based on best empirical performance; (4) a benchmark based on desired performance.

There is considerable debate about the best basis for making performance comparisons among entities, although little empirical evidence exists on the extent to which these choices result in differing conclusions. Those who favor national comparison argue that it underscores the goal of having equal quality of care throughout the country. Those who favor using regional or market comparison argue that some variation nationally is unavoidable and fundamentally people can select only from local providers. Austin has shown that using peer groups for comparison affects the number of hospitals identified as mortality outliers and that the choice of comparison groups may depend on the intended use of the results (Austin, Alter, Anderson, & Tu, 2004). Those who favor using benchmarks (rather than relative performance) prefer to emphasize the importance of a goal rather than grading on a curve. Benchmarks can be established either by observed best practices or by reference to preestablished goals. These arguments often assume that the best observed performance is suboptimal. Those favoring relative performance reporting note that choices are made relative to the available options.

The choices in this area reflect beliefs about the message that a report card is intended to deliver. First, one must consider whether quality is a relative concept or absolute. In reality, there are very few absolutes in medicine (and, by extension, in quality). Process quality, for example, in Donabedian's (1980) conceptualization incorporates both technical excellence (providing the right service competently) and interpersonal excellence (doing so humanely and with reference to the patient's preferences). This suggests there are few interventions that are clinically appropriate and acceptable to all patients all the time. Most quality measures are designed with the idea that a higher rate of performance is desirable, but unless techniques for incorporating informed patient refusal and rare clinical contraindications are factored into the measurement method, excellent quality performance should rarely reach 100 percent.

One of the policy implications of using an absolute level of performance as the metric of comparison is that entities may be encouraged to deliver care that is either clinically inappropriate or unacceptable to patients in order to raise their level of performance. Alternatively, using relative performance as a basis of comparison could fail to establish adequate incentives to improve performance. A particular concern about using relative performance is that the best observed performance may not be very good.

The second consideration among the relative comparison options is whether to make national or regional comparisons. Using national standards establishes a policy of expecting equal excellence in delivery of health services nationally. For many measures, there is no strong rationale for expecting substantially different performance by region. We observe differences in the quality of care received by people in urban and rural areas, by racial or ethnic group, by income or insurance coverage, but in most instances there is no clinical justification for these differences. The proponents of risk or case-mix adjustment suggest that these techniques be applied to quality measurement to account for differences in performance that reflect the populations served. Using national standards may foster greater incentive for quality improvement than using regional standards. This varies with the market.

The third consideration is whether to make comparison relative to the average or best performance. Any number of cut points could be chosen within the distribution of actual performance. Reference to the average would seem to promote substantially less quality improvement activity than reference to the best. Using the best performance as an anchor may yield a conceptually clearer way of distinguishing the top and bottom performers.

Finally, it is common to use a 0.05 significance level in determining whether observed differences are statistically significant. The choice of significance level carries with it a choice about the relative importance of false negative versus false positive results. The costs of the resulting errors in classification will vary with the user of the information. Consumers would prefer to reduce the likelihood of information causing them to choose a facility or provider that was incorrectly labeled as good, whereas facilities and providers would prefer to limit the chance of being falsely labeled as providing poor quality. A study of the implications of the choice of significance level for consumers versus hospitals in reporting mortality rate found that the optimal choice varied by user, the underlying rate of poor quality, and the size of an institution (Austin & Anderson, 2005).

Summary of Methodological Issues in Reporting

This section summarizes some of the methodological choices that report card developers must make in designing public reporting. Many proprietary systems may not make their choices clear. In most instances, report card developers have made varying choices even while using the same basic data source. This has the potential to produce apparently different results and may contribute to consumers' confusion and subsequent unwillingness to use this information to guide choices. The main message from this discussion, however, is that there is no unambiguously correct way to produce public information. Since the methodological choices may affect the results, transparency of method should be highly valued.

What is Known About the Impact of Public Reporting?

Although transparency in health care performance is ethically defensible on its own (Shahian et al., 2011), it is worth considering whether public reporting has resulted in any change in the health care system. Two major pathways for change have been suggested: (1) selection and (2) improvement (Berwick et al., 2003). The first pathway includes consumer choice of health plans, hospitals, and doctors as well as physician referrals to hospitals and other doctors. The second pathway includes quality improvement activity, as well as improvements in care processes and outcomes. In both pathways, we consider what is known about the effects of public reporting alone and with the addition of financial incentives.

The Effect of Public Reporting on Selection

A recent AHRQ systematic review found that almost all identified studies conclude that public reporting has had little effect on selection (Totten et al., 2012). An earlier systematic review of eight studies of the effect of public reporting on health plan selection found mixed results (Fung, Lim, Mattke, Damberg, & Shekelle, 2006). Two studies found no effect of providing CAHPS data on health plan selection among Medicaid beneficiaries, although there was a somewhat greater effect among those who read the report and selected plans with dominant market share. Studies employing hypothetical selection choices found participants were willing to make trade-offs on the basis of quality information (for example, selecting a less expensive plan with higher quality ratings or accepting narrower physician panels if a plan had higher quality ratings). In observational studies of different employer groups, some increased likelihood of selecting or changing plans based on quality information was observed.

A study of the effect of report cards on federal employees' choice of health plans found that quality scores (based on consumer ratings of quality) significantly affected the choice of health plan, with the strongest effects seen among new employees (Wedig & Tai-Seale, 2002). A national survey of consumers found that most relied on family, friends, and their own doctor to make decisions about where to go for care (Robinson & Brodie, 1997). About 40 percent of people surveyed had seen comparative information on health plans, and about one-third of those who saw the information used it (about 13 percent overall).

About half of the employees of companies in St. Louis and Denver who received health plan report cards as part of open enrollment remembered the report (Fowles, Kind, Braun, & Knutson, 2000). Among those who remembered seeing the report, 95 percent found it trustworthy, 82 percent found it helpful for learning about plan quality, 66 percent found it somewhat or very helpful in deciding whether to stay in or switch plans, and 50 percent were more confident in the decision that they made.

Nine studies of the effects of public reporting on choice of hospital found no consistent effect (Fung et al., 2006). These studies looked at changes in market share, utilization, occupancy, and growth. The studies focused on a few reporting systems, including the Medicare hospital mortality reports, the New York Cardiac Reporting System, and the California Cardiac Reporting System. Romano and Zhou (2004) found that hospitals in California that had significantly better or worse outcomes for heart attack patients did not experience any change in the number of patients obtaining care for that condition. A survey of patients who underwent CABG surgery in one of four hospitals in Pennsylvania found that only 20 percent of patients were aware of the information on hospital mortality rates for that procedure; among those who were aware, less than 25 percent said the results influenced their choice of surgeon (Schneider & Epstein, 1998). They also found that hospitals in California with a low complication rate following back surgery experienced a small increase in volume and that hospitals in New York with better and worse outcomes for CABG surgery experienced a change in volume shortly after publication of the results. They observed the strongest effects among patients enrolled in HMOs in California and among patients with Medicare in New York. An earlier quasi-experimental study of the impact of the New York state report on mortality following CABG surgery found that hospitals and physicians with better performance experienced a gain in market share and prices, although this effect diminished over time (Mukamel & Mushlin, 1998). An evaluation of Nursing Home Compare found no effect of reports on patient choice of higher-performing nursing homes (Grabowski & Town, 2011).

A study of hospital mortality rates published by the federal government found that consumers were more influenced by press reports of high-profile problems at local hospitals than by the data on risk-adjusted mortality (Mennemeyer, Morrisey, & Howard, 1997). A study of New York general acute hospitals found no changes in occupancy rate after release of the federal reports on mortality rates (Vladeck, Goodwin, Myers, & Sinisi, 1988).

A review of seven studies on the effect of public reporting on choice of physician found some effects. Five studies, for example, showed an effect of the New York State Cardiac Reporting System on choice of surgeon. Two studies also found that poorer-performing providers were more likely to stop practicing (Hannan, Siu, Kumar, Kilburn, & Chassin, 1995; Jha & Epstein, 2006).

The Impact of Public Reporting on Improvement

Providers' primary use of public reports is for quality improvement. Most of the peer-reviewed studies in this area focus on hospital report cards. A recent AHRQ Evidence Report found that public reporting was associated with improvements in mortality as well as care processes (Totten, Wagner, Tiwari, O'Haire, Griffin, & Walker, 2012). The strength of evidence for the nineteen mortality studies was moderate, whereas the strength of evidence for the nineteen process improvement studies was high.

An earlier synthesis of eleven studies found that report cards stimulated quality improvement activities (Fung et al., 2006). One of the few studies to use an experimental design assigned hospitals to one of three conditions (public reports on quality, private reports on quality, and no reports—the control) and observed whether there were differences among the hospitals in the number of quality improvement projects initiated within nine months after the reports (Hibbard, Stockard, & Tusler, 2003). They found that public reporting was associated with a significantly higher rate of quality improvement projects in hospitals with public reports and low initial performance. Making reports public generated considerable negative reaction on the part of participating hospitals. A study of the long-term effects of reporting found significant improvement in performance among the public report group compared to the private report and no report groups (33 percent, 25 percent, 11 percent of hospitals demonstrating improvement, respectively) (Hibbard, Stockard, & Tusler, 2005). More recently, these conclusions have been challenged, and the authors suggest that when appropriate statistical methods were used, little difference was found between public and private reporting (Shahian et al., 2011). There was a relationship between the number of quality improvement projects initiated and improvement in performance (average of 5.7 projects among hospitals showing significant improvement, compared to 2.6 among hospitals with no change). No significant change in market share was observed. Hafner and colleagues found that public reporting increased the involvement of leadership in performance improvement activities and created a sense of accountability among providers (Hafner et al., 2011).

Two studies have been conducted on the Pennsylvania CABG surgery mortality report card. One found that whereas most cardiologists and all surgeons in the state were aware of the report, few thought it was important or discussed it with their patients (Schneider & Epstein, 1996). Most were critical of the methods, particularly the adequacy of risk adjustment and the reliability of the data. A study of organizations in the state found that the information was a stimulus to development of marketing materials, provider monitoring, benchmarking, and collaborative improvement activities within the hospital (Bentley & Nash, 1998).

Five studies have been conducted on the New York cardiac reporting system. One study found considerably greater acceptance of the reports among physicians in New York than what was reported in Pennsylvania; 67 percent reported that they found the content very useful or somewhat useful, 22 percent said they routinely discussed the results with their patients, and 38 percent said the report affected referral patterns (Hannan, Stone, Biddle, & DeBuono, 1997). A case study in a poor-performing hospital reported that after an initial negative reaction to the report the institution used the results productively to improve collaboration and identify sources of high mortality (Dziuban, McIlduff, Miller, & Dal Col, 1994). A survey of hospital executives found that most were knowledgeable about the methods used in the New York reports and that high-mortality hospitals were more likely to be critical of the results (Romano, Rainwater, & Antonius, 1999). Outcomes appear to have improved in the state following release of the information; risk-adjusted mortality rates in the state declined from 4.17 percent to 2.45 percent (Hannan, Kilburn, Racz, Shields, & Chassin, 1994). This exceeded the rate of decline nationally, but some critics suggested this resulted from fewer high-risk procedures being done or from patients going out of state for care. In fact, a study found that fewer residents of New York went out of state for CABG surgery following the release, and the likelihood of having the surgery following a heart attack (one of the most high-risk reasons for surgery) increased (Peterson, DeLong, Jollis, Muhlbaier, & Mark, 1998). The findings of studies conducted on other hospital report cards are similar (Marshall, Shekelle, Leatherman, & Brook, 2000).

The evaluation of Nursing Home Compare found that nursing homes in competitive markets were more likely to improve on two of the five quality measures than nursing homes in noncompetitive markets (Grabowski & Town, 2011).

Future Directions

Although the evidence on use of report cards by various audiences—consumers, purchasers, and providers—suggests that the information is not widely used and appears to have only a small effect on performance, the trend is clearly in the direction of releasing more information on more entities. This seems unlikely to change in the near future. Studies of the rate at which innovation diffuses suggest that it takes a long time for a new approach to be widely accepted (Rogers, 1995). The literature on making documents useful for various audiences suggests that a key problem for many of these reports may be related to poor presentation of the information (Hibbard et al., 2002). We have more information on quality available today than we have ever had, but the measures available represent a small portion of the reasons people become ill or seek care—so failure to find widespread effects may be consistent with assessment of the meaningfulness or relevance of the information. Expansion of the measures available, increased attention to the methods that are used to construct report cards, better use of communication techniques that are known to be effective, and more formal evaluation of such efforts are required before we have the information necessary to draw conclusions about the utility of public reporting.

SUMMARY

Despite the high level of interest in report cards on quality performance by organizations and the increased number that are being released, there are relatively few well-designed studies of the effects of public reporting on consumer, purchaser, and provider behavior. NCQA has the widest geographic reach and longest experience in producing performance reports on managed care plans. California and Minnesota have the most information available across levels in the health care system (health plans, hospitals, and medical groups). New York's program, which routinely reports risk-adjusted mortality data on one procedure, has been subject to the most extensive evaluation. Wisconsin's hospital reports benefited from the greatest attention to display issues and have been subjected to the most rigorous evaluation.

KEY TERMS

Accreditation A formal designation given to a facility or organization by a recognized entity that indicates the institution meets preestablished standards.

Mandatory reporting A requirement that an entity report performance on specific quality measures to a specific entity (usually the government).

Outcomes Generally used in quality measurement to refer to dimensions of health status such as mortality, functioning, clinical status (such as blood pressure), or patient satisfaction.

Pay-for-performance Reimbursement or compensation is tied to achievement of specific results on quality measures, such as the ninetieth percentile among reporting entities. Generally only a portion of total reimbursement is subject to these conditions.

Pay-for-reporting Entities are paid an incentive (or a penalty is imposed if the entity fails to act) for reporting results on specific quality measures. The payment is not linked to the level of performance, just to the act of reporting.

Performance Refers to the results of a quality (or other type) of measure.

Process A type of quality measure that indicates whether or not a particular action was taken, such as screening for certain cancers, measuring clinical status, counseling, and other similar types of health care services.

Reliability The confidence with which one can distinguish between the performances of two or more entities.

Risk adjustment A statistical process that takes into account any differences in the populations served by different entities, and removes those differences from performance scores so that a comparison of performance between those entities is fair.

Transparency The practice of making information about performance publicly available.

Value-based purchasing Reimbursement or compensation is linked to performance on both quality and cost measures.

Voluntary reporting Entities may choose whether or not to publicly report their performance on standardized measures of quality.

DISCUSSION QUESTIONS

1. Measures of quality of care for comparing providers are often divided into structure, process, and outcomes. Which of these measures are most important? Does the answer vary by type of user (such as purchasers or consumers)? Does the answer vary by provider type?

2. Report card developers often trade off displaying detailed information versus summarized information. How should we think about the right level of detail for comparing providers? Does the answer vary by type of user?

3. It is sometimes argued that "any information is better than no information." How low a reliability is acceptable for public reporting? Should the answer vary by provider type? Should the answer vary by audience (purchasers or consumers)?

4. What is the most effective way to present comparisons between and among providers? How much detail can consumers handle in support of their decision making?

5. How should we trade off the competing goals of fairness to providers and transparency for consumers?

6. How much responsibility does a report card effort have to minimize potential consumer misinterpretation of the report card? In particular, should the report card suppress information that might be misunderstood, or is transparency more important?

FURTHER READING

Fung, C. H., Lim, Y-W., Mattke, S., Damberg, C., & Shekelle, P. G. (2006). Systematic review: The evidence that publishing patient care performance data improves quality of care. *Annals of Internal Medicine, 148*, 111–123.

This is an excellent systematic evidence review that is organized around different proposed uses of publicly reported information on quality. The reference section contains many of the classic references in this area.

National Committee on Quality Assurance. (2011). *Continuous improvement and the expansion of health care quality: The state of health care quality 2011.* Washington, DC: Author.

NCQA has the longest running experience with public reporting of quality performance by health plans. They issue an annual report, which can be found on their website, summarizing some of the key issues in quality reporting and changes in performance among health plans.

Shahian, D. M., Edwards, F. H., Jacobs, J. P., Prager, R. L., Normand, S-L.T., Shewan, C. M., . . . Grover, F. L. (2011). Public reporting of cardiac surgery performance: Part 1—history, rationale, consequences. *Annals of Thoracic Surgery, 92,* S2–S11.

This article provides an excellent historical and philosophical perspective on public reporting. Although it was prepared to explain to the membership of the Society of Thoracic Surgeons why registry results were going to be made publicly available, the foundation of this argument is generally applicable.

Totten, A. M., Wagner, J., Tiwari, A., O'Haire, C., Griffin, J., & Walker, M. (2012). *Public reporting as a quality improvement strategy. Closing the quality gap: Revisiting the state of the science* (Evidence Report No 208). Rockville, MD: Agency for Healthcare Research and Quality.

This systematic review updates the Fung systematic review with more recent studies and some new analyses of the evidence.

In addition to these readings, two websites are particularly worth looking at:

www.cms.gov is the starting point for all of the federal government's "Facility" Compare reports (such as Hospital Compare and Nursing Home Compare).

www.ncqa.org has a variety of information about public reporting at different levels.

REFERENCES

Adams, J. L., Mehrotra, A., Thomas, J. W., & McGlynn, E. A. (2010). Physician cost profiling: Reliability and risk of misclassification. *New England Journal of Medicine, 362*(11), 1014–1021.

America's best health plans. (2009, November 12). *U.S. News & World Report.*

Asch, S. M., McGlynn, E. A., Hogan, M. M., Hayward, R. A., Shekelle, P., Rubenstein, L., . . . Kerr, E. A. (2004). Comparison of quality of care for patients in the Veterans Health Administration and patients in a national sample. *Annals of Internal Medicine, 141*(12), 938–945.

Austin, P. C., Alter, D. A., Anderson, G. M., & Tu, J. V. (2004). Impact of the choice of benchmark on the conclusions of hospital report cards. *American Heart Journal, 148*(6), 1041–1046.

Austin, P. C., & Anderson, G. M. (2005). Optimal statistical decisions for hospital report cards. *Medical Decision Making, 25,* 11–19.

Bentley, J. M., & Nash, D. B. (1998). How Pennsylvania hospitals have responded to publicly released reports on coronary artery bypass graft surgery. *Joint Commission Journal on Quality Improvement, 24,* 40–49.

Berwick, D. M., James, B., & Coye, M. J. (2003). Connections between quality measurement and improvement. *Medical Care, 41*(1 Suppl.), I30–I38.

Committee on Quality Health Care in America, Institute of Medicine. (2001). *Crossing the quality chasm: A new health system for the 21st century.* Washington, DC: National Academy Press.

Crofton, C., Lubalin, J. S., & Darby, C. (1999). Consumer Assessment of Health Plans Study (CAHPS). (Foreword.) *Medical Care, 37,* MS1–MS9.

Donabedian, A. (1980). *Explorations in quality assessment and monitoring. Vol. I: The definition of quality and approaches to its assessment.* Ann Arbor, MI: Health Administration Press.

Dziuban, S. W., McIlduff, J. B., Miller, S. J., & Dal Col, R. H. (1994). How a New York cardiac surgery program uses outcomes data. *Annals of Thoracic Surgery, 58,* 1871–1876.

Fowles, J. B., Kind, E. A., Braun, B. L., & Knutson, D. J. (2000). Consumer responses to health plan report cards in two markets. *Medical Care, 38,* 469–471.

Fung, C. H., Lim, Y-W., Mattke, S., Damberg, C., & Shekelle, P. G. (2006). Systematic review: The evidence that publishing patient care performance data improves quality of care. *Annals of Internal Medicine, 148,* 111–123.

Grabowski, D. C., & Town, R. J. (2011). Does information matter? Competition, quality, and the impact of nursing home report cards. *Health Services Research, 46*(6), 1698–1719.

Hafner, J. M., Williams, S. C., Koss, R. G., Tschurtz, B. A., Schmaltz, S. P., & Loeb, J. M. (2011). The perceived impact of public reporting hospital performance data: Interviews with hospital staff. *International Journal of Quality in Health Care, 23*(6), 697–704.

Hannan, E. L., Kilburn, H., Jr., Lindsey, M. L., & Lewis, R. (1992). Clinical versus administrative data bases for CABG surgery: Does it matter? *Medical Care, 30*(10), 892–907.

Hannan, E. L., Kilburn, H., Jr., Racz, M., Shields, E., & Chassin, M. R. (1994). Improving the outcomes of coronary artery bypass surgery in New York State. *Journal of the American Medical Association, 271,* 761–766.

Hannan, E. L., Siu, A. L., Kumar, D., Kilburn, H., Jr., & Chassin, M. R. (1995). The decline in coronary artery bypass graft surgery in New York State. The role of surgeon volume. Journal of the American Medical Association, *273,* 209–13.

Hannan, E. L., Stone, C. C., Biddle, T. L., & DeBuono, B. A. (1997). Public release of cardiac surgery outcomes data in New York. *American Heart Journal, 134,* 55–61.

Hibbard, J. H., Slovic, P., & Jewett, J. J. (1997). Informing consumer decisions in health care: Implications from decision-making research. *Milbank Quarterly, 75*(3), 395–414.

Hibbard, J. H., Slovic, P., Peters, E., & Finucane, M. L. (2002). Strategies for reporting health plan performance information to consumers: Evidence from controlled studies. *Health Services Research, 37,* 291–313.

Hibbard, J. H., Stockard, J., & Tusler, M. (2003). Does publicizing hospital performance stimulate quality improvement efforts? *Health Affairs, 22*(2), 84–94.

Hibbard, J. H., Stockard, J., & Tusler, M. (2005). Hospital performance reports: Impact on quality, market share, and reputation. *Health Affairs, 24*(4), 1150–1160.

Hofer, T. P., Hayward, R. A., Greenfield, S., Wagner, E. H., Kaplan, S. H., & Manning, W. G. (1999). The unreliability of individual physician "report cards" for assessing the costs and quality of care of a chronic disease. *Journal of the American Medical Association, 281*(22), 2098–2105.

Jha, A. K., & Epstein, E. M. (2006). The predictive accuracy of the New York State coronary artery bypass surgery report-card system. *Health Affairs, 25,* 844–855.

Kohn, L. T., Corrigan, J. M., & Donaldson, M. S. (Eds.). (1999). *To err is human: Building a safer health system.* Washington, DC: National Academy Press.

Longo, D. R. (2004). Health care consumer reports: An evaluation of employer perspectives. *Journal of Health Care Finance, 30*(3), 85–92.

Mangione-Smith, R., DeCristofaro, A. H., Setodji, C. M., Keesey, J., Klein, D. J., Adams, J. L., . . . McGlynn, E. A. (2007). The quality of ambulatory care delivered to children in the United States. *New England Journal of Medicine, 357*(15), 1515–1523.

Marshall, M. M., Shekelle, P. G., Leatherman, S., & Brook, R. H. (2000). The public release of performance data: what do we expect to gain? A review of the evidence. *Journal of the American Medical Association, 283,* 1866–1874.

McGlynn, E. A. (1998). The outcomes utility index: Will outcomes data tell us what we want to know? *International Journal for Quality in Health Care, 10*(6), 485–490.

McGlynn, E. A., Adams, J., Hicks, J., & Klein, D. (1999a). *Creating a coordinated autos/UAW reporting system for health plan performance* (Publication no. DRU-2123-FMC). Santa Monica, CA: RAND.

McGlynn, E. A., Adams, J., Hicks, J., & Klein, D. (1999b). *Developing health plan performance reports: responding to the BBA* (Publication no. DRU-2122-HCFA). Santa Monica, CA: RAND.

McGlynn, E. A., Asch, S. M., Adams, J., Keesey, J., Hicks, J., DeCristofaro, A., & Kerr, E. A. (2003). The quality of health care delivered to adults in the United States. *New England Journal of Medicine, 348*(26), 2635–2645.

Mennemeyer, S. T., Morrisey, M. A., & Howard, L. Z. (1997). Death and reputation: How consumers acted upon HCFA mortality information. *Inquiry, 34,* 117–128.

Mukamel, D. B., & Mushlin, A. I. (1998). Quality of care information makes a difference. *Medical Care, 36,* 945–954.

National Committee on Quality Assurance. (2011). *Continuous improvement and the expansion of health care quality: The state of health care quality 2011.* Washington, DC: Author.

Peterson, E. D., DeLong, E. R., Jollis, J. G., Muhlbaier, L. H., & Mark, D. B. (1998). The effects of New York's bypass surgery provider profiling on access to care and patient outcomes in the elderly. *Journal of the American College of Cardiology, 32,* 993–999.

Robinson, S., & Brodie, M. (1997). Understanding the quality challenge for health consumers: The Kaiser/AHCPR survey. *Joint Commission Journal on Quality Improvement, 23,* 239–244.

Rogers, E. M. (1995). *Diffusion of innovations.* New York: Free Press.

Romano, P. S., Rainwater, J. A., & Antonius, D. M. (1999). Grading the graders: How hospitals in California and New York perceive and interpret their report cards. *Medical Care, 37,* 295–305.

Romano, P. S., & Zhou, H. (2004). Do well-publicized risk-adjusted outcomes reports affect hospital volume? *Medical Care, 42*(4), 367–377.

Schneider, E. C., & Epstein, A. M. (1996). Influence of cardiac-surgery performance reports on referral practices and access to care. *New England Journal of Medicine, 335,* 251–256.

Schneider, E. C., & Epstein, A. M. (1998). Use of public performance reports. *Journal of the American Medical Association, 279*, 1638–1642.

Scholle, S. H., Roski, J., Adams, J. L., Dunn, D. L., Kerr, E. A., Dugan, D. P., & Jensen, R. E. (2008). Benchmarking physician performance: Reliability of individual and composite measures. *American Journal of Managed Care, 14*(12), 833–838.

Shahian, D. M., Edwards, F. H., Jacobs, J. P., Prager, R. L., Normand, S-L.T., Shewan, C. M., . . . Grover, F. L. (2011). Public reporting of cardiac surgery performance: Part 1—history, rationale, consequences. *Annals of Thoracic Surgery, 92*, S2–S11.

Slovic, P. (1982). Toward understanding and improving decisions. In W. C. Howell & E. A. Fleishman (Eds.), *Human performance and productivity. Vol. 2: Information processing and decision making.* Hillsdale, NJ: Erlbaum.

Totten, A. M., Wagner, J., Tiwari, A., O'Haire, C. Griffin, J., & Walker, M. (2012). *Public reporting as a quality improvement strategy. Closing the quality gap: Revisiting the state of the science* (Evidence Report No. 208). Rockville MD: Agency for Healthcare Research and Quality.

Ulmer, C., Bruno, M., & Burke, S. (Eds.). (2010). *Future directions for the national healthcare quality and disparities reports.* Committee on Future Directions for the National Healthcare Quality and Disparities Reports, Board on Health Care Services. Washington, DC: National Academies Press.

Vladeck, B. C., Goodwin, E. J., Myers, L. P., & Sinisi, M. (1988). Consumers and hospital use: The HCFA "death list." *Health Affairs, 7*, 122–125.

Wedig, G. J., & Tai-Seale, M. (2002). The effect of report cards on consumer choice in the health insurance market. *Journal of Health Economics, 21*, 1031–1048.

Zaslavsky, A. M., Zaborski, L., & Cleary, P. D. (2000). Does the effect of respondent characteristics on consumer assessments vary across health plans? *Medical Care Research and Review, 57*(3), 379–394.

CHAPTER FOURTEEN

HEALTH CARE INFORMATION SYSTEMS

Jeff Luck
Leah J. Vriesman
Paul Fu Jr.

Learning Objectives

- Gain a basic appreciation of the evolution of health care information systems and technology so that the rapid pace of adoption and change can be measured against other industries
- Determine the areas of improvement that HIT can make in the three critical areas of health care access, cost, and quality
- Examine the application of information systems in service delivery, public health, and biomedical informatics
- Improve understanding about legislative initiatives influencing trends for HIT adoption

After five decades of use in administrative and financial applications at large health care providers, payers, and government health agencies, recent years have seen information systems used more widely in clinical applications, in smaller organizations, and increasingly by patients themselves. These broader applications of information systems hold the promise of better health care system performance: improved quality, increased efficiency, and enhanced access. They must also ensure the privacy and security of personal health information stored and transmitted electronically. This chapter provides an overview of key information technology applications that are affecting the U.S. health care system.

Information Systems and Informatics

A health care information system comprises computerized data as well as procedures to collect, store, analyze, transfer, and retrieve that data. Information technology underlies these systems and consists of computers, the networks and telecommunications systems that connect them, and the software that operates the computers and networks. Information systems support financial management as well as administrative applications such as scheduling and claims processing. As shown in Figure 14.1, biomedical informatics is the "interdisciplinary field that studies and pursues the effective uses of biomedical data, information, and knowledge for scientific inquiry, problem solving, and decision making, driven by efforts to improve human health" (Kulikowski et al., 2012) "Clinical informatics" comprises subfields such as medical, nursing, and dental informatics. Public health informatics is the "systematic application of information and computer science and technology to public health practice, research, and learning" (Yasnoff & Miller, 2000).

Benefits, Implementation Barriers, and Federal Policy Responses

Applications of information technology, including the Internet and web-based applications, have transformed many sectors of the global economy, making work processes more efficient, faster, and in many respects more responsive to customers. It is therefore hoped that health information technology can also improve the performance of the U.S. health care system, by improving quality and patient safety, reducing costs, and potentially enhancing access. For example, one analysis estimated a potential $78 billion annual saving based on a standardized national system for health care information exchange and interoperability among providers and payers (Walker et al., 2005). A widely cited RAND analysis estimated

FIGURE 14.1. FIELDS OF BIOMEDICAL INFORMATICS AND DOMAINS OF APPLICATION

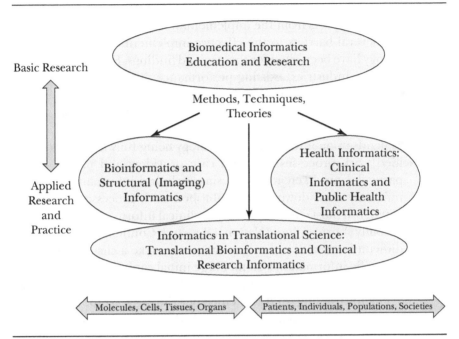

Source: Kulikowski et al., 2012.

that annual efficiency savings from 90 percent adoption of EHRs could exceed $75 billion (Hillestad et al., 2005).

These expected benefits can be manifested in several ways, including: reduced duplication of services due to health information exchange; better management of chronic disease with use of patient registries and support for patient self-management; reduction of medical errors and inappropriate tests and treatments with the help of computerized clinical decision support; and streamlining of administrative tasks and quality measurement. These changes are affecting all domains of the U.S. health care system: providers, payers, patients, life science firms, and public health agencies. Yet until quite recently, HIT implementation in the United States lagged well behind many other OECD countries, especially in the outpatient care arena (Jha et al., 2008).

The current evidence regarding the actual impact of HIT is somewhat mixed. For example, the degree of HIT adoption by U.S. hospitals is not yet significantly related to improvements in existing measures of quality or efficiency (DesRoches, Campbell, et al., 2010). However, systematic reviews of the literature show an increasing proportion of published studies reporting positive impacts from the implementation of HIT (Buntin et al., 2011).

Several barriers to the effective implementation of information technology have been cited for these mixed findings. First, as has been observed in other industries, existing performance measures may not capture the real benefits of information technology, and there is a time lag between widespread information technology adoption and broad performance improvements (Jones et al., 2012). Second, performance improvement depends upon information technology being fully incorporated into modified work processes at health care providers and payers. Physicians in particular are likely to resist using a clinical information system if it significantly slows down their established work processes (McDonald et al., 2004), but most currently available clinical information systems have severe usability shortcomings (National Research Council, 2009). Third, it is often difficult for health care organizations to make a clear "business case" for a specific information system. Large initial capital investment are required not only for hardware and software but also for planning, project management, training, and lost efficiency during startup; offsetting financial returns may take years to accrue. And U.S. provider organizations often face limited incentives to invest in information systems. For example, most of the cost savings from providers' information system investments accrue to payers and purchasers. Fully integrated health care organizations such as HMOs the Veterans Health Administration can see a return on investment more clearly, because long-term quality and efficiency benefits accrue to them (Baker et al., 2008).

In 2004, the federal government established the Office of the National Coordinator (ONC) to accelerate implementation of health information technology. Five years later, as part of the American Recovery and Reinvestment Act of 2009 (ARRA), the Health Information Technology for Economic and Clinical Health Act (HITECH) greatly expanded the scope of ONC's activities and included several provisions that aimed to address directly several of the implementation barriers just described (Blumenthal, 2011a, 2011b). Billions of dollars in subsidies, plus future eventual penalties for lack of adoption, were enacted to help overcome provider organizations' financial reluctance to invest in HIT. Requirements for the "meaningful use" of information technology (MU) were intended to ensure the actual use of these systems in care delivery and for quality measurement. Certification was required to help ensure that information systems met MU standards, but do not guarantee that clinicians will find those systems user-friendly. Both the HITECH Act and the Affordable Care Act of 2010 (ACA) also contain provisions to improve health care quality, safety, cost-effectiveness, and access through secure electronic exchange of health information. ONC has therefore promulgated standards for health information exchange (HIE). Finally, ONC provides support for training the expanded workforce that broader HIT implementation will necessitate.

Applications of Information Systems by Health Care Providers

Health information technology systems have been actively deployed within U.S. health care institutions for more than four decades. The earliest health care applications emerged during the late 1960s and were enabled by two developments. First, computing power began to increase rapidly, and the advent of minicomputers made the use of technology affordable, whereas mainframes were cost-prohibitive. Second, development of health-care-specific structured programming languages made it possible to focus on the complex data environment that defined the health care encounter. The Massachusetts General Hospital Utility Multi-Programming System (MUMPS), developed in the 1960s, was a tree-structured database and programming language well suited to representing the medical record. It became the basis on which many successful commercial and noncommercial health care applications were created. The Veterans Administration developed a fourth-generation programming language (4GL) based on MUMPS called File Manager, which was used to develop the VistA electronic health record suite of applications used today. From the success of VistA, the Indian Health Service and the U.S. Department of Defense adopted File Manager for development of their own health information systems.

Initially, health care provider applications focused on automating administrative operations such as simple patient accounting and payroll in order to achieve the efficiency and productivity gains seen in other economic sectors. By the 1970s, there were a far greater number of administratively focused software packages available, including accounts payable and receivable, general ledger, patient accounting and billing, and resource scheduling, as well as emergence of the first clinical information systems for laboratory, radiology, and medication management.

The continued increase in microprocessor speed and power and the arrival of networking technologies transformed the ability of health care institutions to more effectively use HIT. During the 1980s and 1990s, hospital information management systems were designed to run the entirety of hospital operations, including admission, discharge, and transfers as well as patient appointments and scheduling, order control and results reporting, billing and accounts. Isolated terminals were eventually replaced by desktop workstations connected to facility-wide networks, making it possible to broaden the number of individuals using the system at a given time.

Practice management systems were also being developed as the physician-office counterpart to hospital information systems, combining appointment scheduling and accounting and billing in a single application specifically focused on outpatient management. Development of the first widely available personal computers during the mid-1980s (IBM PC and Apple Macintosh) significantly increased market penetration, although it was still relatively minor owing to the high cost of new technology adoption.

Clinical information systems also expanded in scope during this time. Earlier iterations focused on automating manual capture of data, such as collecting lab instrument data into a single digital location. Improvements in digital acquisition of data, as from automated laboratory instruments or CT scanners, allowed development of "silo" systems that aggregated data from multiple domain-specific subsystems. These domain-specific silo systems included laboratory, pharmacy, radiology, and emergency department information systems. It was not uncommon for early adopter health care facilities to have multiple workstations adjacent to one another, each accessing a silo system. At the micro level, clinical monitoring systems that focus on aggregation of biological signal collection (vital signs, input and output, invasive catheter readings) can transmit data continuously to upstream health information systems. At the macro level, large integrated delivery networks can consolidate data into warehouses to facilitate data mining and process improvement activities across the entire enterprise.

Over the past decade, significant developments in information technology have made it possible to collect more data than ever on the detailed encounters that make up the provider-patient care delivery process and present it more effectively to a range of users. In accordance with Moore's Law, microprocessor capacity continues to double approximately every eighteen months, with handheld personal digital assistants now having more processing power than the first supercomputers. Data storage capacity is measured in terabytes and petabytes. Networks have evolved from wired to wireless. The Internet has transformed how people look for information, and more important how they expect to have data and information presented.

The ability to aggregate data and information from multiple health information systems into a single system along with a strong national focus on improving the quality and safety of health care delivery has yielded several health care applications with the potential to significantly affect the U.S. health care system.

Clinical Decision Support Systems (CDSS)

The modern era of medicine presents three challenges for information processing and decision making. The sheer volume of clinical data produced annually, even within a single subspecialty domain, is beyond the ability of any individual clinician to master in its entirety on an ongoing basis. The National Library of Medicine indexed more than 700,000 new items in 2010 (NLM, 2012), Initiatives to improve the safety and quality of health care have led to development and promulgation of evidence-based clinical guidelines and best practices; research reveals that a substantial percentage (30 to 60 percent) of clinical decisions may change if the evidence-based recommendations are presented in context with patient data at the point of care (Pestotnik, 2005). Finally, the complexity of the care delivery process creates the potential for errors wherever there is insufficient time to fully evaluate all potential linkages (see Figure 14.2)

To address these challenges, information systems that assist in the process of decision making, known as decision support systems, have been developed to use rules and straightforward representations of knowledge to assist in the decision-making process. Decision support systems that model very complex sets of rules and facts are known as expert systems (Yasnoff & Miller, 2003) According to the Centers for Medicare and Medicaid (CMS), clinical decision support is an "HIT functionality that builds upon the foundation of an EHR to provide persons involved in care processes with general and person-specific information, intelligently filtered and organized, at appropriate times, to enhance health and healthcare" (CMS, 2010). Clinical decision support systems (CDSS) are systems or groups of systems that integrate patient-specific data along with computer-represented clinical knowledge (for example, guidelines or antibiotic resistance sensitivity) in order to frame point-of-care alerting, reporting, and order or care plan recommendations.

CDSS range in complexity and integration from simple knowledge base tools to sophisticated but passive and standalone decision aids, to

FIGURE 14.2. HIT LINKAGES BETWEEN EVIDENCE-BASED MEDICINE AND QUALITY IMPROVEMENT

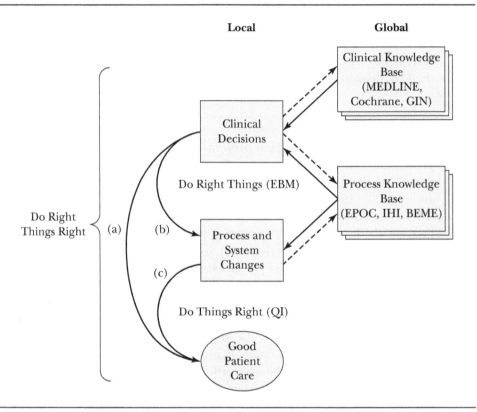

Source: Glasziou, Ogrinc, & Goodman, 2011.

complex systems integrated into electronic medical records or computerized physician order entry systems. Simple online knowledge bases help to furnish validated or standardized clinical information for the provider; they include journal and textbook tools such as MD Consult (from an eponymous company in St. Louis) and NIH PubMed, evidence-based practice guidelines such as UpToDate (Waltham, Massachusetts) and the Cochrane Library (Oxford, United Kingdom), and reference data resources such as Micromedex (Greenwood Village, Colorado) and Medispan (Indianapolis). More sophisticated knowledge base tools such as Gideon (Los Angeles) can aid the diagnostic process by using images and decision-tree logical paths to assist with infectious disease identification. Passive CDSS require that clinicians first identify the need for such a utility and, secondarily, engage the system to obtain necessary feedback. Typical use of passive decision support tools is to broaden or refine a differential diagnosis or validate a decision against a clinical database. Aside from alerts and reminders, passive to moderate CDSS may include templates, order sets, data displays that highlight important information, reference information, and other tools to support optimal care within the clinical experience (Healthcare Information and Management Systems [HIMSS], 2011)

Complex CDSS engage the user in continuous dialogue, integrated into the actual clinical workflow through intuitive human-computer interaction in a real-time fashion. Effective recommendations are patient-specific, evidence-based, and presented to the clinician consultatively, to avoid inadvertent elimination of clinical judgment. It is essential that these CDSS be integrated into the computer documentation (electronic medical and health records) and ordering (computerized physician order entry) workflow if one is to obtain the highest yield impact (Pestotnik, 2005). Active CDSS make available all six of the generic functions of clinical decision support systems: alerting, interpreting, assisting, critiquing, diagnosing, and managing decision support (Pryor, 1990). Using integration or messaging with underlying electronic medical record systems, the active CDSS permits continuous data surveillance, alerting clinicians when predefined rules built on clinical evidence are triggered (such as an abnormal result or adverse trend). Even though they offer the highest level of benefit to the end user, active CDSS are the most difficult to design and implement because these systems pose the greatest intrusion into the clinical decision-making workflow. However, as messaging standards evolve and the HIT industry standardizes on methods to consistently represent clinical information and knowledge across platforms, active systems will become increasingly available.

Computerized Physician Order Entry (CPOE)

Computerized physician order entry (CPOE) systems automate the manual process by which physician orders are communicated to other health care providers, including nursing, pharmacy, and ancillary departments such as dietary, respiratory therapy, occupational therapy, and physical therapy. Basic CPOE systems achieve improvements in safety and quality by enabling entry of standardized and complete physician orders and eliminating errors that are due to illegibility or use of confusing or unfamiliar terms, expressions, or names (Kaushal & Bates, 2001). More advanced CPOE systems integrate decision support tools into the ordering workflow, as in producing related laboratory results, local microbiologic sensitivities for appropriate antibiotic ordering, diagnosis and medication guidelines, and formulary guidance (Niazkhani et al., 2009).

The majority of emphasis has been on use of CPOE systems to improve the medication ordering process. An early study described a decrease in serious medication errors of 55 percent following CPOE introduction, with some reports ranging as high as an 80 percent effect on error prevention (Bates et al., 1998). In a 2008 meta-analysis of 25 studies that analyzed the effects on medication error rate, 23 showed a significant relative risk reduction of 13 percent to 99 percent (Ammenwerth, Schnell-Inderst, Machan, & Seibert, 2008). An additional study has found that hospitals issued nearly 1.76 billion medication orders in 2008 and that about 26.1 percent of the medication orders issued in acute care hospitals were processed using CPOE systems (Radley et al., 2013). After conducting a meta-analysis of published studies, the authors determined that the use of a CPOE system reduced the risk of making a prescription error by 48 percent. Considering the rate of CPOE adoption in 2008, the researchers estimated that the technology contributed to a 12.5 percent decline in medication errors that year, meaning that a total of about 17.4 million prescription errors were avoided. CPOE systems have also shown a milder reduction in charges and costs (Kaushal et al., 2006).

Recognizing the potential almost a decade ago, organizations as diverse as the Institute of Medicine and the Leapfrog Group (a health care quality assessment coalition) have identified adoption of CPOE as a recommended safety practice (Adams & Corrigan, 2003). However, only 10 to 20 percent of hospitals have CPOE (Ash et al., 2012), the large majority of which are academic hospitals with teaching programs or hospitals with large numbers of employed physicians, such as Veterans Affairs or Kaiser Permanente hospitals (Ash et al., 2012). And while more than 80 percent of the nation's hospitals are community hospitals, less than 10 percent currently report having even a basic CPOE system (Ash et al., 2012). While computerized physician order entry systems (CPOE) can reduce the number of medication errors and adverse drug events (ADEs) in health care institutions, recent reports suggest that CPOE systems may augment medication errors or increase mortality if not properly implemented (Han et al., 2005; Koppel et al., 2005). Unfortunately, they tend to produce a large number of partly irrelevant alerts, in turn leading to alert overload with the potential for causing alert fatigue (Riedmann et al., 2011).

CPOE remains an effective tool for improving patient safety if implemented appropriately. Although government and nonprofit hospitals lead the curve in adopting CPOE systems, cost and reimbursement issues are being addressed in order to speed more widespread adoption. In 2012, over 6 in 10 physicians had capability to use computerized provider order entry for lab orders and nearly three-quarters had capability to record electronic notes in patient records. This represents 66 percent and 68 percent growth, respectively, since 2009 (King, Patel, & Furukawa, 2012).

Imaging

Medical imaging can be the most IT-intensive aspect of a health care provider organization. Because the utilization and precision of medical imaging are continually increasing, provider organizations must make significant capital investments in systems to store and distribute imaging data.

Digital images are generated and used by many medical specialties. Traditionally film-based images such as X-rays and mammograms are becoming digitized, and inherently digital modalities—computed tomography (CT), magnetic resonance (MR) imaging, ultrasound, and positron emission tomography (PET) scanning—generate huge amounts of data (Greenes & Brinkley, 2006). Images are also central to pathology, nuclear medicine, cardiology, and other specialties.

In the traditional process, radiologists interpret images at an imaging facility and dictate reports that are transcribed and provided to the referring physician in support of diagnostic decisions. A radiology information system (RIS) supports this process by handling patient scheduling, reporting, and other administrative functions; these systems can also incorporate sophisticated voice recognition software for radiologists to generate reports.

Increasingly, radiologists are interpreting images remotely from where they are captured. Other specialists, such as orthopedists, also require direct access to the underlying images, which can be logistically cumbersome for film-based modalities. Specialists, such as cardiologists, generate and use images (angiography, echocardiography) directly in support of their diagnostic and therapeutic decision making.

These demands have led providers to implement picture archiving and control system (PACS) technology, which comprises components that allow electronic acquisition, storage, viewing, and distribution of images. The

Digital Imaging and Communications in Medicine (DICOM) standard was developed to facilitate sharing of imaging data from multiple modalities and imaging equipment vendors (DICOM, 2012). Because digital image files are so large, PACS requires a large investment in data servers, digital archiving, viewing workstations, and high-bandwidth networks, as well as IT staff. Overall, PACS is a relatively mature technology implemented in most imaging-intensive provider organizations, particularly hospitals (Dorenfest Institute, 2010).

Electronic Medical Record (EMR) and Electronic Health Record (EHR)

In 2003, the electronic health record (EHR) was defined by the Institute of Medicine's Committee on Data Standards for Patient Safety as being a system that includes:

1. A longitudinal collection of electronic health information for and about persons, where health information is defined as information pertaining to the health of an individual or health care provided to an individual
2. Immediate electronic access to person- and population-level information by authorized, and only authorized, users
3. The provision of knowledge and decision-support that enhance the quality, safety, and efficiency of patient care
4. Support of efficient processes for health care delivery (Tang, 2003)

A growing amount of data has been captured in electronic systems, ranging from clinical to administrative and financial. Typically, the data are scattered across source systems that usually span an organization. Even if they remain within a single health care delivery system, data may originate from multiple sources that do not interface with a single repository. This makes access to the complete medical "record" of any individual a challenge for all patients and providers. The Health Information Management Systems Society (HIMSS) has developed a 7-level Electronic Medical Record Adoption Model that categorizes hospital EMR systems on the basis of their informatics capabilities and data integration. At the end of 2012, 61.7 percent of U.S. hospitals were at Stage 3 or lower, while only 10.1 percent of hospitals were at Stage 6 or 7, providing comprehensive clinical functionalities and data access (HIMSS, 2012).

The task of creating a longitudinal medical record for an individual is made even more difficult as a patient transitions between systems of care, for financial or personal reasons. Shifting public program eligibilities

(Access for Infants and Mothers, Medicaid, and SCHIP) may result in involuntary movement between health plans and providers. As a result, care may be disrupted and documentation scattered among providers and systems. At the traditional and safety net provider level, providers operate with thin margins and often do not have the resources to deploy or support more sophisticated electronic clinical or back office systems.

Reliable and widespread health data availability has been shown to be a key factor for the domains of clinical decision-making, health system management, care process improvement, health policy analysis, and health services research (Brailer, Augustinos, Evans, & Karp, 2003). However, there are additional, distinct, quantifiable benefits from use of electronic health records that can form the core business drivers initiating intra-organizational change. The IOM Committee on Data Standards for Patient Safety defined five criteria to guide identification of core EHR system functionalities that also serve as logical focus areas for assessment and planning activities (Tang, 2003). There is a significant body of literature documenting the ability of clinical information systems to positively affect all of these focus areas:

1. *Improve patient safety.* The IOM noted that between 44,000 and 98,000 individuals die annually from preventable adverse events in the health care setting (Kohn et al., 2000; Brennan, 2000). Use of relatively simple interventions such as clinical information systems that provide physician and patient reminders, treatment planners, and patient education have been shown to be effective at preventing some adverse events, but evidence on reduction of serious medical errors needs to receive more scientifically rigorous study. More sophisticated tools such as decision support systems for drug dosing and preventive care have also been shown to benefit providers and patients (Ammenwerth et al., 2008; Cutler, Feldman, & Horwitz, 2005). Clinical test results ordered by one physician may not be available to subsequent providers; this can lead to reordering of tests or missed critical values. Medication errors (adverse drug events) may also result from prescription by one provider (for instance, during an inpatient stay) and subsequent treatment (after discharge) by another where the patient is unable (or unwilling) to disclose the current active medication list, and ADEs were most strongly positively associated with the number of medications on the patient was currently taking (Sarkar, Lopez, Massalli, & Gonzalez, 2011).

2. *Support delivery of effective patient care.* The need for access to knowledge resources, especially subspecialty topics, arises frequently during office practice. Not all information needs encountered during clinical

visits are met through existing resources, however (Tang, Fafchamps, & Shortliffe, 1994). But lack of information can lead to lower-quality patient care. Appropriate medical care consistent with evidence-based practice guidelines are received by only 55 percent of Americans (McGlynn et al., 2003). Some of these issues may be addressed through availability of online resources such as journals and texts, as well as the medical references optimized for online reference that are now increasingly accessible. Pubmed.gov makes many journals available in a full-text format. Health care systems frequently license content systemwide. Other areas, such as the effectiveness of disease management protocols and systems, show great promise but require additional study before conclusive recommendation and adoption (Morris, 2003; Eccles et al., 2002). Redundant laboratory tests and other ancillary services may be reduced if previously ordered results are made available for review during subsequent encounters. Communication failures between providers (as during transition in patient care settings, or between care teams, or when moved through insurance plan coverage changes) can result in an event of omission no less adverse for a lack of malice, but systems can be implemented to standardize the exchange of information and reduce risk.

3. *Facilitate management of chronic conditions.* People with chronic conditions account for more than 75 percent of all health care spending, and physicians caring for these patients also report that the lack of care coordination leads to poor outcomes; almost half of all people with chronic medical conditions have more than one (Partnership for Solutions, 2004). Computer-based and mobile patient education applications are increasingly becoming popular for education and management of chronic care conditions. Implementation of a patient-controlled health record may allow context-sensitive delivery of patient education materials in a "push" format to the patient, but also as a way of "pinging" the provider, supplying updates on medication compliance or behavior protocols like exercise or weigh-in reporting. From 2011 to 2012, growth in physician adoption of EHR technology to engage patients and families in their health care was especially strong; the share of physicians with computerized capability to provide patients with clinical summaries after each visit increased by 46 percent (King et al., 2012).

4. *Improve efficiency.* A General Accounting Office (GAO) study released in 2003 noted that in a 1,951 bed teaching hospital more than $8.6 million in yearly savings was accrued through replacement of paper medical charts with electronic medical records system (GAO, 2003). A study by the San Francisco-based nonprofit Health Technology Center cited statistics

showing that up to 20 percent of laboratory and X-ray tests are repeated because prior results are unavailable for review, and that one in seven hospitalizations occurs because prior patient information is unavailable (HTC & Phelps & Phillips LLP, 2003). And a new report by the Office of the National Coordinator of Health Information Technology stated that physician adoption of eight computerized capabilities to improve quality, safety, and efficiency grew substantially, with increases ranging from 21 percent to 42 percent (King et al., 2012). Of the 72 percent of office-based physicians that have EHRs currently in place, nearly three-quarters—73 percent—of those surveyed said their EHRs could write prescriptions electronically, while 68 percent could keep a list of a patient's medication allergies (King et al., 2012).

5. *Feasibility of implementation.* Over the past three decades, there have been multiple efforts to coordinate these sources of data. Community health information networks developed during the 1980s were not highly successful because of organizational challenges in dealing with interorganizational competition, data ownership and control governance, confidentiality, and high up-front costs.

On the other hand, large integrated health delivery networks have acknowledged the importance of data sharing across facilities and providers by making significant, long-term investment in health information technology. The Veterans Health Administration made an investment of $600 to $700 million to take a decentralized, basic hospital information system (DHCP) and transform it into VistA and CPRS, a sophisticated electronic medical records system that allows transmission and access of patient health information between regions and hospitals across the entire network and yields sources for an enterprise data warehouse used for performance management. Kaiser Permanente recently completed a multiyear, $6 billion investment over a decade in implementing the EpicCare EMR (Madison, Wisconsin) electronic medical record system. Kaiser Permanente has long been a pioneer in deploying information technology solutions to its clinicians throughout multiple regions, and this initiative is the capstone that ties all regions together into a single EMR system called HealthConnect®.

Although there is a growing body of literature documenting distinct, quantifiable benefits from use of EHR systems within multihospital integrated delivery networks, there are an increasing number of EHR systems targeted toward the medium- and small-provider group level, and demonstrated benefits (and barriers to success) at that scale (CMS, 2012). Provider associations are becoming aware of the importance of electronic documentation and are stepping up the level of involvement and interaction with members. The American Academy of Family Physicians (AAFP) Center for Health Information Technology is working to educate small- and medium-sized physician offices on EHR systems and to assist in acquisition and implementation of these systems (AAFP, 2011). The American Academy of Pediatrics initiated a working group to assess the role of the organization in recommending specific EHR systems that support the unique health care needs of the pediatric population (Berkowitz, personal communication, September 2004). The "downward" push of technology into the smaller health care provider environment is enabling potential capture of even greater quantities of health care information in the future.

"Meaningful Use" Criteria

Under the 2009 federal economic stimulus package (ARRA), health care providers who demonstrate meaningful use of certified electronic health record systems can qualify for Medicaid and Medicare incentive payments. Meaningful use criteria for certified electronic health record technology incorporate such core objectives as improving quality, safety, and efficiency; engaging patients and family; improving care coordination and public health; and, maintaining privacy and security of patient health information (Hsiao et al., 2011). There are three stages for hospital implementation and compliance in establishing these criteria have been met—Stage 1 (2011–2012) "Data capture and sharing," Stage 2 (2014) "Advance clinical processes," and Stage 3 (2016) "Improved outcomes"—tied to financial incentive payments for compliance.

In December 2012, CDC's National Center for Health Statistics released a report finding that 27 percent of office-based physicians had EHR systems capable of supporting thirteen of the Stage 1 core objectives for the meaningful use program. To qualify for Stage 1, eligible professionals must meet fifteen core objectives and five additional objectives from a menu of 10 options. A report in the *New England Journal of Medicine* found that only 12.2 percent of the 509,328 eligible professionals had attested to the Medicare portion of the meaningful use program as of May 2012 (Wright et al., 2013). That percentage included 17.8 percent of eligible primary care providers and 9.8 percent of specialists. Primary care providers accounted for 44 percent of the Medicare meaningful use attestations, the report found. The median Medicare attestation rate for states was 7.7 percent of eligible professionals. Medicare attestation rates varied from 1.9 percent of eligible professionals in Alaska to 24.2 percent of eligible professionals in North Dakota, according to the report. The researchers noted that if EHR adoption rates continue at the same pace, many physicians could face federal penalties for not meeting meaningful use criteria by 2015.

Provider Adoption Rates of HIT and EMR

There is widespread acknowledgement of substantial barriers for physician HIT adoption. Decker, Jamoom, and Sisk (2012) found that although trends in adoption of electronic health record systems across geographic regions converged from 2002 through 2011, adoption continued to lag for nonprimary care specialists, physicians age fifty-five and older, physicians in small practices (one to two providers), and physician-owned practices. The significant impact on physician workflow constitutes the greatest risk for implementation failure, and yet the greatest opportunity for substantive improvement through eliminating workflow steps subject to a high rate of possible error. Perceived negative impact, such as decreased efficiency, can be used as a rallying point around which dissatisfied medical staff might effectively bring an implementation to a halt. This can be mitigated to some extent through strong administrative and medical leadership throughout the implementation, as well as extensive use of physician champions drawn from medical staff or house staff (in a teaching hospital) (Poon et al., 2004; Weeger, Gewald, & Vriesman, 2011). Another possible barrier to HIT adoption is the high cost of procurement and implementation, although analysis of Leapfrog data suggests that hospital ownership type may have a greater impact on the decision to commit to hospital HIT (such as CPOE) than positive net income or membership in a large integrated delivery network (Cutler et al., 2005).

Gaps in rates of adoption of at least a basic record system have increased substantially over the past four years based on hospital size, teaching status, and location. Small, nonteaching, and rural hospitals continue to adopt electronic health record systems more slowly than other types of hospitals (DesRoches, Worzala, Joshi, Kralovec, & Jha, 2012). Using national survey data on U.S. hospitals from 2011, the year federal incentives for the meaningful use of electronic health records began, this same study found that the share of hospitals with any electronic health record system increased from 15.1 percent in 2010 to 26.6 percent in 2011, and the share with a comprehensive system rose from 3.6 percent to 8.7 percent. The proportion able to meet criteria for meaningful use also rose; in 2011, 18.4 percent of hospitals had these functions in place in at least one unit and 11.2 percent had them across all clinical units.

Electronic Data Exchange Standards and Networks

The need to exchange clinical information between providers and provider organizations and hospitals is not novel. Information technology has been deployed to attain this goal for decades, the earliest notable examples being the Community Health Information Networks (CHIN) implemented in the 1980s. Though the vast majority of the CHINs failed from problems with funding sustainability or technical infrastructure, there are small handfuls that remain. As with most health information technology, the significant advances in computing power and networking capacity over the past fifteen years have reinvigorated the vision of fully portable clinical information.

In 2004, a presidential executive order was issued that endorsed incentives for use of HIT and formally established the Office of the National Coordinator for Health Information Technology (ONC) (Bush, 2004). Dr. David Brailer was appointed to ONC and tasked with coordinating programs and policies in order to achieve within ten years the goal of the National Health Information Infrastructure that supported access to an EHR for all Americans. The July 2004 ONC report titled "The Framework for Strategic Action" stated that patient health information should be portable and accessible from all points of care, and that both deployment of electronic health record systems and EHR interoperability were mandatory for seamless flow of information from clinical setting to clinical setting. Widespread adoption of EHR systems has many challenges, but interoperability between regional collaboratives is seen as more achievable.

Health Information Exchange (HIE)

Health information exchange (HIE) refers either to the electronic secured movement of clinical and business data or to an organization that provides data exchange services to a set of health care clients. Most health business data exchange can be categorized into three transactions: eligibility determinations, claim status inquiries, and claims submission and payment. The first two types of transactions are being used by hospitals at extremely low rates (11.6 percent and 16.1 percent, respectively in 2011), but are on the rise. Claims submission and payment were among the first to be implemented, and because of their impact on improving hospital cash flow, they have been adopted more extensively (70.6 percent in 2011) (Stone & Yoder, 2012).

Interoperability is critical for HIE to succeed regionally and nationally. Hospital-owned, internally developed HIE has more flexibility due to fewer stakeholders, allowing local hospitals and providers to tailor technical infrastructure, membership details, bundled payment analysis, and governance of the data being exchanged. But hospital-owned HIE must ensure and pursue a role of shared standards between unaffiliated providers to support myriad patients, public health reporting, and disease surveillance. This type of data and its exchange will be the "strategic lever" CEOs can use to position their organizations for long-term sustainability as they take on more risk in coordinated care and bundled payment arrangements (Stone & Yoder, 2012).

Regional Health Information Exchange

Regional health information organization (RHIO) was an earlier term used to describe regional collaborations among health care entities to allow access to electronic patient health information that was securely stored within the local community. The RHIO model emphasized flexibility, allowing customization of governance, technology, and policy depending on regional needs.

Perhaps the most successful demonstration of the RHIO concept began in 1991, when the Regenstrief Institute established a data sharing network for hospital emergency departments in the greater Indianapolis region. It uses a centralized clinical repository to afford access to results and other clinical data across the city. A centralized repository model refers to a method of access to clinical information where an end user queries a single data source for clinical information. This single source is created and fed either real-time from partner entities or batch data transmission and upload. In 2004, the Indiana Health Information Exchange (IHIE) was brought into existence with the goal of broadening the Regenstrief infrastructure and involving a greater number of providers across the state. Today, the IHIE serves more than 19,000 doctors and 80 hospitals, with data on more than 7 million patients, connecting hospitals, rehabilitation centers, long term care facilities, laboratories, imaging centers, clinics, community health centers and other health care organizations (IHIE, 2012).

A less successful RHIO example was the Santa Barbara County Care Data Exchange (SBCCDE), begun in 1998 with a $10 million investment from the California HealthCare Foundation and through CareScience (now part of the Premier health care alliance). Aiming to be a national demonstration model, it used a peer-to-peer approach to allow data sharing among disparate vendor systems. In this method of access to clinical information, an end user client pulls down data residing on a host server operated by the data owner (the entity that generated the clinical data). In Santa Barbara, a central server operated by coordinated security and messaging but did not contain any clinical data. After eight years of software development delays, design changes, and governance challenges, SBCCDE was unable to develop a sustainable financing model and shut down (Miller & Miller, 2007).

Although more limited in scope, the New England Healthcare Exchange Network (NEHEN) is an example of success in establishing the necessary framework for exchange of data among multiple organizational entities (Glaser, DeBor, & Stuntz, 2003). It also focuses on a peer-to-peer approach for sharing information, and now includes more than 50 participating organizations. The most recent annual survey by the eHealth Initiative (2012) found that over two hundred regional health information exchange projects are now in some stage of development across the nation.

All regional health information exchange efforts share several challenges (Halamka et al., 2005). Whether deployed peer-to-peer or using a central repository technical approach, successful interoperability requires both data and messaging standards and adoption of common standards by all participating parties. Patients and organizations furnishing data must be confident of the measures taken to safeguard the privacy and security of sensitive information, from source through to destination. Identifying the appropriate governance and leadership model is essential for a successful transition to operations, but this structure is likely to be highly regionalized. Without defined return-on-investment metrics for all participants, it is difficult for regional exchanges to transition from initial startup funding to ongoing financial viability.

Nationwide Health Information Network (NwHIN)

The National Committee on Vital and Health Statistics (NCVHS) first described a vision and plan for a National Health Information Infrastructure (NHII) in 2001 (HHS, 2001). The NHII was not a specific technology solution. Rather, it was the "set of organizing principles, systems, standards, procedures, and policies" that described the framework around which to achieve the concept of complete patient-specific health information availability for patient care where and when it is needed (Yasnoff et al., 2000). It incorporated advances in health information technology, electronic medical and health records, and the growing number of regional health information exchange organizations to project a realistic and achievable goal. Federal initiatives surrounding public health preparedness and personal health records used the NHII as a foundation for national implementation.

Although the concept remained the same, the terminology began to evolve with the release of the Institute of Medicine (IOM) report *Crossing the Quality Chasm*, in which the need for a National Health Information Network (NHIN) was suggested (IOM, 2001). The 2004 ONC "Framework for Strategic Action" report also references the NHIN, and subsequent federal initiatives such as the AHRQ-funded prototype demonstration models, referenced the NHIN in describing the physical interoperability of regional networks and electronic health information technology systems spanning personal health, public health, and clinical medicine.

One estimate placed the capital expenditure for such a network at $156 billion, with $48 billion in annual operating costs; two-thirds of estimated capital costs were allocated toward achieving functionality (results reporting, CPOE, EHR, ANSI X.12 270/271, patient communication, e-prescribing) and the remaining costs for interoperability programming (Kaushal et al., 2005). However, it has also been suggested that the implementation of an HIE on a national scale could also lead to significant cost savings, close to $78 billion per year, to counteract the initial cost of implementation (Walker et al., 2005). These types of financial estimates helped to facilitate the funding provided for HIE in the HITECH Act.

ONC now defines the Nationwide Health Information Network (NwHIN) as "a set of standards, services, and policies that enable the secure exchange of health information over the Internet." Central to this vision of interoperable health information systems, which will allow organizations to share information easily within regional health information exchanges, are standards for the diverse types of clinical and administrative information generated in the provision and financing of health care. Terminology standards, such as ICD-9 coding for medical diagnoses, common procedural terminology (CPT) codes, or the Systematized Nomenclature of Medicine (SNOMED), assign standard codes to several hundred thousand specific clinical concepts. Messaging standards such as Health Level 7 (HL-7) define the format of messages within which clinical or administrative data can be exchanged among information systems within an organization or across organizations. A health information standard can be created and maintained by a nonprofit consortium, such as Health Level Seven (www.hl7.org), or it may be a proprietary product such as SNOMED (owned by the College of American Pathologists). Government actions may accelerate adoption of particular standards, as occurred when HIPAA mandated use of several standards, including ICD-9 and CPT, or when the ONC contracted for SNOMED to be made publicly available.

Public Health Informatics

Public health informatics has been defined as systematic application of information and computer science and technology to public health practice, research, and learning (Yasnoff et al., 2000). It broadens the focus from the patient-clinician dyad to larger issues of how information systems can assist in analysis of data on the multiple determinants of health to improve disease prevention and population health. It differs from other biomedical informatics domains in its complex dependency on federal, state, and local government regulations. As with information systems aimed at health care delivery, the IOM has supported greater adoption of informatics tools and techniques within public health (Gebbie, Rosenstock, & Hernandez, 2003).

Public health professionals have long used information technology to facilitate public health practice in areas such as communicable disease surveillance and collection and dissemination of population health information, but such systems have historically been designed and implemented in isolation (Friede & O'Carroll, 1996). Federal legislation and initiatives following the September 11, 2001, World Trade Center attack led to coordination between previously separate funding and operational silos, and funding was allocated to enhancement of the public health infrastructure. In April 2012, an IOM Committee on Public Health Strategies to Improve Health, recommended that Congress double public health infrastructure spending from 2011 levels of $12 billion to $24 billion if we are to achieve a minimum package of public health targets for the nation (IOM, 2012) Although NwHIN discussions focus on direct benefit to the individual patient, provider, and payer, the public health information infrastructure (PHII) component is an integral part of reaching population health goals.

The pool of data used for public health assurance activities is very broad, especially when viewed in light of a model that incorporates multiple determinants of health (Evans & Stoddart, 1990). Clinical data are usually supplied through automated reporting of laboratory, radiology, or other ancillary test results. Trigger events, such as reportable diseases, may require follow-up manual chart review to yield necessary information. Unfortunately, where manual effort is required, clinicians may not complete the reporting process, whether mandatory or not. Electronic health records and health information exchange have the potential to greatly increase the efficacy and accuracy of public health systems by automating reporting of detailed patient information. For example, real-time emergency department chief complaint data can be obtained through messaging feeds from provider EHR systems and sent directly to decision support systems. Notably, the Health Insurance Portability and Accountability Act (HIPAA) Privacy Rule supports essential public health objectives by permitting disclosure of protected health information (PHI) for specific public health purposes, such as mandated reporting for disease prevention or control. In addition, the rule permits covered entities to make disclosures when required by laws other than those governing public health purposes.

Other sources are environmental data, which can include air quality and particulate measurements, water quality, animal deaths, and testing data (for example, West Nile virus, Lyme disease, and other tick-borne diseases); and survey data, which are critical for assessment of the health of populations. Survey datasets range from national clinical studies (National Health and Nutrition Evaluation Survey, http://www.cdc.gov /nchs/nhanes.htm) to statewide random-digit phone surveys (California Health Interview Survey, http://healthpolicy.ucla.edu/chis/Pages/default .aspx) and to local and regional interviews (Los Angeles County Health Survey, http://publichealth.lacounty.gov/ha/hasurveyintro.htm).

The CDC has articulated the Public Health Information Network (PHIN) as its vision for an interoperable, multi-organizational business and technical architecture that supports public health activities and improves public health outcomes. Specifically, the PHIN spans all sources of data and targets (1) disease surveillance, (2) national health status indicators, (3) data analysis, (4) public health decision support, (5) alerting and communications, and (6) management of public health response through support for development of necessary messaging standards and common software solutions (CDC, n.d.-c). Using a group of common services (public health conceptual data model; standards for messaging and vocabulary; public health directory of people, organizations, and jurisdictions), PHIN brings together several existing programs and activities that were separately organized, including the Health Alert Network (HAN) and the National Electronic Disease Surveillance System (NEDSS); defines a new, common architecture; and sets the framework for existing application migration and future application development as part of the PHIN.

- HAN is an Internet and broadcast communications system that disseminates emergent health information, alerts, and advisories to key public health officials and first responders at the state and community levels (CDC, n.d.-a)

- NEDSS focuses on implementation of integrated disease surveillance systems at the federal, state, and local levels (CDC, n.d.-b). It aims to capitalize on movement within the health care delivery system toward electronic documentation to permit more timely and comprehensive information while not overly burdening providers.

In 2011, the American Medical Informatics Association convened experts from the public health and health informatics communities to develop an informatics agenda for public health. Sixty-two recommendations were generated and were clustered into three key thematic areas. (Massoudi et al., 2012).

The first theme was enhancing the communication and information sharing capacity within the public health community. The advances in information and computing technologies, such as high bandwidth networking, computational clusters, high-density disk arrays, and cloud computing, make it possible to aggregate, store, and analyze vast quantities of data in near-real-time. The infusion of post-9/11 and ARRA funding also led to the development of many new applications and frameworks. Meeting participants noted that there was substantial experience from these efforts, yet very little formal sharing within the public health informatics community. A key recommendation was to develop and maintain a comprehensive and detailed repository of available public health data sources and data elements.

The second theme focused upon the need to improve the way data and information is shared across the public health informatics landscape. Specifically, given a limited resource environment, participants focused upon the need to maximize future investments in public health informatics initiatives. Increasing dependence upon increasing quantities of electronically collected data suggests that the development and use of a common framework of public health processes and use cases developed around evidence-based public health practices could promote more effective development of systems and data sets. Similarly, it was noted that there were many public health data and vocabulary standards available, such as the terminology resources at the National Library of Medicine, but there was little understanding and use. There was strong consensus that the level of research and evaluation for public health informatics needed to be elevated. It was recommended that formal program evaluations be augmented with measures informed and adapted from work in other fields, such as social and behavioral science, health outcomes, and comparative effectiveness research. Paired with workforce development and academic training programs using defined competencies, it will be possible to foster the development of continuously learning communities within public health informatics.

The final key theme focused upon the need to have more effective coordination and leadership within the field of public health informatics. Although informatics tools are inseparable from the delivery of current public health services, and there exists a very substantial investment in existing public health informatics infrastructures, there is insufficient "coherent governance" at a national level (Yasnoff et al., 2004) to coordinate activities spread across federal, state, territorial, and local levels. It was strongly recommended that a coordinating agency be designated to provide public health informatics leadership and to serve as the convener for the development of a strategic plan for public health infrastructure and informatics investment. One model of such a coordinating agency is ONC, which, in collaboration with CMS funding incentives, has accelerated the meaningful adoption of electronic health record and health information exchange.

Disease Registries

Chronic conditions cause significant morbidity and mortality and account for as much as 75 percent of health care spending (Metzger, 2004). Disease registries deployed in conjunction with other care management enhancements can assist both individual patients and populations in maintaining health status. Although the first disease registries were deployed during the early 1980s at institutions such as Group Health of Puget Sound (Seattle) and Lovelace Health System (Albuquerque, New Mexico), adoption has accelerated significantly in recent years. At the micro level, disease registries track patients with chronic diseases with the goal of consolidating data from external electronic sources and manually entered records into a single repository from which the chronic condition can be more effectively managed and better preventive care delivered through reduction in omissions and gaps in care (Kilo, 2005). At the population level, registries can assist in identifying best practices and can generate data for reporting on the health of larger population groups, or provider performance.

Disease-specific registries are also used for program administration. However, some diseases have multiple funding streams associated with service delivery; as a result, there may be proliferation of information systems each focusing on a single aspect. For example, regarding HIV/AIDS, there are HIV registries, AIDS registries, the Ryan White program registry, and drug assistance program registries (Lumpkin & Richards, 2002). This complexity of enrolling and maintaining multiple registries can lead to data synchronization problems in reporting across multiple systems. In parallel with PHIN and federal efforts to adopt common standards, state and local agencies are starting the process of closer integration and coordination to reduce errors of omission and of commission.

Immunization Registries

Immunization registries are databases covering population groups defined by geography or payer or provider that contain information about children and adults who receive immunization. Although focused registries were developed in the late 1980s for institutions such as Kaiser Permanente (the Kaiser Immunization Tracking System), it was not until the early 1990s that sufficient national effort and funding was focused into implementing broader immunization registries. Healthy People 2010 notes specific target immunization rates for the general population and defines the goal of having 95 percent of children age six or younger having at least two immunizations recorded in a regional registry (Saarlas, Edwards, Wild, & Richmond, 2003).

These registries may include decision support tools to assist in identifying needed immunizations at the point of care, analytical tools to assist in reporting rates, and care delivery tools to assist in sending electronic or paper mail reminders. Mature registries offer both process benefits (reminders and decision support) and cost benefits associated with reducing manual medical record pulls, researching past history across multiple patient documents, and overimmunizing. These efficiencies are gained only if the majority of individuals within the database have up-to-date records and virtually all providers are using the system to enter immunization data. As with disease registries, the compliance rate for data completeness improves considerably if submission is automated and originates from EHR or practice management software that captures the requisite demographics and immunization and vaccine detailed information (including manufacturer, lot number, and expiration date).

Applications of Information Systems by Health Plans and Payers

Managed care organizations (MCOs) and government health care payers (Medicare and Medicaid) use large transaction-oriented information systems—often referred to as "legacy systems"—to support their core administrative activities. One such system supports the claims adjudication process, where claims submitted by providers are approved for payment or denied on the basis of the MCO's rules and applicable contracts with providers and purchasers. These systems can handle millions of claims per month in a large MCO. The member database contains demographic data about persons covered by the MCO, as well as information about the group each member belongs to and the associated benefits for which she or he is eligible. Another database contains data about providers (such as physicians and hospitals), as well as contracted payment rates and network membership (such as PPO or HMO). Other information systems support premium billing and payments to providers (both capitation and fee for service).

Other information systems support care management activities such as case management for high-risk members, utilization management, or disease management. Because these systems contain more clinical data than the legacy administrative systems, they play a larger role in supporting population health improvement activities. Integrative activities such as external reporting, provider profiling, and decision making (such as premium pricing) require data from multiple information systems to be extracted into a data warehouse. Increasingly, MCOs are replacing fragmented legacy systems with more integrated enterprise systems. In addition, EHR adoption by providers and information sharing via HIEs may also make clinical data for population health management more readily available to MCOs.

Fully electronic interchange of information, claims, and payments between providers and MCOs is expected to improve the efficiency of the U.S. health care system, but progress toward that goal remains mixed. Although HIPAA mandates standards for information "transactions," it does not require that all such transactions actually be performed electronically. A substantial majority of provider claims are now submitted electronically (Emdeon Business Services, 2010), often via "clearinghouse" organizations that assist providers in complying with submission requirements across multiple MCOs. The majority of payment transactions are electronic (InstaMed, 2012), although small providers lag well behind on this dimension. Fully automated real-time claims adjudication is offered by some MCOs, but relatively few providers and clearinghouses are yet able to submit all required information electronically at the time services are provided.

Changes in the health insurance market, such consumer-directed health plans (CDHPs), significantly expand the required scope and complexity of MCO information systems. The goal of CDHPs is to reduce spending by making members more aware of the costs of care and encouraging them to choose lower-cost providers (Haviland et al., 2012). CDHPs feature high deductibles, usually coupled with tax-free health savings accounts (HSAs). MCOs therefore offer CDHP members online portals to access information about providers, plus decision support systems to inform their choices. Claims and financial systems must also be linked to member HSAs.

Quality measurement and quality improvement (QI) are core MCO activities that rely heavily on information systems. (See Chapter Eleven for an overview of health care quality measurement and improvement concepts and techniques.) The most widely used set of quality indicators for MCOs is the Health Plan Employer Data and Information Set (HEDIS), a mandatory component of the National Committee for Quality Assurance (NCQA) accreditation process for MCOs. HEDIS consists of over seventy-five measures assessing preventive care, management of specific clinical conditions, member satisfaction, and service utilization (NCQA, n.d). To construct these measures, MCOs collect and aggregate data from providers who serve their members.

Providers face an increasing scope of payer requirements for external quality and performance reporting. For example, physicians face a small financial penalty for not reporting data to Medicare's Physician Quality Reporting Initiative (PQRI), and achieving PCMH certification requires submission of dozens of performance measures. Physicians are also often eligible for MCOs' pay-for-performance (P4P) programs that give physicians financial incentives for improved performance. The Integrated Healthcare Association (IHA), sponsored by California MCOs, pays out approximately $50M annually to over 200 physician organizations based on indicators of quality, member satisfaction, and IT use (IHA, 2012). For hospitals, avoidance of Medicare financial penalties leads to near-universal reporting of CMS Core Measures of quality. Medicare's Value Based Purchasing program will use these quality measures, plus additional measures of patient satisfaction and efficiency, as the basis of more comprehensive hospital P4P. And HITECH's MU criteria require both physicians and hospitals to report performance on several Clinical Quality Measures.

It is hoped that EHRs will help providers meet these expanding requirements more efficiently at a time when reimbursements are also being tightened. Calculation of a single performance measure requires multiple data elements, including disease-specific inclusion and exclusion criteria that define the patients to which the measure applies. Extracting these data elements electronically from an EHR is much less labor-intensive than manual chart abstraction—but also requires that clinical staff accurately document the care they provide. In addition, standardizing measures across external stakeholders streamlines data capture and extraction. The National Quality Forum (NQF) endorses hundreds of nationally standardized quality measures and is developing measure specifications to facilitate automated electronic extraction of necessary data elements from EHRs (NQF, 2011).

Future Directions

Some emerging applications of informatics hold significant potential to affect clinical practice and medical science, particularly telemedicine and bioinformatics.

Telemedicine

Telemedicine systems use information technology and telecommunications links to enable expert clinicians to interview patients, make diagnoses, and recommend treatment at a distance (Craig & Patterson, 2005). Telemedicine is most widely used in radiology and pathology, where images are transmitted from remote sites to a specialist, who then produces a written interpretation. Such applications can operate effectively in asynchronous, or "store-and-forward," mode. Applications are also growing in other specialties where remote interpretation of images can effectively yield diagnoses or treatment recommendations, especially dermatology, ophthalmology, and cardiology. High-speed internet connections facilitate telemedicine applications that require real-time communication between the patient's location and the remote specialist, such as mental health care.

Telemedicine promises a range of benefits. It can enhance access to specialty care for isolated populations (rural residents, prisoners, the disabled, or urban residents with limited access to specialist physicians). It can also increase efficiency by reducing transportation costs or taking advantage of economies of scale in use of specialized medical expertise. For example, telemedicine plays a growing role in providing care for the most acutely ill patients, such as remote intensivist monitoring of ICU patients ("eICU") (Cummings et al., 2007) or the remote assessment of stroke patients (Mitka, 2009).

Several factors could be expected to foster expanded use of telemedicine: growing availability of broadband internet connections, increasing electronic capture of health information available via EHRs, and ongoing cost pressures. However, successful, telemedicine programs require not just technology but also organizational networks within which this technology can be effectively used in clinical care (Krasnow & Rodrigues, 1998). For example, the VA, which serves a large number of rural patients and has established clinician relationships and technical infrastructure, has perhaps the nation's largest scale implementations of telemedicine (Hill et al., 2010). Non-technological restrictions remain the most significant barriers to broader telemedicine use in the U.S.: varying reimbursement standards across payers (Whitten & Buis, 2006) and medical licensing laws that restrict consultation across state lines.

Bioinformatics

Bioinformatics can be broadly defined as "the study of how information technologies are used to solve problems in biology (Altman, 1998)." Bioinformatics often focuses on molecular biology, particularly molecules such as the DNA that encodes the genetic information for all organisms (the subject of genomics) and the proteins produced from that genetic information (whose structure and function are the subject of proteomics).

The sequencing of the human genome has opened a new era in medical science and, it is hoped, in clinical medicine (Feero et al., 2010). Bioinformatics is central to realizing this promise, and is itself a rapidly evolving discipline. Broadly speaking, bioinformatics systems perform two major types of application. First, large databases organize and afford access to the huge and growing amount of data about genomes, proteins, and their associated biological and medical (phenotypic) manifestations. Second, sophisticated algorithms are needed to derive useful scientific and clinical knowledge from those data (Schadt et al., 2010).

Bioinformatics is at the frontier of applying "big data" approaches to biology and medicine (Manyika et al., 2011). For example:.

- Public databases house genomic and proteomic data for humans and other organisms, and incorporate powerful search tools (National Center Biotechnology Information [NCBI], n.d.).
- Genomewide association studies aim to correlate specific genetic variations with the incidence of human disease (Manolio, 2010).
- Informatics tools are central to proteomic investigations, such as identifying biomarkers for specific diseases (Lisacek et al., 2006).

- Projects such as The Cancer Genome Atlas (2012) compare genomic variation with the pathology and clinical manifestations of specific diseases.
- Pharmacogenomics, which studies the relationships between genetic variation and response to drugs, is expected to accelerate drug discovery and identify treatments tailored to individual patients. Specialized databases and algorithms support these areas (McDonagh et al., 2011).

The availability of inexpensive genome sequencing raises hopes for truly "personalized medicine" (Chan & Ginsburg, 2011). Informatics tools will be essential to help physicians identify which genetic variations are clinically relevant, as well as to remain current with rapidly evolving knowledge of tailored diagnostics and treatment. Practical solutions to this vast knowledge management need will be important future challenges for bioinformatics and clinical informatics.

Privacy and Security of Electronic Health Information

Electronic collection, storage, and transmission of health information poses risks of unauthorized information use, modification, or disclosure that did not exist when health information was mostly stored in paper form. For example, information about a person's medical conditions could more easily be inappropriately disclosed to an employer or used for marketing purposes. The American public expresses ongoing concern about such risks (Markle Foundation, 2011). Growth of HIEs and wider adoption of EHRs makes these risks ever more salient.

Patients expect their health care providers and health plans, as well as those organizations' business partners, to protect the privacy of their personal health information, including detailed demographic data, medical history and conditions, and medications or treatments received. More specifically, privacy can be defined as "an individual's claim to control the circumstances in which personal information is collected, used, and transmitted" (Gostin, 1997).

Protecting the privacy of personal health information depends on strong security, that is, "the technological, organizational, and administrative safety practices, policies, and procedures designed to protect data systems against unwarranted disclosure, modification, or destruction and to safeguard the system itself" (Gostin, 1997). Security technologies and practices have a direct impact on the design and operation of health information systems.

At the federal level, HIPAA mandates broad privacy protection standards for health care providers, payers, and clearinghouses (HHS, 2012a). These "covered entities" are given wide latitude to use personal health information for "treatment, payment, and health care operations," but they must obtain patients' specific authorization to use the information for marketing or other purposes. Use and disclosure of information is permitted for several activities, such as public health, law enforcement, and research; HITECH strengthened requirements that covered entities notify patients in the event of "breaches" to the privacy or security of their protected health information. HIPAA mandates that providers allow patients access to the information in their own medical records. HIPAA preempts weaker state laws, but states are free to enact more stringent privacy protection standards.

HIPAA also mandates security standards that covered entities must meet to protect personal health information (HHS, 2012b). Rather than specifying particular technologies that organizations must adopt, the standards offer guidance in several areas (administrative, physical, and technical safeguards). Within a fundamental framework of risk analysis and management, organizations have wide latitude in choosing how to implement the standards. For example, they may choose to use biometrics in addition to passwords for user identification.

Individuals' concern for the privacy of their health information must be balanced against growing needs to access and aggregate health information about populations of patients. For example, personal health information must be used in a public health investigation of a disease outbreak. Research, policy analysis, and quality improvement efforts often aggregate and analyze data about large numbers of patients. Data for these purposes can be "de-identified" by removing personal data elements such as names, addresses and dates of birth. However, such data may remain identifiable thanks to unique patterns in individuals' detailed demographic and clinical data and therefore must still be kept secure.

It has become clear that HIPAA, drafted when internet use and EHR adoption were much lower than now, has severe shortcomings (Gostin & Nass, 2009). For example, its reliance on informed consent has no impact on inadequate security or unauthorized disclosures, at the same time as it poses unnecessary barriers to information-based health research. More robust frameworks have been developed that comprise both better privacy protection policies and better technical standards for protecting health information that is exchanged among organizations (Connecting for Health, 2012). The need for broader implementation of such frameworks will only grow as movements toward personalized medicine capture larger volumes of highly sensitive personal health information.

SUMMARY

Information technology continues to transform many sectors of the economy and society, and increasingly the U.S. health care system as well. Applications of information systems in clinical practice are growing. Information technology is also central to the vision of personalized medicine, patients' engagement in chronic disease prevention and management, and broad information sharing across the diverse U.S. system of payers and provider organizations. However, realizing improved quality, efficiency, and access from information technology implementation will require supportive national health policies, ongoing reforms in health care financing, and effective management of health care provider organizations.

KEY TERMS

Biomedical informatics The interdisciplinary field that studies and pursues the effective uses of biomedical data, information, and knowledge for scientific inquiry, problem solving, and decision making, driven by efforts to improve human health.

Clinical decision support system (CDSS) Systems or groups of systems that integrate patient-specific data along with computer-represented clinical knowledge (for example, guidelines or antibiotic resistance sensitivity) in order to frame point-of-care alerting, reporting, and order or care plan recommendations.

Computerized provider order entry (CPOE) Systems that automate the manual process by which physician orders are communicated to other health care providers, including nursing, pharmacy, and ancillary departments such as dietary, respiratory therapy, occupational therapy, and physical therapy. Advanced CPOE systems integrate decision support tools into the ordering workflow.

Disease registry Systems that incorporate data from multiple sources about patients with chronic diseases or other health conditions (such as receipt of implants), so as to reduce omissions and gaps in care.

Electronic medical record (EMR) A longitudinal collection of electronic health information about persons, providing authorized, and only authorized, users immediate electronic access to health information and decision support, as well as support of efficient processes for health care delivery.

Health information exchange The electronic secured movement of clinical and business data among health care providers, payers, and public health agencies.

Health information technology Systems of computers and software and networks and telecommunications to connect them, as well as computerized clinical and administrative data and procedures to collect, store, analyze, transfer, and retrieve those data.

Meaningful use The 2009 HITECH Act and subsequent regulation define Meaningful Use as: the use of certified EHR [electronic health record] technology in a meaningful manner (for example electronic prescribing); ensuring that the certified EHR technology is connected in a manner that provides for the electronic exchange of health information to improve the quality of care; and that in using certified EHR technology the provider must submit to the Secretary of Health & Human Services (HHS) information on quality of care and other measures.

Telemedicine Systems that use information technology and telecommunications links to enable expert clinicians to interview patients, make diagnoses, and recommend treatment at a distance.

DISCUSSION QUESTIONS

1. Why has implementation of information technology in health care and public health been so slow compared to other industries? Discuss the relative importance of factors such as financial incentives or disincentives, organizational culture, complex clinical workflows, information technology capabilities and change, and information exchange complexity.

2. How does the structure of the health care financing system affect information technology implementation? Why are integrated systems like the Veterans Health Administration more likely to implement comprehensive clinical information technology solutions?

3. How have the financial incentives of the HITECH Act influenced the adoption of information technology by health care providers? Do you believe further federal action would be helpful or overly burdensome?

4. How will more widespread implementation of clinical information technologies (EMR, CPOE, CDSS) change the provision of care? Explore a few scenarios at the patient level.

5. How can public health agencies benefit from advances in health information technology and data sharing among providers and payers, given the agencies' limited resources?

6. How can payers, including Medicare and Medicaid, most effectively engage with provider organizations to maximize the quality improvement impact of information technology?

7. Give some examples of populations that could be helped by telemedicine (e.g., rural, homebound, poor, imprisoned). What types of physicians would each population most benefit from accessing?

8. What are some steps provider and payer organizations should take to protect the privacy of personal health information? What steps should be taken by a HIE that receives data from multiple providers and payers in a community?

FURTHER READING

Blumenthal, D. (2011). Wiring the health system: Origins and provisions of a new federal program. *New England Journal of Medicine, 365*(24), 2323–2329.

Blumenthal, D. (2011). Implementation of the federal Health Information Technology Initiative. *New England Journal of Medicine, 365*(25), 2426–2431.

Former national coordinator for HIT provides an overview of key challenges and opportunities in implementing HIT, as well as the federal incentives put in place by the HITECH Act.

Shortliffe, E. H., & Cimino, J. J. (Eds.). (2006). *Biomedical informatics: Computer applications in health care and biomedicine* (3rd ed.). New York: Springer.

A very comprehensive book describing clinical applications of information technology.

O'Carroll, P. W., Yasnoff, W. A., Ward, M. E., Ripp, L. H., & Martin, E. L. (Eds.). (2003). *Public health informatics and information systems*. New York: Springer.

The most comprehensive book describing the full range of public health informatics. Office of the National Coordinator (ONC) for HIT provides background as well as regularly updated information about key issues and Federal government policies regarding HIT, interoperability, information exchange standards, and privacy/security. See http://www.healthit.gov.

Wager, K. A., Lee, F. W., & Glaser, J. P. (2009). *Managing health care information systems: A practical approach for health care management*. San Francisco: Jossey-Bass.

Another book that describes the organizational and management issues surrounding the implementation of health information technology.

This website provides comprehensive basic information about bioinformatics, as well as links to other sites offering more in-depth information: http://bioinformatics .org/wiki/Main_Page.

The Center for Democracy and Technology's Health Privacy Project provides information from a patient-oriented perspective regarding risks to health information privacy as well as Federal and state initiatives to protect it. See https://www.cdt.org /issue/health-privacy.

REFERENCES

Adams, K., & Corrigan, J. M. (Eds.). (2003). *Priority areas for national action: Transforming healthcare quality.* Washington, DC: National Academies Press.

Altman, R. B. (1998). Bioinformatics in support of molecular medicine. *Proceedings of AMIA Symposium,* 53–61.

American Association of Family Physicians. (2011). Center for Health IT: HER adoption. Retrieved from http://www.centerforhit.org/online/chit/home/ehr-adoption.html

Ammenwerth, E., Schnell-Inderst, P., Machan, C., & Seibert, U. (2008). The effect of prescribing on medication errors and adverse drug events: A systematic review. *Journal of American Medical Informatics Association, 15*(5), 585–600.

Ash, J. S., Sittig, D. F., Guappone, K. P., Dykstra, R. H., Richardson, J., Wright, A., . . . Middleton, B. (2012). Recommended practices for computerized clinical decision support and knowledge management in community settings: A qualitative study. *BMC Medical Informatics and Decision Making, 12*(6).

Baker, G., Macintosh-Murray, A., Porcellato, C., Dionne, L., Stelmacovich, K., & Born, K. (2008). InterMountain Healthcare. *High-performing healthcare systems: Delivering quality by design* (pp. 151–178). Toronto: Longwoods.

Bates, D. W., Leape, L. L., Cullen, D. J., Laird, N., Petersen, L. A., Teich, J. M., . . . Seger, D. L. (1998). Effect of computerized physician order entry and a team intervention on prevention of serious medication errors. *Journal of the American Medical Association, 280*(15), 1311–1316.

Blumenthal, D. (2011a). Wiring the health system: Origins and provisions of a new federal program. *New England Journal of Medicine, 365*(24), 2323–2329.

Blumenthal, D. (2011b). Implementation of the federal health information technology initiative. *New England Journal of Medicine, 365*(25), 2426–2431.

Brailer, D. J., Augustinos, N., Evans, L. M., & Karp, S. (2003). *Moving toward electronic health information exchange: Interim report on the Santa Barbara County data exchange.* Oakland: California HealthCare Foundation.

Brennan, T. A. (2000). The Institute of Medicine report on medical errors: Could it do harm? *New England Journal of Medicine, 342*(15), 1123–1125.

Buntin, M. B., Burke, M. F., Hoaglin, M. C., & Blumenthal, D. (2011). The benefits of health information technology: A review of the recent literature shows predominantly positive results. *Health Affairs 30*(3), 464–471.

Bush, G. W. (2004, May). Executive order 13335: Incentives for the use of health information technology and establishing the position of the National Health Information Technology Coordinator. Retrieved from http://nodis3.gsfc.nasa.gov/displayEO.cfm?id=EO_13335

Chan, I. S., & Ginsburg, G. S. (2011). Personalized medicine: Progress and promise. *Annual Review of Genomics and Human Genetics, 12*, 217–244.

Centers for Disease Control and Prevention. (n.d.-a). Health alert network. Retrieved from http://emergency.cdc.gov/HAN

Centers for Disease Control and Prevention. (n.d.-b). National electronic disease surveillance system. Retrieved from http://wwwn.cdc.gov/nndss/script/nedss.aspx

Centers for Disease Control and Prevention. (n.d.-c). Public health information network. Retrieved from http://www.cdc.gov/phin/about/index.html

Centers for Medicare and Medicaid Services. (2010). Eligible professional meaningful use core measures. Retrieved from http://www.cms.gov/Regulations-and-Guidance/Legislation/EHRIncentivePrograms/downloads/11_Clinical_Decision_Support_Rule.pdf

Centers for Medicare and Medicaid Services. (2012). *The CMS EHR incentive programs: Small-practice providers and clinical quality measures.* Retrieved from http://www.cms.gov/EHRIncentivePrograms

Connecting for Health. (2012). *The common framework: Overview and principles.* New York: Markle Foundation. Retrieved from http://www.markle.org/health/markle-common-framework

Craig, J., & Patterson, V. (2005). Introduction to the practice of telemedicine. *Journal of Telemedicine and Telecare, 11*(1), 3–9.

Cummings, J., Krsek, C., Vermoch, K., & Matuszewski, K. (2007). Intensive care unit telemedicine: Review and consensus recommendations. *American Journal of Medical Quality, 22*(4), 239–250.

Cutler, D. M., Feldman, N. E., & Horwitz, J. R. (2005). U.S. adoption of computerized physician order entry systems. *Health Affairs, 24*(6), 1654–1663.

Decker, S. L., Jamoom, E. W., & Sisk, J. E. (2012). Physicians in nonprimary care and small practices and those age 55 and older lag in adopting electronic health record systems. *Health Affairs, 31*(5), 1108–1114.

DesRoches, C. M., Campbell E. G., Rao, S. R., Donelan, K., Ferris, T. G., Jha, A. K., ... Blumenthal, D. (2008). Electronic health records in ambulatory care; A national survey of physicians. *New England Journal of Medicine, 359*(1), 50–60.

DesRoches, C. M., Campbell, E. G., Vogeli, C., Zheng, J., Rao, S. R., Shields, A. E., ... Jha, A. K. (2010). Electronic health records' limited successes suggest more targeted uses. *Health Affairs, 29*(4), 639–646.

DesRoches, C. M., Worzala, C., Joshi, M. S., Kralovec, P. D., & Jha, A. K. (2012). Small, nonteaching, and rural hospitals continue to be slow in adopting electronic health record systems. *Health Affairs, 31*(5), 1092–1099.

Digital Imaging and Communications in Medicine. (2012). Retrieved from http://medical.nema.org

Dorenfest Institute. (2010). *Picture archiving and communication systems: A 2000–2008 study.* Chicago: HIMSS Foundation.

Eccles, M., McColl, E., Steen, N., Rousseau, N., Grimshaw, J. Parkin, D., & Purves, I. (2002). Effect of computerised evidence based guidelines on management of asthma and angina in adults in primary care: Cluster randomised controlled trial. *British Medical Journal, 325*(7370), 941.

eHealth Initiative. (2012). *2012 report on health information exchange: Supporting healthcare reform.* Retrieved from http://www.ehealthinitiative.org/resources /viewcategory/48-health-information-exchange.html

Emdeon Business Services (2010). *National progress report on healthcare efficiency.* Retrieved from http://www.ushealthcareindex.org/resources/USHEINationalProgress Report.pdf

Evans, R. G., & Stoddart, G. L. (1990). Producing health, consuming healthcare. *Social Science and Medicine, 31*(12), 1347–1363.

Feero, W. G., Guttmacher, A. G., & Collins, F. S. (2010). Genomic medicine: An updated primer. *New England Journal of Medicine, 362*(21), 2001–2011.

Friede, A., & O'Carroll, P. W. (1996). CDC and ATSDR electronic information resources for health officers. *Journal of Public Health Management Practice, 2*(3), 10–24.

Gebbie, K. M., Rosenstock, L., & Hernandez, L. M. (Eds.). (2003). *Who will keep the public healthy? Educating public health professionals for the 21st Century.* Washington, DC: National Academies Press.

General Accounting Office. (2003). *Report to the ranking minority member, Committee on Health, Education, Labor, and Pensions, U.S. Senate, information technology, benefits realized for selected healthcare functions.* Washington, DC: Author.

Glaser, J. P., DeBor, G., & Stuntz, L. (2003). The New England healthcare EDI network. *Journal of Healthcare Information Management, 17*(4), 42–50.

Glasziou, P., Ogrinc, G., & Goodman, S. (2011). *BMJ Quality and Safety, 20*(Suppl 1), i13–i17.

Gostin, L. O. (1997). Personal privacy in the healthcare system: Employer-sponsored insurance, managed care, and integrated delivery systems. *Kennedy Institute of Ethics Journal, 7*(4), 361–376.

Gostin, L. O., & Nass, S. (2009). Reforming the HIPAA privacy rule: Safeguarding privacy and promoting research. *Journal of the American Medical Association, 301*(13), 1373–1375.

Greenes, R., & Brinkley, J. (2006). Imaging systems. In E. Shortliffe & J. J. Cimino (Eds.), *Medical informatics: Computer applications in healthcare and biomedicine.* New York: Springer-Verlag.

Halamka, J., Overhage, J. M., Ricciardi, L., Rishel, W., Shirky, C., & Diamond, C. (2005). Exchanging health information: Local distribution, national coordination. *Health Affairs, 24*(5), 1170–1179.

Han, Y. Y., Carcillo, J. A., Venkataraman, S. T., Clark, R. S., Watson, R. S., Nguyen, T. C., . . . Orr, R. A. (2005). Unexpected increased mortality after implementation of a commercially sold computerized physician order entry system. *Pediatrics, 116*(6), 1506–1512.

Haviland, A. M., Marquis, M. S., McDevitt, R. D., & Sood, N. (2012). Growth of consumer-directed health plans to one-half of all employer-sponsored insurance could save $57 billion annually. *Health Affairs, 31*(5), 1009–1015.

Health Technology Center & Phelps & Phillips, LLP. (2003). *Spending our money wisely: Improving America's healthcare system by investing in healthcare information technology.* San Francisco: Health Technology Center.

HHS. (2012a). *Summary of the HIPAA privacy rule.* Retrieved from http://www.hhs .gov/ocr/privacy/hipaa/understanding/summary/index.html

HHS. (2012b). *Summary of the HIPAA security rule.* Retrieved from http://www.hhs .gov/ocr/privacy/hipaa/understanding/srsummary.html

Hill, R. D., Luptak, M. K., Rupper, R. W., Bair, B., Peterson, C., Dailey, N., & Hicken, B. L. (2010). Review of Veterans Health Administration telemedicine interventions. *American Journal of Managed Care, 16*(12 Suppl HIT), e302–e310.

Hillestad, R., Bigelow, J., Bower, A., Girosi, F., Meili, R., Scoville, R., & Taylor, R. (2005). Can electronic medical record systems transform healthcare? Potential health benefits, savings, and costs. *Health Affairs, 24*(5), 1103–1117.

HIMSS. (2011, February). *Clinical decision support (CDS) and meaningful use frequently asked questions.* Retrieved from http://www.himss.org/content/files/CDS _MU_FAQ.pdf

HIMSS. (2012, December). *Electronic Medical Record Adoption Model (EMRAM).* Retrieved from http://www.himssanalytics.org/emram/index.aspx

Hsiao, C. J., Hing, E. Socey, T. C., & Cai, B. (2011). *Electronic health record systems and intent to apply for meaningful use incentives among office-based physician practices: United States, 2001–2011.* Hyattsville, MD: National Center for Health Statistics. Retrieved from http://www.cdc.gov/nchs/data/databriefs/DB79.pdf

IHA. (2012). *IHA pay for performance report of results for measurement year 2010.* Oakland, CA: Integrated Healthcare Association.

IHIE. (2012). *Indiana Health Information Exchange.* Retrieved from http://www.ihie .org/home

InstaMed. (2012). *Trends in healthcare payments annual report: 2011.* Philadelphia: InstaMed.

Institute of Medicine. (2001). *Crossing the quality chasm: A new health system for the 21st Century.* Washington, DC: National Academies Press.

Institute of Medicine. (2012). *For the public's health: Investing in a healthier future.* Washington, DC: National Academies Press.

Jha, A. K., Doolan, D., Grandt, D., Scott, T., . . . Bates, D. W. (2008). The use of health information technology in seven nations. *International Journal of Medical Informatics, 77*(12), 848–854.

Jones, S. S., Heaton, P. S., Rudin, R. S., & Schnieder, E. C. (2012). Unraveling the IT productivity paradox: Lessons for healthcare. *New England Journal of Medicine, 366*(24), 2243–2245.

Kaushal, R., & Bates, D. W. (2001, July). Computerized physician order entry (CPOE) with clinical decision support systems (CDSSs). In *Making healthcare safer: A critical analysis of patient safety practices.* Evidence Report/Technology Assessment: Number 43 (AHRQ Publication No. 01-E058). Rockville, MD: Agency for Healthcare Research and Quality. Retrieved from http://www.ahrq.gov/clinic/ptsafety /chap6.htm

Kaushal, R., Blumenthal, D., Poon, E. G., Jha, A. K., Franz, C., Middleton, B., . . . Bates, D. W. (2005). The costs of a national health information network. *Annals of Internal Medicine, 143*(3), 165–173.

Kaushal, R., Jha, A.K., Franz, C., Glaser, J., Shetty, K. D., Jaggi, T., . . . Bates, D. W. (2006). Brigham and Women's Hospital CPOE working group. *Journal of the American Informatics Association, 13*(3), 261–266.

Kilo, C. M. (2005). Transforming care: Medical practice design and information technology—how one innovative medical practice has eliminated many office visits and improved continuity of care for patients with chronic conditions. *Health Affairs, 24*(5), 1296–1301.

King, J., Patel, V., & Furukawa, M. (2012). Physician adoption of electronic health record technology to meet meaningful use objectives: 2009–2012 (Data Brief No. 7). Washington, DC: Office of the National Coordinator for Health Information Technology.

Kohn, L. T., Corrigan, J. M., & Donaldson, M. S. (Eds.). (2000). *To err is human: Building a safer health system.* Washington, DC: National Academies Press.

Koppel, R., Metlay, J. P., Cohen, A., Abaluck, B., Localio, A. R., Kimmel, S. E., & Strom, B. L. (2005). Role of computerized physician order entry systems in facilitating medication errors. *Journal of the American Medical Association, 293*(10), 1197–1203.

Krasnow, D., & Rodrigues, R. J. (1998). International perspectives. In S. F. Viegas & K. Dunn (Eds.), *Telemedicine: Practicing in the information age.* Philadelphia: Lippincott-Raven.

Kulikowski, C. A., Shortliffe, E. H., Currie, L. M., Elkin, P. L., Hunter, L. E., Johnson, T. R., . . . Williamson, J. J. (2012). AMIA board white paper: Definition of biomedical informatics and specification of core competencies for graduate education in the discipline. *Journal of the American Informatics Association, 19,* 931–938.

Lisacek, F., Cohen-Boulakia, S., & Appel, R. D. (2006). Proteome informatics II: Bioinformatics for comparative proteomics. *Proteomics, 6*(20), 5445–5466.

Lumpkin, J. R., & Richards, M. S. (2002). Transforming the public health information infrastructure. *Health Affairs, 21*(6), 45–56.

Manolio, T. A. (2010). Genomewide association studies and assessment of the risk of disease. *New England Journal of Medicine, 363*(2), 166–176.

Manyika, J., Chui, M., Brown, B., Bughin, J., Dobbs, R., Roxburgh, C., & Byers, A. H. (2011). *Big data: The next frontier for innovation, competition, and productivity.* Retrieved from http://www.mckinsey.com/insights/mgi/research/technology_and _innovation/big_data_the_next_frontier_for_innovation

Markle Foundation. (2011). *The public and doctors overwhelmingly agree on health IT priorities to improve patient care.* New York: Markle Foundation.

Massoudi, B. L., Goodman, K. W., Gotham, I. J., Holmes, J. H., Lang, L., Miner, K., . . . Fu P. C. (2012). An informatics agenda for public health: Summarized recommendations from the 2011 AMIA PHI Conference. *Journal of the American Medical Informatics Association, 19*(5), 688–695

McDonagh, E. M., Whirl-Carrillo, M., Garten, Y., Altman, R. B., & Klein, T. E. (2011). From pharmacogenomic knowledge acquisition to clinical applications: The PharmGKB as a clinical pharmacogenomic biomarker resource. *Biomarkers in Medicine, 5*(6), 795–806.

McDonald, C. J., Overhage, J. M., Mamlin, B. W., Dexter, P. D., & Tierney, W. M. (2004). Physicians, information technology, and healthcare systems: A journey, not a destination. *Journal of the American Medical Informatics Association, 11*(2), 121–124.

McGlynn, E. A., Asch, S. M., Adams, J., Keesey, J., Hicks, J., DeCristofaro, A., & Kerr, E. A. (2003). The quality of healthcare delivered to adults in the United States. *New England Journal of Medicine, 348*(26), 2635–2645.

Metzger, J. (2004). *Using computerized registries in chronic disease care.* Oakland: California Healthcare Foundation.

Miller, R. H., & Miller, B. S. (2007). The Santa Barbara County care data exchange: What happened. *Health Affairs, 26*(5), w568–w580.

Mitka, M. (2009). Groups back telemedicine for stroke care. *Journal of the American Medical Association, 302*(1), 20–21.

Morris, A. H. (2003). Treatment algorithms and protocolized care. *Current Opinion on Critical Care, 9*(3), 236–240.

National Committee for Quality Assurance (NCQA). (n.d.). *HEDIS and quality measurement.* Retrieved from http://www.ncqa.org/tabid/59/Default.aspx

National Library of Medicine: National Institutes of Health. (2012). *MEDLINE fact sheet.* Retrieved from http://www.nlm.nih.gov/pubs/factsheets/medline.html

National Research Council. (2009). *Computational technology for effective healthcare.* Washington, DC: National Academies Press.

NCBI. (n.d.). *National Center for Biotechnology Information.* Retrieved from http://www.ncbi.nlm.nih.gov

Niazkhani, Z., Pimejad, H., Berg, M., & Aarts, J. (2009). The impact of computerized provider order entry systems on clinical workflow: A literature review. *Journal of American Medical Informatics Association, 16*(4), 539–549.

NQF. (2011). *Electronic quality measures (eMeasures).* Retrieved from http://www.qualityforum.org/Projects/e-g/eMeasures/Electronic_Quality_Measures.aspx

Partnership for Solutions. (2004). *Chronic conditions: Making the case for ongoing care.* Baltimore: Johns Hopkins University.

Pestotnik, S. L. (2005). Expert clinical decision support systems to enhance Antimicrobial Stewardship Programs: Insights from the Society of Infectious Diseases Pharmacists. *Pharmacotherapy, 25*(8), 1116–1125.

Poon, E. G., Blumenthal, D., Jaggi, T., Honour, M. M., Bates, D. W., & Kaushai, R. (2004). Overcoming barriers to adopting and implementing computerized physician order entry systems in U.S. hospitals. *Health Affairs, 23*(4), 184–190.

Pryor, T. A. (1990). Development of decision support systems. *International Journal of Clinical Monitoring and Computing, 7*(3), 137–146.

Radley, D. C., Wasserman, M. R., Olsho, L.E.W., Shoemaker, S. J., Spranca, M. D., & Bradshaw, B. (2013). Reduction in medication errors in hospitals due to adoption of computerized provider order entry systems. *Journal of the American Medical Informatics Association, 20*, 470–476.

Riedmann, D., Jung, M., Hackl, W. O., Stühlinger, W., van der Sijs, H., & Ammenwerth, E. (2011). Development of a context model to prioritize drug safety alerts in CPOE systems. *Medical Informatics and Decision Making, 11*(35).

Saarlas, K. N., Edwards, K., Wild, E., & Richmond, P. (2003). Developing performance measures for immunization registries. *Journal of Public Health Management Practice, 9*(1), 47–57.

Sarkar, U., Lopez, A., Masalli, J., & Gonzales, R. (2011). Adverse drug events in U.S. adult ambulatory medical care. *Health Services Research, 46*(5), 1517–1533.

Schadt, E. E., Linderman, M. D., Sorenson, J., Lee, L., & Nolan, G. P. (2010). Computational solutions to large-scale data management and analysis. *Nature reviews. Genetics, 11*(9), 647–657.

Stone, A. H., & Yoder, L. H. (2012). Strategic considerations during electronic health record implementation. *Journal of Nursing Administration, 42*(4), 208–214.

Tang, P. (2003). *Key capabilities of an electronic health record system: Letter report.* Washington, DC: National Academies Press.

Tang, P. C., Fafchamps, D., & Shortliffe, E. H. (1994). Traditional medical records as a source of clinical data in the outpatient setting. *Proceedings of the Annual Symposium on Computing Applications in Medical Care, 575*–579.

The Cancer Genome Atlas (TCGA). (2012). Retrieved from http://cancergenome.nih.gov/abouttcga/overview

U.S. Department of Health and Human Services. (2001). *Information for health: A strategy for building the national health information infrastructure.* Washington, DC: National Committee on Vital and Health Statistics.

Walker, J., Pan, E., Johnston, D., Adler-Milstein, J., Bates, D. W., & Middleton, B. (2005). The value of healthcare information exchange and interoperability. *Health Affairs,* (Suppl), W5-10–W5-18.

Weeger, A., Gewald, H. & Vriesman, L. (2011, October). *Adoption or resistance: Hospital physicians' acceptance of electronic medical records.* WHITE Conference Paper.

Whitten, P., & Buis, L. (2006). *Private payer reimbursement for telemedicine services in the United States.* East Lansing, MI: Michigan State University.

Wright, A., Henkin, S., Feblowitz, J., McCoy, A. B., Bates, D. W., & Sittig, D. F. (2013). Early results of the meaningful use program for electronic health records. *New England Journal of Medicine, 368,* 779–780.

Yasnoff, W. A., Humphreys, B. L., Overhage, J. M., Detmer, D. E., Brennan, P. F., Morris, R. W., . . . Fanning, J. P. (2004). A consensus action agenda for achieving the national health information infrastructure. *Journal of the American Medical Informatics Association, 11*(4), 332–338.

Yasnoff, W. A., & Miller, P. L. (2003). Decision support and expert systems in public health. In P. W. O'Carroll, W. A. Yasnoff, M. E. Ward, L. H. Ripp, & E. L. Martin (Eds.), *Public health informatics and information systems.* New York: Springer-Verlag.

Yasnoff, W. A., O'Carroll, P. W., Koo, D., Linkins, R. W., & Kilbourne, E. M. (2000). Public health informatics: Improving and transforming public health in the information age. *Journal of Public Health Management and Practice, 6*(6), 67–75.

CHAPTER FIFTEEN

PERFORMANCE MEASUREMENT OF NURSING CARE

Jack Needleman
Ellen T. Kurtzman
Kenneth W. Kizer

Learning Objectives

- Understand that nursing performance measurement has become a major area of quality measurement
- Examine major systems and initiatives in nursing performance measurement
- Gain an understanding of the challenges of developing effective performance measurement systems for nursing care

Why Measure Nursing Performance?

There are over 3 million nurses in the United States: of these, 2.6 million are employed in nursing positions, with over 1.6 million, or 62 percent, are employed in hospitals (U.S. Department of Health and Human Services. Health Resources and Services Administration, 2010). Nurses are the largest health profession in the United States and largest employee group in hospitals.

In the 1980s and 1990s, many *registered nurses* (RNs) reported that because of hospital mergers and the process of care restructuring directed at lowering costs in the 1990s, they were working harder than ever, spending less time taking care of increasingly ill patients, and, consequently, that the safety and quality of patient care was deteriorating (Aiken, Sochalski, & Anderson, 1996; Brider, 1996; Gilliland, 1997; Peter D. Hart Research Associates, 1997; Shindul-Rothschild, 1996). A 1996 Institute of Medicine (IOM) report, while sympathetic to those concerns, found a "paucity of objective research on the relationships among restructuring, staffing, and quality" and called for "development of a research agenda in this area and for the articulation of reliable, valid, and practical measures of structure, process, and outcome to be used in quality-of-care research as well as quality assurance and improvement programs" (Wunderlich, Sloan, & Davis, 1996).

Partly in response to that report, and to broader concerns about quality of care as reflected in the 2001 IOM report *Crossing the Quality Chasm* (IOM, 2001), the degree to which the availability of nurses, the organization of the nursing workforce, and work environment in which nurses practice contribute to the growing health care quality chasm gained increased attention by providers, researchers, payers, and consumer organizations.

Together, the concerns about nurse staffing in hospitals, nursing's influence on patient safety and health care outcomes, and the condition of the nursing workforce have led to increased interest in measuring and reporting nursing's performance and in developing and using nursing-sensitive performance measures. Nursing-sensitive performance measures are processes and outcomes—and structural proxies for these processes and outcomes (such as skill mix and nurse staffing hours)—that are affected, provided, and/or influenced by nursing personnel, although nursing may not be exclusively responsible. It is possible to identify multiple interrelated goals or purposes for such measurement and reporting:

- To quantify nursing's influence on patient safety and health care outcomes with a special focus on promoting the highest levels of quality in acute care hospitals.
- To enhance the clinical practice of nursing personnel and nursing-related quality improvement projects.
- To promote provider accountability to the public, including, but not limited to, public reporting and financial incentives.
- To identify levels of staffing—including appropriate standards—and approaches to organizing nursing in hospitals to be implemented by hospitals and supported by payers and other public and private parties.

- To facilitate the identification of priority areas for research needed in measuring nursing-sensitive care.
- To address the need to educate and train the current and future workforce.
- To support benchmarking and sharing of best practice.
- To promote the translation of the state of science of nursing care into the delivery of nursing care.

This chapter reviews recent efforts and issues involved in identifying a set of nursing-sensitive performance measures.

The Scope of Nursing's Contribution to Inpatient Hospital Care

Establishing the scope—or boundaries—of nursing practice is a critical step in both understanding nursing's contribution to patient safety and health care outcomes and measuring those aspects of practice that are most relevant to inpatient hospital quality.

Nurses' Work

To measure nursing performance, it is useful to begin with an understanding of the work that nurses do. The conceptualization of nurses' work has been subject to extensive debate over an extended time, as nurses attempt to define their sphere of practice and attempt to integrate models of nursing as a scientific discipline and as an art (Hilton, 1997).

The variety of alternative descriptions of nurses' work can make it difficult for nurses to talk to one another about their work, to develop computerized nursing information systems (since these require choices to be made on frameworks and concepts), and to communicate with policymakers and the public about nursing (Snyder, Egan, & Nojima, 1996). A range of activities has sought to standardize the language used to define nursing diagnosis, interventions, and outcomes. An early effort to define a standard structure for nursing diagnosis was put forward in 1973 by the North American Nursing Diagnosis Association (NANDA), and that system has been updated on an ongoing basis (NANDA, 1999). Separately, the Center for Nursing Classification in the University of Iowa Nursing School developed systems of classifying nursing interventions (McCloskey & Bulecheck, 2000) and nursing outcomes (Johnson, Moorhead, & Maas, 2000). Since 1994, NANDA and researchers at the University of Iowa have been working jointly to refine, integrate, and extend these systems (Aquilino & Keenan, 2000).

Three alternative systems of classifying nurses' work suggest the range of activities involved in nursing. The Omaha system puts nurses activities into four broad categories: (1) health teaching, guidance, and counseling; (2) treatments and procedures, (3) case management; and (4) surveillance (Martin & Scheet, 1992).

Another classification, by Hendrickson and colleagues, divides nurses' activities into patient care activities at the bedside and other patient care (Hendrickson, Doddato, & Kovner, 1990). *Bedside activities* include feeding; bathing, cleaning, and dressing; procedure therapies; medications; education and support of the patient; education and support of the family; assessment and rounds; and transfers and mobility. *Nonbedside patient care* includes charting, orders, other documentation, interactions with others on the telephone or in person, coordination at shift changes, and preparing therapies. This list of activities adds concreteness to the conceptual categories in the Omaha system. This list of activities can be nested within the Omaha system, though not unambiguously. Assessment and rounds, for example, might fall into both case management and surveillance, an example that underscores the multitasking implicit in nurses' work. The list also illustrates the significant amount of time required for nonbedside patient care and nonpatient care activities. Hendrickson and colleagues found in their study that only 31 percent of nurses' time was spent with patients.

A third classification system by Irvine, Sidani, and Hall classifies nurses' roles into independent, dependent, and interdependent functions (Irvine, Sidani, & Hall, 1998). They define nurses' independent roles as assessment, diagnosis, intervention, and follow-up care, while nurses' dependent functions include the execution of medical orders and physician-initiated treatments. Interdependent functions, those that nurses engage in that are partially or totally dependent on the functions of other health care providers, include communication, case management, coordination of care, continuity and monitoring, and reporting.

All classifications underscore the important work of nurses outside of carrying out treatments or procedures ordered by others and their active role in monitoring patient condition, managing and coordinating care, and educating patients and preparing them and their families to care for themselves. To be fully effective, performance systems should capture the impact of nurses' work in each of these domains.

As patients in hospitals have become more acutely ill, and as hospitals have attempted to redesign how nurses' work is carried out, the mix of activities conducted by nurses has shifted. Table 15.1 presents an illustration of the shift over a three-year period in the top ten activities of nurses at a large community hospital in Pennsylvania as work was redesigned. Notable among these changes was the increase in professional judgment, patient education, and assessing data on patients, and the reduction in time spent bathing and turning patients, and intake and output—a shift to tasks requiring more training and judgment.

Despite these changes, a recent study found a substantial portion of nurses' time remains spent on documentation and indirect care (see Table 15.2).

Organizing to Accomplish Nurses' Work

Hospitals organize their nursing functions in a variety of ways, and the approaches may vary over time and across units within hospitals. Brennan

TABLE 15.1. COMPARISON OF CHANGES IN TOP TEN RN ACTIVITIES DURING THREE YEARS OF WORK REDESIGN

Activity	1993 Rank	%	1994 Rank	%	1995 Rank	%
Charting	1	7.9	2	8.7	4	7.6
Patient assessment	2	7.3	3	7.9	1	10.3
Medication administration	3	6.9	1	8.8	3	8.5
Bathing	4	6.7	4	6.7		
Report	5	4.9	5	5.2	5	5.1
Respond to patient's requests	6	3.9	6	4.5	7	3.3
Close observation	7	3.4	7	4.4	6	4.6
Vital signs	8	3.2	8	3.1	8	3.3
Turning	9	3.0	9	2.9		
Intake and output	10	2.7	10	2.9		
Professional judgment					2	9.5
Patient education					9	2.9
Assessing patient data					10	2.5
Percent of time captured		50		55		58

Source: Pederson, 1997.

TABLE 15.2. NURSES' TIME, BY CATEGORY, 2008

Category	Percent
Direct care	47.05
Indirect care	18.10
Administration	4.94
Documentation	19.00
Personal	4.75
Waste	2.65
Other	3.50

Source: Yee, Needleman, Pearson, Parkerton, & Wolstein, 2012.

and colleagues, using a modified Delphi technique, identified eleven dimensions along which nursing models vary (Brennan, Anthony, Jones, & Kahana, 1998). Among the models that have been defined are

Team. Under the leadership of a professional nurse, a group of staff work together to fulfill the full functions of professional nurses for a group of patients. The team consists of an RN and unlicensed assistive personnel and may include a licensed practical nurse.

Primary. One primary nurse is assigned to care for all of the patient's needs for the duration of the patient's hospital stay.

Functional. A task-oriented method in which a function is assigned to a staff member. One nurse is responsible for administering medications and another for treatments.

Case management. Care coordinated by a case manager who may or may not provide the nursing care. A care map or pathway is used to guide care.

Total patient care. Provision of patient care whereby each nursing staff member is assigned to give complete care to a group of patients during a given shift.

Patient-centered (or patient-focused) care. Organization for the provision of as many elements of patient care as possible by caregivers closest to the patient. Implementation of patient-centered care includes the development of multiskilled workers through extensive cross-training of caregivers.

These definitions have overlapping elements and are not always used in a consistent manner. Minnick has found that when nurse managers were asked about the specific practice behaviors of nurses on their units, there was little correspondence to the goals of the stated "nursing model," and concludes that a questionnaire that identifies specific practices rather than asking about models may be necessary to accurately capture information on the organization of nursing in a hospital.

Issues in Constructing Nursing-Sensitive Performance Measures

In addition to the scope of nursing practice, the characteristics of performance measures need to be defined before identifying candidate measures. Not all candidate measures deserve equal consideration.

Balancing Structure, Process, and Outcome Measures in the Performance System

The classic *Donabedian model of quality measurement* identifies structure, process, and outcome as three dimensions along which quality can be analyzed. Existing nursing performance measurement systems have adopted a mix of measures from the structure-process-outcome dimensions. The ANA indicators, for example, include registered nursing hours per patient day (a structural measure), nurse satisfaction (a process measure), and nosocomial infection (an outcome measure). Outcome measures are frequently preferred for measuring system performance, but, because many factors can influence outcomes besides nursing care, correctly interpreting outcome measures requires appropriate controls for these other factors, controls that can be difficult to implement. At the other end of the spectrum, structural measures are often viewed as too rigid and an imperfect proxy for how the system is performing. Process measures, like structural measures, are often easier to measure, but their connection to patient outcomes must be validated.

Linkage to Nursing Care

There are a substantial number of quality or performance measures in health care that are clear and clearly documented. Did the patient receive beta-blockers after a heart attack if there were no contraindications?

Did the patient receive prophylactic antibiotics within a fixed time before surgery? For some nursing care, problems or lapses in performance should be observable in charts—failure to give a drug on time, for example. Other lapses in care may not be documented. Inadequate or rushed catheter care will not be charted. Where lapses in care cannot be charted, it may be impossible to tie specific outcomes to inadequate nursing. Establishing links between nursing care and many outcomes will be based on an understanding of the likely etiology of the adverse event or complication rather than direct evidence abstracted from a chart.

One interesting approach to this problem is the development of instruments to directly measure missed care. Kalisch and colleagues, for example, have constructed an instrument for measuring missed care and examined the association of missed care, staffing levels, and patient outcomes (Kalisch, Tschannen, & Lee, 2011, 2012; Kalisch & Williams, 2009).

Measuring at the Unit or Hospital Level

Studies of nursing have been conducted at both the nursing unit level and the hospital level. The nursing unit is a natural level at which to conduct measurement and assess performance. Hospital nursing is organized and delivered within units. The count of patients and count of nurses can be precise, while at the hospital level there are issues of averaging across varying units and inpatient and outpatient activities. Nurse staffing and performance can vary across units within hospitals, and there is more variability in nursing or patients within hospitals than across them (Minnick, Roberts, Young, Kleinpell, & Marcantonio, 1997). It is at this level that ANA has organized its principal data collection.

There are several drawbacks to measurement at the unit level, however. It is expensive, requiring either special data collection or chart abstracting. Hospital-level data can be collected in the same way, but often hospital-level analysis is conducted using administrative data such as hospital discharge data sets, American Hospital Association survey data, or Medicare cost reports. Because administrative data are relatively inexpensive compared to unit-level data, the number of hospitals from which data can be collected and analyzed and whose performance can be compared can be much larger. Second, over the course of an admission, patients may move among units. In these cases, attributing complications or adverse outcomes to care in a specific unit may be difficult. In addition, confidentiality and privacy for both patients and nurses may diminish the usefulness of unit-level reporting. There are clear trade-offs among scope, cost, precision, and privacy that must be addressed in defining a nursing performance system.

Availability and Comparability of Data

The issue of using administrative datasets or custom datasets is one of cost, but two other issues also emerge in making a choice among alternative sources of data. The first is that nursing records are generally not available through administrative datasets. Discharge data are abstracted from physician notes, and nurses' notes are not used for diagnosis or procedures. Second, the data systems for nursing diagnosis, intervention, and outcomes that nurses have developed are not standardized. Lack of standardization and lack of automation discourage use of nursing data from patient charts. As electronic health records are standardized and nursing informatics becomes more strongly established (Bakken, Stone, & Larson, 2008), this problem may be reduced.

Measuring Nursing Performance

Nursing performance measurement is an emerging "enterprise." While Florence Nightingale, the legendary architect of professional nursing, is quoted as saying, "To understand God's thoughts, we must study statistics, for these are the measure of His purpose" (Salsburg, 2001), it is a relatively recent phenomenon to measure, analyze, and report nursing's impact on care.

An Overview of Factors Believed to Influence Nursing's Performance

A wide range of factors has been put forward as influencing the performance of nursing. These factors fall into four broad categories: nurse training and competencies, physical plant and structure, nursing organization, and work environment and culture.

Nurse training and competencies reflect the skills individual nurses bring to the hospital and the bedside. Formal training—levels of education, advanced practice training, knowledge of specific equipment and patient conditions—are a part of this factor. Research on factors influencing successful nurse decision making add additional competencies that are partly provided by training and partly by experience. The models put forward vary, but have included such factors as clinical skills, knowledge and understanding, interpersonal skills, problem-solving skills, clinical judgment, and moral sensibility (Norman, 1985; Taylor, 1995; Yura & Walsh, 1967).

Physical plant and structure can influence workload, but they can also contribute to performance. Computerization can reduce errors in order entry and retrieval and charting. Nursing unit layout can influence the ability to quickly respond to patient needs or obtain needed supplies or drugs quickly and without error. Standardization in design of patient rooms and equipment may also contribute to reduced errors by nurses (Reiling, Breckbill, Murphy, McCullough, & Chernos, 2003).

Presence of some types of equipment can also reduce the risk of drug errors or risk of a nurse injuring herself or himself. The U.S. nursing workforce has been aging, and while there is some evidence that younger workers are increasingly considering nursing (Auerbach, Buerhaus, & Staiger, 2011), efforts to retain older nurses and reduce nursing shortages will require taking ergonomics into account to assure that older nurses can do their work accurately and effectively.

Nursing organization should influence nursing performance, but its impact is not well established. The absence of consistently applied definitions and rigor in the design of research on work organization makes it hard to draw strong conclusions. Studies that focus on the proportion of RNs in the nursing workforce in hospitals, without regard to the specific model used to organize nursing, consistently find a positive impact of a higher mix of RNs on a range of patient outcomes. Thomas and Bond report several studies that suggest that primary nursing produces better outcomes, but the designs are weak and none examines the factors that influence why hospitals select specific models (Thomas & Bond, 1995).

The impact of nursing work environment and culture has been more widely studied, using a variety of instruments and alternative data sets. Many of these studies focus on nurse satisfaction with their work, but others examine the association of patient outcomes with various aspects of work environment and culture, either individually or collectively. Among the factors that have been associated with good nursing performance are flattening of organizational structures, increased professional status for staff nurses associated with shared governance and increased autonomy over practice and the practice environment, and effective communication among nurses, physicians, and administrators (Havens & Aiken, 1999; Stone, Hughes, & Dailey, 2008).

Recent Activities and Efforts to Measure and Publicly Report Nursing Care Performance

In response to known lapses in health care quality and safety, generally, and a national call to action from the President's Advisory Commission on Consumer Protection and Quality in the Health Care Industry (President's Advisory Commission on Consumer Protection and Quality in the Health Care Industry, 1998), the Institute of Medicine, (IOM, 2001; Kohn, Corrigan, & Donaldson, 1999), and other health care stakeholders, there has been a growing demand for measuring and publicly reporting health care performance. A number of initiatives and organizations have emerged as leaders in measuring nursing performance and assumed various roles in the "quality enterprise"—terminology typically used to describe the tools and infrastructure that support transparency in cost and quality, accountability for performance, and performance-based incentives to stimulate quality improvement (Farquhar, Kurtzman, & Thomas, 2010; Kurtzman & Johnson, 2012).

The examples in the sections that follow have been organized by function (setting national standards, measuring performance, and publicly reporting performance results) and level of impact (national, regional or state, or system), are illustrative of advancements in this area, and represent the most notable contributions. The list is not comprehensive or inclusive of all that has been achieved in measuring and portraying nursing's contribution to inpatient hospital care.

Setting National Standards for Nursing Care Performance

In this section we look at three entities tasked with setting national standards for nursing care performance: the National Quality Forum, The Joint Commission, and the Centers for Medicare and Medicaid Services.

National Quality Forum. The National Quality Forum (NQF) is a voluntary consensus standards-setting organization that was created in 1999 to develop and implement a national strategy for health care quality measurement and reporting. Established as a public-private partnership, the NQF is a private, nonprofit membership organization represented by diverse constituencies including consumer organizations; public and private health care purchasers; physicians, nurses, hospitals, and other provider organizations; accrediting and certifying bodies; and health care research and quality improvement organizations, among others. NQF's mission is to improve the quality of American health care by building consensus on national priorities and goals for performance improvement, endorsing national consensus standards for measuring and publicly reporting health care performance, and promoting the attainment of national goals through education and outreach.

Voluntary Consensus Standards are defined as "common and repeated use of rules, conditions, guidelines or characteristics for products or related processes and production methods, and related management systems practices; the definition of terms; classification of components; delineation of procedures; specification of dimensions, materials, performance, designs, or operations; measurement of quality and quantity in describing materials, processes, products, systems, services, or practices; test methods and sampling procedures; or descriptions of fit and measurements of size or strength." In addition to having broad acceptability because of the reputation of the organization setting the standards, voluntary consensus standards can be adopted by the federal government without the comment and review process otherwise required under the Administrative Procedures Act because they have been deemed to have received comparable vetting by the standards organization (U.S. Office of Management and Budget, 1998).

In February 2003, the NQF undertook a fourteen-month project to study the relationship between nursing personnel and quality and the degree to which national voluntary consensus standards for nursing-sensitive care could be established. The project surveyed the field to identify the range of measures in use and critically assessed the evidence base supporting those measures.

The NQF's process involved a large and highly diverse group of stakeholders in a structured process—referred to as its consensus development process (CDP)—and was directed at endorsing a set of national nursing-sensitive performance measures (National Quality Forum, 2010). In conducting its work, the NQF sought to identify measures that met its four sets of standard evaluation criteria (importance to measure and report, scientific acceptability of measure properties, usability, and feasibility) and reflected the contribution of nursing personnel to providing quality care. To this end, a unique assessment of "nursing sensitivity" was conducted. Specifically, measures that were recommended as proposed consensus standards had to represent structural, process, and outcome measures that are linked by evidence to nursing variables. To be designated as a "nursing-sensitive consensus standard," the measure had to directly measure some element of nurse staffing that has been associated with better-quality care or be quantifiably influenced by nursing personnel, although the relationship did not need to be shown to be causal or exclusive to nursing. The culmination of this effort was the endorsement of fifteen national voluntary consensus standards for nursing-sensitive care (see Table 15.3) and eleven related research and implementation recommendations (see Table 15.4) by the NQF Board of Directors in April 2004 (National Quality Forum, 2004).

TABLE 15.3. NQF-ENDORSED NATIONAL VOLUNTARY CONSENSUS STANDARDS FOR NURSING-SENSITIVE CARE

Framework Category	Measure	Description
Patient-centered outcome measures	1. Death among surgical inpatients with treatable serious complications (failure to rescue)	Percentage of major surgical inpatients who experience a hospital-acquired complication (i.e., sepsis, pneumonia, gastrointestinal bleeding, shock/cardiac arrest, deep vein thrombosis/ pulmonary embolism) and die
	2. Pressure ulcer prevalence	Percentage of inpatients who have a hospital-acquired pressure ulcer (stage 2 or greater)
	3. Falls prevalence[1]	Number of inpatient falls per inpatient days
	4. Falls with injury	Number of inpatient falls with injuries per inpatient days
	5. Restraint prevalence (vest and limb only)	Percentage of inpatients who have a vest or limb restraint
	6. Urinary catheter-associated UTI for intensive care unit (ICU) patients[1]	Rate of UTI associated with use of urinary catheters for ICU patients
	7. Central line catheter-associated blood stream infection rate for ICU and high-risk nursery (HRN) patients[1]	Rate of blood stream infections associated with use of central line catheters for ICU and HRN patients
	8. Ventilator-associated pneumonia for ICU and HRN patients[1]	Rate of pneumonia associated with use of ventilators for ICU patients and HRN patients
Nursing-centered intervention measure	9. Smoking cessation counseling for acute myocardial infarction (AMI) [1,2]	Percentage of AMI inpatients with history of smoking within the past year who received smoking cessation advice or counseling during hospitalization

(continued)

TABLE 15.3. NQF-ENDORSED NATIONAL VOLUNTARY CONSENSUS STANDARDS FOR NURSING-SENSITIVE CARE (Continued)

Framework Category	Measure	Description
	10. Smoking cessation counseling for heart failure (HF) [1,2]	Percentage of HF inpatients with history of smoking within the past year who received smoking cessation advice or counseling during hospitalization
	11. Smoking cessation counseling for pneumonia [1,2]	Percentage of pneumonia inpatients with history of smoking within the past year who received smoking cessation advice or counseling during hospitalization
System-centered measures	12. Skill mix (RN, LVN/LPN, UAP, and contract)	Percentage of registered nursing (RN) care hours of total nursing care hours Percentage of licensed vocational/practical nursing (LVN/LPN) care hours of total nursing care hours Percentage of unlicensed assistive personnel (UAP) care hours of total nursing care hours Percentage of contract hours (RN, LVN/LPN, and UAP) of total nursing care hours
	13. Nursing care hours per patient day (RN, LVN/LPN, and UAP)	Number of RN care hours per patient day Number of nursing staff hours (RN, LVN/LPN, UAP) per patient day
	14. Practice Environment Scale—Nursing Work Index (composite and five subscales)	Composite score and mean presence scores for each of the following subscales derived from PES-NWI: Nurse participation in hospital affairs Nursing foundations for quality of care Nurse manager ability, leadership, and support of nurses Staffing and resource adequacy Collegial nurse-physician relations
	15. Voluntary turnover	Number of voluntary uncontrolled separations during the month for RNs and advanced practice nurses, LPNs and nurse assistants/aides

TABLE 15.4. NQF-ENDORSED RECOMMENDATIONS FOR RESEARCH AND IMPLEMENTATION

Research Recommendation	General Description
Development of workforce measures and empirical base to support them	Research should be undertaken on the relationship between nursing variables and patient outcomes.
Development of pain assessment and management measures	Research should be undertaken to identify measures that specifically explore nursing's contribution to the assessment and management of pain.
Development of nurse-centered intervention process measures	Research should be undertaken to determine the relationship between patient outcomes and process measures.
Sufficiency of measures against evaluation criteria	Research should be initiated that investigates and documents each measure's adequacy against the NQF evaluation criteria.
Development of measures where gaps in consensus exist	Additional research should be undertaken to address a broad range of important areas for which no measures exist.

Implementation Recommendation	General Description
Recommendation Related to Data Issues	Providers, researchers, and information system vendors need to develop better data systems to support nursing care monitoring functions.
Use for Quality Improvement	Measures should be collected and analyzed by providers at the hospital unit-level.
Implementation	The readiness of provider organizations to implement these consensus standards is an overall indication of their commitment to quality.
Scope of Consensus Standards	The NQF-endorsed consensus standards for nursing-sensitive performance should be viewed by health care stakeholders as a constellation of measures (i.e., measure set).
Improving the Set	Review of the initial set of its voluntary consensus standards for nursing-sensitive care should be conducted on a regular basis.

In the course of this work, NQF found that confidence in many proposed or previously used measures was limited by an inadequate research base or absence of validating studies, issues of data reliability, or questions about how closely the measure was associated with nursing and nursing care. As a result, most of the measures included in the dataset require primary data collection or chart abstraction, activities involving significant effort or cost. The research and implementation recommendations call for efforts to broaden the range of available measures, conduct validation studies for existing measures for which the evidence base is limited, systematize data collection, and incorporate collection and construction of measures into ongoing systems to reduce the cost of measuring nursing and nursing-related work.

Since their original endorsement, the national voluntary consensus standards for nursing-sensitive care have been reviewed by NQF under its "maintenance" efforts—reviews undertaken every three years to reevaluate measures against standard criteria and in comparison to new and previously endorsed measures. Maintenance efforts are intended to ensure the currency of NQF measures as a reflection of their evidentiary basis and specifications as well as to ensure harmonization and the best available measures have been endorsed. NQF's approach to maintenance follows its CDP (National Quality Forum, 2010). In its review of the fifteen measures originally endorsed in 2004, NQF "retired" three measures—smoking cessation counseling for acute myocardial infarction, heart failure, and pneumonia. The decision to retire the smoking cessation measures was based on specification concerns that drew into question the measures' reliability and validity. NQF retained their endorsement of the remaining twelve measures.

Beyond measure maintenance, however, the NQF national voluntary consensus standards for nursing-sensitive care have been implemented by a variety of stakeholders and in a variety of ways. For example, they have served as the basis for and been incorporated into a number of voluntary and mandatory measurement and reporting activities. They have been incorporated into federal transparency and performance-based payment programs (Medicare's Reporting Hospital Quality Data for Annual Payment Update program) and accreditation requirements. The measures have also been used by researchers to study hospital quality and disparities and to pursue other scientific inquiries.

The Joint Commission. The Joint Commission (TJC) accredits and certifies more than 19,000 health care organizations and programs in the United

States, including hospitals, doctor's offices, nursing homes, office-based surgery centers, behavioral health treatment facilities, and providers of home care services. Accredited organizations can also earn certification for programs devoted to chronic diseases and conditions, such as asthma, diabetes, and heart failure. TJC has played a significant role in setting national standards for nursing care performance by developing uniform technical specifications for the NQF National Voluntary Consensus Standards for nursing-sensitive care and establishing staffing effectiveness requirements as part of its hospital accreditation program. In November 2009, TJC's Standards & Survey Procedures Committee approved new requirements that became effective July 1, 2010. These new requirements replaced the original staffing effectiveness standard, which had been suspended in June 2009. Under these requirements, at least once a year an analysis of undesirable patterns and trends must include an analysis of the adequacy of staffing, identified issues related to the adequacy of staffing must be reported to leaders of and those responsible for the safety program, and leaders must provide hospital governance with written reports on all results of analyses related to the adequacy of staffing.

Centers for Medicare and Medicaid Services. As the nation's largest health care payer, the Center for Medicare and Medicaid Services (CMS) has promulgated a number of rules and regulations that address transparency and accountability (Centers for Medicare and Medicaid Services, n.d.). Among their value-based purchasing programs is the Reporting Hospital Quality Data for Annual Payment Update (RHQDAPU) program. Hospitals that do not comply with performance reporting requirements under RHQDAPU receive a reduction of their annual payment update—currently set at 2 percent. Initially, hospitals had to report ten performance measures to CMS to meet RHQDAPU reporting requirements. This number has grown, and hospitals report a range of measures that address patient outcomes, process of care, and structural features. As of fiscal year 2010 (FY2010), hospitals that participated in RHQDAPU were required to submit data on a structural measure—whether the hospital participates in a systematic clinical database registry for nursing-sensitive care.

In addition to its initiatives reporting outcomes and process measures, CMS partnered with the Agency for Healthcare Research and Quality to develop a series of surveys of consumer assessments of their health care experience. The hospital survey (Hospital Consumer Assessment of Healthcare Providers and Systems, or HCAHPS), a twenty-seven-item instrument, includes four questions on nursing care (questions about being treated with courtesy and respect, being listened to, having things explained, and responsiveness to call buttons) and questions on pain management, assistance with toileting, noise, preparation for discharge, and others that are also associated with nursing care. HCAHPS scores for individual hospitals are made available to consumers and others through the CMS Hospital Compare website (Centers for Medicare and Medicaid Services, 2012).

Measuring Nursing Care Performance

Organizations that have developed systems for measuring and monitoring nursing care performance include the American Nurses Association, Collaborative Alliance for Nursing Outcomes, Department of Defense, and Department of Veterans Affairs.

American Nurses Association. In 1994, in response to reductions in staff that resulted from workforce redesign, the American Nurses Association (ANA) began its Patient Safety and Quality Initiative, which was established to build evidence linking nurse staffing and patient outcomes. The initiative involved the development of hospital quality indicators and the recruitment of hospitals and their nurses to collect these quality indicators along with staffing data in seven states (Arizona, California, Minnesota, North Dakota, Ohio, Texas, and Virginia). What began as an effort to build a seven-state database pilot resulted in the establishment, in 1998, of ANA's National Center for Nursing Quality® (NCNQ®) and its measurement repository—the National Database of Nursing Quality Indicators® (NDNQI®) (Montalvo, 2007).

Based on Donabedian's quality framework (structure, process, and outcomes), the seven state pilots, an extensive literature review, and expert panel consensus, twenty-one performance measures were initially identified and ten performance measures ultimately selected, which included a mix of structure, process, and outcomes:

Outcome measures:
- Nosocomial infection rate (bacteremia)
- Patient injury rate
- Patient satisfaction with nursing care
- Patient satisfaction with pain management
- Patient satisfaction with educational information
- Patient satisfaction with care

Process measures:
- Maintenance of skin integrity (pressure ulcers)
- Nurse staff satisfaction

Structure measures:
- Proportion of nursing care hours provided by registered nurses
- Total nursing care hours per patient day

In parallel with these ANA measurement efforts, analyses were conducted to determine the nature and strength of association between nurse staffing and four outcomes that were derived from patient discharge abstracts—pressure ulcers, pneumonia, urinary tract infections, and postoperative infections. Associations were found between each of the four outcomes and the proportion of licensed nursing hours provided by registered nurses and three measures (pressure ulcers, postoperative infections, and length of stay) and licensed nursing hours per day. This initial work laid the foundation for rapid expansion and informed implementation efforts.

Since its inception, NDNQI—whose mission is to aid the registered nurse in patient safety and quality improvement efforts by providing research-based national comparative data on nursing care and the relationship to patient outcomes—has grown. By 2011, over 325,000 nurses were actively participating by responding to the annual RN survey. As of 2012, the database, which originally pooled data for the original thirty pilot hospitals, aggregated data for over 1,800 hospitals. During any given quarter, close to 19,000 nursing units contribute data to NDNQI. The measures that are collected and analyzed now number eighteen and address the following constructs:

- Nursing staff skill mix[*]
- Nursing hours per patient day[*]
- Nurse turnover[*]
- Assault or injury assault rates
- Catheter-associated urinary tract infections[*]
- Central line–associated bloodstream infections[*]
- Fall or injury fall rates[*]
- Hospital- or unit-acquired pressure ulcer prevalence[**]
- Pain assessment, intervention, or reassessment cycle
- Peripheral IV infiltrations
- Restraint prevalence[*]
- RN education or certification

- Ventilator-associated pneumonia*

    *Indicators endorsed by National Quality Forum (NQF)

    **Indicator endorsed by NQF, but NDNQI collects Stage I and greater, while the NQF measure is defined as Stage II and greater

NDNQI is the largest nursing quality database domestically and internationally. Reports are used by hospital leaders, administrators, and representatives from state and national organizations to examine care, identify opportunities to improve that care, and gauge progress against those benchmarks. To facilitate these efforts and provide meaningful comparisons, units can be classified by patient population, acuity or service line, and specialty. Comparisons are available for the adult, pediatric, and neonatal populations. In addition to the standard service lines (critical care, step-down, medical, surgical, and medical-surgical) and to accommodate meaningful "apples-to-apples" comparisons, NDNQI stratifies and compares blended acuity units to one another.

A number of measure development efforts and programmatic enhancements are planned. Measures are being developed and tested: staffing measures for perioperative, perinatal, and emergency departments; expansion of the fall measures to address populations on pediatric units; and a measure of physical assault that assesses the safety of the nursing work environment that applies to every hospital unit. Additionally, NDNQI has introduced an analysis of its top performers and begun making annual awards for nursing quality at its annual conference. Most recently, the Nursing Quality Network—a collaborative of nurses dedicated to creating and disseminating knowledge about the quality of care through an online member community, learning voyages, and educational resources—was founded.

Research has been foundational to the establishment and ongoing enhancement of NDNQI. Numerous studies and a growing body of evidence have relied on its data, all pointing to important associations between staffing—measures of structure—and a variety of outcomes.

Collaborative Alliance for Nursing Outcomes (CALNOC). The Collaborative Alliance for Nursing Outcomes (CALNOC) was launched in 1996 as one of ANA's pilot projects that ultimately contributed to development of the ANA's NDNQI. Built on a foundation of grassroots collaboration between founding partners, the California constituent of the American Nurses Association (ANA) and the Association of California Nurse Leaders, CALNOC has become a self-sustaining nonprofit corporation independent of NDNQI that provides nearly three hundred participating hospitals in seven states with facility-specific and group benchmarks for nursing-sensitive structure, process, and outcome data.

CALNOC offers participating hospitals direct website access to comparative performance reports at the level of unit, unit type (surgical or ICU, for example), facility, corporate system, geographic location and hospital type. CALNOC web-based reports can be used by providers to set priorities for performance improvement projects, monitor the effect of the improvement activities over time, and meet the American Nurses Credentialing Center's Magnet Recognition Program® reporting data display specifications. CALNOC also provides consultation and education services to optimize strategic use of CALNOC data.

CALNOC measures have been adapted for and adopted by a variety of uses and settings (such as pediatric, obstetric, and emergency acute care; long-term care; and acute rehabilitation). Notably, CALNOC supplied its data to the California Hospitals Assessment and Reporting Taskforce (CHART) from 2007 until its strategic change in measures in 2012. CHART has produced a public report card for more than two hundred hospitals—approximately 83 percent of admissions—in the state (CalHospitalCompare.org, n.d.). Additionally, CALNOC serves as a measure developer—credited for developing two of the NQF-endorsed measures (pressure ulcer and restraint use prevalence)—and indicators of medication administration, patient safety, and RN education and experience. Along with these contributions, CALNOC has pursued a robust intramural and extramural research agenda funded by the Robert Wood Johnson Foundation, Agency for Healthcare Research and Quality, and Gordon and Betty Moore Foundation examining the impact of hospital, patient, and staffing characteristics on patient care quality, safety, costs, processes, and outcomes.

Military Nursing Outcomes Database (MilNOD). The Military Nursing Outcomes Database (MilNOD), a database of staffing and adverse event indicators from fifty-six units in thirteen hospitals over four years, was created to address a need for evidence-based management and for research (Loan, Patrician, & McCarthy, 2011). The goals of MilNOD were to enable targeted patient care improvements through data measurement and sharing and to examine the associations between staffing and outcomes at the shift level. MilNOD replicated and adapted methods developed by CALNOC to provide chief nurses, directors, and nurse managers with standardized, timely, and relevant information for decision making. MilNOD provided nurse executives with data from their own facilities, comparisons to like hospitals in the military system, and external comparisons from CAL-NOC. Military nursing leaders used information from MilNOD to evaluate nurse staffing effectiveness as related to safety and quality of patient care, thus supporting intentions of TJC's staffing effectiveness standards.

The MilNOD database provided a rich source of shift-level data for research. Indicators that were collected at the shift level were nursing hours, patient census, acuity, and admissions, discharges, and transfers. The research conducted has revealed associations between staffing numbers, skill mix, and staff category (a proxy for experience) at the shift level and falls, medication errors, and nurse needlestick injuries (Patrician, Loan, et al., 2011; Patrician, Pryor, Fridman, & Loan, 2011). In addition, the research team documented a decrease in adverse events over time, not only of falls and medication errors, but also of hospital-acquired pressure ulcers. Nurse managers and executives reported using the data for daily operations, quality improvement, and reporting to external agencies.

The MilNOD system no longer exists as it was originally designed, but has transitioned into a Deputy Commander for Nursing (DCN) Dashboard, embedded within standard operations of nearly all U.S. Army Medical Command hospitals. This dashboard has evolved into a system whereby data collection is automated and pulled from other existing systems, but retains most of the standardized definitions of the original MilNOD system.

Veterans Affairs Nursing Outcomes Database (VANOD). The Veterans Affairs Nursing Outcomes Database (VANOD) was launched in 2002 as a national database of nursing-sensitive quality indicators. Not unlike its CALNOC and MilNOD counterparts, VANOD was initially used to monitor, evaluate, and improve nursing-sensitive outcomes in the context of hospital staffing and their work environments.

Using the NQF-endorsed measures as its basis, VANOD has developed into a web-based interoperable data warehouse and decision support resource that goes beyond the original functionality. All VA medical centers contribute data that are derived from existing sources and as a by-product of care to the VANNOD database. Comparative reports can be generated by unit, unit type, and hospital. Ultimately, the VA's goal is to make data electronically available in standard formats and generate meaningful reports that can be used to improve quality and safety, assess the relationships between nursing and patient safety and health care quality, and drive strategic and data-based decisions such as staffing projections.

A variety of reports are available in three areas: administrative (such as demographic and financial, nursing staff injury, nursing turnover, and patient turnover), clinical (such as skin breakdown risk and outcomes, and medication scanning failures), and satisfaction (RN satisfaction, skill mix satisfaction, and patient satisfaction). These reports drive operations in a range of areas such as credentialing and privileging, staff performance reviews, quality improvement, team-based care, workload management, and forecasting. Additionally, data from VANOD "feeds" various other databases and registries including the VA's ASPIRE, an online quality dashboard that publicly reports VA medical center performance on a variety of outcomes and processes of care (VA Hospital Compare, 2011).

Publicly Reporting Nursing Care Performance

Public reporting of nursing care performance has become an area of increasing interest at the state level. Public reporting systems have been developed in Massachusetts and Maine.

Massachusetts (PatientsCareLink). In 2005, the Massachusetts Hospital Association and the Organization of Nurse Leaders (ONL)—formerly the Massachusetts Organization of Nurse Executives—implemented *PatientsCareLink (PCL)* (previously Patients First). PCL is a voluntary, statewide transparency collaborative that serves Massachusetts hospitals and their nursing leaders (Smith & Jordan, 2008). All acute care, long-term care, and rehabilitation hospitals in the commonwealth submit staffing, quality, and patient safety data, which are publicly reported on PCL's website (PatientCareLink, 2012). Measures, which draw from the NQF national voluntary consensus standards for nursing-sensitive care as specified by TJC and the CMS RHQDAPU program, include staffing plans and actual staffing reports by unit type (such as critical care, medical-surgical, and emergency department), hospital-level outcomes such as pressure ulcer prevalence, falls and falls with injuries, readmissions, mortality, condition-specific composite quality-of-care measures (such as heart failure), and state-level performance for several outcomes including mortality, readmissions, and central-line associated bloodstream infections.

Since it was established, PCL has pursued its mission to "help participating hospitals provide transparent staffing and patient safety information to the public and other health care stakeholders, and also offer valid and reliable information on quality and safety to patients and healthcare workers alike." While public reporting was its original pursuit, PCL's principles and goals underlie a more robust suite of quality and safety tools and services. For example, a patient and family section of the website houses information that supports patients' and families' interpretation of hospital performance results and provides tools and links to useful patient safety resources. A more recently added "success stories" page provides quality improvement best practices and case studies.

Maine (Nurse Sensitive Indicator Data). In 2003 then-Governor Baldacci and the Maine Legislature established Dirigo Health as an independent executive agency to arrange for the provision of comprehensive, affordable health care coverage to eligible small employers and individuals on a voluntary basis. At the same time, the Maine Quality Forum, as an independent division of Dirigo Health, was established to provide consumers with a reliable resource for information about health maintenance, health care, and quality of health care services and health information. The Maine Health Data Organization (MHDO), an independent executive agency established by the Maine legislature to collect health care performance information and make it publicly accessible, promulgates the rules to mandate and collect the health care quality data from health care practitioners and facilities, as adopted by the Maine Quality Forum. Under state statute since 2006, all hospitals in Maine are required to submit uniform health care quality data, including measures of nursing performance, to MHDO. The acute care and rehabilitation hospitals submit both the Nursing-Sensitive Patient-Centered and Nursing-Sensitive System-Centered Health Care Quality Data Sets, while the psychiatric hospitals submit only the Nursing-Sensitive System-Centered Health Care Quality Data Set. The first of these datasets includes measures of pressure ulcer prevalence, falls and falls with injuries, and restraints. The second includes staffing mix, nursing care hours per patient day, and voluntary turnover. Since June 2009, Maine hospitals' performance results have been publicly reported on a MQF/MHDO website.

Since its initiation, the data gathered and submitted to MHDO has been used for quality improvement including collaboratives such as those focused on pressure ulcer prevention. Nursing-Sensitive System-Centered measures (staffing-level data) have also been used to drive nurse-to-patient staffing legislation, policy analysis, and research.

Measuring Nursing Performance: The State of the Science

Given the imperative to better understand nursing's influence on patient outcomes, a growing body of empirical research has been undertaken to quantify nursing performance and its impact. This emerging research has primarily focused on examining the association between measures of the process and structure of nursing care and patient outcomes.

Research on Outcomes Influenced by Nursing

Outcome measurement is one of the cornerstones of performance measurement, and a wide range of outcomes have been tested for an association with nursing. There is evidence of an association of nurse staffing with mortality, hospital-acquired pneumonia, a range of hospital-acquired infections, falls, medication errors, pain management, shock and cardiac arrest, pulmonary failure, upper gastrointestinal bleeding, and length of stay (which may influence costs of care). Evidence for other outcomes, most notably pressure ulcers and deep vein thrombosis, is mixed. Additionally, registered nurse (RN) hours as a proportion of all nursing staff hours are associated more strongly and with more outcomes than RN hours per patient day (Kane, Shamliyan, Mueller, Duval, & Wilt, 2007; Needleman, Kurtzman, & Kizer, 2007).

A meta-analysis by Kane and colleagues published in 2007 estimated the impact of nurse staffing on a variety of outcomes. The results summarized in Table 15.5 are drawn from their published results.

Issues in Measuring Outcomes

Collectively, this research finds a variety of outcomes associated with nurse staffing. What should we make of the failure to consistently find an association between nursing and mortality or other outcomes that one might expect to be associated with nursing? There are several possible explanations, and these have implications for the design of nursing performance systems.

Are the data captured and retrieved? To associate an outcome with nursing, or to use an outcome as an indicator, one must have confidence that the outcome is reported in the dataset used with sufficient frequency and regularity that the rate is a good measure of nursing's performance. For unit-based studies, with data collection in real time from charts on the floor, with staff sensitized to identify and record specific events, data capture and retrieval may not be an issue. For studies in which these conditions are not met, problems in the data-generating process may undercut the confidence that can be placed in measures. As noted in a study of the implementation of the ANA indicators in one medical center, "the extent to which databases are in place to capture any of these indicator data reduces the need for labor-intensive chart abstraction and thus enhances the ease of retrievability" (Jennings, Loan, DePaul, Brosch, & Hildreth, 2001).

TABLE 15.5. POOLED ODDS RATIOS OF PATIENT OUTCOMES CORRESPONDING TO AN INCREASE OF ONE REGISTERED NURSE FULL-TIME EQUIVALENT PER PATIENT DAY

Outcome	Studies	Odds Ratio (95% CI)	Attributable to Nurse Staffing of Events (%)	No. Avoided Events/1,000 Hospitalized (95% CI)
All patients				
Mortality, hospital level analysis, all patients	5	0.96 (0.94; 0.98)	4.2	3 (2; 4)
Mortality, intensive care units	5	0.91 (0.86; 0.96)	9.2	5 (2; 8)
Mortality, surgical patients	8	0.84 (0. 8; 0.89)	16	6 (4; 8)
Mortality, medical patients	6	0.94 (0.94; 0.95)	5.6	5 (4; 5)
Hospital-acquired pneumonia	4	0.81 (0.67; 0.98)	19.1	1 (0; 2)
Pulmonary failure	5	0.94 (0.94; 0.94)	6	1 (1; 1)
Cardiopulmonary resuscitation	5	0.72 (0.62; 0.84)	27.6	2 (1; 2)
Intensive care units				
Hospital-acquired pneumonia	3	0.7 (0.56; 0.88)	30.2	7 (3; 10)
Pulmonary failure	4	0.4 (0. 27; 0.59)	60.3	7 (5; 9)
Unplanned extubation	5	0.49 (0. 36; 0.67)	50.9	6 (4; 8)
Cardiopulmonary resuscitation	3	0.72 (0.62; 0.84)	27.6	2 (1; 2)
Relative change in length of stay	4	0.76 (0.62; 0.94)	24	7 (2; 11)
Surgical patients				
Failure to rescue	5	0.84 (0.79; 0.9)	16	26 (17; 35)
Surgical wound infection	1	0.15 (0.03; 0.82)	84.5	7 (1; 8)
Cardiopulmonary resuscitation	1	0.72 (0.62; 0.84)	27.6	1 (1; 2)
Nosocomial bloodstream infection	5	0.64 (0.46; 0.89)	36	4 (2;5)
Relative change in length of stay	3	0.69 (0.55; 0.86)	31	14 (6;21)

Note: An increase of one registered nurse full-time equivalent per patient day would result in eight additional registered nurse hours per patient day at an increased cost of $24.57/hour × 8 hours, or $196.56/patient day. Attributable to nurse staffing fraction of events and number of avoided events per one thousand hospitalized patients were estimated assuming causality in the association.

Source: Kane, Shamliyan, Mueller, Duval, & Wilt, 2007.

How specific or linkable is the outcome to nursing? Many factors may contribute to an outcome, of which nursing is only one, and it may not be the most important. Variations in the rates unrelated to nursing add noise to the data and make observing an association more difficult. Variations due to other factors associated with nursing can also make statistical inference difficult. For example, Jennings and colleagues question the use of bacteremia as a nursing-related infection, noting, "nosocomial infections may be less relevant if the focus remains on bacteremia from central lines. Physicians usually insert these lines, and the possibility of contamination on insertion cannot be discounted" (Jennings et al., 2001).

Infrequent events. There are two problems in demonstrating that infrequently occurring events are associated with nursing in statistical analysis. First, the power of the analysis is reduced. Second, a substantial number of hospitals will have no cases of infrequent events, even if nurse staffing is low and nursing is associated with the event, simply because most hospitals are small and the pool of patients in which the complication can occur is small. Large numbers of hospitals with no events also reduce the power of the analysis. If one believes in the link between a specific complication and nurse staffing based on clinical judgments, then one can use it, but we should not expect such events to be validated in cross-sectional statistical analyses of hospital experience.

Risk adjustment. Risk adjustment (formal adjustment of outcome rates to reflect differences in risk across patient populations) is critical for comparing rates of adverse events across hospitals. Inadequate risk adjustment may have weakened results in some studies and may be especially difficult to do in unit-level analyses.

Overall, there are multiple reasons why no association might have been observed in these studies, and the reasons will influence the design of a nursing performance system. There is a need for continued efforts to refine and improve measures and data used to generate them.

Issues in Measuring Processes of Care and Structural Proxies

In examining measures of process and structure, one needs to question whether the nurse staffing is adequate when compared to patient needs and whether other organizational factors amenable to change influence nursing performance. Several measurement problems stand in the way of finding answers to these two questions: variations in nursing case mix, differences in physical plant, differences in organization and culture across nursing units or hospitals, and counting nurses within the hospital.

Patient-Level Adjustment: Nursing Case Mix. Case mix makes a difference in the adequacy of nurse staffing on a unit or in a hospital. Frailer patients, bed-bound patients, and those requiring closer monitoring all require more nursing time. One hospital may be adequately staffed for its patient acuity at six hours per patient day while another is short-staffed. Adjustment is necessary if comparisons are to be made across hospitals or over time.

The adjustment should be made based on nursing need, not general patient acuity or need for all services. A number of studies have used the average diagnosis-related group (DRG) case-mix index for the hospital to adjust estimates of nursing hours or nursing FTEs per patient day. There are many advantages to using the DRG case-mix index; for instance, it is a standardized measure that can be calculated from the discharge abstract data and has been widely used in prior research. However, it also has a number of weaknesses. Most significantly, studies show that DRGs are poorly correlated with patient nursing need (Halloran, 1985; Halloran & Kiley, 1987).

An alternative measure would be the staffing projection that emerges from nursing workload or nurse staffing systems such as the Quadramed AcuityPlus or GRASP Workload Management systems. All accredited hospitals are supposed to have such systems, although approximately half of U.S. hospitals use a system developed at that hospital. In principle, the staffing that emerges from these systems is adjusted to the physical plant and nursing model used at the hospital. A potential performance measure would be the ratio of actual to projected staffing or gap between staffing targets and actual staffing, as estimated from the system (Needleman et al., 2011).

There are several important limitations of these systems as they currently exist. The large number of hospital-specific systems preclude comparisons across hospitals; there is no gold standard for measuring staffing. Systems can differ in the staffing need they would project in the same case mix in the same hospital (Carr-Hill & Jenkins-Clarke, 1995; O'Brien-Pallas, Cockerill, & Leatt, 1992). Systems require validating, updating, and recalibration if the estimates are to remain valid. Hospitals may also adjust their projection system to staff tightly or generously. While the potential to use data from these systems in performance measurement is high, these validation and calibration issues need to be addressed before reliable comparisons can be made across hospitals.

For studies that attempt to compare outcomes and staffing across hospitals or acuity-adjusted staffing over time, systems that are codable in administrative datasets are needed, but no such systems currently exist. As noted previously, DRG case-mix indexes are poorly correlated with needed nurse staffing. Several researchers have, however, used the DRG patient classification framework to construct patient nursing acuity measures. One approach has been to group DRGs into clusters based on anticipated nursing needs or to divide DRGs into more homogenous categories relative to nursing levels, using measures such as number of secondary diagnoses or number of MDCs into which secondary diagnoses fall (Diers & Bozzo, 1997; Soeken & Prescott, 1991). Another approach is to estimate the nursing workload for each DRG and construct a nursing case mix from this DRG weight (Ballard, Gray, Knauf, & Uppal, 1993).

Physical Plant Impacts on Nurse Staffing Needs and Organization. Research has found a range of factors that influence the efficiency with which nurses carry out their work, including physical layout, communications systems, and computerization. The physical layout of hospital nursing units can influence nurse staffing needs and the ability of nursing staff to observe patients closely.

Physical layout, communications systems, and computerization all vary widely among hospitals, and systems to measure adequacy of nursing must take such differences into account. In theory, creation of hospital-specific staff projection systems or customization of commercial systems such as Quadramed's or GRASP's should take such differences into account. Data to incorporate such information into hospital-level monitoring systems or to adjust staffing per patient day from hospital-level measurement are currently not available.

Work Organization's Impact on Nursing Need. The least studied dimension of factors that influence need for nursing and nursing effectiveness are those associated with work organization. These include characteristics of the nurses themselves, the composition of the nursing team, scheduling and coordination, and culture and work environment. Studies have demonstrated that each has an impact on nursing performance and outcomes (Carr-Hill & Jenkins-Clarke, 1995; O'Brien-Pallas, Irvine, Peereboom, & Murray, 1997).

Minnick and Pabst found that there was a tendency in hospitals to underassign nurses on units in which the suggested hours of care from the acuity or workload system were high (Minnick & Pabst, 1998). These units have high staffing, but not as high as needed. They note that if adjustment for acuity is not adequate in analysis, it will appear that higher nurse staffing is associated with poorer outcomes. They also suggest that if nurse administrators assign more experienced staff to these understaffed units, the greater experience might offset some of the increased risk of poor outcomes due to insufficient staffing.

Since nursing models are likely to be chosen in response to the mix of staff and staff skills available (and, in turn, hospitals are likely to hire staff that fit their nursing model), knowing the nursing model in use should provide information about the staff structure in a hospital. Unfortunately, as noted earlier, definitions of models are not used in a consistent manner. This is another issue that must be addressed in designing performance measurement systems.

Organizational Culture. Elements of *organizational culture* related to nurses' autonomy, ability to exercise professional judgment and participate in nursing unit decision making, and social support and stress have all been found to be associated with nurse satisfaction and nursing performance. Many studies use direct surveys of staff nurses to obtain information about organization and culture. A number of different instruments have been used, including the Nursing Work Index (Aiken & Patrician, 2000), Insel and Moos' Work Environment Scale (WES) (Avallone & Gibbon, 1998), McCloskey/Mueller Satisfaction Scale (MMSS), (10 ANA quality indicators for acute care settings, 1999), and *Job Content Questionnaire* (JCQ) (Karasek, 1985). Surveys are expensive to undertake, and overworked nurses may resist responding to requests to participate. The domains and focus of the instruments are different, and one must decide for what dimensions of the work environment it is most important to obtain information.

Counting Nurses. Counting the size and composition of the nursing staff in hospitals would appear to be straightforward, but this proves not to be the case either conceptually or operationally. One issue is who to count. Are nursing managers part of the nursing staff for purposes of counting nurses? If it is a unit study, how should staff who work in several units be counted? While interest is usually in productive hours of care to inpatients in all nursing categories, data systems do not provide the information needed to construct these measures with great precision. Nursing staff are often reported in full-time equivalents (FTEs), but nursing hours and shifts vary across hospitals, making the translation of FTEs into hours of care imprecise. Aide data are absent in many national databases. They have never been collected by Medicare and were dropped from the American Hospital Association Annual Survey for several years. Agency and contract staff are incompletely reported in staffing surveys. Inpatient nurse staffing (with the exception of a few state datasets) must be estimated from hospital-level staffing, which is always imprecise. Information on overtime, an emerging issue in nurse staffing, is available from only a few state datasets.

The interpretation of nursing hours per day will also be influenced by the scope of nurses' work in the hospital and the impact of nonnurse direct patient care providers on nursing. Nurses operate in teams within nursing units and in coordination with other services, such as transport, pharmacy, phlebotomy, and dietary. There are no good measures in most systems of labor in these areas, only overall staffing. Analysis of the adequacy of nurse staffing and nursing performance needs to take into account the availability of support services in these other areas.

Future Directions

Measuring the performance of hospital nursing care has become an increasingly important aspect of quality improvement and provider accountability and will continue to grow in importance. Over the next decade, several forces will combine to increase the demand for more precise mechanisms for measuring and reporting nursing's contribution to patient safety and health care outcomes. The most important among these factors is the *Patient Protection and Affordable Care Act (ACA)*.

The ACA expands health insurance coverage and encourages greater quality and efficiency in the delivery of health care, strengthens the performance measurement and public reporting enterprise, and "ups the ante" for nurses. Specifically, the law includes a variety of provisions that authorize the identification of measurement gaps, development of measures to fill those gaps, and public reporting of performance data. Overall, the ACA institutionalizes a federal infrastructure for performance measurement and reporting. In doing so, the public's expectation of a fully transparent and accountable health care system, including one that holds nurses accountable for high-quality care, has been established.

Implementation of the ACA affects the quality enterprise in another way—it shifts the nature of nurses' work and alters their roles, necessitating adjustments to the information that is measured and reported. As demand for accessible, affordable primary care grows, nurses will spend more of their time integrating services and coordinating care, enhancing transitions, reducing hospital readmissions, and providing health promotion and disease prevention. At the same time, hospital care will become exceedingly sophisticated, complex, and information-rich.

Nurses will need to possess and demonstrate state-of-the-art clinical expertise, advanced decision making, and effective communication skills. Suitable measures that reflect these shifts in emphasis—including measures that reflect care delivered outside of the hospital—will need to be developed and integrated into measurement and reporting systems.

At the same time that health care reform is shaping nurses' work, so too will trends in the delivery of interprofessional care. It is widely recognized that patients benefit when health care providers work collaboratively, communicate closely, and foster a cooperative practice environment (Kizer, 2010). For that reason, leaders in nursing, medicine, and other health care professions are committed to new models of team-based education and practice. Interprofessional care emphasizes unique skills and competencies—trusting relationships, reliable communication systems, strong and flexible partnerships, and smooth handoffs. When interprofessional teams that include nurses, but are not comprised exclusively of nurses, assume accountability for care, disentangling nurses' contributions becomes difficult. Future performance measurement and reporting systems will need to acknowledge the shared accountabilities of teams while honoring the unique contributions of each team member, including the influence of hospital nurses.

SUMMARY

Measuring the performance of hospital nursing care is becoming increasingly important in order to assess the impact of nurse staffing levels in hospitals and to support hospital nursing-related quality improvement activities. Developing effective performance measurement systems enables health care stakeholders to better understand and monitor the degree to which nursing care influences patient safety and health care quality. The work of the NQF, NDNQI and CalNOC, among others, builds on a growing body of research and can serve as the core for further development of nursing performance measurement systems. The implementation of value-based payment methods by Medicare and private payers and implementation of the ACA will lead to more assessment of nursing performance.

Having fully functional systems of nursing-sensitive performance measurement requires developing measures that address all the domains of nursing which should be monitored and all aspects of health care quality. This task requires addressing technical issues needed to effectively analyze the impact of nursing (risk adjustment and other hospital-to-hospital and longitudinal variations), developing data systems that will provide the information needed to implement the model system, regularly improving the set of endorsed standards so that they reflect the most current science and empirical evidence, and persuading all health care stakeholders (such as consumers, purchasers, and providers) that measurement and reporting nursing-sensitive standards are important to improving the quality of care that is delivered. Each of these tasks requires substantial development work and construction and maintenance of the infrastructure to sustain the performance measurement efforts.

KEY TERMS

Donabedian model of quality measurement Avedis Donabedian, one of the early leaders in defining quality and quality improvement in health care, organized the discussion of quality into structure (organizational design and physical characteristics of the work environment), process (how work was carried out), and outcomes.

Organizational culture There is no single definition of organizational culture, a term used in many settings and by many disciplines. In general, organizational culture refers to the knowledge, values, and beliefs of those in an organizational setting and the work environment they engender.

Registered nurse A graduate nurse who has passed the state registration exam; the licensure and education requirements and scope of practice are more substantial than for licensed practical nurses (licensed vocational nurses in California and Texas).

Risk adjustment Formal adjustment of outcome rates to reflect differences in risk across patient populations. Risk adjustment may control for age, gender, health status, or other factors believed to affect the outcome being measured. A wide range of risk adjustment methodologies are employed in practice.

DISCUSSION QUESTIONS

1. Florence Nightingale, the legendary architect of professional nursing, is quoted as saying, "To understand God's thoughts, we must study statistics, for these are the measure of His purpose." On the earthly plain,

there are multiple audiences for nursing performance measurement. Who are these audiences, what would each use nursing measurement for, and what types of measures are most useful to them?

2. Performance measures for nursing and other quality-related activities are often classified, following Donabedian, as measuring structure, process, or outcomes. What are the strengths and weaknesses of each type of measure for monitoring and improving nursing care?

3. What is the appropriate level at which to measure nursing performance?

4. What are the biggest obstacles in practice to implementing structural measures of nursing care? Process measures? Outcome measures?

5. The National Quality Forum develops voluntary consensus standards for health care quality, with wide participation of consumers, employers, insurers, health care providers, and other critical stakeholders. What are the strengths and weaknesses of this approach?

6. Value-based payment is becoming more widespread in the United States. How should nursing care be incorporated into these systems? Which of the measures described in this chapter would you use in a value-based payment system? What new measures would you develop as additional or alternative value-based payment measures?

FURTHER READING

Auerbach, D. I., Buerhaus, P. I., & Staiger, D. O. (2011). Registered nurse supply grows faster than projected amid surge in new entrants ages 23–26. *Health Affairs, 30*(12), 2286–2292.

The current discussion of nursing performance comes against a backdrop of an ongoing chronic shortage of nurses in the United States. This article discusses recent short-term changes and long-term trends in the nursing workforce.

Committee on the Robert Wood Johnson Foundation Initiative on the Future of Nursing, Institute of Medicine. (2011). *The future of nursing: Leading change, advancing health.* Washington, DC: National Academies Press. Also available on the National Academy of Sciences website at http://www.iom.edu/Reports/2010/The-Future-of-Nursing-Leading-Change-Advancing-Health.aspx

Building on the two revolutionary Institute of Medicine reports *To Err Is Human* and *Crossing the Quality Chasm, Keeping Patients Safe* lays out guidelines for improving patient safety by changing nurses' working conditions and demands. *The Future of Nursing* addresses major issues related to the current and future issues of the nursing workforce.

Kane, R. L., Shamliyan, T. A., Mueller, C., Duval, S., & Wilt, T. J. (2007). The association of registered nurse staffing levels and patient outcomes: Systematic review and meta-analysis. *Medical Care, 45*(12), 1195–1204.

A synthesis of the research on nurse staffing levels that complements the work cited in the Institute of Medicine reports *Keeping Patients Safe* and *The Future of Nursing*.

Kurtzman, E. T., & Kizer, K. W. (2005). Evaluating the performance and contribution of nurses to achieve an environment of safety. *Nursing Administration Quarterly*, *29*(1), 14–23.

The leader of the NQF project on nursing performance standards and then-head of the National Quality Forum discuss the NQF work and challenges of measuring the contribution of nurses to safety.

Page, A., & Institute of Medicine Committee on the Work Environment for Nurses and Patient Safety. (2003). *Keeping patients safe: Transforming the work environment of nurses*. Washington, DC: National Academies Press. Also available on the National Academy of Sciences website at http://www.iom.edu/CMS/3809/4671.aspx

REFERENCES

Aiken, L. H., & Patrician, P. A. (2000). Measuring organizational traits of hospitals: The Revised Nursing Work Index. *Nursing Research, 49*(3), 146–153.

Aiken, L. H., Sochalski, J., & Anderson, G. F. (1996). Downsizing the hospital nursing workforce. *Health Affairs, 15*(4), 88–92.

Aquilino, M. L., & Keenan, G. (2000). Having our say: Nursing's standardized nomenclatures. *American Journal of Nursing, 100*(7), 33–38.

Auerbach, D. I., Buerhaus, P. I., & Staiger, D. O. (2011). Registered nurse supply grows faster than projected amid surge in new entrants ages 23–26. *Health Affairs, 30*(12), 2286–2292.

Avallone, I., & Gibbon, B. (1998). Nurses' perceptions of their work environment in a Nursing Development Unit. *Journal of Advanced Nursing, 27*(6), 1193–1201.

Bakken, S., Stone, P. W., & Larson, E. L. (2008). A nursing informatics research agenda for 2008–18: Contextual influences and key components. *Nursing Outlook, 56*(5), 206–214, e203.

Ballard, K. A., Gray, R. F., Knauf, R. A., & Uppal, P. (1993). Measuring variations in nursing care per DRG. *Nursing Management, 24*(4), 33–36.

Brennan, P.F.P., Anthony, M. P., Jones, J.M.S., & Kahana, E. P. (1998). Nursing practice models: Implications for information system design. *Journal of Nursing Administration October, 28*(10), 26–31.

Brider, P. (1996). Morale skidding with restructuring. *American Journal of Nursing, 96*(2), 62–64.

CalHospitalCompare.org. (n.d.). *Rating hospital quality in California*. Retrieved from www.calhospitalcompare.org

Carr-Hill, R. A., & Jenkins-Clarke, S. (1995). Measurement systems in principle and in practice: The example of nursing workload. *Journal of Advanced Nursing, 22*, 221–225.

Centers for Medicare and Medicaid Services. (2012). *HCAHPS: Hospital quality information from the consumer perspective*. Retrieved from http://www.hcahps online.org/home.aspx

Centers for Medicare and Medicaid Services. (n.d.). *Roadmap for implementing value-driven healthcare in the traditional Medicare fee-for-service program.* Baltimore: Author.

Diers, D., & Bozzo, J. (1997). Nursing resource definition in DRGs: RIMS/Nursing Acuity Project Group. *Nursing Economics, 15*(3), 124–130, 137.

Farquhar, M., Kurtzman, E. T., & Thomas, K. A. (2010). What do nurses need to know about the quality enterprise? *Journal of Continuing Education in Nursing, 41*(6), 246–248.

Gilliland, M. (1997). Workforce reductions: Low morale, reduced quality care. *Nursing Economics, 15*(6), 320–322.

Halloran, E. J. (1985). Nursing workload, medical diagnosis related groups, and nursing diagnoses. *Research in Nursing and Health, 8*(4), 421–433.

Halloran, E. J., & Kiley, M. (1987). Nursing dependency, diagnosis-related groups, and length of hospital stay. *Health Care Financing Review, 8*(3), 27–36.

Havens, D. S., & Aiken, L. H. (1999). Shaping systems to promote desired outcomes: The magnet hospital model. *Journal of Nursing Administration, 29*(2), 14–20.

Hendrickson, G., Doddato, T. M., & Kovner, C. T. (1990). How do nurses use their time? *Journal of Nursing Administration, 20*(3), 31–37.

Hilton, P. A. (1997). Theoretical perspectives of nursing: A review of the literature. *Journal of Advanced Nursing, 26*(6), 1211–1220.

Institute of Medicine. (2001). *Crossing the quality chasm: A new health system for the 21st century.* Washington, DC: National Academy Press.

Irvine, D., Sidani, S., & Hall, L. M. (1998). Linking outcomes to nurses' roles in health care. *Nursing Economics, 16*(2), 58–64, 87.

Jennings, B. M., Loan, L. A., DePaul, D., Brosch, L. R., & Hildreth, P. (2001). Lessons learned while collecting ANA indicator data. *Journal of Nursing Administration, 31*(3), 121–129.

Johnson, M., Moorhead, S., & Maas, M. L. (Eds.). (2000). *Nursing outcomes classification (NOC)* (2nd ed.). St. Louis, MO: Mosby.

Kalisch, B. J., Tschannen, D., & Lee, K. H. (2011). Do staffing levels predict missed nursing care? *International Journal for Quality in Health Care, 23*(3), 302–308.

Kalisch, B. J., Tschannen, D., & Lee, K. H. (2012). Missed nursing care, staffing, and patient falls. *Journal of Nursing Care Quality, 27*(1), 6–12.

Kalisch, B. J., & Williams, R. A. (2009). Development and psychometric testing of a tool to measure missed nursing care. *Journal of Nursing Administration, 39*(5), 211–219.

Kane, R. L., Shamliyan, T. A., Mueller, C., Duval, S., & Wilt, T. J. (2007). The association of registered nurse staffing levels and patient outcomes: Systematic review and meta-analysis. *Medical Care, 45*(12), 1195–1204.

Karasek, R. A. (1985). *The job content questionnaire and user's guide (Version 1.1).* Los Angeles: University of Southern California.

Kizer, K. W. (2010). What is a world-class medical facility? *American Journal of Medical Quality, 25*(2), 154–156.

Kohn, L., Corrigan, J., & Donaldson, M. (1999). *To err is human: Building a better health care.* Washington, DC: National Academy Press.

Kurtzman, E. T., & Johnson, J. E. (2012). Quality and safety in healthcare: Policy issues. In D. J. Mason, J. K. Leavitt, & M. W. Chaffee (Eds.), *Policy and politics in nursing and health care* (6th ed.). Philadelphia: Elsevier.

Loan, L. A., Patrician, P. A., & McCarthy, M. (2011). Participation in a national nursing outcomes database: monitoring outcomes over time. *Nursing Administration Quarterly, 35*(1), 72–81.

Martin, K. S., & Scheet, N. J. (1992). *The Omaha System: Applications for community health nursing.* Philadelphia: Saunders.

McCloskey, J. C., & Bulecheck, G. M. (Eds.). (2000). *Nursing interventions classification (NIC): Iowa intervention project* (3rd ed.). St. Louis, MO: Mosby.

Minnick, A. F., & Pabst, M. K. (1998). Improving the ability to detect the impact of labor on patient outcomes. *Journal of Nursing Administration, 28*(12), 17–21.

Minnick, A., Roberts, M. J., Young, W. B., Kleinpell, R. & Marcantonio, R. (1997). What influences patients' reports of three aspects of hospitals' services? *Medical Care, 35*(4), 399–409.

Montalvo, I. (2007). The National Database of Nursing Quality Indicators (NDNQI®). *Online Journal of Issues in Nursing, 12*(3), Manuscript 2.

National Quality Forum. (2003). National Voluntary Consensus Standards for Hospital Care: An initial performance measure set. Washington, DC: Author.

National Quality Forum. (2004). *National voluntary consensus standards for nursing-sensitive care: An initial performance measure set.* Washington, DC: Author.

National Quality Forum. (2010). Consensus standards maintenance and endorsement cycle process. Washington, DC: Author.

Needleman, J., Buerhaus, P., Pankratz, V. S., Leibson, C. L., Stevens, S. R., & Harris, M. (2011). Nurse staffing and inpatient hospital mortality. *New England Journal of Medicine, 364*(11), 1037–1045.

Needleman, J., Kurtzman, E. T., & Kizer, K. W. (2007). Performance measurement of nursing care: State of the science and the current consensus. *Medical Care Research and Review, 64*(2 Suppl), 10S–43S.

Norman, G. R. (1985). Defining competence: A methodological review. In V. R. Neufeld & G. R. Norman (Eds.), *Assessing clinical competence* (pp. 15–35). New York: Springer.

North American Nursing Diagnosis Association. (1999). *Nursing diagnoses: definitions and classification, 1999–2000* (3rd ed.). Philadelphia: Author.

O'Brien-Pallas, L., Cockerill, R., & Leatt, P. (1992). Different systems, different costs? An examination of the comparability of workload measurement systems. *Journal of Nursing Administration, 22*(12), 17–22.

O'Brien-Pallas, L., Irvine, D., Peereboom, E., & Murray, M. (1997). Measuring nursing workload: Understanding the variability. *Nursing Economics, 15*(4), 171–182.

PatientCareLink. (2012). Retrieved from http://www.patientcarelink.org

Patrician, P. A., Loan, L., McCarthy, M., Fridman, M., Donaldson, N., Bingham, M., & Brosch, L. R. (2011). The association of shift-level nurse staffing with adverse patient events. *Journal of Nursing Administration, 41*(2), 64–70.

Patrician, P. A., Pryor, E., Fridman, M., & Loan, L. (2011). Needlestick injuries among nursing staff: Association with shift-level staffing. *American Journal of Infection Control, 39*(6), 477–482.

Pederson, A. (1997). A data-driven approach to work redesign in nursing units. *Journal of Nursing Administration, 27*(4), 49–54.

Peter D. Hart Research Associates. (1997). *Health professionals' view of quality: A national survey.* Washington, DC: Author.

President's Advisory Commission on Consumer Protection and Quality in the Health Care Industry. (1998). Quality first: Better health care for all Americans. Final report to the President of the United States. Washington, DC: Author.

Reiling, J., Breckbill, C., Murphy, M., McCullough, S., & Chernos, S. (2003). Facility designing around patient safety and its effect on nursing. *Nursing Economics, 21*(3), 143–147.

Salsburg, D. (2001). *The lady tasting tea: How statistics revolutionized science in the twentieth century.* New York: W. H. Freeman.

Shindul-Rothschild, J. (1996). Patient care: How good is it where you work? *American Journal of Nursing, 96*(3), 22–24.

Smith, D. P., & Jordan, H. S. (2008). Piloting nursing-sensitive hospital care measures in Massachusetts. *Journal of Nursing Care Quality, 23*(1), 23–33.

Snyder, M., Egan, E. C., & Nojima, Y. (1996). Defining nursing interventions. *Image: The Journal of Nursing Scholarship, 28*(2), 137–141.

Soeken, K. L., & Prescott, P. A. (1991). Patient Intensity for Nursing Index: The measurement model. *Research in Nursing and Health, 14*(4), 297–304.

Stone, P. W., Hughes, R., & Dailey, M. (2008). Creating a safe and high-quality health care environment. In R. G. Hughes (Ed.), *Patient safety and quality: An evidence-based handbook for nurses.* Rockville, MD: Agency for Healthcare Research and Quality.

Taylor, C. (1995). Rethinking nursing's basic competencies. *Journal of Nursing Care Quality, 9*(4), 1–13.

10 ANA quality indicators for acute care settings. (1999). *Healthcare Benchmarks, 6*(12), 138–139.

Thomas, L. H., & Bond, S. (1995). The effectiveness of nursing: A review. *Journal of Clinical Nursing, 4*(3), 143–151.

U.S. Department of Health and Human Services. Health Resources and Services Administration. (2010). *The registered nurse population: Findings from the 2008 National Sample Survey of Registered Nurses.* Rockville, MD: Retrieved from http://bhpr.hrsa.gov/healthworkforce/rnsurveys/rnsurveyfinal.pdf

U.S. Office of Management and Budget. (1998). *Federal participation in the development and use of voluntary consensus standards and in conformity assessment activities (Circular A-119).* Retrieved from http://www.whitehouse.gov/omb/circulars_a119

VA Hospital Compare. (2011). Retrieved from http://www.hospitalcompare.va.gov

Wunderlich, G. S., Sloan, F. A., & Davis, C. K. (1996). *Nursing staff in hospitals and nursing homes: Is it adequate?* Washington, DC: National Academy Press.

Yee, T., Needleman, J., Pearson, M., Parkerton, P., & Wolstein, J. (2012). The influence of integrated electronic medical records and computerized nursing notes on nurses' time spent in documentation. *Computers, Informatics, Nursing, 30*(6), 287–292.

Yura, H., & Walsh, M. (1967). *The nursing process: Assessing, planning, implementing, evaluating.* Norwalk, CT: Appleton Century Crofts.

PART FOUR

SPECIAL POPULATIONS

CHAPTER SIXTEEN

LONG-TERM SERVICES AND SUPPORTS FOR THE ELDERLY POPULATION

Steven P. Wallace
Nadereh Pourat
Linda Delp
Kathryn G. Kietzman

Learning Objectives

- Describe the range of institutional and noninstitutional long-term services and supports (LTSS) that constitute the long-term care system
- Understand the basic organization and financing of LTSS nationally
- Explain how gender, race or ethnicity, and class patterns of LTSS use reflect inequities in access and quality
- Predict how changing demographics in the coming thirty years will affect the need and use of LTSS

Americans, and people throughout the world, are living longer and healthier than at any time in human history. Nevertheless, the human body and mind often become compromised at some point in life and can lose functional capacity due to accidents, disease, or accumulated wear and tear. When people face difficulties with personal care or otherwise living independently, they usually come to depend on the help of others. About 12.5 million persons of all ages in the United States need this type of assistance, almost half of whom are under age sixty-five (Kaye, Harrington, & LaPlante, 2010).

The set of health and social services delivered over a sustained period to people who have lost (or never acquired) some capacity for personal care is called long-term care (LTC) or long-term services and supports (LTSS). The latter term is increasingly being used because it emphasizes the fact that most of the care is supportive and collaborative. Ideally, LTSS enable recipients to live with as much independence and dignity as possible in the least restrictive environment that they desire. LTSS can be provided in institutional, community, or home settings and can involve assistance with such daily activities as walking, bathing, cooking, managing medications, and overseeing finances. It can be furnished by paid providers (*formal care*), unpaid family and friends (*informal care*), or by a combination of the two. LTSS can also include creating conditions that facilitate independent living, such as home modifications, accessible transportation, and special equipment like a motorized wheelchair. LTSS differs from most topics discussed in this volume because it depends heavily on social services and less on medical services.

The demand for LTSS will grow rapidly in the coming years due to the aging of the population overall, as well as increased lifespans. Reductions in infectious diseases have contributed to an increase in life expectancy, from 49.2 years in 1900 to 78.5 years in 2009. This, combined with falling birthrates, leads to elderly people constituting a growing segment of the population. By 2030, when most Baby Boomers will have reached age sixty-five, one in five Americans (72 million people) will be elderly. Those ages eight-five and older will increase from about six million today to nineteen million by 2050 (Federal Interagency Forum on Aging-Related Statistics, 2012). While LTSS needs can exist at any age, older adults are the most likely to experience personal care disabilities. Adults aged eighty-five years and older are the most likely to need assistance with routine household activities, with about one-third needing help with routine needs compared to 14 percent of those ages 75 to 84, 6 percent of those ages 65 to 74, and 4 percent of those ages 45 to 64; women have higher rates of disability at all ages (see Table 16.1). The rapidly increasing older population and their high rates of disability highlight the growing relevance of long-term services and supports issues.

TABLE 16.1. INDIVIDUALS WITH IMPAIRMENTS NEEDING HELP CARRYING OUT ROUTINE HOUSEHOLD ACTIVITIES BY AGE AND SEX, UNITED STATES, 2010

	Total Number Needing Help (% of Age Group)	Men Number Needing Help (% of Age Group)	Women Number Needing Help (% of Age Group)
Age 18–44	1,510,211 (1.4)	670,179 (1.2)	840,032 (1.5)
45–64	2,963,623 (3.7)	1,089,542 (2.8)	1,874,081 (4.6)
65–74	1,386,888 (6.5)	407,048 (4.2)	979,840 (8.6)
75–84	1,729,578 (13.7)	524,212 (9.9)	1,205,366 (16.5)
85 and over	1,556,964 (32.0)	382,071 (22.7)	1,174,893 (37.0)

Source: U.S. National Health Interview Survey, 2011.

This chapter summarizes the current status of the LTSS system, describing the services and policy issues for institutional care (such as nursing homes), home and community care, informal unpaid care, and the workforce in those sectors. It highlights how financial considerations have framed the dominant policy debates and research agenda. Policymakers frequently consider community services and family care as less expensive substitutes for nursing home care, making quality-of-life issues a secondary priority. Older adults and disability advocates, however, prioritize independence and quality of life over costs. Complicating the debate between independence and the costs of care is the diversity by gender, race or ethnicity, and income among older Americans.

Institutional Care

When most people think about long-term care or LTSS, the first service that comes to mind is nursing home care. But only 4.2 percent of older adults live in nursing homes, with an additional 2.7 percent living in community housing that offers supportive services (Federal Interagency Forum on Aging-Related Statistics, 2012). Nevertheless, the high cost of nursing home care, averaging $73,000 per year for double occupancy and $81,030 for a private room (Genworth Financial, 2012), make it a top policy priority.

Institutions that deliver long-term care services can be classified by the extent of medical or nursing care they provide. At one end are subacute facilities and skilled nursing homes that provide intensive posthospital care, twenty-four-hour skilled nursing, and often rehabilitation. At the other end are residential facilities with little or no medical or nursing care, but that offer assistance for functional activities like cooking and bathing, typically in board-and-care or assisted-living facilities. Regardless of the level of medical care, institutionalized populations have some level of disability that require care and supervision.

Public policy first encouraged the establishment of private long-term care institutions when Old Age Assistance (public aid for low-income elderly) was established in 1935 and specifically barred residents of publicly owned facilities from receiving this aid. The program allowed local governments to close their unpopular almshouses for the poor and ill, transferring the care of the ill and dependent elderly to private facilities, and shifting the costs to the states and federal government. The federal government later gave funds directly for the construction of more medicalized nursing homes in the 1950s to solve a hospital bed shortage and to save money by discharging hospital patients to a less intensive level of care (Wallace, 2012).

Public funding for nursing homes expanded dramatically after the passage of Medicare and Medicaid in 1965, fueling a rapid growth in the number of facilities. Both programs defined nursing homes as predominantly medical institutions, emphasizing the nursing over the home. Prospective payment for hospital care (through diagnosis-related groups, or DRGs), starting in 1984, provided strong incentives to hospitals to reduce the length of hospital stay and discharge patients to nursing homes for the last stages of treatment and recovery. In response, some nursing homes increased their emphasis on medical services so they could capture well-paid, Medicare-funded, posthospital patients. Growing governmental spending on nursing homes led to a number of initiatives to reduce the reliance on nursing homes, which has resulted in declining rates of nursing home use and increasing use of alternatives, including assisted living (Stevenson & Grabowski, 2010).

The 1999 U.S. Supreme Court decision in *Olmstead v. L.C.* also affected long-term care policy. The court ruled that the Americans with Disabilities Act (ADA) applied to public programs and that states had to administer their Medicaid (and other) programs in a way that provides assistance in the least restrictive setting possible when desired by recipients (Teitelbaum, Burke, & Rosenbaum, 2004). The decision further pushed states and the federal government to promote home and community services over nursing homes and has provided a reference point for aging and disability advocates when they promote LTSS alternatives that offer greater autonomy and independence.

The two primary types of LTC institutions in the United States are freestanding *nursing homes* and *assisted living facilities (ALFs)*. Nursing homes provide residential and medical services to residents who require subacute and rehabilitative care after a trauma or major medical event such as stroke. They also provide these services to those at the end of life or those with long-term chronic care needs such as dementia. About 19 percent of elderly persons admitted to nursing homes stay for less than three months, 24 percent stay three months to a year, and the rest stay for more than a year (Jones, Dwyer, Bercovitz, & Strahan, 2009). While those with long stays used to be primarily individuals who simply needed help with daily activities (like meals or medication management), the growth of alternatives to nursing homes has led to an increase in the acuity (illness severity and disability) of residents.

The sixteen thousand nursing homes nationally are frequently privately owned (61.5 percent), relatively small (averaging 105 beds per facility), certified by both Medicare and Medicaid (87.6 percent), and part of a chain (54.2 percent). In 2004, there were about 1.7 million nursing home beds and 1.5 million residents, creating an occupancy rate of 87.3 percent (Jones et al., 2009).

The other major type of long-term care institution is assisted living facilities (ALFs), known in some states as residential care facilities for the elderly (RCF-E) or board-and-care facilities. Over 15,700 ALFs were operating in the United States in 2010, reflecting a 16 percent growth from 2005 (Sanofi-Aventis, 2011). ALFs are disproportionally located in more affluent areas and in California, Pennsylvania, and Florida (Stevenson & Grabowski, 2010). The facilities typically offer twenty-four-hour custodial care including assistance with basic activities of daily living, medication assistance, two to three meals per day in a common room, light housekeeping, social activities, and some transportation. Rooms are more likely to be private and more homelike than nursing homes and allow residents more autonomy over daily routines. In some cases they are individual apartments that have access to services as needed. The average AFL size is about seventy-five beds, and the median annual cost for one bedroom single occupancy is estimated at $39,000 in 2010 (Genworth Financial, 2012). Their occupancy rate in 2009 was estimated at 88.4 percent (Assisted Living Federation of America, 2009).

Although most people assume that Medicare pays for most nursing home stays, it will only pay for a maximum of one hundred days of posthospital recovery care ("postacute care") and provides no coverage for custodial care (after recovery-oriented treatment has ended). Medicaid, by contrast, pays for custodial as well as postacute care. In 2007, nursing home expenditures accounted for 8 percent of all Medicare and 19 percent of all Medicaid expenditures (Ng, Harrington, & Kitchener, 2010). In addition, Medicaid pays more in the aggregate for nursing home care than any other source, followed closely by the residents themselves. Because the annual costs of nursing homes usually exceed the median income of $31,410 of householders age sixty-five years of age and older (Federal Interagency Forum on Aging-Related Statistics, 2012), many individuals who start paying out of pocket for care become eligible for Medicaid after "spending down" or depleting their resources. Nursing home spend-down has attracted policy attention because those who spend down account for a significant proportion of Medicaid nursing home expenditures and because the phenomenon is a demonstration of the catastrophic costs of long-term care. Impoverishment due to the high cost of home care has received little policy attention, but is also highly associated with spending down (Wiener, Anderson, Khatutsky, Kaganova, & O'Keeffe, 2013). The high cost of nursing home care has also led to policies that protect some of the income of spouses when one member of a couple is institutionalized under Medicaid. As a result, if one member of a couple needs nursing home care, the spouse who remains in the community is allowed to keep a modest amount of income that is not deemed available to pay for nursing home care, along with the home they remain in.

The ways that nursing homes are paid for is extremely complex. Medicare nursing home payment rates are generally higher than Medicaid rates, encouraging the growth of facilities that provide Medicare reimbursable subacute and rehabilitative services. Both programs pay per diem rates, but differ in how they calculate those rates and in what additional services may be billed. Reimbursement methods affect access to and quality of nursing home care. Low Medicaid rates can reduce both access to and quality of care, although simply increasing payments to nursing homes does not guarantee that the nursing home will spend the additional revenue in ways that improve patient outcomes rather than on increasing profits. To discourage nursing homes from taking only the least disabled (and least expensive) Medicaid patients, some states have tried reimbursement formulae that pay more for the care of the most disabled (Miller, Mor, Grabowski, &

Gozalo, 2009). But this system may have the unintended consequence of reducing access for those needing only lower-level custodial care.

Although forty-two states have provisions for providing Medicaid home care services to assisted living facility (ALF) residents, in most states Medicaid-eligible residents must pay privately for the room-and-board component of care. Government regulation and market oversight tend to be much looser for ALFs than nursing homes since they are regulated solely by state licensing laws. Supplemental security income (cash assistance for the lowest-income aged, blind, and disabled) can be used to pay for ALF, but it is rarely enough (Stevenson & Grabowski, 2010). In addition, some government-subsidized senior housing buildings have added LTSS services to allow residents to remain living independently longer, creating enriched housing (Stone, Harahan, & Sanders, 2008).

Widespread concern about the treatment of nursing home residents has focused attention on quality-of-care issues. Of the three main aspects of quality of care—structure, process, and outcomes—the first two measures are most often studied. Research has shown a direct relationship between structure measures such as staffing levels and quality of care, leading to some states mandating minimum staffing levels for nursing homes above the federal standard (Harrington, 2005). Process and medical outcome measures frequently include the reduction of urinary incontinence, pressure sores, malnutrition, and pain. However, data and research on patient quality of life in facilities from the older person's perspective are sparse. Other characteristics of nursing homes, such as for-profit status, have also been linked to quality, with better quality of care in not-for-profit nursing homes compared to for-profit institutions (Hillmer, Wodchis, Gill, Anderson, & Rochon, 2005).

One tool used to monitor nursing home quality is the federally mandated minimum data set (MDS) that provides information on every resident of a facility. The MDS contains assessment items for each resident covering seventeen areas, such as mood and behavior, physical functioning, and skin conditions. The data are aggregated at the facility level and used to identify potential quality-of-care problems when indicators like rates of pressure sores and weight loss are higher than average. The introduction of this monitoring system contributed to an improvement in quality of care, although much room for quality improvement remains (Wunderlich & Kohler, 2001).

Public policies seek to improve nursing home quality through both market mechanisms and regulatory means. Web sites such as www.medicare.gov/NhCompare provide information on quality of care including staffing levels, clinical outcomes, and complaints. The utility of such information is limited, particularly because prospective residents and their families frequently search for a nursing home in urgent and less-than-ideal circumstances and make decisions largely on criteria like distance, cost, and immediate availability. Unlike consumer goods and services, prospective residents and their families infrequently have the knowledge or the peace of mind to rationally peruse these complex data to balance cost, quality, and other relevant nursing home characteristics to make optimum decisions.

Community-Based Services

For many, long-term care conjures up the image of bedridden elderly residents in nursing homes. But older people with functional limitations usually prefer to remain at home, and most do so, often receiving assistance from family and friends as well as community agencies. The most severe limitations that require help from another person or special equipment are usually classified as *activities of daily living* (ADLs), which are personal care activities necessary to remain living at home, such as getting out of a bed or chair, dressing, and bathing.

Recent estimates indicate that as many as 5.4 million adults over sixty-five years of age who receive assistance with daily activities live in the community. As many older adults continue to live in the community and receive assistance with moderate or more severe disabilities (two or more ADLs) as there are older adults in nursing homes (Khatutsky, Wiener, Anderson, & Porell, 2012).

Community-based long-term services and supports (LTSS) include a wide array of programs such as home care, adult day care, transportation, and congregate meals. Home care is provided by visiting nurses, home health aides with some training who can provide basic personal care such as help with bathing, and homemakers or untrained workers who assist with housecleaning and some personal care. Adult day care is supportive care provided outside the home that often includes some therapies and nurse monitoring and may also assist family caregivers by providing a respite in caring and/or allow the family caregiver to remain employed when the elder needs constant monitoring. In addition to hands-on care, older adults may also use assistive devices such as walkers and grab bars, health and medication monitoring, and home-delivered meals. We refer to both in-home and out-of-home services as "community-based" long-term services and supports in this chapter.

Medicare pays for limited community-based care since it emphasizes medically oriented, postacute home care, not the ongoing social support services many people need to live independently in the community. Medicare recipients must be homebound, under the care of a physician, and in need of part-time or intermittent skilled nursing care, or physical, speech, or occupational therapy. Despite its limited scope, the high skill level of those providing Medicare home care and its frequent use make Medicare the largest source of home care expenditures, covering two-fifths of all LTSS spending (Kassner, 2011). Medicare expenditures for home health care have steadily increased, from $18.2 billion in 2005 to $31.5 billion in 2010, and are projected to grow to $50.7 billion by 2020 (Centers for Medicare and Medicaid Services, 2011).

An exception to Medicare's acute and postacute care bias is the Program for All-Inclusive Care of the Elderly (PACE), which was added as a permanent Medicare benefit in 1997. PACE combines Medicare and Medicaid funding in a capitated program that provides all needed medical and LTSS to low-income older persons who are disabled enough to qualify for Medicaid nursing home care. The integrated delivery model offers a continuum of community-based social and medical services, usually built around the extensive use of adult day care, to maintain elders in their own homes. Yet a number of barriers, including the requirement that disabled elders must leave their personal physicians and switch to the program's physicians, have limited this program to serving only about 23,000 elders nationally.

Medicaid, unlike Medicare, does not limit community-based LTSS to posthospital care. The government's concern with reducing Medicaid nursing home spending encouraged the expansion of Medicaid coverage of community-based services. The growth in both the availability and popularity of LTSS has led Medicaid funding for home health, personal care, and related services to grow from $17 billion in 1999 to $45 billion in 2008, when it served 3.1 million disabled low-income persons of all ages. Medicaid is the second largest payer of community-based LTSS after Medicare, accounting for about one-quarter of all LTSS spending (Kassner, 2011). Medicaid spending exceeds Medicare spending only when high-cost nursing home care is included. States have a wide discretion in enacting policies to cap the costs of many community-based long-term care services that are offered as "waiver" services, including limiting the number of persons who can receive services. As a result, more than 511,000 people were on waiting lists for these services in 2011, with an average wait time of twenty-five months (Kaiser Family Foundation, 2012).

There are nine million Medicaid beneficiaries who are disabled (all ages) or elderly who are also enrolled in the Medicare program. Known as the "dual eligible" population, these individuals are among the sickest and poorest of beneficiaries covered by either program. They are also among the most expensive, representing 15 percent of total Medicaid enrollment while accounting for 39 percent of expenditures, and comprising 21 percent of Medicare enrollment while accounting for 36 percent of Medicare costs. The Affordable Care Act of 2010 (ACA) includes a number of provisions that aim to improve care for the "dual eligibles" while reducing costs through better integration and coordination, improved quality, and increased access to community-based services. Notably, the ACA has established a Federal Coordinated Health Care Office charged with leading these integration efforts and improving coordination between the Center for Medicare and Medicaid Services (CMS) and the states that administer the Medicaid.

Another federal program that funds services to help maintain older adult independence at home and in the community is the Older Americans Act (OAA). Title III of the OAA spent $1.5 billion in 2010 for supportive services such as transportation and information or referral (25 percent of funds), congregate meals in locations such as senior centers (29 percent), home-delivered meals (15 percent), preventive health programs (1 percent), and caregiver support programs (10 percent) (Administration on Aging, 2012). The OAA also funds the nursing home ombudsman program that places trained volunteers in willing facilities to act as advocates for patients in those facilities. The OAA receives a fixed allocation of funds each year, in contrast to Medicaid and Medicare funding, which uses formula-driven budgets based on actual use and charges. The cap on OAA spending, and its relatively unchanged budget from year to year, creates a situation where some of its programs run out of money before the end of the year and are forced to refuse new clients. Moreover, the amount of assistance provided to each recipient tends to be even lower than that furnished by Medicaid programs.

The policy focus on cost containment has shaped the direction of research on community care. Community-based services are usually cheaper than nursing home care for a single individual, and services can delay institutionalization (Gaugler, Kane, Kane, & Newcomer, 2005), but total costs tend to be higher because more persons are served by community-based care than would have been served by nursing homes (Weissert, Chernew, & Hirth, 2003). In an effort to reduce spending during the recession of 2008 to 2012, many states attempted to restrict Medicaid LTSS eligibility or services to only those who were in imminent risk of institutionalization. Limiting Medicaid home care to individuals with high disability levels and high institutionalization risk, however, ignores the facts that functional decline often develops gradually and the need for home care exists along a continuum (Kietzman et al., 2012). Thus, persons who would benefit from a modest amount of help remain ineligible, and those who need substantial help bump up against arbitrary dollar or hour limits that exist primarily to reduce home care costs. A more client-focused paradigm makes all disabled persons eligible for some home care, with the quantity of care varying in a continuous fashion based on need (Weissert et al., 2003).

Another body of research examines the policy concern that publicly funded care will begin to substitute for care provided "free" by family and friends. Such a concern is based on the premise that formal (paid) and informal (unpaid) services are interchangeable and that an hour of paid care results in one less hour of care by family members. Most studies of the intersection of formal and informal services focus exclusively on allocating tasks between family caregivers and formal providers. Family members, however, often describe caregiving as a complex relationship, not simply as a set of discrete tasks. If a paid homemaker assumes the task of bathing a disabled parent, the care recipient's children are likely to continue to express their concern for the parent through other supportive actions. It is thus not surprising that researchers find that formal services supplement rather than supplant informal care (McMaughan Moudouni, Ohsfeldt, Miller, & Phillips, 2012).

A similar line of research arises from the fear that large numbers of elderly people will come out of the woodwork to use new services because community-based services such as household cleaning, unlike nursing homes, are believed to be universally desired at high levels of service. This fear, too, appears to be misdirected. Some elderly people postpone assistance until they are extremely disabled in order to maintain a sense of independence (Kane, Kane, & Ladd, 1998). Having absorbed a value system that glorifies self-sufficiency, they may be reluctant to rely on others even when they are very needy. Those who fear that the expansion of community services will generate additional demand implicitly acknowledge that the elderly are drastically underserved.

Consumer Direction

As the demand for community-based services has increased, programs funded by the Older Americans Act (OAA) and Medicaid have developed innovative approaches to how these services are delivered. One important emerging trend is the advent and growth of consumer-directed services that offer more flexible benefits and consumer involvement in decision making than traditional agency-directed services. The growing popularity of consumer direction may partly be attributed to the aging of the Baby Boomers (the large post–World War II cohort born between 1946 and 1964), who are more likely to want to take an active role in decisions about their own care. LTSS are increasingly assessing consumer preferences and satisfaction with services and incorporating this feedback into service planning and delivery, and promoting consumer choice and control through programs that deliver personal care, respite care, and family caregiver support (Kunkel & Lackmeyer, 2010).

Consumer-directed personal care services typically allow low-income consumers to directly hire a caregiver of their choosing through public programs, including family members. Many states have adopted consumer direction as a way to improve the quality and reach of Medicaid-funded personal care services, while also driving down the costs. The national Cash and Counseling demonstration program used a controlled experimental design to compare the effectiveness of a consumer-directed versus traditional agency-managed service approach to personal care. In some cases savings were found from reduced nursing home use that offset the higher costs associated with increased access to personal care services; participants in the consumer-directed group were also more satisfied, their unmet needs were reduced, and no adverse effects were generated with regard to participant health and safety (Carlson, Foster, Dale, & Brown, 2007). The positive results of the consumer-directed model for consumers and for their informal and paid caregivers were similar for both older adults and younger disabled persons (Simon-Rusinowitz, Loughlin, Ruben, Garcia, & Mahoney, 2010).

Challenges to Expanding Community Care

The 2010 Affordable Care Act (ACA) is known primarily for a small number of key provisions that expand health insurance. One rarely discussed component of the ACA is a significant new program that would have expanded support for personal care and other home care services. For over twenty years policymakers and advocates have discussed ways of expanding community-based long-term care insurance using a social insurance model, extending beyond the welfare model of Medicaid. The Community Living Assistance Services and Supports (CLASS) Act was added as a component of the ACA to establish a voluntary national insurance system that would collect premiums from working adults and then provide them with cash assistance (about $50 a day) to pay for home-care expenses if they become disabled, at any age. The general outlines of the program had high levels of public support, but the specific law had exceptionally low levels of public awareness. The program was never implemented because the law specified financing parameters that turned out to be unfeasible, and modifying the law was impossible because of political changes in Congress (Gleckman, 2011). In the end, a policy that would have assisted the middle class with help at home floundered on a combination of financial and partisan complications, leaving this need unmet.

The most fundamental critique of the long-term care "system" is that it does not look or work like a system. There is a wide variety of community and institutional services that have different systems of eligibility, financing, philosophies, and capacities. In addition, each state has different licensing and financial incentives for different types of long-term services and supports. Some states promote consumer direction and support families who provide caregiving, while others do not. The balance of state financing for community versus institutional care ranges from 15 percent community versus 85 percent institutional, to 60 percent community versus 40 percent institutional. And with public financing available mostly for the poorest and most disabled, the working poor and middle class are unable to afford to pay for LTSS, but also are not eligible for public support until they become destitute (Reinhard, Kassner, Houser, & Mollica, 2011).

Informal Care

Research refutes the enduring myth that families abandon their elderly relatives. Ethel Shanas was one of the first scholars to show that elderly people remain in close contact with surviving kin (Shanas, 1979), and more recent studies demonstrate that this contact translates into assistance during times of crisis. At least 90 percent of older adults who receive care at home get at least some help from their family or friends, and only 28 percent of those receiving family care also receive formal (paid) in-home assistance (Houser, Gibson, & Redfoot, 2010). In 2009, an estimated 61.6 million people in the United States provided some form of unpaid care to an adult with limitations, at an economic value of approximately $450 billion (Feinberg, Reinhard, Houser, & Choula, 2011).

Informal care continues to be allocated on the basis of gender. Women account for about two-thirds of those caring for an older person. Compared with men caregivers, women caregivers tend to be older, married, and the primary caregiver. Women provide more intensive and complex care, they are more likely to report difficulty with care provision and balancing caregiving with other family and employment responsibilities, and are more likely than men to suffer from poor emotional health secondary to caregiving (National Alliance for Caregiving, 2009).

Although informal caregivers often report feeling personally rewarded by the caregiving experience, most research on informal care focuses primarily on the burden it imposes. Studies have found that caregivers experience a range of physical, emotional, social, and financial problems. In many cases, caregiving responsibilities reignite family conflict, impose financial strain, and encroach on both paid employment and leisure activity (Pinquart & Sörensen, 2007; Savundranayagam, Montgomery, & Kosloski, 2011).

Despite the prevalence of informal caregiving and extensive documentation of the physical, emotional, and financial burdens experienced by so many, limited assistance is available. Informal caregivers often express the need for temporary relief from their caregiving responsibilities, and many interventions have been developed that improve caregiver outcomes, yet most caregivers continue to be underserved and have unmet needs (Gitlin & Schultz, 2012).

A dominant concern of policymakers is that caregivers will pass the responsibilities of care, and associated costs, on to the state. As a result, policymakers may support social services and financial assistance for caregivers to the extent that these programs are expected to encourage informal caregivers to continue to assume the greatest responsibility for care, postpone or prevent care recipient institutionalization, and save money. Such responses may be shortsighted, however, if they do not account for the economic consequences that accrue from losses in workplace productivity or from caregivers who withdraw from the workforce completely.

While many caregivers struggle to balance their caregiving and workplace responsibilities, policies that advance effective solutions have been limited. The Family and Medical Leave Act (FMLA), passed with widespread acclaim in 1993, provides leaves of no more than twelve weeks, but unlike policies in almost all other industrialized countries the leave is unpaid, it excludes part-time and contingent workers and those employed in small firms, and defines family narrowly. As such, the FMLA is available to fewer than 60 percent of workers and has resulted in notable inequities, as workers who are white, middle-class, and married are those most likely to be able to afford and use it (Wisensale, 2006).

A number of states have independently engaged in efforts to establish paid family leave programs. In 2002, California became the first state to offer paid family leave through the short-term disability system; Washington followed suit in 2007 and New Jersey in 2009. A study of the California experience finds positive effects for both workers and businesses. Policy-makers and advocates alike are increasingly taking interest in the promise of these new programs (Appelbaum & Milkman, 2011).

Another policy initiative enacted to address the needs of informal caregivers is the National Family Caregiver Support Program (NFCSP). This program was established in 2000 through the Older Americans Act (OAA), which uses a social services model to provide services to all persons over age sixty (and now their caregivers as well), with no required means test. The NFCSP marks a significant paradigm shift as informal caregivers are now viewed as an OAA service population in their own right. States are charged with providing five services to caregivers: information about available services; assistance in gaining access to the services; individual counseling, organization of support groups, and caregiver training; respite care; and supplemental services (such as home modifications and emergency response systems). However, funding for the NFCSP is quite limited and, since its inception in 2000, has remained relatively flat, with an annual budget of about $153 million for each of the fiscal years 2008 through 2011 (Administration on Aging, 2012). This significantly constrains the scope of service coverage and the NFCSP's capacity to provide more costly services like respite care to many caregivers. Future funding decisions will determine whether the program remains largely symbolic or if it grows into a significant source of support for caregivers nationwide.

Recent developments in health policy acknowledge the needs of informal (family) caregivers and have also begun to recognize the important and integral role they play as providers in the system of care—whether the care recipient is at home in the community, in acute or institutional care, or transitioning between these settings. The Affordable Care Act of 2010 (ACA) includes provisions that involve individuals and their caregivers as decision makers about care options, introduce new models of care that recognize family caregivers as partners in the caregiving process, and better support and prepare family caregivers to effectively assume the caregiver role (Reinhard, Kassner, & Houser, 2011).

Workers in the Long-Term Care System

An estimated four million direct care workers, funded primarily by Medicaid and Medicare, provide paid long-term care and personal assistance services for the elderly and for others living with disabilities. Almost 40 percent work as nursing aides, orderlies, and attendants in institutions such as nursing homes. The others care for residents in the community, half of them elderly, in homes and other community-based settings. Projected increases in the population of elderly and those living alone create an expanding need for community-based personal care and home health aides, which are currently the fastest growing occupations nationwide. Together with other long-term direct care workers, they will become the largest occupational group in the country, reaching five million workers by 2020 (Kaye et al., 2010; Seavey & Marquand, 2011).

Workers may enter the workforce for the intrinsic rewards of care work; they like their work when they are provided with resources and support to provide quality care and to cope with the physical and emotional demands of care work (Delp, Wallace, Geiger-Brown, & Muntaner, 2010). But fiscal and bureaucratic constraints, work overload, time pressure, lack of respect, discrimination and abuse, role ambiguity, and job insecurity, combined with the financial strain of low wages and limited health benefits, create stress and dissatisfaction. Turnover rates range from 35 to 65 percent among aides in community and home care settings and are even higher in long-term care institutions (National Institute for Occupational Safety and Health, 2009; Seavey & Marquand, 2011). Direct care workers in long-term care are predominantly middle-aged women of diverse racial or ethnic backgrounds. While women are a minority of other occupations (46 percent), they make up 87 percent of nursing aides, home health aides, and personal home care aides (see Table 16.2). These direct care workers are also more likely to be immigrants, and almost one-third are African American. Nearly half (45.9 percent) of these direct care workers live in or near poverty, about twice the rate of all other workers.

Home care workers earn as little as minimum wage, and half earn $9.44 an hour or less, while the median nursing home wages are only slightly higher, at $11.54 an hour. Total income may be considerably less for the many workers able to obtain only part-time employment; annual median earnings for home care aides in 2009 were $12,000. Only 52 percent of nursing home and residential care workers and 32 percent of home health care workers have access to employer-sponsored health insurance (Seavey & Marquand, 2011).

Home health care workers and personal care aides must often patch together multiple clients to obtain sufficient hours of care work to earn a minimal income and, in some cases, to be eligible for health insurance. They do so by traveling from one client to another, often without payment for the costs of that travel, which can be substantial. The need to travel between clients in all types of weather and traffic results in a high risk

TABLE 16.2. CHARACTERISTICS OF SELECTED DIRECT CARE AND ALL OTHER OCCUPATIONS, UNITED STATES, 2008–2010

	Nursing and Home Health Aides and Personal Home Care Workers (occupational codes 3600 and 4610)	All Other Occupations
Men	12.9	53.7
Women	87.1	46.3
Native born	78.0	84.0
Immigrant	22.0	16.0
Latino	14.5	14.9
African American (non-Latino)	30.1	11.0
Asian American (non-Latino)	5.4	5.1
White (non-Latino)	47.2	66.9
Near poor (<199% FPL)	45.9	23.5
Not poor (200%+ FPL)	54.1	76.5

Source: Ruggles et al., 2012.

for traffic accidents and injuries, on top of injuries sustained in clients' homes from heavy lifting, needle punctures, assaults, and trips and falls. Over 48,000 annual work-related injuries and illnesses are reported to the federal government for home care workers (Seavey & Marquand, 2011). Official statistics underestimate the true number of injuries, since workers may continue to work while injured or ill. Workers without sick leave may be unable to afford the loss of paid work days, and those without substitute workers may be forced to choose between caring for the consumer or for their own health (Delp et al., 2010).

Aides in nursing homes have the highest injury rates of any occupation, exceeding even construction workers and truck drivers, with as many as 60 percent reporting an injury in the previous year and, among those injured, 24 percent unable to work. Mandatory overtime, frequent job changes, lack of respect, and low wages were key predictors of injury (Khatutsky et al., 2012).

Demographic trends present critical questions to policymakers and society at large. As we confront the growing need for workers, how do we avoid low wages and poor working conditions that lead to high turnover and labor shortages, and create quality jobs that are sustainable for workers and that enhance quality care for the elderly? While society increasingly depends on workers who provide personal assistance to the elderly at home, the outdated 1938 Fair Labor Standards Act excludes those workers from basic minimum wage and overtime pay protection. The act was amended in 1974 to protect domestic workers, but continues to exclude workers who provide "companionship services to individuals who because of age or disability are unable to care for themselves." Many states have enacted laws to provide minimum wages for home care work, although exclusions often remain for workers who live with the consumer they care for and for those who are family members. Inadequate data limit the ability to assess the impact of these policy decisions. National surveys do not accurately capture the number of workers who provide long-term care in the home, especially paid family members, and only limited research exists to assess the impact on worker health when unrelated providers live with the consumer. At the federal level, the Department of Labor proposed eliminating the "companionship exemption" in 2012 and will clarify when basic minimum wage and overtime protections apply to home care workers.

Other policy debates surround the issue of how employment relations are structured in the unique setting of the home. A growing trend toward publicly funded, consumer-directed care—in which consumers have a voice in choosing who will care for them—addresses gender and class inequities by enabling low-income family members to receive payment for providing home care services. This policy challenges the traditional belief that women should provide unpaid care, an expectation that places an undue burden on women and on low-income families that must juggle paid work outside the home and unpaid care for family members. Many states have structured consumer-directed care to extend a voice to home care workers through unionization, raising wages, providing benefits, and creating a mechanism for workers to collectively advocate for improved home care services. Other initiatives include implementing worker cooperatives, defining key competencies and appropriate training to promote direct care worker retention and career advancement, and passing legislation to require that a minimum percentage of revenues generated from direct care services be expended on the workforce providing those services; as a result of this policy, wage increases led to a decline in turnover rates among Illinois workers employed by a private national home care company (Seavey & Marquand, 2011; Stone & Harahan, 2010). Coalitions of workers and consumers will be critical to advocate for quality jobs and quality care and to ensure policy changes that meet the growing demand for long-term care.

Gender, Race, and Class in Long-Term Services and Supports

Long-term services and supports are generally designed around functional needs and reimbursement types, not around population groups. Nonetheless, different populations have varying patterns of LTSS use that are sometimes the result of preferences and other times the result of inequitable policies and practices. In American society, inequities are most likely to occur along the lines of gender, race, and class.

The impact of gender on nursing home use is most evident among the oldest old (age eighty-five and over), where the institutionalization rate for women is almost twice that of men (14.1 percent versus 7.9 percent in 2010). Some of the reasons for this trend are that women are more likely to be widows than men, they have higher levels of disability in advanced ages, and they are poorer and so are less able to afford to pay for alternative services. Policies that provide better incomes for women in old age, such as better Social Security coverage for periods when women leave the workforce to care for young children or aging parents, would provide more resources if they become disabled in old age. In addition, bolstering community care resources for low-income seniors will disproportionately assist older women who want to remain in their own homes.

Race and ethnicity also define sharp differences in institutional use, and there is an interaction with immigration. The highest institutionalization rate among the oldest old is by African Americans (see Table 16.3), followed closely by non-Latino whites and then by U.S.-born Latinos. The lowest rates are mostly among immigrants.

The trend over time has been for non-Latino whites to use nursing homes less and ALFs and community care more, while the use of nursing homes for African Americans has been rising steadily over the years. Nursing homes have also been found to mirror the racial segregation of the communities they are in. This results in African Americans and Latinos disproportionately residing in facilities with worse quality of care as measured by licensing inspection deficiencies and staffing levels (Fennell, Feng, Clark, & Mor, 2010; Smith, Feng, Fennell, Zinn, & Mor, 2007). It is unlikely that the growth in minority nursing home use has been driven by

TABLE 16.3. INSTITUTIONALIZATION RATES BY NATIVITY, RACE, AND ETHNICITY, AGE SIXTY-FIVE AND OVER, UNITED STATES, 2010

	Total population age 65+ (thousands)	% Institutionalized age 65–74	% Institutionalized age 75–84	% Institutionalized age 85+
Immigrants				
Latino	1,333	0.7	2.4	6.0
Asian	1,182	0.4	1.6	7.0
U.S.-Born				
Latino	1,173	1.6	3.9	11.9
Non-Latino Asian	222	0.8	2.0	8.3
Non-Latino African American	3,090	2.3	5.4	13.2
Non-Latino white	30,147	1.0	3.4	12.7
American Indian or Alaska Native	350	1.8	3.6	8.3

Source: Ruggles et al., 2012.

preferences, given the fact that most older adults of all races and ethnicities report a preference to remain living at home as long as possible.

The rising rates of African Americans in nursing homes have been interpreted as the result of access barriers to community LTSS that are needed for African American elders to remain at home, combined with increasing options such as assisted living for older adults with more income (who are more often non-Latino white), which allow them to avoid nursing homes (Feng, Fennell, Tyler, Clark, & Mor, 2011). In addition, African Americans have significantly higher levels of disability than non-Latino whites, and the increasing levels of disability in nursing homes result in somewhat more African Americans entering that level of care. Similar dynamics may be operating for older Latinos, who also have higher levels of disability than older non-Latino whites (Markides & Wallace, 2007). Recent public policies that are designed to improve the quality of care in nursing homes have attempted to use market principles to improve quality—such as higher reimbursements for better process and outcome measures. The unintended consequence, however, appears to disadvantage nursing homes with high percentages of minority residents, which further reinforces the quality-of-care gap between the nursing homes most often used by minority elderly and those most often used by non-Latino white elders (Konetzka & Werner, 2009). These findings suggest that not examining the impact of "color-blind" LTSS policies on racial and ethnic minority elders can exacerbate racial inequities in care.

There is much less research on the use of community-based LTSS by race or ethnicity, in part because there is less administrative data on the subject. There is some evidence that African Americans and Latinos receive less community-based LTSS when levels of needs are accounted for, but higher levels of informal (unpaid) assistance (Konetzka & Werner, 2009). It is unclear how much of this is due to barriers in obtaining formal support versus preferences for family assistance. In states where family members can be paid by public programs for providing care, the barriers may be somewhat less.

Specific research on class factors in long-term care is sparse and primarily deals with the problems faced by Medicaid recipients. The quality of life of Medicaid nursing home residents appears to be especially poor. Medicaid recipients tend to be relegated to institutions that, according to some measures, offer the worst-quality care. Some observers argue that social policy for older persons in the United States creates a two-class system. Low-income elderly rely on Medicaid and other poverty programs, while those who are better off benefit from tax preferences, employment-based retiree benefits and privately purchased long-term care policies. Poverty programs are the most vulnerable to cuts because their constituency lacks political and economic clout.

The greatest difference by class may lie in services provided outside the bounds of established organizations. Although most studies ignore the vast network of helpers recruited through ad hoc, informal arrangements, some evidence suggests that disabled elderly people rely disproportionately on this type of assistance. A national survey found about one-third of unpaid caregivers reported that their care recipient also had paid help from aides, housekeepers, or others, with whites and high-income caregivers the most likely to have this additional assistance (National Alliance for Caregiving, 2009). The help from such workers typically is not included in government statistics; however, it constitutes a major source of assistance to the affluent that is not available to others.

Future Directions

It is estimated that about 70 percent of persons who reach age sixty-five will have some long-term care needs during the rest of their lives. On average, they will need functional or other assistance for three years, two-thirds of that in their own homes, with mostly unpaid assistance from friends and family. Their final year, on average, will be spent in a nursing home or assisted living facility (Kemper, Komisar, & Alecxih, 2005). Nevertheless, the set of services available is largely uncoordinated, the financing inadequate, and public knowledge about available services woefully inadequate. The rapid growth of the older population will put new strains on our long-term care system, especially when the Baby Boom generation reaches age eighty-five, beginning around 2030. We can confidently predict that this cohort will be disproportionately widowed women with high rates of disability and poverty; a growing number will be members of racial and ethnic minorities.

Although the priority in both policy and research is typically on cost containment, the most critical issue is how we can provide adequate and high-quality long-term care services equitably to this growing and diverse population. The limited financial resources of many older people create a need for a universal Medicare-type of social insurance for long-term care. The failure of the federal government to implement the CLASS Act in 2011 was not because of the lack of need; it merely delays the day when public policy will have to provide adequate attention to the growing elderly population and the organization and financing of long-term services and supports in a way that provides adequate-quality, equitable services to the population in need.

SUMMARY

The rapidly growing older population is the most likely to need assistance with living independently. A wide variety of different formal services have developed to help families provide the care needed by those with disability, but their organizing and financing is not coordinated. Most Americans do not know enough about their likely needs for long-term services and supports during their lifetimes, nor about how to get help when they need it. Public policy has focused for many years on ways to restrain the rising costs of LTSS to government. The Baby Boom generation will likely push policy to also better address affordability, adequacy, and quality in the coming years.

NOTE

This chapter includes sections drawn from earlier editions of the chapter that were written by Emily Abel. Partial support of Wallace and Kietzman for this work was provided by The SCAN Foundation.

KEY TERMS

- **Activities of daily living (ADLs)** Personal care activities needed to maintain independent living, usually includes transferring out of a bed or chair, dressing, bathing, eating, using the toilet, and often walking. The number of these activities that a person needs assistance with is used as a measure of disability and as eligibility criteria in some policies and programs.
- **Assisted living facility (ALF)** A facility that offers supportive care (such as help with bathing), but not medical care in a more homelike environment than nursing homes.
- **Formal care** Long-term services and supports that are provided by paid workers. May be in any setting (such as a nursing home or a personal home).

- **Informal care** Long-term services and supports that are provided by family and friends without pay. The type and intensity of care can be the same as formal care.
- **Nursing home** A licensed facility with nursing care and relatively high levels of staffing. These facilities are highly regulated and often have the appearance of low-intensity hospitals.

DISCUSSION QUESTIONS

1. Where and from whom would *your* parents or grandparents want to receive assistance with daily activities if they became disabled? How would they pay for it?
2. What is the relative emphasis in public policy on different types of long-term services and supports, especially nursing homes, formal home care, and informal home care? What are some of the reasons for this different emphasis?
3. Who are the primary providers of informal care? What issues do these providers face, and what policy solutions can address those issues?
4. What arguments can be made to increase funding for community-based service?
5. Discuss the impact of a person receiving long-term care at home versus in an institution on the individual's quality of life and the financing of long-term services and supports.
6. What would improve working conditions for employees in the long-term care system? How are those changes similar to or different from policy changes that would improve the situation of informal (unpaid) caregivers?
7. How and why does long-term care need and receipt of care differ by race, class, and gender?
8. To what extent does the United States have a two-class system of long-term care? How does this affect issues of access and quality for those who need services?
9. What would be important elements of any future efforts to assure that most or all Americans can pay for their own needed long-term care?

FURTHER READING

The SCAN Foundation. Policy Briefs on Long-Term Services and Supports. http://www
.thescanfoundation.org/publications/policy-briefs

AARP Public Policy Institute. Long-Term Care. http://www.aarp.org/research/ppi/ltc

Family Caregiver Alliance. Fact Sheets and Publications. http://www.caregiver.org

Pratt, J. (2009). *Long-term care: Managing across the continuum* (3rd ed.). Sudbury, MA: Jones & Bartlett.

Wolf, D. A., & Folbre, N. (Eds.). (2012). *Universal coverage of long-term care in the United States: Can we get there from here?* New York: Russell Sage Foundation.

REFERENCES

Administration on Aging. (2012). *FY 2011 AoA budget table*. Washington, DC: Author. Retrieved from http://www.aoa.gov/AoARoot/About/Budget/DOCS/FY_2012_AoA_CJ_Feb_2011.pdf

Appelbaum, E., & Milkman, R. (2011). *Leaves that pay: Employer and worker experiences with paid family leave in California*. Washington, DC: Center for Economic and Policy Research.

Assisted Living Federation of America. (2009). *2009 Overview of assisted living*. Retrieved from http://www.alfa.org/News/1924/Assisted-Living-Occupancy-Rates-Remain-Unchanged

Carlson, B. L., Foster, L., Dale, S. B., & Brown, R. (2007). Effects of cash and counseling on personal care and well-being. *Health Services Research, 42*(1 Part 2), 467–487.

Centers for Medicare and Medicaid Services. (2011). *Projections based on the National Health Expenditures (NHE) released in January 2011*. Baltimore, MD: Author. Retrieved from http://www.cms.gov/Research-Statistics-Data-and-Systems/Statistics-Trends-and-Reports/NationalHealthExpendData/Downloads/proj2010.pdf

Delp, L., Wallace, S. P., Geiger-Brown, J., & Muntaner, C. (2010). Job stress and job satisfaction: Home care workers in a consumer-directed model of care. *Health Services Research, 45*, 922–940.

Federal Interagency Forum on Aging-Related Statistics. (2012). *Older Americans 2012: Key indicators of well-being*. Retrieved from http://www.agingstats.gov

Feinberg, L., Reinhard, S. C., Houser, A., & Choula, R. (2011). Valuing the invaluable: 2011 update: The growing contributions and costs of family caregiving. *Insight on the Issues, 51*. Retrieved from http://assets.aarp.org/rgcenter/ppi/ltc/i51-caregiving.pdf

Feng, Z., Fennell, M. L., Tyler, D. A., Clark, M., & Mor, V. (2011). Growth of racial and ethnic minorities in US nursing homes driven by demographics and possible disparities in options. *Health Affairs, 30*(7), 1358–1365.

Fennell, M. L., Feng, Z., Clark, M. A., & Mor, V. (2010). Elderly Hispanics more likely to reside in poor-quality nursing homes. *Health Affairs, 29*(1), 65–73.

Gaugler, J. E., Kane, R. L., Kane, R. A., & Newcomer, R. (2005). Early community-based service utilization and its effects on institutionalization in dementia caregiving. *The Gerontologist, 45*(2), 177–185.

Genworth Financial. (2012). *Genworth 2012 cost of care survey*. Retrieved from http://www.genworth.com/content/etc/medialib/genworth_v2/pdf/ltc_cost_of_care.Par.40001.File.dat/2012%20Cost%20of%20Care%20Survey%20Full%20Report.pdf

Gitlin, L., & Schultz, R. (2012). Family caregiving of older adults. In T. R. Prohaska, L. A. Anderson, & R. H. Binstock (Eds.), *Public health for an aging society* (pp. 181–204). Baltimore, MD: Johns Hopkins University Press.

Gleckman, H. (2011). Requiem for the CLASS Act. *Health Affairs, 30*(12), 2231–2234.

Harrington, C. (2005). Nurse staffing in nursing homes in the United States. *Journal of Gerontological Nursing, 31*(2), 18–23.

Hillmer, M. P., Wodchis, W. P., Gill, S. S., Anderson, G. M., & Rochon, P. A. (2005). Nursing home profit status and quality of care: Is there any evidence of an association? *Medical Care Research and Review, 62*(2), 139–166.

Houser, A., Gibson, M. J., & Redfoot, D. L. (2010). *Trends in family caregiving and paid home care for older people with disabilities in the community: Data from the National Long-Term Care Survey.* Retrieved from http://assets.aarp.org /rgcenter/ppi/ltc/2010–09-caregiving.pdf

Jones, A., Dwyer, L. L., Bercovitz, A. R., & Strahan, G. W. (2009). The National Nursing Home Survey: 2004 overview. *Vital and Health Statistics, 13*(167).

Kaiser Family Foundation. (2012). *Medicaid home and community-based services programs: Data update.* Retrieved from http://www.kff.org/medicaid/7720.cfm

Kane, R. A., Kane, R. L., & Ladd, R. C. (1998). *The heart of long-term care.* New York: Oxford University Press.

Kassner, E. (2011). *Home and community-based long-term services and supports for older people.* Washington, DC: AARP Public Policy Institute.

Kaye, H. S., Harrington, C., & LaPlante, M. P. (2010). Long-term care: Who gets it, who provides it, who pays, and how much? *Health Affairs, 29*(1), 11–21.

Kemper, P., Komisar, H. L., & Alecxih, L. (2005). Long-term care over an uncertain future: What can current retirees expect? *Inquiry, 42*(4), 335–350.

Khatutsky, G., Wiener, J. M., Anderson, W. L., & Porell, F. W. (2012). *Work-related injuries among certified nursing assistants working in US nursing homes.* Research Triangle Park, NC: RTI Press.

Kietzman, K. G., Wallace, S. P., Durazo, E. M., Torres, J. M., Soon Choi, A., Benjamin, A. E., & Mendez-Luck, C. (2012). A portrait of older Californians with disabilities who rely on public services to remain independent. *Home Health Care Services Quarterly, 31*(4), 317–336.

Konetzka, R. T., & Werner, R. M. (2009). Review: Disparities in long-term care. *Medical Care Research and Review, 66*(5), 491–521.

Kunkel, S. R., & Lackmeyer, A. E. (2010). The role of aging services network in balancing and transforming the long-term care system. *Public Policy and Aging Report, 20,* 16–21.

Markides, K. S., & Wallace, S. P. (2007). Minority elders in the United States: Implications for public policy. In R. Pruchno & M. Smyer (Eds.), *Challenges of an aging society: Ethical dilemmas, political issues* (pp. 193–216). Baltimore, MD: Johns Hopkins University Press.

McMaughan Moudouni, D. K., Ohsfeldt, R. L., Miller, T. R., & Phillips, C. D. (2012). The relationship between formal and informal care among adult Medicaid personal care services recipients. *Health Services Research, 47*(4), 1642–1659.

Miller, E. A., Mor, V., Grabowski, D. C., & Gozalo, P. L. (2009). The devil's in the details: Trading policy goals for complexity in Medicaid nursing home reimbursement. *Journal of Health Politics, Policy and Law, 34*(1), 93–135.

National Alliance for Caregiving. (2009). *Caregiving in the U.S., 2009.* Retrieved from http://www.caregiving.org/data/Caregiving_in_the_US_2009_full_report.pdf

National Institute for Occupational Safety and Health. (2009). *State of the sector/ healthcare and social assistance: Identification of research opportunities for the next decade of NORA (National Occupational Research Agenda).* Atlanta: Centers for Disease Control and Prevention. Retrieved from http://www.cdc.gov/niosh/docs/2009–139/pdfs /2009–139.pdf

Ng, T., Harrington, C., & Kitchener, M. (2010). Medicare and Medicaid in long-term care. *Health Affairs, 29*(1), 22–28.

Pinquart, M., & Sörensen, S. (2007). Correlates of physical health of informal caregivers: A meta-analysis. *The Journals of Gerontology Series B: Psychological Sciences and Social Sciences, 62*(2), P126–P137.

Reinhard, S. C., Kassner, E., & Houser, A. (2011). How the Affordable Care Act can help move states toward a high-performing system of long-term services and supports. *Health Affairs, 30*(3), 447–453.

Reinhard, S. C., Kassner, E., Houser, A., & Mollica, R. (2011). *Raising expectations: A state scorecard on long-term services and supports for older adults, people with physical disabilities, and family caregivers.* Retrieved from http://www.longtermscorecard .org/Report.aspx

Ruggles, S., Alexander, J. T., Genadek, K., Goeken, R., Schroeder, M. B., & Sobek, M. (2012). Integrated Public Use Microdata Series: Version 5.0 [Machine-readable database]. American CommunitySurvey 2008–2010. Minneapolis: University of Minnesota.

Sanofi-Aventis. (2011). Managed Care Digest Series 2011–2012. *Public Payer Digest, 2012.* Bridgewater, NJ: Author.

Savundranayagam, M. Y., Montgomery, R.J.V., & Kosloski, K. (2011). A dimensional analysis of caregiver burden among spouses and adult children. *The Gerontologist, 51*(3), 321–331.

Seavey, D., & Marquand, A. (2011). *Caring in America: A comprehensive analysis of the nation's fastest-growing jobs—home health and personal care aides.* Retrieved from http://www.directcareclearinghouse.org/download/caringinamerica-20111212.pdf

Shanas, E. (1979). The family as a social support system in old age. *The Gerontologist, 19*(2), 169–174.

Simon-Rusinowitz, L., Loughlin, D. M., Ruben, K., Garcia, G. M., & Mahoney, K. J. (2010). The benefits of consumer-directed services for elders and their caregivers in the Cash and Counseling demonstration and evaluation. *Public Policy and Aging Report, 20*, 27–31.

Smith, D. B., Feng, Z., Fennell, M. L., Zinn, J. S., & Mor, V. (2007). Separate and unequal: Racial segregation and disparities in quality across U.S. nursing homes. *Health Affairs, 26*(5), 1448–1458.

Stevenson, D. G., & Grabowski, D. C. (2010). Sizing up the market for assisted living. *Health Affairs, 29*(1), 35–43.

Stone, R., & Harahan, M. F. (2010). Improving the long-term care workforce serving older adults. *Health Affairs, 291*, 109–115.

Stone, R. I., Harahan, M., & Sanders, A. (2008). Expanding affordable housing with services for older adults: Challenges and potential. In S. M. Golant & J. Hyde (Eds.),

The assisted living residence: A vision for the future (pp. 329–350). Baltimore, MD: Johns Hopkins Press.

Teitelbaum, J., Burke, T., & Rosenbaum, S. (2004). *Olmstead v. L.C.* and the Americans with Disabilities Act: Implications for public health policy and practice. *Public Health Reports, 119*(3), 371–374.

U.S. National Health Interview Survey. (2011). *Health data interactive.* Retrieved from http://www.cdc.gov/nchs/hdi.htm

Wallace, S. P. (2012). Long-term care policy and older Latinos. In J. L. Angel, F. Torres-Gil, & K. Markides (Eds.), *Aging, health, and longevity in the Mexican-origin population* (pp. 243–258). New York: Springer.

Weissert, W., Chernew, M., & Hirth, R. (2003). Titrating versus targeting home care services to frail elderly clients. *Journal of Aging and Health, 15*(1), 99–123.

Wiener, J. M., Anderson, W., Khatutsky, G., Kaganova, Y., & O'Keeffe, J. (2013). *Medicaid spend down: New estimates and implications for long-term services and supports financing reform.* Washington, DC: RTI International.

Wisensale, S. K. (2006). What role for the Family and Medical Leave Act in long-term care policy? *Journal of Aging and Social Policy, 18*(3/4), 79–93.

Wunderlich, G. S., & Kohler, P. O. (Eds.). (2001). *Improving the quality of long-term care.* Washington, DC: Institute of Medicine, National Academy Press.

CHAPTER SEVENTEEN

HIV AND AIDS IN THE TWENTY-FIRST CENTURY

Erin G. Grinshteyn
William E. Cunningham

Learning Objectives

- Comprehend the changing nature of the HIV/AIDS epidemic
- Learn how the disease is treated and what treatment barriers still exist
- Learn the range of services that are needed to care for people living with HIV/AIDS
- Understand how the approaches to treatment and prevention of HIV/AIDS have converged
- Be aware of current policy issues affecting the prevention and treatment of HIV/AIDS
- Identify areas of research and intervention that still need to be addressed in the future

The epidemic of HIV infection and associated acquired immune deficiency syndrome (AIDS) presents to the health care system myriad challenges, which have changed over time. In the 1980s and early 1990s, there were few highly effective treatments. However, advancements in treatment since then have demonstrated longer survival and improved quality of life for people with *human immunodeficiency virus (HIV)* disease.

New treatments have resulted in lower morbidity and mortality (Palella et al., 1998), as well as fewer side effects and once a day formulation of antiretroviral regimens (Wainberg & Friedland, 1998). As a result of highly potent antiretroviral treatments, HIV infection has been transformed from an acute infectious disease into a chronic disease that people live long lives with, when well managed with antiretroviral therapy. Nonetheless, HIV infection remains contagious, often disabling, and potentially fatal if untreated. Of particular concern for managers and policymakers is evidence of a lack of equity in the treatment of HIV disease among minorities, women, the uninsured and Medicaid-insured, and heterosexual and injection drug users, compared to other groups (Andersen et al., 2000; Shapiro et al., 1999). Such challenges increasingly force health care policymakers, planners, and administrators to reevaluate the organization, delivery, and financing of HIV/AIDS health services.

Recently, a new paradigm for HIV/AIDS has emerged that intends to combine prevention and treatment into one system of services. This new Seek, Test, Treat, and Retain model (also called Testing, Linkage, and Care, or TLC+) aims to merge HIV prevention with HIV care by targeted testing of high-risk groups, aggressive engagement of those who are not yet diagnosed HIV-positive in order to support early and ongoing HIV care, leading to better retention in a long-term treatment regimen, reduced HIV viral load in the broader community, and thus markedly reduced transmission of HIV to uninfected persons, as well as better health for infected persons (Andersen et al., 2000; Shapiro et al., 1999). This model marks an important break from past approaches because it sees treatment as part of prevention, rather than a separate, often competing interest.

Health services providers, researchers, and policy leaders must understand the changing needs of people infected with HIV, as well as accessibility to care, cost of care, quality of services and the relationship of these to HIV policy strategies efforts. First, important characteristics of the changing epidemiology and treatment patterns of HIV/AIDS should be understood in the context of real-life health care delivery in order to effect reduced incidence of HIV infections. Second, providers and managers must integrate emerging data on the accessibility, costs, and quality of services in this era of more effective AIDS treatments. At the same time, the existing trends of disparities in care for diverse subpopulations and service systems should be addressed more rigorously. Third, issues of access to care, quality, and costs have to be addressed not only within the arena of formal medical services, but more broadly within the continuum of care, from community outreach to ambulatory medical and psychosocial services to hospital and long-term care. Fourth, the implications and research needs for policy, planning, and program administration in health services should be utilized to a greater extent by leaders who have the power to act on the findings that have been so arduously ascertained. Developing an understanding of these issues broadly within the context of national and local health policy for HIV, as well as other chronic diseases, is paramount.

In this chapter, existing knowledge about critical issues of HIV/AIDS is discussed. The purpose is to provide the necessary background for addressing the challenges of the disease and for developing health policy, planning, and program implementation. Approaches to critical policy problems are suggested, and crucial areas for new investigation are identified to guide future HIV/AIDS health policy.

The Changing Epidemiology and Clinical Treatment of HIV/AIDS

AIDS (acquired immunodeficiency syndrome) is the result of a chronic infection with the HIV virus, which when untreated is characterized by progressive failure of the immune system and development of opportunistic infections or cancers and a high risk of death. HIV is a special type of virus (known as a retrovirus) that causes immune suppression leading to severe, life-threatening illnesses, together known as AIDS. Individuals infected with HIV develop antibodies within a short period of time after infection and may exhibit no symptoms for many years. Typically, the immune system weakens gradually and the blood level of *CD4 cells* (a type of white blood cell known as a T-helper or inducer lymphocyte) declines from a normal level of 1,200 to 1,400 cells per cubic millimeter. People with few CD4 cells are prone to opportunistic infections and certain cancers. Symptoms such as persistent fever, night sweats, diarrhea, and weight loss begin to occur more frequently once the CD4 count drops below 500 cells per cubic millimeter. It is unclear whether everyone with asymptomatic HIV infection and CD4 count greater than 200 will eventually go on to develop AIDS; a small proportion of those infected have shown no sign of immune failure after more than two decades (Losina & Freedberg, 2011). In addition to the CD4 count, the most powerful predictor of survival is the quantity of HIV RNA in the blood stream (known as viral load) (Mellors et al., 1996; O'Brien et al., 1996). The natural history of progression to AIDS has been estimated at a mean of eleven years from time of HIV infection

(Pantaleo et al., 1995). Newer HIV treatment regimens have significantly improved survival; for those individuals under care, HIV has become a chronic disease like heart disease or diabetes, which are generally not fatal or disabling when appropriately managed. New treatments such as integrase inhibitors, fusion inhibitors, and immune modulators, as well as more convenient dosing of these and other medications have recently been added to clinician armamentariums, leading to additional hope and additional challenges (Hong et al., 1998). For instance, side effects of medications—such as lipid abnormalities—can contribute to medical comorbidities like heart disease that also require chronic therapy (Currier & Havlir, 2004, 2005; Havlir & Currier, 2003).

Epidemiology

By 2008 (the most recent year for which data are available), global HIV infections had reached approximately 60 million infections. More than 33 million people were living with HIV infection, and more than 25 million had died of AIDS. It is estimated that in the single year 2008, 2.7 million people became infected with HIV, and 2 million died of AIDS (Joint United Nations Programme on HIV/AIDS & World Health Organization, 2009). In the United States, an estimated 1.2 million Americans are living with HIV infection, including a disproportionate number of persons of color (Centers for Disease Control and Prevention [CDC], 2011b). By the end of 2009, 1.14 million people were diagnosed with AIDS (see Table 17.1), and by the end of 2008, the cumulative number of deaths for those with an AIDS diagnosis was 617,025 (Table 17.2). In 2009, there were 34,993 new cases of AIDS reported in the United States and five U.S. dependent areas (with 34,247 of those occurring in the fifty states) (CDC, 2011a). However, based on extrapolations from 2006 data, there were an estimated 56,300 new HIV infections that year (since not all infections are known and thus reported) (Hall et al., 2008). By the end of 2008, the majority of those diagnosed as HIV-positive were male (75 percent). The prevalence for blacks or African Americans was eight times the rate for whites, and the prevalence for Hispanics or Latinos was two and a half times the rate for whites (CDC, 2011c). For the overall adult population, HIV has not been in the list of the leading causes of death since 1997; since 1995, there have been consecutive years of decrease in the adjusted death rate due to HIV. While the death rate decreased an average of 33 percent per year during the years 1995, 1996, 1997, and 1998 and continued to drop by 5.1 percent from 1999 through 2008, women and persons of color account for an

TABLE 17.1. CUMULATIVE AIDS CASES IN THE UNITED STATES THROUGH DECEMBER 2009[a]

	N	Percentage
Age at diagnosis (years)		
<13	9,448	1
13–14	1,321	0
15–24	50,134	5
25–34	343,788	31
35–44	427,812	39
45–54	198,707	18
55–64	59,658	5
>65	17,743	2
Race and ethnicity		
Non-Hispanic white	426,102	38
Non-Hispanic black	466,351	42
Hispanic or Latino	190,263	17
Asian	8,324	1
Native Hawaiian or other Pacific Islander	3,700	0
Multiple races	12,726	1
Transmission category		
Male adult or adolescent		
Male-to-male sexual contact	529,908	48
Injection drug use	273,444	25
Male-to-male sexual contact and injection drug use	77,213	7
Heterosexual contact	72,183	6
Other[b]	12,774	1
Subtotal	965,522	81
Female adult or adolescent[e]		
Injection drug use	87,126	7
Heterosexual contact	126,637	11
Other[b]	7,023	1
Subtotal	220,786	19

(continued)

TABLE 17.1. CUMULATIVE AIDS CASES IN THE UNITED STATES THROUGH DECEMBER 2009[a] (*Continued*)

	N	Percentage
Child (<13 years at diagnosis)[e]		
Perinatal	8,640	91
Other[c]	807	9
Subtotal	9,447	1
U.S. dependencies, possessions, and associated nations	34,103	3
Total[d]	1,142,714	100

[a]Includes persons with a diagnosis of AIDS from the beginning of the epidemic through 2009.

[b]Includes hemophilia, blood transfusion, perinatal, and risk factor not reported or not identified.

[c]Includes hemophilia, blood transfusion, and risk factor not reported or not identified.

[d]Includes persons of unknown race or ethnicity. Because totals for the estimated numbers were calculated independently of the values for the subpopulations, the subpopulation values may not equal the totals.

[e]Percentages are calculated for within-group comparisons; subtotal percentage calculated relative to the total cases.

Source: Data for this table were taken from Centers for Disease Control and Prevention, *HIV Surveillance Report Vol. 21* (2010). These numbers do not represent reported case counts. Rather, they are point estimates, which result from adjustments of reported case counts. The reported case counts are adjusted for reporting delays and for redistribution of cases in persons initially reported without an identified risk factor. The estimates do not include adjustment for incomplete reporting.

increasing proportion of AIDS-related deaths relative to earlier years (see Table 17.2). The reduction in mortality is largely due to improvements in treatment, although the availability of new medications has not improved health as much for women as for men, or for persons of color compared to whites. Further evidence of the overall improvement of the health of persons with HIV in the United States is the reduction in age-adjusted mortality for HIV, which declined by 9.1 percent from 2008 to 2009. However, as discussed later in this chapter, an inequitable distribution of treatment to persons of color, women, and other disadvantaged groups probably accounts for the corresponding disparities in health improvements for these groups.

Widely recognized risk factors for transmission of HIV are male-to-male sexual contact, male-to-female sexual contact, injection drug use (IDU), blood product exposure, and perinatal transmission from mother to infant (during pregnancy and delivery). Frequently, individuals are

TABLE 17.2. ESTIMATED DEATHS OF PERSONS WITH AIDS IN THE UNITED STATES, 2006–2008[a]

	Year Of Death		
	2006	2007	2008
Age at death (years)			
< 13	13	7	5
13–14	5	11	0
15–24	239	209	212
25–34	1,463	1,384	1,330
35–44	5,534	5,012	4,393
45–54	6,564	6,306	6,162
55–64	2,777	2,668	3,293
> 65	1,004	1,012	1,212
Race and ethnicity			
Non-Hispanic white	5,017	4,722	4,769
Non-Hispanic black	8,786	8,531	8,182
Hispanic or Latino	3,224	2,884	3,029
Asian	105	76	81
American Indian and Alaska Native	80	76	79
Native Hawaiian or other Pacific Islander	7	10	13
Multiple races	421	431	449
Transmission category			
Male adult or adolescent[b]			
Male-to-male sexual contact	6,190	6,080	5,959
Injection drug use	3,450	3,045	3,008
Male-to-male sexual contact and injection drug use	1,452	1,303	1,275
Heterosexual contact	1,745	1,692	1,808
Other[b]	143	122	116
Subtotal	12,979	12,243	12,166
Female adult or adolescent[c]			
Injection drug use	1,888	1,778	1,758
Heterosexual contact	2,621	2,577	2,541
Other	92	77	79
Subtotal	4,601	4,432	4,377

(*continued*)

TABLE 17.2. ESTIMATED DEATHS OF PERSONS WITH AIDS IN THE UNITED STATES, 2006–2008^a (Continued)

	Year Of Death		
	2006	2007	2008
Region of residence			
Northeast	4,692	4,197	4,004
Midwest	1,641	1,614	1,656
South	8,123	8,149	8,332
West	2,562	2,267	2,096
U.S. dependencies, possessions, and associated nations	623	504	517
Total[d]	17,641	16,730	16,605

Notes:

[a]Includes persons who died with AIDS during the years 2006 through 2008.

[b]Includes hemophilia, blood transfusion, and risk factor not reported or not identified.

[c]Includes hemophilia, blood transfusion, perinatal, and risk factor not reported or not identified.

[d]Includes persons of unknown race or multiple races and persons of unknown sex. Cumulative total includes 640 persons of unknown race or multiple races. Because column totals were calculated independently of the values for the subpopulations, the values in each column may not sum to the column total.

Source: Data for this table were taken from Centers for Disease Control and Prevention, *HIV Surveillance Report Vol. 21* (2010). These numbers do not represent reported case counts. Rather, they are point estimates, which result from adjustments of reported case counts. The reported case counts are adjusted for reporting delays and for redistribution of cases in persons initially reported without an identified risk factor. The estimates do not include adjustment for incomplete reporting.

exposed through multiple infection routes, and so the actual mode of HIV transmission may be unclear. A substantial portion of HIV-infected persons are unaware of their underlying HIV infection. Many cases of HIV infection remain underreported in the United States, because they may not meet the Centers for Disease Control (CDC) definition of AIDS. However, as of 2008, all fifty states, the District of Columbia, and six dependent areas (American Samoa, Guam, the Northern Mariana Islands, Palau, Puerto Rico, and the U.S. Virgin Islands) have used the same confidential reporting standards for HIV infection. Still, the accuracy of diagnosing and reporting HIV/AIDS varies by geographic location and affected population. The growth of the HIV/AIDS epidemic is, however, in large part due to changes in the modes of transmission and the sociodemographic characteristics of the groups in which the epidemic is growing fastest. The numbers of people with AIDS were highest in the South (46 percent) while significantly lower in the Northeast (25 percent), West (17 percent), and Midwest (11 percent) at the end of 2007. Unlike the early epidemic, the rate of increase in HIV transmission is slower among whites and men who have sex with men (MSM) than communities of color and heterosexuals. In addition, the incarcerated population has some of the highest rates of infection. HIV prevalence is estimated to be five times higher in state and federal correctional systems than among the general population in the United States (Flanigan & Beckwith, 2011).

Treatment

The most widely used drugs for people living with HIV/AIDS are *antiretroviral therapies (ARTs)*, which slow the progress of HIV infection and boost immune system function. The earliest developed antiretrovirals used to treat HIV disease were in the class of drugs known as nucleoside reverse transcriptase inhibitors (NRTI), including zidovudine (ZDV/AZT), didanosine (ddI), and zalcitabine or dideoxycitidine (ddC). Other classes of antiretrovirals include nucleoside reverse transcriptase inhibitors, non-nucleoside reverse transcriptase inhibitors, protease inhibitors, entry and fusion inhibitors, and integrase inhibitors.

Several medications in different classes are frequently combined in "cocktails," which constitute highly potent or *highly active antiretroviral therapy (HAART)*. It is well established that consistent, appropriately managed combination antiretroviral therapy initiated before severe loss of immune function is very effective for improving survival and reducing complications among patients with HIV infection (Thompson et al., 2010). Delay in diagnosis of HIV or institution of therapy is thought to represent poor access to care and/or poor quality of care. Difficulties with adherence to medication regimens have been eased with the introduction of simplified dosing regimens. Despite gains in development of HAART medications and regimens, problems continue. Bothersome side effects and complications sometimes affect persons taking ARTs, which may influence adherence. More important, HIV sometimes develops resistance to antiretroviral therapy, creating circumstances of (1) potential treatment failure and (2) development of HIV that is resistant to current medications (Little et al., 2002). An increasing rate of HIV resistant to current medications, especially among those newly infected, may be the next crisis in the treatment of HIV infection.

Antibiotics are used to prevent or to treat a previously common pneumonia (pneumocystis carinii or PCP) or other opportunistic infections that develop in persons with AIDS. Introduction of HAART has changed the need for prophylactic treatment in many patients. Primary and secondary prophylaxis of opportunistic infections (for example, against PCP and mycobacterium avium complex, or MAC) may be discontinued for patients with restored immune function as a result of receiving combination antiretroviral therapy (Zellweger et al., 2004).

Most other clinical services are directed toward monitoring for immune system decline (CD4 count tests), development of specific HIV complications (PCP, infectious diarrhea, or central nervous system infection), the effectiveness of treatment (viral load tests and resistance testing), reduction of treatment side effects and, increasingly, monitoring and treating comorbidities such as hypertension and heart disease. This monitoring involves use of the full range of medical services from physical examination to radiology to laboratory tests. Ongoing monitoring is also important because concomitant infectious diseases (for example, STDs, tuberculosis, and hepatitis) and metabolic complications of treatment (diabetes and lipid disorders) remain common problems. Laboratory testing of infecting HIV specimens for resistance to ARTs has become an important part of clinical care for HIV-infected persons. In the absence of a complete cure from traditional medical treatment, some people with HIV/AIDS may also resort to alternative medicine, which may affect medical care.

Access to, Linkage to, and Retention in Regular Medical Care. Having a regular source of medical care is recognized as important for the general population, as well as for those with various chronic diseases. Problems in access to care for people with HIV may be reflected in the degree to which they are in regular care. The HIV Cost and Services Utilization Study (HCSUS) estimated that about half (between 36 and 63 percent) of all nonmilitary, nonincarcerated adults in the contiguous United States with known or unknown HIV infection see a provider outside of an emergency room at least every six months (Bozzette et al., 1998). In terms of initial linkage to care, or ongoing retention in care, more recent estimates for some measures are available through the Medical Monitoring Project, an ongoing surveillance system. For 77 percent of those diagnosed as HIV-positive, the first visit to a health care provider occurred in three or fewer months after being diagnosed. Of those who had ever had a CD4 T-lymphocyte test, 83 percent reported having had three or more CD4 T-lymphocyte tests during the previous year; the percent is exactly the same for those who had ever had an HIV viral load test and those who had three or more in the previous year (Blair et al., 2011).

Insurance coverage is a crucial factor affecting access to care and related factors for persons living with HIV/AIDS, as it is in other conditions. Overall, much of the HIV-infected population is covered by public insurance. It is estimated that 45 percent of the population in care is covered by Medicaid, and 30 percent is covered by Medicare. Private insurance covers 37 percent of the population, while 16 percent of persons with HIV disease have no health insurance coverage (Blair et al., 2011). Public insurance also finances the majority of HIV-related care. Although public insurance covers about half of the HIV population, it accounts for 62 percent of HIV-related costs. Private insurance accounts for only 28 percent of HIV-related costs, while the uninsured account for 11 percent of HIV-related costs (Bozzette et al., 1998).

Barriers to Care. Lack of insurance and underinsurance represent formidable financial barriers to HIV/AIDS care (Andersen et al., 2000; Shapiro et al., 1999). Persons with HIV/AIDS are more likely than the general population to be uninsured or to have Medicaid insurance. Among the insured, substantial disparities in access persist because of other barriers to care, such as competing subsistence needs. For example, HCSUS found that more than one-third of people went without or postponed medical care because of one or more subsistence needs and that minorities, women, and drug users were most likely to report these problems. Going without or postponing care for one of the four subsistence needs was associated with significantly greater multivariate odds of never receiving ARTs and having low overall access to care (Cunningham, Andersen, et al., 1999a). Thus, addressing social needs may actually compete (in terms of time, energy, and money) with obtaining medical care. Other important barriers may include disability from HIV/AIDS disease, loss of employment, and social stigma, resulting in the avoidance of needed medical care (Sayles et al., 2007; Sayles et al., 2009).

Lack of insurance, poverty, and underutilization of ambulatory services often coincide within the groups in which the epidemic is spreading most rapidly. The groups that are most likely to face disparities in service delivery and outcomes overwhelmingly include racial and ethnic minorities, women, and injection drug users (Cunningham et al., 2006; Puskas et al., 2011). Research conducted since the advent of HAART has found that blacks, Latinos, and women often have trouble accessing important HIV treatment (Shapiro et al., 1999). While HAART led to dramatically lowering mortality rates for whites—from 53 percent to 29 percent between 1990 and 2006—deaths among Latinos remained steady and increased from 29 percent to 56 percent among African Americans (Cavaleri et al., 2010). In addition, injection drug users also have lower levels of HAART use compared to noninjection drug using populations (Anderson & Mitchell, 2000; Cunningham et al., 2000; Knowlton et al., 2010).

Understanding the reasons behind nonreceipt of antiretroviral therapy is important. The high costs associated with newly developed AIDS medications (not all of which are covered by insurance) may also serve as a barrier to treatment for disadvantaged groups. Studies of the diffusion of AIDS treatments such as zidovudine show that when new AIDS treatments are first developed they take time to diffuse through the population, but often do so unevenly (Crystal, Sambamoorthi, & Merzel, 1995). Big gaps tend to be found between advantaged and disadvantaged groups in the use of new treatments, particularly a short time after they are introduced into the population, but the gap tends to close over time, although it does not disappear (Cunningham et al., 2000). One reason blacks and other disadvantaged groups may have delayed access to the newest, most effective treatments may be that they are less likely to participate in clinical trials of new treatments because of access barriers, mistrust, or poorer health status (Cunningham et al., 1995; Gifford et al., 2002).

Stability and continuity of care are particularly important for persons with HIV infection. However, discontinuity in HIV care has been identified as a problem in obtaining appropriate access to care and improved health outcomes (Gwadz et al., 2010). A cohort study in one low socioeconomic status urban population found that failure to suppress viral load with HAART was associated with higher rates of missed clinic appointments, nonwhite ethnicity, and drug use (Lucas, Chaisson, & Moore, 1999). Similar findings were found in a second cohort, which also demonstrated a clinical consequence: men with longer interruption and HAART discontinuers had a significantly higher rate of HIV RNA and lower CD4 cell counts (Li et al., 2005). From a health services standpoint, a potential consequence of discontinuity is greater use of the emergency department for nonemergency medical services. Inadequate access is often cited as the reason for inappropriate ER use (Josephs et al., 2010; Magnus et al., 2001; Reichmann et al., 2011). While annual inpatient hospitalization rates for HIV-infected adults declined from 2002 to 2007—from 35 to 27 per 100 persons—women, those over fifty years of age, African Americans, injection drug users, and those without private insurance had higher hospitalization rates.

Other nonfinancial barriers to access to care are language barriers, cultural competence, and illiteracy. For example, one study found that Latinos had poorer survival compared to whites, even after controlling for insurance status, socioeconomic status, and having a regular source of care. Another study found that lower acculturation levels among Latinos were associated with lower levels of access to care. These findings suggest that Latinos may face access barriers related to language and culture that result in suboptimal treatment and worse outcomes (Cheng, Chen, & Cunningham, 2007; Cunningham et al., 2000; Kinsler et al., 2009).

Access to care may also be related to the costs of HIV care, prevention, and health outcomes. In the HCSUS, expenditures on ARTs were inversely related to expenditures on hospital care. Another study showed that better access to comprehensive community-based services was associated with fewer hospitalizations for HIV disease. Together, these and other studies suggest that costs may be reduced with adequate access to care (Bozzette et al., 2001; Cunningham et al., 1996). Better access to treatment for HIV leads to better health outcomes, whether measured in mortality, quality of life, reduction in transmission of HIV to others, and that treatment appears cost-effective relative to other existing alternatives (Cohen et al., 2011; Cunningham et al., 1995; Cunningham et al., 1998; Gallant et al., 2011). Thus, improving access to high-quality HIV care may prevent spread of the disease and improve outcomes without excessive costs. This hypothesis is now being tested in a variety of different studies of different subpopulations all over the world, as it holds the very best promise for controlling HIV at the present time.

Costs

Current federal funding for HIV/AIDS in fiscal year 2012 is estimated to total $28.4 billion, with 53 percent for care and treatment, 10 percent for research, 10 percent for cash and housing assistance, 4 percent for prevention, and 24 percent for combating the international epidemic. In the beginning of the epidemic, the largest category of direct HIV/AIDS care costs has been hospital utilization. However, there has been an overall reduction in this proportion since the advent of HAART medications. Thus, overall AIDS costs are not as great as they were feared to become earlier in the epidemic, and there is little reason to expect that AIDS costs will become disproportionate to other chronic diseases and threaten the financing system. However, costs vary greatly as a function of the population served, the type of provider, and the region of the country (Bozzette et al.,

2001). Because it is known that sicker patients cost more regardless of the disease, there is concern that much of this variation is related to the adequacy of outpatient care provided to various populations. Inadequate outpatient care could result in delayed initiation of HAART treatment or treatment with less effective medications and result in higher morbidity and mortality, development of preventable opportunistic infections, and more rapid progression of the disease. Available data suggest that HIV/AIDS patients from groups with lower socioeconomic status and less access to care (minorities, drug users, and women) use costlier sources of care (such as emergency rooms and hospitals) for longer duration, raising the concern that these variations in cost are due to variations in provider quality. Hence the costs of HIV/AIDS care should be examined in the context of the quality of care as well.

Quality of Care

Consistent with the general conceptual model of quality of care in health services, the emphasis of HIV/AIDS quality of care assessment centers on whether persons with HIV/AIDS receive appropriate clinical treatment specific to their stage of HIV disease. In addition, evaluation and comparisons of outcomes of treatment between relevant groups are used to draw inferences about the quality of HIV care, although concerns about adequate case mix or severity adjustment plague this approach just as much as they do any other area of quality-of-care analysis (Bozzette, 2010).

Underuse of Therapy. Despite available clinical guidelines to inform HIV providers, certain subpopulations are less likely to receive these treatments. In HCSUS, blacks and women were less likely to receive HAART therapy compared to whites and white men, respectively (Andersen et al., 2000). In addition, blacks and Hispanics were less likely to receive appropriate PCP and MAC prophylactic therapies compared to whites (Asch et al., 2001). Other research found that public insurance (compared to private insurance) may be associated with poorer level of quality or inappropriate care.

Hospital and Physician Experience and Specialization. Experience in treating HIV disease is another important predictor of better quality of care. Studies have found that hospitals and staffs with greater experience in treating HIV/AIDS have lower inpatient mortality (Cunningham, Tisnado, et al., 1999b). Greater physician experience in treating HIV/AIDS also predicts longer survival. The preponderance of evidence in AIDS indicates that the critical factor in producing better-quality care is experience with a sufficient volume of patients with AIDS, rather than specialty certification in infectious disease, immunology, or oncology. In addition to experience (volume or caseload), self-reported expertise in HIV/AIDS also makes a difference. While general medicine physicians with expertise in HIV/AIDS and infectious disease specialists have similar rates of HAART prescribing patterns, patients who see generalists without expertise in HIV/AIDS are less likely to be on HAART (Landon et al., 2003). Although experience fosters the knowledge to provide quality care, physician attitude toward patients (for instance, regarding perceived reliability to follow treatment regimens) also influences optimal prescribing of HAART for patients (King, Wong, Shapiro, Landon, & Cunningham, 2004; Wong, Asch, Andersen, Hays, & Shapiro, 2004).

Adherence to Treatment. Adherence is essential for successful treatment of persons with HIV because inadequate dosing of antiretroviral therapy may not suppress viral replication and may allow HIV to form new genetic variants of the virus. These variants can be resistant to entire classes of drugs, rendering certain combinations of drugs ineffective. Drug-resistant strains of HIV are also transmittable to others, creating an alarming public health threat. The reasons for nonadherence are multifaceted, but they must be understood in order to develop effective interventions (Simoni, Amico, Pearson, & Malow, 2008). Long-term adherence to treatment with antiretroviral regimens is critical to survival with HIV infection, but problems in adhering are commonly reported. In HCSUS, only 57 percent of those who were taking antiretroviral therapy reported that they actually took all their medications as they were prescribed. Barriers to adherence include fear of disclosure, substance abuse, forgetfulness, treatment suspicions, complicated regimens, quality-of-life impediments, responsibilities related to work and family, and access to medication. Alternatively, facilitators have been reported that encourage adherence, including having a sense of self-worth, health benefits of antiretrovirals, accepting seropositivity status, understanding why strict adherence is important, using reminder tools, and having a simple regimen (Mills et al., 2006).

Health-Related Quality of Life Outcomes. The goal of providing medical care is to improve outcomes. Thus, outcomes are a marker of quality of care. One important outcome of HIV care is *health-related quality of life (HRQL)*. HRQL is increasingly recognized as an important facet of health status and health service delivery for those with HIV disease, one that consists of physical and mental functioning and well-being from the perspective of individuals. HRQL is perhaps one of the most important health outcomes to examine in HIV disease because of the disease's bothersome symptomatology, high mortality, and the resultant need for regular and urgent medical services. Various drug treatments for HIV may also affect HRQL differently than they affect disease progression and physiologic markers of outcomes. Both clinical trials and observational studies of HIV disease now commonly include generic measures of HRQL outcomes to evaluate the simultaneous effects of clinical interventions, treatment side effects, and disease impact over time (Cunningham, Wong, & Hays, 2008; Hays et al., 2000). HRQL measures have been shown to be associated with CD4 count, symptom severity, length of hospital stay, and disease progression (from asymptomatic HIV infection to symptomatic infection to AIDS) (Cunningham et al., 2008). The associations between HRQL and the clinical indicators of health status of patients support the hope that astute diagnostic evaluation and targeted treatment of abnormalities may improve function and patients' sense of well-being.

Prevention and Education

Most experts agree that a multicomponent strategy to HIV prevention that includes behavioral, structural, and biomedical approaches is the best way to reduce new infections (Padian, Buve, Balkus, Serwadda, & Cates, 2008). Controlling the AIDS epidemic depends on this "*combination prevention*," which includes behavior change to reduce high risk with biomedical interventions and structural changes; one approach will not adequately reduce new infections, but the combination of approaches will do a better job of controlling the rate of infection. Groups with high incidence are targeted for intervention: MSM, IDUs, women who have partners with risk factors, adolescents, and minority ethnic groups. Education and outreach have been the major approaches to risk reduction, although the approaches outlined next are the newest methods of prevention.

Opt-Out Testing

Opt-out testing is a policy of routine HIV screening unless a patient explicitly refuses testing and has been advocated by the CDC since 2006. Starting then, the CDC advised that everyone between the ages of thirteen and sixty-four years of age and all pregnant women should be tested routinely for HIV infection. Opt-out screening is believed to have a multitude of benefits. Not only will it increase awareness of HIV status among many who otherwise may not know that they are HIV-positive, but it also helps to inform those who are infected about their infection status earlier in the disease course, when treatment is most effective. In addition, it can lower the incidence of mother-to-child transmission to 2 percent or less, thereby reducing the number of babies born HIV-positive. Finally, opt-out testing reduces the stigma that is associated with being tested for HIV (a stigma that reduces the likelihood of high-risk individuals being tested), since it makes testing universal. Overall, the ambition of the CDC's 2006 recommendations for HIV testing is to improve detection, promote earlier treatment of infection, and thereby reduce the numbers of new infections (Branson et al., 2006).

Biomedical Prevention Technology

While behavioral interventions (such as condom use) have previously made up the majority of the public health approach in the past, these alone have not been wholly successful and, thus, biomedical interventions are now being added to the behavioral interventions for a more comprehensive approach to prevention (Chovnik, 2011). Research shows that even a partially effective biomedical intervention could dramatically reduce the incidence of HIV transmission. Biomedical interventions that aim to reduce HIV transmission include diaphragms, pre-exposure prophylaxis (PrEP), postexposure prophylaxis (PEP), drug suppression of concurrent STDs, microbicides (vaginal and rectal), vaccination against other viral infections, condom use, antiretroviral treatment for currently infected persons, male circumcision, and an HIV vaccine (Imrie, Elford, Kippax, & Hart, 2007). Despite a long history of disappointing results with respect to developing an HIV vaccine, there has recently been progress in HIV vaccine research, with demonstration of modest protection in the RV 144 trial in Thailand, where there was a marginal but statistically significant reduction in HIV incidence (Chovnik, 2011; Rerks-Ngarm et al., 2009). While there still is no vaccine in general use, as of September 2010 there were twenty-two ongoing trials of preventive HIV vaccines, so work is still being done to advance this effort (Chovnik, 2011). Yet, since a vaccine for HIV prevention does not currently exist, current biomedical interventions that do work to prevent HIV infection, which are discussed next, include using antiretroviral drugs as well as using microbicides to reduce infection for those who are high risk and to prevent mother-to-child transmission.

While *microbicides* have not been shown to be extremely effective at preventing vaginal or rectal HIV transmission, there are promising areas of research that may prove to be effective. Newer antimicrobial products contain antiretroviral compounds that inhibit HIV replication (Padian et al., 2008). This could have a stronger impact on HIV transmission than traditional microbicides. Another trend in microbicide research is examining the effect of long-acting dispersal methods that (1) are not reliant on being applied during sex and (2) do not require frequent application (Padian et al., 2008). Ideally, any microbicide use should be combined with condom use to decrease the likelihood of transmission; however, use of microbicides alone will likely reduce transmission rates as opposed to no intervention at all (Eaton & Kalichman, 2007).

Antiretrovirals are also now being used not just as a method for treatment but as a way to prevent new infections as well. Antiretrovirals are being given to both the infected person and the uninfected person as a manner of prevention. For HIV-infected individuals, taking antiretrovirals may not only help manage their own disease, but it has been shown to reduce infection to others as well. Mother-to-child transmission has been reduced through these types of interventions since the 1990s, and now this strategy is being examined for other types of transmission as well. Antiretroviral therapy given to an uninfected person as pre-exposure prophylaxis (PrEP) could help reduce the likelihood of infection, and when given to an HIV-positive person could reduce infectiousness (Padian et al., 2008). Finally, postexposure prophylaxis (PEP) has also been used to prevent HIV infection by administering antiretrovirals after a person has already been exposed to HIV. This strategy was first developed for health care workers who have been exposed to HIV due to an occupational hazard. The positive findings for health care workers who had good results with PEP have now been extrapolated to other segments of the population, and PEP is being administered as HIV prevention for nonhealth care workers who have been exposed to the disease through various methods of transmission (Workowski & Berman, 2010).

Yet, while these biomedical interventions seem quite promising, there are challenges that must be acknowledged as well. Scale-up costs and behavioral consequences of the interventions are still unknown, and the first-generation technologies will not be 100 percent effective (Chovnik, 2011; Girard, Osmanov, & Kieny, 2006). *Risk compensation*—the idea that some individuals may increase their high-risk sexual behaviors due to a decrease in perceived risk while using biomedical products—is a cause for concern and may actually decrease the overall effectiveness of the intervention.

Seek, Test, Treat, Retain

As part of the Seek, Test, Treat, Retain strategy, many of these same medications are now being used to prevent primary or secondary transmission of HIV (Gardner, McLees, Steiner, Del Rio, & Burman, 2011). *Pre-exposure prophylaxis (PrEP)* entails high risk HIV- persons taking daily antiretroviral medications in an attempt to lower their chances of infection should they be exposed to the virus. *Postexposure prophylaxis (PEP)* has also been used to prevent HIV infection after a person has already been exposed to the virus. Health care workers who have been exposed to HIV due to an occupational hazard have been advised to employ PEP based on a study showing reduced risk of acquiring the disease after exposure. These findings have been extrapolated to other segments of the population, and PEP is now administered as HIV prevention for nonhealth care workers who have been exposed to the virus through various methods of transmission (Workowski & Berman, 2010).

The *Seek, Test, Treat, Retain* strategy combines treatment and prevention and is being focused especially on certain high-risk populations, such as injection drug users and incarcerated persons (Volkow & Montaner, 2010). This model emphasizes the importance of first seeking out those in high-risk populations who may already be HIV-positive but are unaware of it, then testing them for HIV status based on CDC recommendations for annual testing. For those who test HIV-positive at any time, the next step is treating them with HAART, and then continuing to retain them in continuous and comprehensive HIV care, which includes not only ART medications but ideally also monitoring for and treatment of the full range of comorbidities, from STDs to substance use to diabetes and heart disease, in a patient-centered way (Volkow & Montaner, 2010). Increased access to testing enhances treatment uptake, and comprehensive treatment programs increase adherence to medication regimens, which reduce morbidity and mortality and also reduce new infections by lowering the level of viral load in the community that could be transmitted to uninfected persons. While the Seek, Test, Treat, Retain strategy was previously advocated for higher-risk populations such as injection drug users or incarcerated populations, the most recent research and advocacy are calling for widespread implementation of this approach as a means to control HIV transmission, morbidity, and mortality more broadly (Nosyk & Montaner, 2012). Overall, the Seek, Test, Treat, Retain approach is dependent on early detection and appropriate treatment and has been shown to lower the rates of new infections (Das et al., 2010). Thus, prevention and treatment are now concurrently and inextricably linked in this new paradigm, with high expectations of promising results for both aspects of the strategy's approach. This paradigm is illustrated in Figure 17.1, which shows the importance of both treatment and prevention in the continuum of care (Cheever, 2007; Gardner et al., 2011).

Mental Health and Drug Use

The prevalence of psychiatric disorders (major depression, dysthymia, generalized anxiety disorders, and panic attacks) and substance abuse is disproportionately high among people with HIV disease (Weaver et al., 2008). Similar to the general population, psychiatric and substance abuse disorders within the HIV population may impair quality of life, adversely affect access to appropriate health care, and compromise adherence with medication regimens. Psychiatric and substance abuse disorders may also be associated with sexual behavior and drug-using activity, which endanger others with the risk of HIV infection.

Consequently, there is substantial need for drug and alcohol abuse treatment. Reducing substance abuse can improve HIV prevention, as well as appropriate use of services. Many HIV-infected people need treatment for psychiatric disorders, with or without concomitant treatment for HIV. To the extent that mental health, substance abuse, and medical services are all needed, patients will benefit from coordination of these services—for example, through sharing of medical records, streamlining assessment of benefits eligibility, and providing the services in close proximity to reduce transportation barriers and inconvenience.

FIGURE 17.1. CONTINUUM OF ENGAGEMENT FOR HIV CARE

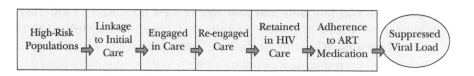

Source: Gardner et al., 2011.

Policy Implications and Research Needs for Management, Planning, and AIDS Policy

The HIV/AIDS epidemic has spread out from its initial demographic and risk groups to much broader communities of the socially and economically disadvantaged. Concurrently, the range of medical treatments for HIV and AIDS complications has grown more effective, as well as more complex. HIV/AIDS is only one of many public health problems and social issues that confront the United States as it begins the twenty-first century. The initial impetus for action has waned, as the epidemic enters its fourth decade and the populations most affected by HIV/AIDS change. Within the HIV/AIDS community, allocation of scarce resources is politically charged. Should more funds be directed toward risk-reduction behavior, or should treatment and biomedical prevention take priority? How can research funds make the greatest impact? Through a return to basic science or improved service delivery and outcomes research? What is the appropriate funding relationship between medical services and social services? Similarly vexing questions plagued the debate about proper allocation of resources between HIV/AIDS and other diseases. Certainly no easy answers exist for these questions, and powerful interest groups can be found on every side. A debate about priorities is healthy, but there is potential for conflict that may do a disservice to people living with HIV infection. Developing partnerships and networks to effectively organize and deliver health and social services is paramount.

Health Policy Issues and Options

As HIV infection increases in communities of color and among the poor, the financial burden on public payers and health care providers continues to be heavy. Reliance on Medicaid has profound implications for people with HIV/AIDS as public support for Medicaid wanes. In addition, federal eligibility mandates have increased the cost of Medicaid to states. As a result, many state legislatures are searching for ways to effectively control the costs of the program. Rate setting of provider payments is one way states have attempted to control their Medicaid costs. Moving persons into managed Medicaid health plans has also become common. In many states, the reimbursement level has not kept up with inflation; Medicaid generally pays providers less than their cost of care. As providers limit the number of Medicaid patients they serve, access to care may deteriorate for those dependent on Medicaid. These factors will be affected by the expansion of Medicaid under the ACA (discussed further in the upcoming section on the ACA).

Medicare currently pays for a smaller portion of AIDS expenditures than Medicaid, although the proportion of HIV-positive individuals on Medicare has increased greatly since the 1990s, probably because people are living longer with the infection. It is important to note that Medicare eligibility is only a partial solution for persons with AIDS because Medicare outpatient prescription drug benefit has a costly "donut hole." However, with the implementation of the Affordable Care Act (see the upcoming section on the ACA), the donut hole will be phased out and medications should become more affordable. In 2011, beneficiaries who reached the donut hole received a 50 percent discount on brand-name drugs, while benefits received through AIDS Drug Assistance Program (ADAP) were counted as contributions toward donut hole spending (Department of Health and Human Services [DHHS], 2010).

Ryan White CARE Act and ADAP Programs

The *Ryan White CARE Act* was originally signed in 1990, as a federal program designed to improve the quality and availability of care for persons with HIV/AIDS and their families. A variety of medical and supportive services are covered: primary health care, case management, home health, food services, hospice care, housing, transportation, and prevention and education services (Bowen et al., 1992). The main target populations for these services were the poor and the uninsured. Over 500,000 people with HIV/AIDS in the United States are served by this act. In 2009, the Ryan White HIV/AIDS Treatment Extension Act of 2009 was adjusted and reauthorized to continue this legislation through 2013.

ART medication support, through the *ADAP (AIDS Drug Assistance Program)*, is an important component of the CARE Program (Buchanan & Smith, 1998). Under the ADAP, uninsured and underinsured persons with HIV disease can access newly developed treatment medications (for example, protease inhibitors). Although expensive, ADAP provides economic benefits by offsetting higher hospitalization costs. Although the CARE Act has been successful in increasing availability of medical and nonmedical services for persons with HIV disease, concern has arisen whether CARE Act funding spent on newly developed medications is too high.

Affordable Care Act

Numerous barriers to care exist for those with HIV and AIDS. In particular, obtaining private health insurance for those living with HIV and AIDS has been arduous. However, the Affordable Care Act (ACA), which was signed into law by President Obama on March 23, 2010, aims to reduce these barriers to care that have long existed for HIV-positive persons and those with AIDS.

First, the ACA aims to improve access to care. Only 17 percent of HIV-positive persons have private insurance, and 30 percent of HIV-positive persons have no insurance at all (DHHS, 2010). As previously discussed, Medicaid, Medicare, and the Ryan White Care HIV/AIDS Treatment Extension Act of 2009 are primarily responsible for funding health and social services for those with HIV/AIDS. With full implementation of the ACA in 2014, insurers will no longer be able to deny coverage to those with HIV/AIDS (or anyone with a preexisting health condition), and they will not be able to rescind coverage unless fraud can be proven. Lifetime caps on insurance benefits will no longer be allowed. In addition, Medicaid eligibility will be expanded to include single adults who meet income eligibility thresholds; thus, an HIV-positive person will not have to wait for an AIDS diagnosis to be eligible for Medicaid if he or she meets the income eligibility, allowing access to treatment before the disease progresses (DHHS, 2010). Access to prescription drugs will also be improved, as the ACA will phase out the aforementioned "donut hole" that can make prescription drug coverage for those with Medicare extremely expensive (DHHS, 2010). Quality of care will also be improved for those with HIV/AIDS under the ACA. This will be achieved for those with private and public insurance first through better information in a more user-friendly manner about what is and is not covered. In addition, improved quality is achieved by providing a new comprehensive benefit package that equals that of a typical employer plan. This package includes prescription drugs, preventive care, chronic disease management, and substance abuse and mental health treatment. Improved access to preventive care also improves quality for those living with HIV/AIDS, and coordinated care will be emphasized, which has been proven to be an effective strategy for those with more complex illnesses such as HIV/AIDS (DHHS, 2010).

Finally, the ACA will expand funding for community health centers, which act as a safety net for many low-income persons and vulnerable populations. Providing increased resources to these centers, which provide much of the care for those most in need, will improve access to and quality of care. Overall, through many areas of change, the ACA will improve access to care and quality of care for those with HIV/AIDS, with full implementation of the program in 2014.

Future Directions

Ideally, policy and planning options are based on evidence of the effectiveness of treatment and acceptable level of cost in delivering such treatment. The completion of the landmark HCSUS study vastly improved policy-relevant AIDS health services data. This study has made available data on a range of issues pertinent to HIV policy, notably costs and utilization, access and barriers to care, adherence, quality of life, social support services, mental health, dental health, and quality of care. New research efforts must continue to include the changing clinical profile of the epidemic. In addition, research efforts must yield insights into national trends, such as regional variation in the patterns of HIV-related disease complications. Changes in treatment patterns and in the price of medication over time make prediction of future costs even more difficult. The many nonmedical costs of HIV/AIDS should be examined: direct costs of transportation, informed support, and housing, as well as indirect costs of disability days from work resulting from treatment or deteriorating health. In response to these needs, in 2004 the Centers for Disease Control and Prevention funded a new HIV/AIDS surveillance project, the Morbidity Monitoring Project (MMP). This ongoing project will recruit each year a nationwide representative sample of more than ten thousand HIV-infected individuals receiving medical care (viral load test, CD4+ counts, or antiretroviral treatment in the past twelve months) for medical record abstraction and patient interview.

Studies of special populations will also be needed: women, children, adolescents, IDUs, persons in rural communities, and the racial and ethnic minorities who constitute a growing proportion of the HIV-infected population. Data collected on cost and utilization will enable policymakers to compare current patterns of cost and utilization across the spectrum of HIV disease across geographical areas, across the range of institutional and individual providers (including managed care settings), and for both insured and uninsured populations, as well as variations in financing and provider arrangements.

Given that side effects are likely to be associated with medications used to treat HIV disease, further research is needed to develop and evaluate interventions to improve adherence with treatment regimens. Such research takes on greater salience with the widespread use of HAART medications. Particular populations of interest for future adherence research include those with mental disorders, substance abusers, or both.

Lack of insurance, poverty, and underuse of ambulatory treatment likely will continue within the groups in which the epidemic is spreading most rapidly. Disadvantaged groups (minorities, women, IDUs, and the poor) experience difficulty more often in obtaining access to outpatient care. In addition, they may not receive appropriate treatment, which can account for greater mortality in those populations. People with impaired access to health services often use costlier sources of medical care and use them for a longer duration. Furthermore, variations in the quality of AIDS care by geographic region, sociodemographic group, and type of provider likely reflect poor-quality care for certain individuals.

In view of these concerns, the important characteristics of the changing epidemiology of AIDS and clinical treatment patterns need to be constantly under review in order to address problems in access, cost, and quality. Health service delivery systems must be developed to address the emerging needs of diverse population groups affected by HIV/AIDS. Additionally, it is important that Ryan White CARE programs also address the emerging needs of diverse population groups affected by HIV/AIDS. Neither the arena of formal medical services nor supportive services can be overlooked. Developing finance and delivery systems within the context of long-range planning and evaluation is paramount. Existing knowledge and critical gaps in information about HIV/AIDS have been reviewed to constitute a basis for addressing the current and future challenges that HIV/AIDS presents for development of relevant health policy and health and social services planning and program implementation.

SUMMARY

With advancements in treatment since the start of the HIV/AIDS epidemic, survival has increased and quality of life has dramatically improved. HIV infection is no longer an acute infectious disease, but is now a chronic condition that can be managed successfully with antiretroviral therapy. When untreated, HIV infection is still a contagious, serious, and possibly fatal disease. Challenges include disparities in care, which lead to poorer outcomes for the most high-risk individuals.

The new paradigm for treatment and prevention of HIV/AIDS combines the two into one system of services. The Seek, Test, Treat, and Retain model attempts to merge HIV prevention with HIV care through targeted testing of high-risk groups and aggressive engagement of those who are not yet diagnosed HIV-positive in order to support early and ongoing HIV care. This combined model of treatment and prevention leads to improved retention in a long-term treatment regimen, reduced HIV viral load in the broader community, and thus markedly reduced transmission of HIV to uninfected persons, as well as better health for infected persons. This model is the changing face of prevention and treatment. No longer regarded as separate issues in the battle against this disease, they are being treated as pieces of one unified issue that must be addressed concomitantly.

Future research efforts must include the changing clinical profile of the epidemic. Future research must provide information about national trends, including detail on regional variation in the patterns of HIV-related disease complications, indirect and nonmedical costs, and how well the new models of treatment and prevention are working. Future research should include studies of special populations, including women, children, adolescents, IDUs, persons in rural communities, and the racial and ethnic minorities who constitute a growing proportion of the HIV-infected population. New research should inform policymakers so that the best decisions are made with respect to legislation enacted that affects those with HIV/AIDS.

As we move forward, the changing epidemiology of AIDS and clinical treatment patterns need to be constantly under review in order to address problems in access, cost, and quality for those affected by HIV/AIDS. Health service delivery systems must be developed to address the emerging needs of diverse population groups affected by HIV/AIDS. Finally, as the Affordable Care Act is enacted in 2014 and beyond, the health services infrastructure and delivery system will change in ways that must be monitored to assess the effect on those with HIV/AIDS.

KEY TERMS

AIDS Acquired immunodeficiency syndrome. The result of a chronic infection with the HIV virus, which when untreated is characterized by progressive failure of the immune system and development of opportunistic infections or cancers and a high risk of death.

AIDS Drug Assistance Program (ADAP) A policy that helps uninsured and underinsured persons with HIV disease access ART they could not otherwise afford.

Antiretroviral therapies (ARTs) The most commonly used drugs for people living with HIV/AIDs. These slow the progress of HIV infection and boost immune function.

CD4 cells A type of white blood cell known as a T-helper or inducer lymphocyte. CD4 cell count levels are used to monitor immune system decline.

Combination prevention A concept of preventing infection through various combinations of behavioral, structural, and biomedical approaches.

Health-related quality of life (HRQL) A multidimensional concept that includes measures of mental and physical well-being that is increasingly recognized as an important facet of health status and outcome of health service delivery for those with HIV disease.

Highly active antiretroviral therapy (HAART) Several medications in different classes are frequently combined in ''cocktails'' to form highly potent or highly active antiretroviral therapy (HAART).

HIV A special type of virus (known as a retrovirus) that causes immune suppression leading to severe, life-threatening illnesses, together known as AIDS.

Microbicide A compound whose purpose is to reduce the infectivity of microbes. To prevent HIV infection, these can be applied vaginally or anally to reduce infection both during sexual intercourse and childbirth.

Opt-out testing A policy of routine HIV screening unless a patient explicitly refuses testing. This policy has been advocated by the Centers for Disease Control and Prevention since 2006.

Post-exposure prophylaxis (PEP) PEP has been used to prevent HIV infection by administering antiretrovirals to a previously uninfected person after they have already been exposed to HIV to help reduce the likelihood of a persistent infection.

Pre-exposure prophylaxis (PrEP) Antiretroviral therapy that is given to an uninfected person as pre-exposure prevention to help reduce the likelihood of infection and can also be given to an HIV-positive person to reduce infectiousness.

Risk compensation The idea that some people may increase their high-risk sexual behaviors due to a decrease in perceived risk as a result of using products designed for prevention.

Ryan White CARE Act A variety of medical and supportive services for people living with HIV/AIDS are covered by this act, including primary health care, case management, care coordination, home health, food services, hospice care, housing, transportation, and prevention and education services. The poor and uninsured in highly affected geographic areas in the United States are the main targets of this act.

Seek, Test, Treat, Retain (STTR) The STTR strategy combines treatment and prevention. This model emphasizes the importance of first seeking out those in high-risk populations who may already be HIV-positive but unaware of it, then testing them for HIV status. For those who test HIV-positive at any time, the next step is treating them with HAART and then continuing to retain HIV-positive persons in continuous and comprehensive HIV care, which includes not only ART medications but ideally also monitoring for and treatment of the full range of comorbidities—from STDs to substance use to diabetes and heart disease—in a patient-centered way.

Seropositivity Showing a positive reaction to a blood serum test for a specific disease.

DISCUSSION QUESTIONS

1. How has the changing epidemiology of the HIV/AIDS epidemic affected the issues facing doctors, patients, and policy makers?
2. What groups are now most at risk for contracting HIV and what barriers to care do these groups face?
3. How is the Seek, Test, Treat, Retain paradigm different from previous models that addressed prevention and treatment?
4. How will the Affordable Care Act affect those with HIV/AIDS? Will it improve access to care, reduce cost of care, and improve quality of care?
5. What are some examples of future policy issues that need to be addressed moving forward?

FURTHER READING

American Academy of HIV Physicians: http://www.aahivm.org/Default.aspx

> The American Academy of HIV Physicians promotes accessible, quality care for people living with HIV. This organization is devoted to educating and credentialing physicians while also connecting many allied health workers devoted to HIV care. This group also advocates for policies that affect HIV care practice and delivery. A wide range of resources are available for health care workers who specialize in caring for those infected with HIV as well as the latest news related to HIV/AIDS.

CDC's HIV/AIDS website: http://www.cdc.gov/hiv/default.htm

> The Centers for Disease Control and Prevention's website includes information on testing, HIV/AIDS statistics, fact sheets, recommendations and guidelines, and specialized information related to specific populations. This website provides a wealth of information related to treatment and prevention and is especially useful with respect to providing up to date statistics and information for populations of interest.

The Federal Government's HIV/AIDS website: http://www.aids.gov/

> This is the government's website for information about HIV/AIDS. This website is a useful tool for understanding what federal resources are available, where to get tested, and how to engage in treatment. Information related to the Affordable Care Act and the National HIV/AIDS Strategy can be found here.

Gabriel, N. S., & Northridge, M. E. (2013). The social legacy of HIV/AIDS. *American Journal of Public Health, 103*, 199.

> This brief overview exemplifies how public policy and social policy have shaped the course of HIV/AIDS prevention and treatment. Though just an introduction, this article introduces how the concept of stigma in minority communities can be addressed by social policy and how that, in turn, will affect the social legacy of HIV/AIDS in the United States.

Gardner, E. M., McLees, M. P., Steiner, J. F., del Rio, C., & Burman, W. J. (2011). The spectrum of engagement in HIV care and its relevance to test-and-treat strategies for prevention of HIV infection. *Clinical Infectious Diseases, 52*(6), 793–800.

> Test and treat strategies have been employed for HIV positive individuals in an effort to improve outcomes and reduce HIV transmission. This article is an excellent assessment of the spectrum of engagement in care and discusses the deleterious consequences of poor engagement in care for HIV infected persons.

The Joint United Nations Programme on HIV/AIDS website: http://www.unaids.org/en/

> The mission of UNAIDS is to ensure that universal access to HIV prevention, treatment, care, and support is achieved throughout the world. Information provided on this website includes the types of programs UNAIDS supports, data from throughout the world, and the specific targets UNAIDS is committed to addressing.

Stone, V., Ojikutu, B., & Rawlings, M. K. (Eds.). (2009). *HIV/AIDS in U.S. communities of color*. New York, NY: Springer.

This book addresses the reasons why treatment failure occurs and promotes understanding cultural values in an effort to provide patient-centered care for those living with HIV/AIDS. This book is also a valuable resource not only for treatment but also for prevention specifically within minority communities. Both behavioral and clinical aspects of HIV/AIDS in minority communities are discussed with respect to both treatment and prevention.

The World Health Organization's HIV/AIDS website: http://www.who.int/topics/hiv _aids/en/

The WHO HIV/AIDS website provides helpful information on statistics, fact sheets, news, prevention, and treatment. Specialized topics are discussed related to HIV and other health concerns. A large amount of information about statistics, policies, and targets is available for each region throughout the world.

REFERENCES

Andersen, R. M., Bozzette, S. A., Shapiro, M. F., St. Clair, P., Morton, S., Crystal, S., ... Cunningham, W. (2000). Access of vulnerable groups to antiretroviral therapy among persons in care for HIV disease in the U.S. *Health Services Research, 35*(2), 389–416.

Anderson, K. H., & Mitchell, J. M. (2000). Differential access in the receipt of antiretroviral drugs for the treatment of AIDS and its implications for survival. *Archives of Internal Medicine, 160*(20), 3114–3120.

Asch, S. M., Gifford, A. L., Bozzette, S. A., Turner, B., Mathews, W. C., Kuromiya, K., ... McCutchan, J. A. (2001). Underuse of primary Mycobacterium avium complex and Pneumocystis carinii prophylaxis in the United States. *Journal of Acquired Immune Deficiency Syndromes, 28*(4), 340–344.

Blair, J. M., McNaghten, A. D., Frazier, E. L., Skarbinski, J., Huang, P., & Heffelfinger, J. D. (2011). Clinical and behavioral characteristics of adults receiving medical care for HIV infection: Medical Monitoring Project, United States, 2007. *MMWR Surveillance Summaries, 60*(11), 1–20.

Bowen, G. S., Marconi, K., Kohn, S., Bailey, D. M., Goosby, E. P., Shorter, S., & Niemcryk, S. (1992). First year of AIDS services delivery under Title I of the Ryan White CARE Act. *Public Health Reports, 107*(5), 491–499.

Bozzette, S. A. (2010). Quality of care for patients infected with HIV. *Clinical Infectious Diseases, 51*(6), 739–740.

Bozzette, S. A., Berry, S. H., Duan, N., Frankel, M. R., Leibowitz, A. A., Lefkowitz, D., ... Shapiro, M. F. (1998). The care of HIV-infected adults in the United States: Results from the HIV Cost and Services Utilization Study. *New England Journal of Medicine, 339*(26), 1897–1904.

Bozzette, S. A., Joyce, G., McCaffrey, D. F., Leibowitz, A. A., Morton, S. C., Berry, S. H., ... Goldman, D. P. (2001). Expenditures for the care of HIV-infected patients in the era of highly active antiretroviral therapy. *New England Journal of Medicine, 344*(11), 817–823.

Branson, B. M., Handsfield, H. H., Lampe, M. A., Janssen, R. S., Taylor, A. W., Lyss, S. B., & Clark, J. E. (2006). Revised recommendations for HIV testing of adults, adolescents, and pregnant women in health-care settings. *Morbidity and Mortality Weekly Reports, 55*(RR14), 1–17.

Buchanan, R. J., & Smith, S. R. (1998). State implementation of the AIDS drug assistance programs. *Health Care Financing Review, 19*(3), 39–62.

Cavaleri, M. A., Kalogerogiannis, K., McKay, M. M., Vitale, L., Levi, E., Jones, S., ... Flynn, E. (2010). Barriers to HIV care: An exploration of the complexities that influence engagement in and utilization of treatment. *Social Work in Health Care, 49*(10), 934–945.

Centers for Disease Control and Prevention. (2011a). *Basic statistics*. Atlanta: Author. Retrieved from http://www.cdc.gov/hiv/topics/surveillance/basic.htm# aidsdiagnoses

Centers for Disease Control and Prevention. (2011b). *HIV in the United States*. Atlanta: Author.

Centers for Disease Control and Prevention. (2011c). HIV Surveillance: United States, 1981–2008. *Morbidity and Mortality Weekly Reports, 60*(21), 689–693.

Cheever, L. W. (2007). Engaging HIV-infected patients in care: Their lives depend on it. *Clinical Infectious Diseases, 44*(11), 1500–1502.

Cheng, E. M., Chen, A., & Cunningham, W. (2007). Primary language and receipt of recommended health care among Hispanics in the United States. *Journal of General Internal Medicine, 22*(Suppl 2), 283–288.

Chovnik, G. (2011). *Organizational preparedness for future biomedical HIV prevention technologies among a sample of community-based AIDS organizations* (Unpublished dissertation). UCLA, Los Angeles.

Cohen, M. S., Chen, Y. Q., McCauley, M., Gamble, T., Hosseinipour, M. C., Kumarasamy, N., ... Fleming, T. R. (2011). Prevention of HIV-1 infection with early antiretroviral therapy. *New England Journal of Medicine, 365*(6), 493–505.

Crystal, S., Sambamoorthi, U., & Merzel, C. (1995). The Diffusion of innovation in AIDS treatment: Zidovudine use in two New Jersey cohorts. *Health Services Research, 30*(4), 593–614.

Cunningham, W. E., Andersen, R. M., Katz, M. H., Stein, M. D., Turner, B. J., Crystal, S., ... Shapiro, M. F. (1999a). The impact of competing subsistence needs and barriers on access to medical care for persons with human immunodeficiency virus receiving care in the United States. *Medical Care, 37*(12), 1270–1281.

Cunningham, W. E., Bozzette, S. A., Hays, R. D., Kanouse, D. E., & Shapiro, M. F. (1995). Comparison of health-related quality of life in clinical trial and non-clinical trial HIV-infected cohorts. *Medical Care, 33*(4), AS15–AS25.

Cunningham, W. E., Hays, R. D., Ettl, M. K., Dixon, W. J., Liu, R. C., Beck, C. K., & Shapiro, M. F. (1998). The prospective effect of access to medical care on health-related quality-of-life outcomes in patients with symptomatic HIV disease. *Medical Care, 36*(3), 295–306.

Cunningham, W. E., Hays, R. D., Mosen, D. M., Andersen, R. M., & Shapiro, M. F. (1996). Access to community-based medical services and number of hospitalizations among patients with HIV disease: Are they related? *Journal of Acquired Immune Deficiency Syndromes and Human Retrovirology, 13*(4), 341–349.

Cunningham, W. E., Markson, L. E., Andersen, R. M., Crystal, S. H., Fleishman, J. A., Golin, C., ... Wenger, N. S. (2000). Prevalence and predictors of highly active antiretroviral therapy use in persons with HIV infection in the U.S. *Journal of Acquired Immune Deficiency Syndromes, 25*(2), 115–123.

Cunningham, W. E., Sohler, N. L., Tobias, C., Drainoni, M. L., Bradford, J., Davis, C., ... Wong, M. D. (2006). Health services utilization for people with HIV infection: Comparison of a population targeted for outreach with the U.S. population in care. *Medical Care, 44*(11), 1038–1047.

Cunningham, W. E., Tisnado, D. M., Lui, H. H., Nakazono, T. T., & Carlisle, D. M. (1999b). The effect of hospital experience on mortality among patients hospitalized with acquired immunodeficiency syndrome in California. *American Journal of Medicine, 107*(2), 137–143.

Cunningham, W. E., Wong, M., & Hays, R. D. (2008). Case management and health-related quality of life outcomes in a national sample of persons with HIV/AIDS. *Journal of the National Medical Association, 100*(7), 840–847.

Currier, J. S., & Havlir, D. V. (2004). Complications of HIV disease and antiretroviral therapy. Highlights of the 11th Conference on Retroviruses and Opportunistic Infections, February 8–11, 2004, San Francisco, California, USA. *Topics in HIV Medicine, 12*(1), 31–45.

Currier, J. S., & Havlir, D. V. (2005). Complications of HIV disease and antiretroviral therapy. *Topics in HIV Medicine, 13*(1), 16–23.

Das, M., Chu, P. L., Santos, G. M., Scheer, S., Vittinghoff, E., McFarland, W., & Colfax, G. N. (2010). Decreases in community viral load are accompanied by reductions in new HIV infections in San Francisco. *PLoS One, 5*(6), e11068.

Department of Health and Human Services. (2010). *How does the Affordable Care Act impact people living with HIV/AIDS?* Retrieved from http://blog.aids.gov /downloads/how_does_acs_impact_people_living_with_hivaids_for_usca.pdf

Eaton, L. A., & Kalichman, S. (2007). Risk compensation in HIV prevention: Implications for vaccines, microbicides, and other biomedical HIV prevention technologies. *Current HIV/AIDS Reports, 4*(4), 165–172.

Flanigan, T. P., & Beckwith, C. G. (2011). The intertwined epidemics of HIV infection, incarceration, and substance abuse: a call to action. *Journal of Infectious Diseases, 203*(9), 1201–1203.

Gallant, J. E., Adimora, A. A., Carmichael, J. K., Horberg, M., Kitahata, M., Quinlivan, E. B., ... Williams, S. B. (2011). Essential components of effective HIV care: A policy paper of the HIV Medicine Association of the Infectious Diseases Society of America and the Ryan White Medical Providers Coalition. *Clinical Infectious Diseases, 53*(11), 1043–1050.

Gardner, E. M., McLees, M. P., Steiner, J. F., del Rio, C., & Burman, W. J. (2011). The spectrum of engagement in HIV care and its relevance to test-and-treat strategies for prevention of HIV infection. *Clinical Infectious Diseases, 52*(6), 793–800.

Gifford, A. L., Cunningham, W. E., Heslin, K. C., Andersen, R. M., Nakazono, T., Lieu, D. K., ... Bozzette, S. A. (2002). Participation in research and access to experimental treatments by HIV-infected patients. *New England Journal of Medicine, 346*(18), 1373–1382.

Girard, M. P., Osmanov, S. K., & Kieny, M. P. (2006). A review of vaccine research and development: The human immunodeficiency virus (HIV). *Vaccine, 24*(19), 4062–4081.

Gwadz, M. V., Colon, P., Ritchie, A. S., Leonard, N. R., Cleland, C. M., Riedel, M.,. . . Mildvan, D. (2010). Increasing and supporting the participation of persons of color living with HIV/AIDS in AIDS clinical trials. *Current HIV/AIDS Reports, 7*(4), 194–200.

Hall, H. I., Song, R., Rhodes, P., Prejean, J., An, Q., Lee, L. M.,. . . Janssen, R. S. (2008). Estimation of HIV incidence in the United States. *Journal of the American Medical Association, 300*(5), 520–529.

Havlir, D. V., & Currier, J. S. (2003). Complications of HIV infection and antiretroviral therapy. *Topics in HIV Medicine, 11*(3), 86–91.

Hays, R. D., Cunningham, W. E., Sherbourne, C. D., Wilson, I. B., Wu, A. W., Cleary, P. D.,. . . Bozzette, S. A. (2000). Health-related quality of life in patients with human immunodeficiency virus infection in the United States: Results from the HIV Cost and Services Utilization Study. *American Journal of Medicine, 108*(9), 714–722.

Hong, H., Neamati, N., Winslow, H. E., Christensen, J. L., Orr, A., Pommier, Y., & Milne, G. W. (1998). Identification of HIV-I integrase inhibitors based on a four-point pharmacophore. *Antiviral Chemistry and Chemotherapy, 9*(6), 461–472.

Imrie, J., Elford, J., Kippax, S., & Hart, G. J. (2007). Biomedical HIV prevention—and social science. *Lancet, 370*(9581), 10–11.

Joint United Nations Programme on HIV/AIDS & World Health Organization. (2009). *2009 AIDS epidemic update*. Retrieved from http://www.unaids.org/en/media/unaids/contentassets/dataimport/pub/report/2009/jc1700_epi_update_2009_en .pdf

Josephs, J. S., Fleishman, J. A., Korthuis, P. T., Moore, R. D., & Gebo, K. A. (2010). Emergency department utilization among HIV-infected patients in a multisite multistate study. *HIV Medicine, 11*(1), 74–84.

King, W. D., Wong, M. D., Shapiro, M. F., Landon, B. E., & Cunningham, W. E. (2004). Does racial concordance between HIV-positive patients and their physicians affect the time to receipt of protease inhibitors? *Journal of General Internal Medicine, 19*, 1146–1153.

Kinsler, J. J., Lee, S. J., Sayles, J. N., Newman, P. A., Diamant, A., & Cunningham, W. (2009). The impact of acculturation on utilization of HIV prevention services and access to care among an at-risk Hispanic population. *Journal of Health Care for the Poor and Underserved, 20*(4), 996–1011.

Knowlton, A. R., Arnsten, J. H., Eldred, L. J., Wilkinson, J. D., Shade, S. B., Bohnert, A. S.,. . . Purcell, D. W. (2010). Antiretroviral use among active injection-drug users: the role of patient-provider engagement and structural factors. *AIDS Patient Care and STDs, 24*(7), 421–428.

Landon, B. E., Wilson, I. B., Cohn, S. E., Fichtenbaum, C. J., Wong, M. D., Wenger, N. S.,. . . Cleary, P. D. (2003). Physician specialization and antiretroviral therapy for HIV. *Journal of General Internal Medicine, 18*(4), 233–241.

Li, X., Margolick, J. B., Conover, C. S., Badri, S., Riddler, S. A., Witt, M. D., & Jacobson, L. P. (2005). Interruption and discontinuation of highly active antiretroviral therapy in the multicenter AIDS cohort study. *Journal of Acquired Immune Deficiency Syndrome, 38*(3), 320–328.

Little, S. J., Holte, S., Routy, J. P., Daar, E. S., Markowitz, M., Collier, A. C., . . . Richman, D. D. (2002). Antiretroviral-drug resistance among patients recently infected with HIV. *New England Journal of Medicine, 347*(6), 385–394.

Losina, E., & Freedberg, K. A. (2011). Life expectancy in HIV. *British Medical Journal, 343*, d6015.

Lucas, G. M., Chaisson, R. E., & Moore, R. D. (1999). Highly active antiretroviral therapy in a large urban clinic: Risk factors for virological failure and adverse drug reactions. *Annals of Internal Medicine, 131*(2), 81–87.

Magnus, M., Schmidt, N., Park, J., Brown, B., & Kissinger, P. J. (2001). Revisiting the association between ancillary services and emergency department visits and hospitalizations among HIV-infected women. *AIDS Patient Care and STDs, 15*(10), 503–504.

Mellors, J. W., Rinaldo, C. R., Gupta, P., White, R. M., Todd, J. A., & Kingsley, L. A. (1996). Prognosis in HIV-1 infection predicted by the quantity of virus in plasma. *Science, 272*, 1167–1170.

Mills, E. J., Nachega, J. B., Bangsberg, D. R., Singh, S., Rachlis, B., Wu, P., . . . Cooper, C. (2006). Adherence to HAART: A systematic review of developed and developing nation patient-reported barriers and facilitators. *PLoS Medicine, 3*(11), e438.

Nosyk, B., & Montaner, J. S. (2012). The evolving landscape of the economics of HIV treatment and prevention. *PLoS Medicine, 9*(2), e1001174.

O'Brien, W. A., Hartigan, P. M., Martin, D., Esinhart, J., Hill, A., Benoit, S., . . . Hamilton, J. D. (1996). Changes in plasma HIV-1 RNA and CD4+ lymphocyte counts and the risk of progression to AIDS. *New England Journal of Medicine, 334*(7), 426–431.

Padian, N. S., Buve, A., Balkus, J., Serwadda, D., & Cates, W., Jr., (2008). Biomedical interventions to prevent HIV infection: Evidence, challenges, and way forward. *Lancet, 372*(9638), 585–599.

Palella, F. J., Delaney, K. M., Moorman, A. C., Loveless, M. O., Fuhrer, J., Satten, G. A., . . . Holmberg, S. D. (1998). Declining morbidity and mortality among patients with advanced human immunodeficiency virus infection. *New England Journal of Medicine, 338*(13), 853–860.

Pantaleo, G., Menzo, S., Vaccarezza, M., Graziosi, C., Cohen, O. J., Demarest, J. F., . . . Fauci, A. S. (1995). Studies in subjects with long-term nonprogressive human immunodeficiency virus infection. *New England Journal of Medicine, 332*(4), 209–216.

Puskas, C. M., Forrest, J. I., Parashar, S., Salters, K. A., Cescon, A. M., Kaida, A., . . . Hogg, R. S. (2011). Women and vulnerability to HAART non-adherence: a literature review of treatment adherence by gender from 2000 to 2011. *Current HIV/AIDS Reports, 8*(4), 277–287.

Reichmann, W. M., Walensky, R. P., Case, A., Novais, A., Arbelaez, C., Katz, J. N., & Losina, E. (2011). Estimation of the prevalence of undiagnosed and diagnosed HIV in an urban emergency department. *PLoS One, 6*(11), e27701.

Rerks-Ngarm, S., Pitisuttithum, P., Nitayaphan, S., Kaewkungwal, J., Chiu, J., Paris, R., . . . Kim, J. H. (2009). Vaccination with ALVAC and AIDSVAX to prevent HIV-1 infection in Thailand. *New England Journal of Medicine, 361*(23), 2209–2220.

Sayles, J. N., Ryan, G. W., Silver, J. S., Sarkisian, C. A., & Cunningham, W. E. (2007). Experiences of social stigma and implications for healthcare among a diverse population of HIV positive adults. *Journal of Urban Health, 84*(6), 814–828.

Sayles, J. N., Wong, M. D., Kinsler, J. J., Martins, D., & Cunningham, W. E. (2009). The association of stigma with self-reported access to medical care and antiretroviral therapy adherence in persons living with HIV/AIDS. *Journal of General Internal Medicine, 24*(10), 1101–1108.

Shapiro, M. F., Morton, S. C., McCaffrey, D. F., Senterfitt, J. W., Fleishman, J. A., Perlman, J. F., ... Bozzette, S. A. (1999). Variations in the care of HIV-infected adults in the United States: Results from the HIV Cost and Services Utilization Study. *Journal of the American Medical Association, 281*(24), 2305–2315.

Simoni, J. M., Amico, K. R., Pearson, C. R., & Malow, R. (2008). Strategies for promoting adherence to antiretroviral therapy: A review of the literature. *Current Infectious Disease Reports, 10*(6), 515–521.

Thompson, M. A., Aberg, J. A., Cahn, P., Montaner, J. S., Rizzardini, G., Telenti, A., ... Schooley, R. T. (2010). Antiretroviral treatment of adult HIV infection: 2010 Recommendations of the International AIDS Society–USA panel. *Journal of the American Medical Association, 304*(3), 321–333.

Volkow, N. D., & Montaner, J. (2010). Enhanced HIV testing, treatment, and support for HIV-infected substance users. *Journal of the American Medical Association, 303*(14), 1423–1424.

Wainberg, M. A., & Friedland, G. H. (1998). Public health implications of antiretroviral therapy and HIV drug resistance. *Journal of the American Medical Association, 279*, 1977–1983.

Weaver, M. R., Conover, C. J., Proescholdbell, R. J., Arno, P. S., Ang, A., & Ettner, S. L. (2008). Utilization of mental health and substance abuse care for people living with HIV/AIDS, chronic mental illness, and substance abuse disorders. *Journal of Acquired Immune Deficiency Syndrome, 47*(4), 449–458.

Wong, M. D., Asch, S. M., Andersen, R. M., Hays, R. D., & Shapiro, M. F. (2004). Racial and ethnic differences in patients' preferences for initial care by specialists. *American Journal of Medicine, 116*(9), 613–620.

Workowski, K. A., & Berman, S. (2010). Sexually transmitted diseases treatment guidelines, 2010. *MMWR Recommendations and Reports, 59*(RR-12), 1–110.

Zellweger, C., Opravil, M., Bernasconi, E., Cavassini, M., Bucher, H. C., Schiffer, V., ... Furrer, H. (2004). Long-term safety of discontinuation of secondary prophylaxis against Pneumocystis pneumonia: Prospective multicentre study. *AIDS, 18*(15), 2047–2053.

CHAPTER EIGHTEEN

CHILDREN'S HEALTH

Moira Inkelas
Neal Halfon
David Lee Wood

Learning Objectives

- Understand how health services organization in the United States matches the unique health needs of children
- Understand the differences between influences on children's health and influences on adult health
- Understand problems with financing and organization in the current system
- Explain implications of life-course models of health for children's health care organization
- Understand emerging and future models of care

Throughout the past century, expert panels and government commissions have highlighted the importance of certain basic principles for children's health care. Over the past decade, the Maternal and Child Health Bureau's (MCHB) Bright Futures guidelines emphasize that health care for children should be comprehensive, continuous, coordinated, and accountable. Despite great technical advances and development of important programs that have improved the health and changed the lives of many children, the system of care for children in the United States has yet to embody the principles of Bright Futures and the recommendations of these expert panels. Children experience uninsurance, underinsurance, and numerous barriers to receiving appropriate care. The medical, developmental, and environmental threats to children have changed in nature and complexity, and the system of care that has evolved to meet these changing needs is fragmented, disorganized, and difficult to navigate.

As the health care marketplace continues to change, attention should be directed toward how these changes affect the availability and quality of essential child health services. The changing marketplace poses its own set of challenges, but significant changes in organization of and payment for health services create new opportunities to construct a child health system that is more responsive to current and emerging health needs of children and better able to overcome deficiencies in the current system. Some of the specific services that should be included in a higher-performing system of children's health care might not meet the narrower financial goals of many managed care organizations. How can development of a better-quality child health system be supported—a system that emphasizes health and developmental potential through prevention and health promotion, early intervention services for children with developmental delay, preventive mental health services, and comprehensive services to children with special medical needs? How can these and other services be ensured when they may not be profitable to the health care organization in the short term?

Whether ongoing marketplace changes and federal and state health financing policies improve the organization of children's health services and children's health status overall depends on the extent to which these and other questions are addressed. How do children fare under a health system restructuring that is driven primarily by cost considerations? How will access and quality of child health services be affected by financing changes in the public and private sectors? Can current access barriers to comprehensive, coordinated health services be resolved? How can the principles of care guide transformation of children's health services? By what standard should we evaluate the effectiveness of new organizational approaches to delivering child health services?

This chapter examines the key issues underlying some of the incongruities between the needs of children and families and the current and evolving structure of health services in the United States. We describe the unique health needs of children and the rationale for a child standard of care to ensure that emerging systems can meet these needs. Next, we examine characteristics of the U.S. health care system that influence children's access to care, including the disjointed organization of health services and financial and structural barriers to health care. In the context of federal and state health care policy and sweeping reforms in the health system, we present several options for accommodating the unique needs of children. Finally, we describe how emerging models of care can be modified to provide more effective, organized, and family-centered health services for children.

Special Health Needs of Children

The National Research Council and Institute of Medicine (IOM) report *Children's Health, the Nation's Wealth* (2004) defined *health* as "the extent to which individual children or groups of children are able or enabled to (a) develop and realize their potential, (b) satisfy their needs, and (c) develop the capacities that allow them to interact successfully with their biological, physical, and social environments."

The committee went on to specify the domains of health that policies and services are designed to influence: "Health conditions, which capture disorders or illnesses of the body systems; functioning, which focuses on the manifestations of health on an individual's daily life; and health potential, which captures the development of assets and positive aspects of health, such as competence, capacity and developmental potential."

Implicit in this definition and the strategies that the IOM proposes for addressing children's health needs is an understanding that children's health needs and risks differ fundamentally from those of adults and thus require special consideration in structuring, organizing, and delivering health services (Forrest, Simpson, & Clancy, 1997; Halfon, Inkelas, & Hochstein, 2000; Halfon, Inkelas, & Wood, 1995). Among the unique characteristics of childhood that have important implications for health system design are a child's developmental vulnerability, dependency, and differential patterns of morbidity and mortality.

Developmental Vulnerability

Developmental vulnerability refers to rapid and cumulative physical and emotional changes that characterize childhood, and the potential impact that illness, injury, or untoward family and social circumstances can have on a child's life-course trajectory. Physical health conditions (such as low birthweight or asthma) as well as the child's social environment (severe poverty, unstable family, and environmental exposures such as lead) can harm the developmental process. The Life Course Health Development model has been used to elucidate the dynamic relationships between factors that can promote or adversely affect children's capacity to achieve their physical, emotional, and cognitive potential (Bronfenbrenner, 1979; Halfon & Hochstein, 2002; Hertzman, 1994). Studies demonstrate two phenomena: the substantial, cumulative impact of early exposures and adverse social conditions on health status throughout the life course and the role of critical developmental periods in which early insults cause long-term consequences by programming physiological pathways to function in a manner that is harmful over the short run (during childhood) or the entire life span (Hertzman, 1994; Kuh, Ben-Schlomo, Lynch, Hallqvist, & Power, 2003). The brain science revolution and comparable advances in genetics also make clear the role of gene-environment interaction early in life and the potential to intervene early to minimize disparities and optimize outcomes. Research linking the impact of various risks and insults to developmental pathways supports broader conceptualization of health determinants and of health services.

The potential to alter the life-course trajectory is illustrated by studies that demonstrate the effectiveness of timely intervention in modifying adverse biological and social conditions that may harm a child's development. Cognitive development and behavioral competence at preschool age are greater when low-birthweight children receive supportive family and educational services (Brooks-Gunn et al., 1994). As another example, for the estimated 5 to 17 percent of children with dyslexia—a neurological disorder that typically impairs reading ability and school performance and achievement—intervening early can have a dramatic impact on a child's learning trajectories (Shaywitz & Shaywitz, 2003). Such studies support the notion that timely and appropriately organized services can prevent loss of developmental potential. They highlight the mutability of various risks and their life-course effects.

Children's developmental vulnerability also implies that interventions must be sustained over time to appropriately address periodic, recurrent, and ongoing biological and environmental threats. For example, although comprehensive early childhood intervention programs that serve socially disadvantaged children have improved young children's cognitive abilities, postintervention exposure to ongoing social disadvantage may offset earlier gains (Brooks-Gunn et al., 1994). Discontinuities in health care and interrupted eligibility for early childhood intervention programs are examples of modifiable threats to sustained developmental improvement for at-risk children.

Health disparities have an important connection with developmental vulnerability. Eliminating health disparities has become a major national health policy goal. More than ever, it is recognized that many health issues in adults and the elderly have their origin in childhood. Disparities linked to dietary pattern, health behavior, and environmental exposure begin in childhood and are compounded over the life span. This brings greater attention to the role of protective and health-promoting factors in childhood for enhancement of long-term health capacity and functioning, and the role of risks and absence of health-promoting assets in significant health disparities.

New and Differential Morbidities

The declining prevalence in the United States of nutritional and infectious disease and the changing patterns of childhood risk have increased the prominence of other causes of morbidity and mortality. Children are affected by a broad and complex array of conditions termed "new morbidities": drug and alcohol use, family and neighborhood violence, emotional disorders, learning problems, and so on. These new morbidities originate in complex family or socioeconomic conditions, rather than an exclusively biological etiology and cannot be adequately addressed by traditional medical services (Haggerty, Roghmann, & Pless, 1975). Instead, such conditions require a continuum of comprehensive services that include multidisciplinary assessment, treatment, and rehabilitation as well as community-based prevention strategies to sustain positive outcomes (Halfon & Berkowitz, 1993). Such multidisciplinary approaches often incorporate and integrate public- and private-sector services. For example, early intervention, family preservation, and violence prevention programs involve broad-based, multisector approaches that transcend agency and service sector boundaries (Fielding & Halfon, 1994).

The types and patterns of conditions for children are changing, and patterns of morbidity and the manifestation of medical conditions in children fundamentally differ in their pathophysiology and treatment relative to adults. Serious chronic medical conditions are less prevalent in children and usually are related to birth or congenital anomalies, rather than the degenerative conditions that affect adults. Age-specific drug metabolism, disease expression, and health status assessments differentiate children from adults. For example, in children cardiac conditions may result from any number of distinct congenital malformations, whereas in adults they are dominated by a single degenerative disorder (atherosclerotic heart disease). These differences explain why pediatric specialists are more prepared to diagnose and treat many children's chronic and severe conditions. Age-related differences in disease prevalence, expression, and management have important implications for issues such as ensuring appropriate access to care, developing age-specific quality assessment measures, guaranteeing availability of adequately trained providers, and furthering regional distribution of pediatric health professionals and services.

Dependency

Children also have complex and changing *dependency* relationships that affect their development and their use of health services. Children depend on their parents or other caregivers to recognize and respond to their health needs, organize their care and authorize treatment, and comply with recommended treatment regimens. An example of this dependency for children's access to health care is illustrated by studies comparing maternal utilization of health services with children's use of care. Studies find that maternal and child use of care is highly correlated, irrespective of the level of health status (Newacheck & Halfon, 1986). Reports such as those by the National Commission on Children and the Carnegie Commission on Early Childhood further address the interdependency of family and social environments and their impact on children's health and development (Carnegie Task Force on Meeting the Needs of Young Children, 1994).

Health Service Delivery for U.S. Children

Although the principle that children's health services should be organized into a comprehensive, coordinated, continuous, and accessible system of health services is broadly supported, it is not clear how evolution in the health care marketplace and restructuring of the delivery system advance these principles for all children. Using a conceptual framework depicted in Figure 18.1, *Children's Health, the Nation's Wealth* (NRC and IOM, 2004) suggests that effectively addressing health conditions, health functioning, and health potential requires health services that achieve the following:

- Modify predisease pathways by minimizing risk of exposure before it occurs and by actively promoting development of health capacities. For

FIGURE 18.1. WHERE SERVICES CAN EFFECT CHANGE IN HEALTHY DEVELOPMENT

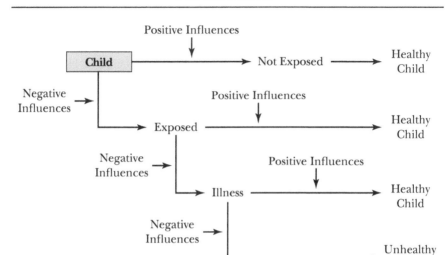

Source: Committee on Evaluation of Children's Health & National Research Council, 2004.

example, young children at risk for poor language development whose parents receive counseling and assistance from pediatric clinicians can have clinically meaningful improvement in language (Needlman & Silverstein, 2004).

- Reduce exposure to health-compromising events. For example, counseling parents on infant sleep position through the national Back to Sleep campaign was accompanied by a 50 percent decline in the incidence of sudden infant death syndrome (SIDS) (Daley, 2004).

- Modify the relationship between exposure and the onset of disease, once the child has been exposed, to alter the exposure-outcome pathway. For example, meningitis can be avoided in children who are exposed but receive prophylactic antibiotics in a timely fashion.

- Modify the disease course and reduce impact through appropriate diagnostic, treatment, rehabilitation, and habilitation services. For example, children with cystic fibrosis who are diagnosed early and given an integrated care management program have dramatically increased life-span and functional capacity (Schechter, 2003).

Children's health care therefore encompasses health promotion and disease prevention services; diagnostic, treatment, and rehabilitation services; health education programs, and other supportive social services. To offer this array in a directed and integrated fashion, health care delivery strategies are necessarily broad and specify multisector service delivery pathways that integrate medical, public health, educational, and social services. For example, to identify developmental delays as early as possible, population monitoring can take place in a child care or Head Start center, while screening may take place at a pediatric office. Diagnostic evaluation and ultimately services for such delays may take place in a variety of settings depending on financing, availability, and how a particular state or region has organized publicly funded services for outreach, diagnosis, and treatment. Given this complexity, achieving the systems outcome of timely identification requires having more defined pathways, multiple types of settings for identification, and collaboration among multiple community agencies and programs. The array of programs and financing streams makes it challenging to consolidate personal medical care services and other services heretofore delivered by the community health sector into vertically integrated delivery systems that follow a medical model. Managed care arrangements can effectively organize primary and specialty medical services for healthy populations and for acute conditions. However, the newer morbidities have complex socioeconomic and environmental determinants that often require intense, sustained, and coordinated health services that neither the current system nor the emerging managed care arrangements are structured to provide (Halfon et al., 2000).

Child Health Service Sectors

The U.S. child health system has been characterized as a patchwork of disconnected programs, each with its own eligibility, administrative, and funding criteria (Schlesinger & Eisenberg, 1990). The three distinct yet interdependent sectors that constitute child health services—the personal medical and preventive services sector, the population-based community health services sector, and the health-related support services sector—have unique histories, mandates, organizational characteristics and constraints, and funding streams (Halfon et al., 1995).

Personal Medical and Preventive Services. Personal medical and preventive health services for children include primary and specialty medical services, which are generally delivered in private and public medical offices, hospitals, and laboratories. Restructuring the organization of the personal health service care sector, where the majority of health care dollars are spent, is the major focus of current health system reform and improvement efforts. Personal medical services are principally funded through private health insurance, public health insurance, and by out-of-pocket payments from families.

Population-Based Community Health Services. The second sector of child health services includes population-based health promotion and disease prevention services, such as lead screening and abatement programs and child abuse prevention. This sector also includes an array of early childhood prevention, health promotion, and developmental optimization programs to promote early learning and health development (Halfon et al., 2000). Other community health services are special child abuse treatment programs and rehabilitative services for children with complex congenital conditions or other chronic debilitating diseases. Community-based programs often have outreach responsibilities for children's health services, such as early intervention and monitoring programs for infants at risk for developmental disability and case management and financing for children with serious chronic diseases. Funding for this sector comes from federal programs such as Medicaid's Early Periodic Screening, Diagnosis, and Treatment program (EPSDT), Title V (Maternal and Child Health) of the Social Security Act, and many other categorical programs.

Health-Related Support Services. The third sector of the child health system includes health-related support services, such as nutrition education, early intervention, rehabilitation, and family support programs. Among the services in this sector are parent education and skill building in families with infants at risk for developmental delay that is due to physiological (low birthweight) or social (very low income) risks, or special education. Funding for these services comes from diverse agencies, among them the U.S. Department of Agriculture (funding the Supplemental Food Program for Women, Infants, and Children, or WIC) and the Department of Education (providing outreach and services through the Individuals with Disabilities Education Act, or IDEA).

Fragmented Delivery System

These three child health sectors evolved separately (Schlesinger & Eisenberg, 1990), and the patchwork nature of the programs that make up each sector poses challenges to forging a continuum of integrated services. Incremental federal and state funding for children's health programs has produced this array of categorical, condition-specific, means-tested programs that are not well integrated within or between the child health service sectors. Many of these programs were developed to fill a gap or address an emerging need (child abuse, HIV, mental health problems, or autism), yet there is often little coordination within federal, state, and local governing authorities, or any attempt to link with private-sector efforts. Program administrative mandates and categorical or block grant criteria often determine the number of children who can be served.

Some states have moved to establish coordinating agencies or administrative councils for children and family services. These include children's cabinets established by governors. The Maternal and Child Health Bureau (MCHB) is the single federal agency charged with improving the health status and organization of service systems for children at the federal level. Some have argued that this federal agency has neither the authority nor sufficient funding to accomplish this ambitious mission. The MCHB has been successful in launching many important initiatives to improve coordination and integration of existing health services. Strategic objectives of the MCHB include ensuring a "medical home" for all children, improving early and ongoing identification of health and developmental concerns, insuring all children, organizing community systems of services that are easy for families to use, promoting family-centered care, and transitioning adolescents with special health care needs successfully into adult systems of care. In 2003 MCHB launched the State Early Childhood Comprehensive Systems initiative to help state health departments focus their efforts on improving healthy development and early learning for young children, by coordinating the efforts of state- and local-level health, mental health, early care and education, family support, and education services.

Integrating Services

Achieving better health outcomes for the growing number of children afflicted with multiple and complex problems requires coordinated health and health-related services that may include primary and specialty medical care, case management, early intervention, and special education (Halfon et al., 2000). Efforts to rationalize the organization and allocation of child health services are exemplified by the infant and toddler portion of the IDEA legislation. The 1986 amendments to this legislation mandate interagency collaboration and regional service integration as part of a state planning process for early childhood intervention services. In many states, this resulted in organized comprehensive and coordinated assessment and treatment services for infants and young children at risk for development disabilities owing to a variety of adverse perinatal outcomes or environmental factors.

Other examples of integrated delivery models developed for children at risk demonstrate efficiency in providing coordinated, multisectoral services for children. The National Institute of Mental Health created the Child and Adolescent Service System Program initiative to increase states' capacity to create coordinated systems of care in mental health for children and youth (Kahn & Kamerman, 1992). Innovative models designed to facilitate service coordination by decategorizing funding streams and creating flexible funding pools include a series of demonstration projects that are taking place in communities in the United States. These projects illustrate some of the strategies used to integrate services and increase children's access to appropriate services by rationalizing provision of public funds.

Part of the difficulty in integrating health services comes from the sheer volume of categorical programs, as well as the scope of eligibility and financial constraints that inhibit greater coordination (Halfon & Berkowitz, 1993). Table 18.1 illustrates part of this challenge. A comprehensive approach to providing preventive, diagnostic, treatment, and rehabilitative services across the physical, emotional, cognitive, and social domains would require integration of many programs and funding sources. The State Early Childhood Comprehensive Systems initiative strives to address state-level policy issues that create complexity and undermine alignment of public programs affecting early childhood, including Medicaid, early care and education, mental health, and family support.

Financing Children's Health Care

Intimately linked to structure and organization of health services is how these services are financed. A range of funding streams currently funds parts of the full continuum of services that children need. Health insurance remains a principal determinant of children's access to medical care. Financial barriers to medical care result primarily from lack of insurance for primary care services (such as well-child care and immunizations) or specialty child health services (such as mental health services and rehabilitative therapy).

Uninsured Children

Public child health insurance eligibility has expanded as studies documented significant differential access to health care for uninsured children.

TABLE 18.1. PUBLIC PROGRAMS IN CHILD HEALTH SERVICE AND HEALTH NEED DOMAINS

Health Service	Health Need				
	Physical	Emotional	Cognitive	Family	Social
Prevention	Title XIX Title XXI Title V Title X WIC MCH block grant	Title X IDEA	Title XIX Title X IDEA Head Start	Title X Head Start TANF IDEA	Title IV TANF
Early identification	Title XIX Title XXI Title V Title X WIC MCH block grant	Title XIX IDEA	Title XIX IDEA	Title XX Title IV	Title IV
Diagnosis	Title XIX Title XXI Title V IDEA	Title XIX IDEA	Title XIX IDEA	Title XX Title IV IDEA	Title IV
Treatment	Title XIX Title XXI Title V IDEA	Title XIX IDEA	Title XIX IDEA		Title IV

Source: Adapted from Halfon & Berkowitz, 1993.

Children without health insurance are less likely to have routine doctor visits or receive care for injuries, and more likely to delay seeking care (Newacheck, Hughes, Hung, Wong, & Stoddard, 2000b). In the National Health Interview Survey (NHIS), parents of uninsured children have reported a higher rate of unmet medical, dental, medication, and vision needs than did parents of privately insured children (Newacheck, Hughes, Hung, Wong, & Stoddard, 2000b). Uninsured families have been more likely to rely on the emergency room to be their regular source of care

(Newacheck, Hughes, & Stoddard, 1996). Unmet needs for medical care during the year are substantially higher not only for uninsured children (with 12.6 percent having an unmet need) but also for children insured for part of the year (13.4 percent) in comparison to full-year-insured children with public insurance (1.4 percent) or private insurance (0.7 percent) (Olson, Tang, & Newacheck, 2005).

The proportion of uninsured children in the United States rose 40 percent between 1977 and 1987 (Employee Benefit Research Institute, 1993), and by 1989 13.3 percent of children were uninsured (U.S. General Accounting Office, 1993). The percentage of children covered by employer-based insurance has dropped steadily for more than twenty years. This decline in private insurance coverage for children resulted from elimination of dependent coverage on the part of some employers, rising costs to employees of optional dependent coverage, and an economic shift toward service jobs without health benefits.

Expansion of the Medicaid program in the 1990s partially compensated for this erosion in employer-based insurance (Newacheck, Hughes, & Cisternas, 1995). The number of children covered by Medicaid rose by approximately half, from 13.6 percent of U.S. children in 1989 (8.9 million children) to 19.9 percent in 1993 (13.7 million) (U.S. General Accounting Office, 1993). By 2003 more than one-quarter of children (25.8 percent) were covered by Medicaid (Kaiser Commission on Medicaid and the Uninsured, 2004). Although Medicaid extends coverage to children in the lowest-income families, about three-quarters of uninsured children (77.1 percent) lived in families with income above the poverty level at this time (Kaiser Commission on Medicaid and the Uninsured, 2004). Enactment of the federal Children's Health Insurance Program (CHIP) further compensated for the decline in private coverage for children.

Medicaid Participation. Extending coverage has not been sufficient to enroll all eligible children. Family awareness and enrollment complexity have been major factors (Halfon, Inkelas, & Newacheck, 1999). About 70.1 percent of uninsured children in 2003 were eligible for Medicaid or CHIP coverage, but were unenrolled (Robert Wood Johnson Foundation, 2005). Children's participation in Medicaid historically has been hampered by eligibility and administrative rules that cause discontinuities in children's enrollment. Complex Medicaid eligibility criteria and fluctuations in family income result in significant turnover in enrollees. In the 1990s the General Accounting Office (renamed the Government Accountability Office in 2004) estimated that 40 percent of Medicaid

TANF (Temporary Assistance for Needy Families) enrollees were losing Medicaid coverage each year (U.S. General Accounting Office, 1993). Reasons that not all eligible children participated included the delinking of Medicaid from cash assistance and complex rules that were difficult for eligibility workers to administer (Ellwood, 1999). Not all parents enrolled their eligible children due to lack of awareness of eligibility given complex and changing rules, age-specific eligibility thresholds that covered younger but not older children in the same household, limited outreach, and parent concerns about enrolling their citizen children in public insurance programs when the parents or other family members have undocumented immigration status. The number of uninsured Medicaid-eligible children nearly doubled between 1993 (an estimated 2.3 million) and 2003 (an estimated 4.1 million) (Tang, 2005). The NHIS showed that unenrolled Medicaid-eligible children would benefit from coverage, as they experienced poorer access to health care than enrolled children, as evidenced by higher rates of unmet need (17.9 versus 6.2 percent) and a higher incidence of lacking regular source of care (23.0 versus 5.6 percent) (Davidoff, Garrett, & Schirmer, 2000).

State Children's Health Insurance Program. Enactment of the Children's Health Insurance Program in 1997 as Title XXI of the Social Security Act extended health insurance to children who had not been eligible for Medicaid or private, employer-based coverage. Specific provisions of the CHIP legislation addressed some historical limitations of Medicaid. States were required to implement outreach programs and ensure that children found not to be eligible for CHIP would be referred to or enrolled in Medicaid if eligible. States also were permitted to extend twelve months of eligibility to a child once Medicaid eligibility was established so that eligibility losses caused by month-to-month income fluctuations could be reduced. State policy choices in CHIP influenced program outcomes. For example, adoption of a six-month waiting period to enroll, use of asset testing, premium requirements, prohibiting self-declaration of income, and lack of a presumptive eligibility policy during the application period are all associated with lower enrollment in states that implement these policies (Kronebusch & Elbel, 2004). State variation in participation, ranging from about 35 to 60 percent in a survey sample, showed the importance of state policies for achieving high participation (Kronebusch & Elbel, 2004).

Private Insurance. Children with employment-based health coverage have been at risk for loss of insurance and disruption of care. Children covered under their parents' employment have often lost health insurance with job loss or job change. As the economy shifted from high-paying, benefit-rich manufacturing jobs to lower-paying, benefit-poor service jobs, dependent coverage declined.

Even those children and families with health insurance have experienced underinsurance for primary or specialty care medical care (Szilagyi, 2012). Over the past twenty years, the introduction of managed care has had a major positive impact in coverage of well-child care and immunizations and specialty care. In 1992, 50 percent of indemnity insurance health plans covered well-child care and 65 percent of preferred provider organizations (PPOs) covered immunizations (U.S. Department of Labor, 1993). Underinsurance for specialty care remained; children with special health care needs caused by a congenital condition, chronic illness, or injury have lacked adequate private medical coverage, especially for speech therapy, behavioral therapy, physical therapy, and other essential services (Szilagyi, 2012). About 58.1 percent of parents self-report that private health insurance adequately covers the service benefits needed by their child with special health care needs (Inkelas, Smith, Kuo, Rudolph, & Igdaloff, 2005). Moreover, despite the demonstrated efficacy of nonmedical social services for health and developmental outcomes, services such as home visitation and health-related consultation have not been benefits for privately insured children. In contrast, Medicaid generally covers these services.

Cost Sharing. Nearly all health plans apply cost-sharing mechanisms to minimize unnecessary use of medical services and thereby limit expenditures. The RAND Health Insurance Experiment found that placing cost-sharing requirements on families for primary and preventive care services reduced children's use of these discretionary services (Valdez, 1986). Although short-term adverse outcomes from reduced use of medical care were not detected in the RAND study, the sensitivity of children's basic ambulatory medical services to cost sharing was demonstrated. With the expansion of managed care, more preventive services such as immunization and well-child care are routinely covered, and administration fees, deductibles, copayments, and other cost-sharing mechanisms are less often applied for preventive and primary care visits. In contrast, cost sharing continues to be applied to acute and chronic care services. For many poor, ar-poor, and even middle-income families, even nominal cost sharing poses a significant barrier to care.

Nonfinancial Barriers to Care

Children's access to medical care has been measured by analyzing utilization patterns for specific services (such as number of annual physician visits), designated populations (adolescents and children in foster care), children with specific conditions (for instance, those with asthma), or specific services (immunization and prenatal care) (Halfon, Inkelas, & Wood, 1995). Such analyses have identified many factors that impede use of care and that appear to account for differential usage (as by ethnicity, income, and residence) when controlling for health need (as measured by health status indicators and number and type of conditions) (Newacheck, 1992; Newacheck & Halfon, 1986; Wood et al., 1992). Nonfinancial barriers to care include structural, environmental, and personal impediments such as bureaucratic complexity in the organization of child health services, cultural barriers based on ethnicity or language, and provider distribution or shortage, among others (Halfon, et al., 1995; Newacheck, 1992; Wood, Corey, Freeman, & Shapiro, 1992).

Race and Ethnicity. In addition to income, differential access has been consistently documented on the basis of race and ethnicity. Differential access and use associated with race and ethnicity may result from varying modes of utilization, insurance barriers, and the cultural competency of providers. Nonwhite children and adolescents have fewer physician visits and are less likely to have continuity of care (Wood et al., 1992). Studies of access to care of Latino children have also indicated a high rate of uninsurance and differential patterns of use that are based on parental immigration status (Holl, Szilagyi, Rodewald, Byrd, & Weitzman, 1995). The quality of care received by Latino children is often lower, with parents reporting receiving less counseling on health promotion topics and having more difficulty obtaining the information they need when their child has a chronic health condition (Inkelas, Smith, Kuo, Rudolph, & Igdaloff, 2005). Problems of care and health outcomes for African American children improve when targeted interventions can overcome organizational barriers (Orr, Charney, & Straus, 1988).

Regular Sources of Care. Barbara Starfield demonstrated in numerous reviews of access to care that, having a regular source of primary care is particularly important for children (Starfield, 2000; Starfield, Cassady, Nanda, Forrest, & Berk, 1998). Children with a regular source of care are more likely to receive needed medical services and immunizations, resulting in a higher level of satisfaction reported by the family (Halfon, Inkelas, & Wood, 1995). Having a regular source of care is principally determined by insurance status, and the insurance effect on access is often mediated by having a regular provider. In several studies, the type and characteristics of the regular care provider have their own independent effect on use, irrespective of type of insurance coverage. Therefore, considering the type of a usual source of care is important in analyzing differences in access among children.

Provider Training. Emerging patterns of morbidity in children, including complex risks, health conditions, and social problems, have posed new challenges to health care providers and delivery systems. Surveys and anecdotal reports document inadequacies in clinical training for health professionals and lack of routine protocols to identify, treat, or refer children suffering from complex medical conditions, mental disorders, developmental problems, complex psychosocial problems, and abuse and neglect (Horwitz et al., 2007). In one study, physicians' assessments identified fewer than 50 percent of emotional problems of the children who were screened (Costello, 1986). These inadequacies are a function of provider training and knowledge, systemic undervaluing of assessment for new morbidities, and a shortage of community-based treatment resources for these problems. Physicians report in national surveys that knowledge about complex, means-tested public programs for children, the time involved, and their familiarity with screening tools are all barriers to children being identified and referred for developmental concerns (Halfon et al., 2004). Despite national recommendations and known disparities, low rates of screening for developmental and mental health problems have persisted, due in part to inadequate service capacities for intervention and treatment.

Distribution of Providers. Geographic access barriers pose problems for both insured and uninsured poor families. For poor children, a limited supply of local physicians is associated with reduced access to preventive care services (Short & Lefkowitz, 1992) and routine emergency room use for nonemergent sick care (Halfon, Newacheck, Wood, & St Peter, 1996). Although the overall number of pediatricians has risen over the past two decades, the geographic distribution of pediatricians relative to the child population has not improved significantly (Chang & Halfon, 1997).

Low reimbursement and administrative requirements of the Medicaid program have been a major influence on children's access because they lead to low participation of physicians in this important program for children. Pediatrician participation in Medicaid has been historically higher in states with higher reimbursement, less use of capitation, and fewer physician-perceived administrative barriers to participation such as paperwork requirements (Berman, Dolins, Tang, & Yudkowsky, 2002).

Improving the Child Health System

The task of integrating personal medical services with complementary community-based health, social, and educational services demands substantial coordination as well as financial incentives. Achieving health system objectives for children requires greater access to health insurance, integration of services, quality measurement, public and community monitoring of performance (including data systems, involvement of communities, and new measures of how well community systems are performing), and tailoring managed care delivery systems to meet the developmental needs of all children and the special needs of vulnerable child populations.

Health Insurance

In the 1990s, state-initiated health insurance expansions for children took center stage. Some states obtained Medicaid demonstration waivers and used this flexibility to convert to managed care systems and expand coverage for previously uninsured groups. Other states embarked on health insurance expansion for children using state funding (such as Pennsylvania's Child Health Insurance Program, or CHIP), or developed programs that combine public and private revenues (such as Colorado's Child Health Plan). Another form of child health insurance expansion covered limited services. Such privately funded programs primarily covered well-child services and care for acute and chronic illness, but not hospitalization. Thus, program costs were relatively modest.

Enactment of CHIP in 1997 strengthened the role of states in administering unique, state-based health insurance programs for children. Children's incomplete participation in Medicaid and their failure to be covered by employer-based insurance when available had challenged CHIP during early implementation (Kronebusch & Elbel, 2004). States have exercised their options to determine benefit package, cost sharing, and enrollment mechanisms, which has led to differences in insurance eligibility and program structure across states (Newacheck, Halfon, & Inkelas, 2000a) as well as differences in participation rates and coverage duration (Kronebusch & Elbel, 2004). Provisions of the 2010 Affordable Care Act (ACA) that improve coverage include prohibiting denial of care for children with preexisting conditions, Medicaid expansions to 133 percent of the federal poverty level (FPL) for children of all ages, and subsidized coverage up to 400 percent of the FPL. Provisions for special populations of children include extension of Medicaid coverage through age twenty-six to young adults graduating from foster care, increased coverage of habilitative therapy services, and higher federal matching for care coordination and related care requirements for children with chronic conditions.

Health System Integration

Expansion of health insurance coverage and system reorganization on the basis of managed care cannot guarantee children's access to a system of health care that is comprehensive and coordinated. Structural and organizational characteristics of the current health system must be addressed to improve allocation and quality of health services for children and families (Halfon et al., 2000).

The principles of comprehensive, continuous, and coordinated care originally embodied in Medicaid's EPSDT program, and reinforced in 1989 amendments to Title XIX, recognize that access to basic ambulatory medical care does not suffice to meet the needs of children with complex health conditions and environmental risks. For such children, screening, diagnostic, and treatment services must be supplemented with a constellation of supportive services, including outreach, comprehensive case management home visiting, and family counseling services (Barnett & Escobar, 1992). Services should address existing health conditions, but should also be sensitive to the functional and developmental capacities of the child as well as to the family's needs and the community environment (Halfon & Hochstein, 2002; Starfield & Newacheck, 1990). This implies a systematic focus on strategically optimizing investment in children's health development.

Programs designed to reduce health risks and promote protective factors have been tested for children at risk of adverse developmental or other outcomes. In a cost-conscious era, initiatives to broaden and integrate child health services and develop linkage across sectors must demonstrate both effectiveness (improved health outcomes, in an applied setting) and efficiency (cost impact). Home visiting and other early intervention programs targeted to at-risk families have proven cost-effective in improving children's health status, cognitive functioning, and academic performance, while decreasing dependence on public assistance (Barnett & Escobar, 1992; Karoly et al., 1998; Olds et al., 1997). Many states developed initiatives in the past twenty years to improve the health and development of all young children. These are broad, population-based health promotion and disease prevention programs in which the medical sector plays a key role. Many of these initiatives fill gaps in services and supports, but few have undertaken system transformation for children. It is not clear to what degree these population-based initiatives will become comprehensive and integrated with traditional children's medical services as they mature.

The potential for integration of services and supports into comprehensive delivery systems is uncertain in the current health care marketplace. Comprehensive approaches to children's health and development, particularly in the early years, are unlikely to reduce the short-term costs of care to a managed care organization by reducing hospitalization or other high-cost medical expenditure. Instead, the savings from these programs may be realized in a lower incidence of special education participation, enhanced family functioning, and lower welfare outlays. Savings are likely to accrue to the education, mental health, and juvenile justice sectors, rather than to the organization that provided the care. Efforts to control state spending also challenge states as they strive to support integrated cross-sector delivery efforts such as early intervention programs, school-based clinics, and public health safety net programs. Over the past decade, many of these services were paid for (in the case of early intervention and school-based clinics) or heavily subsidized (in the case of public clinics and hospitals) with Medicaid funds. When Medicaid funds are managed by commercial health plans, the ability of the state or local community to use these funds for community health programs and health-related support services is reduced. Continued development of integrated continuums poses a fundamental challenge to states and localities that choose not to earmark some portion of their Medicaid funds or identify new revenues for this purpose.

As direct control over Medicaid funds has declined, the range of mechanisms that states are implementing (combined or separate medical and mental health managed systems, service exclusions, and so on) presents an opportunity to test what types of public-private arrangement prove effective. The infrastructure of the managed care organization created new opportunities for coordination, if not integration (Halfon et al., 2000). Greater attention to early childhood development, coupled with the need for health plans covering publicly insured children to forge relationships with existing public programs for children, could spur enhanced integration. For example, statewide population-based early childhood health and development promotion programs in California, North Carolina, and Vermont are linked with initiatives on the part of local health care providers and managed care organizations. There is a tremendous opportunity to understand which managed care mechanisms serve as barriers or facilitators to quality health care, to identify measures that capture the unique objectives of children's health care, and to study the experimentation underway across states.

Measures of Health Care Quality for Children

Government agencies, medical professional organizations, and multidisciplinary expert working groups have developed normative definitions of comprehensive primary care (Starfield & Newacheck, 1990). Standards have been issued by the federal MCHB and the American Academy of Pediatrics for children's medical care, and by the Child Welfare League of America for the health needs of children in foster care (Child Welfare League of America, 1988). The Bright Futures recommendations outline a comprehensive set of standards for the content of well-child services (Green, 1994). The principles embodied in Bright Futures reaffirm the need for an integrated health care system that is comprehensive, continuous, accessible, coordinated, and accountable.

Quality measures of children's health care have largely come from NCQA's health plan quality indicators of effectiveness of care, access, and utilization. HEDIS and other quality assurance systems have not represented all domains of quality that are of interest for children's health care. Family satisfaction information collected from patients can supplement utilization and administrative data, particularly for difficult-to-measure constructs such as perceived access. The Consumer Assessment of Health Plans (CAHPS) consumer satisfaction surveys ask parents about their child's health care and have a supplemental survey for parents of children with special health care needs (CSHCN). The Child and Adolescent Health Measurement Initiative (CAHMI) has developed quality care measures that specifically address the health care needs of children. For example, the CAHMI Promoting Healthy Development Survey (PHDS) examines provision of developmentally relevant services to children from birth to three. These measures were included in national surveys developed and fielded in the past ten years. AHRQ has sponsored children's quality measure development through The 2009 Children's Health Insurance Program Reauthorization Act (CHIPRA), which included provisions to improve measurement in key quality domains for children of all ages (U.S. Department of Health and Human Services, 2010).

There are a number of reasons that developing performance measures and standards of care for children and families has been a unique and challenging undertaking (McGlynn & Halfon, 1998). Because children are constantly developing, it is difficult to attribute positive or negative characteristics of their health care to their functioning and future outcomes. The complexity of some constructs that define quality care for children (comprehensive, family-centered, and integrated) makes it difficult to create valid quality indicators that can be used for performance comparison. Additionally, the relatively small number and heterogeneity within a group of children with a particular kind of complex medical condition is a methodological challenge in creating standards and performance measures associated with those standards.

Public Accountability and Monitoring

Public accountability for ensuring that all children have access to comprehensive health care has not been part of U.S. child health policy. In the European nations that maintain population-based service delivery models and use public health nurses and other providers to track and monitor infants through the preschool years, compliance with immunization schedules and age-appropriate preventive care visits has been higher than in the United States. A combination of universal access to preventive care and integrated health information systems permits such population-based assurance.

Despite recent advances in health information systems, data systems currently are not structured or capable of producing child-focused information on encounters with the broader child health system, including the public health, nutrition, and school-based health sectors. Efforts to introduce model systems that ensure delivery of the most basic of medical services for children include state and local immunization information and monitoring systems. More detailed information on quality of care and health outcomes has emerged through augmentation of existing national surveys as well as new surveys focused on children. National surveys such as NHIS and its supplements on children and on individuals with disabilities, and the Medical Expenditure Panel Survey, have produced much of the national data on children's access, use, and costs of health care. Since 2000 the National Center for Health Statistics fielded three new surveys designed to address this information gap: the National Survey on Early Childhood Health, the National Survey of Children with Special Health Care Needs, and the National Survey of Children's Health.

Community performance monitoring is also important for children's systems of care (McGlynn & Halfon, 1998). Because children's health services are delivered in multiple sectors, investments in children's health are not fully captured by the specific public programs or commercial managed care organizations that provide the services. Such a monitoring process would include evaluating which aspects of the system facilitate or hinder access, using information about best practices to make improvements where necessary, and examining improvement by monitoring children's outcomes.

Ideally, community systems should be organized to respond to the determinants of children's health, in terms of availability of services, providers, and programs (DuPlessis, Inkelas, & Halfon, 1998). Normative standards for children's health care have identified the need for coordination across programs and organizations. To capture the potential contribution to children's health from the sectors responsible for their care, performance should thus be measured at the community level. Consideration of standards of care for children should not neglect administrative and community-level attributes that promote or undermine quality. For example, measures of service and system integration can be applied to evaluate performance within and among the child health service sectors. Defining the critical pathways by which coordination (when successful) takes place constitutes an initial step in developing the measures and the infrastructure for community performance monitoring (DuPlessis et al., 1998). Linking the results to specific organizational attributes would then make it possible to improve those system attributes that affect quality. Monitoring these attributes is important for policy and planning purposes. Population-based measures of determinants of children's health can be monitored and used to mobilize change. Such measurement systems are vital for the population-based accountability that has been lacking for children and families.

Managed Care for Children

Historically, many Medicaid-insured children received medical care in safety-net public health facilities, where provider continuity and comprehensive health care were not always available (St. Peter, Newacheck, & Halfon, 1992). Past difficulties in access and fragmentation of the delivery system, coupled with rapidly rising costs, helped spur the transition in the 1990s from fee-for-service to managed care Medicaid programs. By 2004, 61.3 percent of Medicaid beneficiaries nationally were enrolled in managed care delivery systems, with managed care the predominant arrangement in forty states and only three states maintaining traditional fee-for-service programs (Kaiser Family Foundation, 2004). Most CHIP programs contracted with managed care arrangements for all of their beneficiaries. The effectiveness and improvement of managed care as a delivery system has been an important policy question for both publicly and privately insured children (Hughes & Luft, 1998; Szilagyi, 1998).

Initial studies showed that managed care plans improved access for children. Managed care organizations demonstrated higher preventive care utilization for maternal and child health services (Freund et al., 1989). In an early study that randomized families to managed care or to fee-for-service arrangements, managed care plans successfully reduced emergency room use and ambulatory visits for nonsevere conditions. The authors concluded that managed care can rationalize care for children without inappropriate rationing of care (Mauldon, Leibowitz, Buchanan, Damberg, & McGuigan, 1994). A synthesis of this generation of studies comparing access and use under fee-for-service or managed care arrangements showed that the care models produced mixed results (Szilagyi & Schor, 1998).

Health services researchers have identified ways that managed care organizations' lack of experience with comprehensive delivery systems for children, and their tendency to control rather than coordinate services, could jeopardize care for children with chronic illness (Szilagyi, 2012). Managed care arrangements are largely untested across all states in terms of their ability to cost-effectively manage the care of vulnerable publicly insured children. Many children with special health needs (such as serious medical conditions) or with special circumstances (foster children and homeless children) have been excluded from studies of health outcomes, use, or costs. Even when included in such studies, they often make up such a small proportion of the study sample that evaluation of the impact of managed care on their health outcomes is impossible. In addition, many publicly insured children with complex chronic conditions receive care from multiple public programs, including Medicaid and Title V, that maintain direct public program authorization for health services. It is thus difficult to generalize about how different payment mechanisms influence health care quality for subpopulations of children.

Early studies described the types of access barriers that children with special health needs might confront within a managed care organization. National surveys of pediatricians identified high rates of denied specialty referrals for children (Cartland & Yudkowsky, 1992). Inclusion of pediatric providers in health plans is an ongoing concern. Early studies of managed care for children with special health care needs suggested that managed care plans limit mental health and related services, as well as access to specialists (Szilagyi, 2012). National surveys on health care access and quality for children with special health care needs show that parents experience problems obtaining specialty referrals, although only about 5 percent of children ultimately do not receive the specialty care that parents believe they need (Inkelas, Smith, Kuo, Rudolph, & Igdaloff, 2005).

As managed care expanded in the U.S. health system, priorities for research on the outcomes and effectiveness in such systems were outlined (McGlynn & Halfon, 1998). However, it is not only differences between enrolled populations that make comparison difficult for children. Variation in managed care structures, benefits, and implementation across regions makes it difficult to generalize experience within one region or study to other localities. For example, a survey of state Medicaid programs showed a variety of mixed financing arrangements affecting children's services, including medical and behavioral health contracts, service exclusion, and diagnosis exclusion (Holahan, Rangarajan, & Schirmer, 1999). In the absence of generalizable findings about managed care impact, certain important focus areas for oversight of managed care contractors include specificity of pediatric service benefits, requirements for pediatric providers contracting within networks, medical necessity standards tailored for children, quality indicators for children, appropriate payment rates for pediatric services, and promotion of high-quality care. It is important (but a complex undertaking) to evaluate how contracting arrangements affect care for children. Early studies of Medicaid managed care focused on the difference between fee-for-service and managed care arrangements, rather than on difference within managed care systems (Szilagyi, 1998). As coverage increases for U.S. children, there is greater opportunity to study how organizational approaches influence care processes and health outcomes.

From Managed Care Organizations to HDOs

New forms of managed health care must be created to overcome obstacles to comprehensive and coordinated systems of health services for high-risk children and families. This could take the form of social HMOs, or *health development organizations* (HDOs). The social HMO concept was designed to augment vertically integrated medical services with additional health promotion, social services, and enhanced coordination mechanisms to produce appropriate horizontal integration (Halfon & Berkowitz, 1993). Demonstration project social HMOs for the frail and elderly population offered multifaceted risk assessment and an inclusive set of services, resources, case management, and coordination (Newacheck, Hughes, Halfon, & Brindis, 1997). Evaluation of social HMOs for the elderly produced mixed outcomes (Leutz, Greenlick, & Capitman, 1994), but the

FIGURE 18.2. HOW RISK-REDUCTION AND HEALTH-PROMOTION STRATEGIES INFLUENCE HEALTH DEVELOPMENT

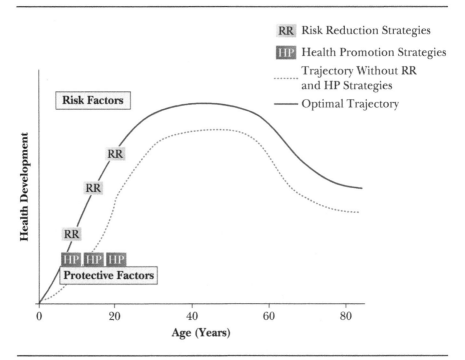

Note: This figure illustrates how risk-reduction strategies can mitigate the influence of risk factors on the developmental trajectory and how health promotion strategies can simultaneously support and optimize the development trajectory. In the absence of effective risk reduction and health promotion, the developmental trajectory is suboptimal (dotted curve). *Source:* Halfon et al., 2000.

social HMO concept represents one approach with the goal of maximizing the fit between the true health needs of children and an appropriately constructed and integrated delivery system.

An extension of the social HMO concept has been termed a health development organization (Halfon et al., 2000). The HDO framework creates a mechanism to integrate services not only vertically and horizontally but longitudinally as well, to optimize the health development trajectory of children. HDOs would actively develop the health of the child population by using principles and practices that optimize health development trajectories. These include minimizing the influence of risk factors during a critical developmental period through targeted risk reduction and strategic use of health promotion and other protective factors. This is illustrated in Figure 18.2. The accountable care organization (ACO) concept is consistent with the goal of the HDO, but the horizontal and longitudinal integration that is necessary to mitigate risks for children is unique to the HDO approach.

Future Directions

There is opportunity during this time of great financial and structural change to fashion more efficient delivery systems. Sufficient attention should be paid to the unique needs of children and to designing a system that meets children's needs. Insurance coverage is important but insufficient to ensure basic health care quality for children generally or for special populations. The move to organizational approaches that emphasize accountability for health outcomes may facilitate some of the changes that are necessary to improve services delivered to children, if essential components and safeguards are included. Care improvement and innovation may occur increasingly through emerging, virtual structures such as national provider collaboratives (Margolis et al., 2010). Policymakers, health care providers, and the public at large have to consider how to ensure that children's unique needs are met under the evolving health system if health outcomes are to be improved.

SUMMARY

Children in the United States experience a system that can offer the latest medical advances but is fragmented, complex, and often means-tested. The evolution of the U.S. health care system into distinct sectors, with fragmented services and categorical funding mechanisms, poses a significant barrier to improved organization of care. Improving the health care delivery system for children means integrating the activities of largely publicly funded community-based health services with privately delivered managed care models. A number of efforts seek to build on growing knowledge to improve the health-promoting and risk-reduction orientation of the child health system. Population-based, integrated models of service delivery systems have been developed in European nations and in localized demonstration projects in the United States. Most European countries offer universal health, developmental, and social services to children beginning at conception, including nationally insured health care, maternity leave and support, and child care and development programs (Kahn & Kamerman, 1992). Because the United States has experienced a more incremental and market-based evolution of service systems, aligning incentives for health promotion among multiple public and private sectors is a more complicated challenge.

The U.S. health care system continues to produce many important innovations in addressing the special medical and developmental needs of children. Using managed care to rationalize delivery of personal medical services may substantially improve children's access to basic medical care. Multiple reports from the IOM suggest that the health care system should not only be focused on diagnostic, treatment, and rehabilitation services but also improve the availability and performance of disease and disability prevention, health promotion, and developmental optimization services. This requires better measurement strategies to document service system needs and performance; service system reform strategies that can reengineer service pathways to better integrate personal health, public health, and population health sector services; financing strategies that can facilitate and incentivize provision of these services; and efforts by states and local communities to implement these strategies.

KEY TERMS

Dependency refers to children's reliance on parents to provide positive environments and on their parents and the health system to identify and respond to concerns

Developmental vulnerability refers to the rapid and cumulative changes that are unique to children and that establish a life-course pattern for health in adulthood.

Differential morbidity refers to less prevalent, congenital, and rare conditions in children and to the range of complex problems with a social component such as foster care and prenatal substance exposure.

Health The Institute of Medicine defines it as the extent to which individuals are able to develop and realize their potential. In contrast to prior definitions of health that focused on an initial endowment of health, this shows the potential of childhood experiences to promote or adversely affect the development of health and well-being, with lifelong impact.

Health development organization is a framework for integrating services vertically (from prevention to treatment), horizontally (between medical and health-related services), and longitudinally (over time), to meet the health development needs of children.

DISCUSSION QUESTIONS

1. Publicly funded medical insurance for children has followed an incremental model. How has this affected public coverage options for children? What challenges does this create for state governments?
2. What particular challenges does the United States face in organizing health care for children, as compared to health care for adults?
3. A major barrier to identifying cost-effective strategies for promoting children's health is the fact that benefits of early investments in health accrue over the life course. What challenges does this create?
4. The Institute of Medicine defines health potential as the development of assets and positive aspects of health. Discuss the challenges that managed care organizations face in promoting health using this definition and outline several financing or organizational options for pursuing such a strategy.

FURTHER READING

Acton, J. D., & Kotagal, U. (2005). Improvements in healthcare: How can we change the outcome? *Journal of Pediatrics, 147*(3), 279–281.

This article presents key principles for improving health care quality and organization of care for children.

Boivin, M., & Hertzman, C. (Eds.). (2012). *Early childhood development: Adverse experiences and developmental health.* Royal Society of Canada: Canadian Academy of Health Sciences Expert Panel (with Ronald Barr, Thomas Boyce, Alison Fleming, Harriet MacMillan, Candice Odgers, Marla Sokolowski, & Nico Trocmé). Ottawa, ON: Royal Society of Canada. Available from https://rsc-src.ca/sites/default/files/pdf/ECD%20Report_0.pdf

This report provides the theory and highlights of the sciences underlying the life-course perspective.

Committee on Evaluation of Children's Health & National Research Council. (2004). *Children's health, the nation's wealth: Assessing and improving child health.* Washington, DC: National Academies Press.

This book presents a conceptual framework for child health, with implications for health measurement, interventions, financing, and organization of care.

REFERENCES

Barnett, W. S., & Escobar, C. M. (1992). Economic costs and benefits of early intervention. In S. J. Meisels & J. P. Shonkoff (Eds.), *Handbook of early childhood intervention.* New York: Cambridge University Press.

Berman, S., Dolins, J., Tang, S. F., & Yudkowsky, B. (2002). Factors that influence the willingness of private primary care pediatricians to accept more Medicaid patients. *Pediatrics, 110*(2), 239–248.

Bronfenbrenner, U. (1979). *The ecology of human development: Experiments by nature and design.* Cambridge, MA: Harvard University Press.

Brooks-Gunn, J., McCarton, C. M., Casey, P. H., McCormick, M. C., Bauer, C. R., Bernbaum, J. C., . . . Meinert, C. (1994). Early intervention in low-birth-weight premature infants: Results through age 5 years from the Infant Health and Development Program. *The Journal of the American Medical Association, 272*(16), 1257–1262.

Carnegie Task Force on Meeting the Needs of Young Children. (1994). *Starting points: Meeting the needs of our youngest children.* New York: Carnegie Corporation of New York.

Cartland, J. D., & Yudkowsky, B. K. (1992). Barriers to pediatric referral in managed care systems. *Pediatrics, 89*(2), 183–192.

Chang, R. K., & Halfon, N. (1997). Geographic distribution of pediatricians in the United States: An analysis of the fifty states and Washington, DC. *Pediatrics, 100*(2 Pt 1), 172–179.

Child Welfare League of America. (1988). *Standards for health care services for children in out-of-home care.* Washington, DC: Child Welfare League of America.

Costello, E. J. (1986). Primary care pediatrics and child psychopathology: A review of diagnostic, treatment, and referral practices. *Pediatrics, 78*(6), 1044–1051.

Daley, K. C. (2004). Update on sudden infant death syndrome. *Current Opinion in Pediatrics, 16*(2), 227–232.

Davidoff, A. J., Garrett, B., & Schirmer, M. (2000, September). Children eligible for Medicaid but not enrolled: How great a policy concern? *(Series A, No. A-41).* Washington, DC: The Urban Institute.

DuPlessis, H. M., Inkelas, M., & Halfon, N. (1998). Assessing the performance of community systems for children. *Health Services Research, 33*(4 Pt 2), 1111–1142.

Ellwood, M. (1999). *The Medicaid eligibility maze: Coverage expands, but enrollment problems persist* (Occasional Paper No. 30). Washington, DC: The Urban Institute. Retrieved from http://newfederalism.urban.org/pdf/occa30.pdf

Employee Benefit Research Institute. (1993). *Sources of health insurance and characteristics of the uninsured: Analysis of the March 1992 Current Population Survey* (Report No. 133). Washington, DC: Author.

Fielding, J., & Halfon, N. (1994). Where is the health in health system reform? *Journal of the American Medical Association, 272*(16), 1292–1296.

Forrest, C. B., Simpson, L., & Clancy, C. (1997). Child health services research: Challenges and opportunities. *Journal of the American Medical Association, 277*(22), 1787–1793.

Freund, D. A., Rossiter, L. F., Fox, P. D., Meyer, J. A., Hurley, R. E., Carey, T. S., & Paul, J. E. (1989). Evaluation of the Medicaid competition demonstrations. *Health Care Financing Review, 11*(2), 81–97.

Green, M. (Ed.). (1994). *Bright futures: National guidelines for health supervision of infants, children, and adolescents.* Arlington, VA: National Center for Education in Maternal and Child Health.

Haggerty, R. J., Roghmann, K. J., & Pless, I. B. (1975). *Child health and the community.* New York: Wiley.

Halfon, N., & Berkowitz, G. (1993). Health care entitlements for children: Providing health services as if children really mattered. In M. A. Jensen & S. G. Goffin (Eds.), *Visions of entitlement: The care and education of America's children.* Albany, NY: SUNY Press.

Halfon, N., & Hochstein, M. (2002). Life course health development: An integrated framework for developing health, policy, and research. *Milbank Quarterly, 80*(3), 433–479.

Halfon, N., Inkelas, M., & Hochstein, M. (2000). The health development organization: An organizational approach to achieving child health development. *Milbank Quarterly, 78*(3), 447–497.

Halfon, N., Inkelas, M., & Newacheck, P. W. (1999). Enrollment in the State Child Health Insurance Program: A conceptual framework for evaluation and continuous quality improvement. *Milbank Quarterly, 77*(2), 181–204.

Halfon, N., Inkelas, M., & Wood, D. (1995). Nonfinancial barriers to care for children and youth. *Annual Review of Public Health, 16*, 447–472.

Halfon, N., Newacheck, P. W., Wood, D. L., & St Peter, R. F. (1996). Routine emergency department use for sick care by children in the United States. *Pediatrics, 98*(1), 28–34.

Halfon, N., Regalado, M., Sareen, H., Inkelas, M., Reuland, C. H., Glascoe, F. P., & Olson, L. M. (2004). Assessing development in the pediatric office. *Pediatrics, 113*(6 Suppl), 1926–1933.

Hertzman, C. (1994). The lifelong impact of childhood experiences: A population perspective. *Proceedings of the American Academy of Arts and Sciences, Daedalus: Health and Wealth, 123*(4), 167–180.

Holahan, J., Rangarajan, S., & Schirmer, M. (1999). Medicaid managed care payment rates in 1998. *Health Affairs, 18*(3), 217–227.

Holl, J. L., Szilagyi, P. G., Rodewald, L. E., Byrd, R. S., & Weitzman, M. L. (1995). Profile of uninsured children in the United States. *Archives of Pediatrics and Adolescent Medicine, 149*(4), 398–406.

Horwitz, S. M., Kelleher, K. J., Stein, R. E., Storfer-Isser, A., Youngstrom, E. A., Park, E. R.,...Hoagwood, K. E. (2007). Barriers to the identification and management of psychosocial issues in children and maternal depression. *Pediatrics, 119*(1), e208–e218.

Hughes, D. C., & Luft, H. S. (1998). Managed care and children: An overview. *The Future of Children, 8*(2), 25–38.

Inkelas, M., Smith, K. A., Kuo, A. A., Rudolph, L., & Igdaloff, S. (2005). Health care access for children with special health care needs in California. *Maternal and Child Health Journal, 9*(2), S109–S116.

Kahn, A. J., & Kamerman, S. B. (1992). *Integrating services integration: An overview of initiatives, issues, and possibilities.* New York: National Center for Children in Poverty, Columbia University School of Public Health.

Kaiser Commission on Medicaid and the Uninsured. (2004, November). *Health insurance coverage in America: 2003 data update.* Washington, DC: Kaiser Family Foundation.

Kaiser Family Foundation. (2004). Medicaid managed care enrollees as a percent of state Medicaid enrollees, as of December 31, 2004. Retrieved from http://www.statehealthfacts.org

Karoly, L. A., Greenwood, P. W., Everingham, S. S., Hoube, J., Kilburn, M. R., Rydell, C. P.,...Chiesa, J. (1998). *Investing in our children: What we know and don't know about the costs and benefits of early childhood interventions.* Santa Monica, CA: RAND Corporation.

Kronebusch, K., & Elbel, B. (2004). Simplifying children's Medicaid and SCHIP. *Health Affairs, 23*(3), 233–246.

Kuh, D., Ben-Shlomo, Y., Lynch, J., Hallqvist, J., & Power, C. (2003). Life course epidemiology. *Journal of Epidemiology and Community Health, 57*(10), 778–783.

Leutz, W. N., Greenlick, M. R., & Capitman, J. A. (1994). Integrating acute and long-term care. *Health Affairs, 13*(4), 58–74.

Margolis, P. A., DeWalt, D. A., Simon, J. E., Horowitz, S., Scoville, R., Kahn, N.,...Miles, P. (2010). Designing a large-scale multilevel improvement initiative: The improving performance in practice program. *Journal of Continuing Education in the Health Professions, 30*(3), 187–196.

Mauldon, J., Leibowitz, A., Buchanan, J. L., Damberg, C., & McGuigan, K. A. (1994). Rationing or rationalizing children's medical care: Comparison of a Medicaid HMO with fee-for-service care. *American Journal of Public Health, 84*(6), 899–904.

McGlynn, E. A., & Halfon, N. (1998). Overview of issues in improving quality of care for children. *Health Services Research, 33*(4 Pt 2), 977–1000.

National Research Council and Institute of Medicine. (2004). *Children's health, the nation's wealth: Assessing and improving child health.* Committee on Evaluation of Children's Health. Board on Children, Youth, and Families, Division of Behavioral and Social Sciences and Education. Washington, DC: The National Academies Press.

Needlman, R., & Silverstein, M. (2004). Pediatric interventions to support reading aloud: How good is the evidence? *Journal of Developmental and Behavioral Pediatrics, 25*(5), 352–363.

Newacheck, P. W. (1992). Characteristics of children with high and low usage of physician services. *Medical Care, 30*(1), 30–42.

Newacheck, P. W., & Halfon, N. (1986). The association between mother's and children's use of physician services. *Medical Care, 24*(1), 30–38.

Newacheck, P. W., Halfon, N., & Inkelas, M. (2000a). Commentary: Monitoring expanded health insurance for children: Challenges and opportunities. *Pediatrics, 105*(4 Pt 2), 1004–1007.

Newacheck, P. W., Hughes, D. C., & Cisternas, M. (1995). Children and health insurance: An overview of recent trends. *Health Affairs, 14*(1), 244–254.

Newacheck, P. W., Hughes, D. C., Halfon, N., & Brindis, C. (1997). Social HMOs and other capitated arrangements for children with special health care needs. *Maternal and Child Health Journal, 1*(2), 111–119.

Newacheck, P. W., Hughes, D. C., Hung, Y. Y., Wong, S., & Stoddard, J. J. (2000b). The unmet health needs of America's children. *Pediatrics, 105*(4 Pt 2), 989–997.

Newacheck, P. W., Hughes, D. C., & Stoddard, J. J. (1996). Children's access to primary care: Differences by race, income, and insurance status. *Pediatrics, 97*(1), 26–32.

Olds, D. L., Eckenrode, J., Henderson, C. R., Kitzman, H., Powers, J., Cole, R.,... Luckey, D. (1997). Long-term effects of home visitation on maternal life course and child abuse and neglect—fifteen-year follow-up of a randomized trial. *Journal of the American Medical Association, 278*(8), 637–643.

Olson, L. M., Tang, S. F., & Newacheck, P. W. (2005). Children in the United States with discontinuous health insurance coverage. *New England Journal of Medicine, 353*(4), 382–391.

Orr, S. T., Charney, E., & Straus, J. (1988). Use of health-services by black children according to payment mechanism. *Medical Care, 26*(10), 939–947.

Robert Wood Johnson Foundation. (2005, August). *Going without: America's uninsured children.* Prepared for the Robert Wood Johnson Foundation by the State Health Access Data Assistance Center and the Urban Institute. Washington, DC: Author.

Schechter, M. S. (2003). Non-genetic influences on cystic fibrosis lung disease: The role of sociodemographic characteristics, environmental exposures, and healthcare interventions. *Seminars in Respiratory and Critical Care Medicine, 24*(6), 639–652.

Schlesinger, M., & Eisenberg, L. (1990). Little people in a big policy world: Lasting questions and new directions in health policy for children. In M. Schlesinger & L. Eisenberg (Eds.), *Children in a changing health system: Assessments and proposals for reform.* Baltimore: Johns Hopkins University Press.

Shaywitz, S. E., & Shaywitz, B. A. (2003). Dyslexia (specific reading disability). *Pediatrics in Review, 24*(5), 147–153.

Short, P. F., & Lefkowitz, D. C. (1992). Encouraging preventive services for low-income children: The effect of expanding Medicaid. *Medical Care, 30*(9), 766–780.

St Peter, R. F., Newacheck, P. W., & Halfon, N. (1992). Access to care for poor children. Separate and unequal? *Journal of the American Medical Association, 267*(20), 2760–2764.

Starfield, B. (2000). Evaluating the State Children's Health Insurance Program: Critical considerations. *Annual Review of Public Health, 21*, 569–585.

Starfield, B., Cassady, C., Nanda, J., Forrest, C. B., & Berk, R. (1998). Consumer experiences and provider perceptions of the quality of primary care: Implications for managed care. *Journal of Family Practice, 46*(3), 216–226.

Starfield, B., & Newacheck, P. W. (1990). Children's health status, health risks, and use of health services. In M. J. Schlesinger & L. Eisenberg (Eds.), *Children in a changing health system.* Baltimore: Johns Hopkins University Press.

Szilagyi, P. G. (1998). Managed care for children: Effect on access to care and utilization of health services. *The Future of Children, 8*(2), 39–59.

Szilagyi, P. G. (2012). Health insurance and children with disabilities. *The Future of Children, 22*(1), 123–148.

Szilagyi, P. G., & Schor, E. L. (1998). The health of children. *Health Services Research, 33*(4 Pt 2), 1001–1039.

Tang, S. S. (2005, July). *Children's health insurance fact sheet.* Elk Grove, IL: American Academy of Pediatrics.

U.S. Department of Health and Human Services. (2010). Connecting kids to coverage: Continuing the progress. 2010 CHIPRA Annual Report. Washington, DC: Author.

U.S. Department of Labor. (1993). *Employee benefits in medium and large establishments* (Bulletin 2422). Washington, DC: Bureau of Labor Statistics.

U.S. General Accounting Office. (1993). *Medicaid: States turn to managed care to improve access and control costs* (GAO/HRD-93-46). Washington, DC: U.S. Government Printing Office.

Valdez, R. (1986). *The effects of cost sharing on the health of children* (RAND Publication No. R-3720-HHS). Santa Monica, CA: RAND Corporation.

Wood, D. L., Corey, C., Freeman, H. E., & Shapiro, M. F. (1992). Are poor families satisfied with the medical care their children receive? *Pediatrics, 90*(1 Pt 1), 66–70.

CHAPTER NINETEEN

HOMELESS PERSONS

Lisa Arangua
Lillian Gelberg

Learning Objectives

- Learn about homeless health status and use of health services
- Understand the health differences between homeless persons and low-income housed persons
- Recognize the reasons the homeless population almost inevitably harbors society's most devastating diseases and emerging diseases at high rates
- Learn that any policy response to the health of the homeless must consider an integrative approach that combines structural factors (situational context in which health is influenced and occurs) and individual factors (risk factors and vulnerabilities, such as risky behavior, that influence health)

Homelessness has reached crisis proportions in the United States today. An estimated 2.3 to 3.5 million people are currently without a home (U.S. Interagency Council on Homelessness, 2010; Cortes et al., 2011). Although the homeless are a growing and especially needy population, they are in some ways disturbingly similar to the rest of us. The majority live in central cities, but 21 percent live in suburban areas and 9 percent in rural areas (Burt et al., 1999). Los Angeles is known as the homeless capital, although some would argue that New York holds this infamous distinction. Most of the homeless persons of Los Angeles are long-time residents of the city and are similar to housed persons in their place of birth, citizenship status, and length of residence in Los Angeles County (with 86 percent living in Los Angeles for ten years or more) (Cousineau, 2001). This chapter profiles the homeless, examines their health status and access to health care, and proposes an integrative approach for homeless health policy.

A Profile of the Homeless

Whereas in the recent past the homeless population consisted primarily of middle-aged alcoholic white men, the distant past has become prologue to the current demographic profile of a homeless population that includes women and children as well as men. About two-thirds of the currently homeless are single men (67 percent) and 20 percent are single women (Burt et al., 1999). Further, 34 percent of homeless women and 8 percent of homeless men are currently married (Koegel & Burnam, 1991). Fifteen percent of homeless persons are parents with children (Burt et al., 1999). Sixty percent of homeless women and 41 percent of homeless men have at least one minor child, but of them only 39 percent of women and 3 percent of men currently have those children with them (Burt et al., 1999).

A majority of the currently homeless are between the ages of twenty-five and forty-four. Most homeless children (62 percent) are under the age of eight. Only 1 percent of the homeless are unaccompanied youths or teen parents under the age of eighteen, and only 2 percent are older than sixty-five (O'Connell et al., 2004). However, recent research suggests that the homeless population is aging. In the 1990s, the average age of the homeless was mid-thirties, whereas in 2003 the average age was mid-forties. Older street-dwelling homeless persons have a high mortality rate (30 percent of these sixty-plus-year-olds died within the four-year observation period), raising issues of competency and guardianship to protect them (O'Connell et al., 2004). With the expected doubling of the elderly in the general population over the next few decades, we can expect a doubling of the elderly in the homeless population as well.

About 23 percent of homeless persons are veterans (Burt et al., 1999). Male veterans are at increased risk for homelessness (male veterans have 1.25 the odds of being homeless relative to male nonveterans) (Gamache, Rosenheck, & Tessler, 2001), and post–Vietnam era male veterans are most at risk for homelessness (Rosenheck, Frisman, & Chung, 1994). Women veterans have a much greater risk of homelessness (two to four times the odds of women nonveterans), and it was the Vietnam-era women veterans who were most at risk for homelessness (Gamache et al., 2003). The effect on onset of homelessness among men and women who have served in the military in more recent wars remains to be determined.

Homeless persons are severely lacking in the educational and financial resources necessary to access health care. Thirty-nine percent have not graduated from high school, 34 percent have a high school diploma or general educational development (GED), and 28 percent have some post–high school education (Burt et al., 1999). Further, in 1996 the mean monthly income for homeless families was $475, 46 percent of the federal poverty line for a family of three. Single homeless persons reported a mean monthly income of $348, 51 percent of the federal poverty level for one person (Burt et al., 1999). Despite their low income, only 28 percent of homeless persons receive income maintenance (Burt et al., 1999). Further, 55 percent do not have medical insurance, compared to 32 percent of formerly homeless persons and 17 percent of the general population (Burt et al., 1999).

From a public policy standpoint, it is important to distinguish between the incidence and the course of homelessness (Phelan & Link, 1999). Half of the homeless population may be considered newly homeless (homeless one year or less), and one-fifth are long-term homeless (more than two years) (Burt et al., 1999). The distinction between homeless and nonhomeless-impoverished is not a clear one, since people cycle in and out of homelessness during their lifetime (Koegel, 1992). However, most preventive policies have focused on the conditions of the long-term homeless (mental illness, substance abuse, and criminal activity), a population overrepresented in enumeration samples of homeless persons. The consequences of focusing on the long-term homeless are not only punitive policies that attribute social problems to individual shortcomings, as the history of homeless policies attests to, but policies that have limited impact on the incidence of homelessness. This distinction between long-term and short-term homelessness redirects policy to focus on variations in the homeless population—why people become homeless, why some cycle in and out of homelessness, and why some remain homeless for a long period of time—rather than focusing on providing housing as a first step (Phelan & Link, 1999). For example, in New York City shelters, even though recurrent shelter stays for homeless women were related to (1) a history of domestic violence, (2) young women giving birth within the past year, (3) having young children, or (4) having children who are not with their mother or who join or leave their mother while she is in a shelter, it was having permanent housing of their own that constituted the strongest protection against cycling back into homelessness (Metraux & Culhane, 1999).

The shortage of adequate affordable housing is the major precipitating factor for homelessness. The theory is that increases in income inequality working through the housing market are the root cause of homelessness, according to economists from the Public Policy Institute of California. A greater number of poor people creates more demand for low-cost and low-quality housing, which drives up the prices of such housing. "The resulting higher rents for abandonment-quality housing imply a higher cut-off income, below which homelessness is preferred to conventional housing" (Quigley, Raphael, & Smolensky, 2001).

Unemployment, personal or family life crisis, rent going up out of proportion to inflation, and reduction in public benefits can also directly result in the loss of a home (Mojtabai, 2005). Early findings on the impact of recent federal welfare reform policies show that reduction or elimination of public assistance benefits resulted in homelessness (Nunez & Cox, 1999). Illness, on the other hand, tends to result from the homeless condition. Evidence has shown that persons with longer percentage of their lifetime spent homeless have worse health, compared to those with less percentage of their lifetime spent homeless (Arangua, Andersen, & Gelberg, 2005). Other indirect precipitants of homelessness are deinstitutionalization from a public mental hospital, substance abuse, and overcrowded prisons and jails from which prisoners who are not self-sufficient are often released (Brickner et al., 1985). Vangeest and Johnson (2002) offer empirical evidence to support this finding that substance abuse is not linked to homelessness directly but rather indirectly through greater disaffiliation from society (less support from family and friends, and lack of employment). Once homeless, substance abusers' social disaffiliation may continue to hamper their ability to become housed again (Zlotnick, Tam, & Robertson, 2003b).

Reasons for homelessness among older adults (age fifty or more) are remarkably stable over various locations (Boston in the United States; England; Melbourne, Australia): their homes were sold or needed repair, they fell behind in rent payments, a close relative died or a relationship was lost, there were tenant-neighbor disputes. As with other homeless populations, indirect causes of older persons' loss of their home included physical, mental, and alcohol problems, along with gambling problems (primarily in Australia). They became homeless through individual vulnerabilities as well as structural vulnerabilities such as welfare policy and gaps in service delivery.

Surprisingly, perceived reasons for homelessness do not differ for those who have mental illness compared to other homeless persons, suggesting that structural solutions, among them low-income housing and income support, might prevent homelessness for the mentally ill, as well as the rest of the homeless population (Mojtabai, 2005). However, on the basis of empirical correlates of homelessness, homeless persons with mental illness have "received a double dose of disadvantage—poverty with the addition of childhood instability [out-of-home placement] and violence [witnessed within the household or personally experienced violence]" (Mojtabai, 2005).

Health Status

Lack of housing affects the health of all homeless people, whether they are newly homeless, long-term homeless, formerly homeless, or episodically homelessness. Even relatively short bouts of homelessness expose individuals to severe deprivation (hunger and lack of adequate hygiene) and victimization (physical assault, robbery, or rape) (Link et al., 1994). The homeless—adults and children—have a high prevalence of untreated acute and chronic medical, mental health, and substance abuse problems. They are exposed to illness because of overcrowding in shelters and exposure to heat and cold (Fischer & Breakey, 1986). Further, sheltered homeless persons with substance abuse, mental health problems, or a physical disability encounter difficulty in successfully exiting the sheltered environment (Culhane & Kuhn, 1998).

A dearth of prospective longitudinal epidemiologic research (Shinn et al., 1998) makes it difficult to identify whether certain health conditions precede, cause, or result from the homeless condition. Some evidence has shown that newly homeless persons report significant medical and psychiatric problems before becoming homeless (Schanzer, Dominguez, Shrout, & Caton, 2007).

Moreover, research has found that unstable housing—such as extreme overcrowding, substandard housing (lack of heat or dilapidated living conditions), or loss of housing—contributes significantly to poor health outcomes, and that stable housing plays a critical role in improving these health conditions (Bauman, 1999).

The significant impact housing has on health produces striking differences in the health outcomes between the homeless and their housed counterparts. A significant gradient in health emerges when we compare the homeless to their poor but stably housed peers. Homeless mothers were more likely than poor but stably housed mothers to experience spousal abuse, child abuse, drug use, and mental health problems (Wood, Valdez, Hayashi, & Shen, 1990). In contrast, when we compare homeless mothers (living on the streets or in shelters) to their marginally housed peers (living temporarily in low-cost residential hotels, apartments, or private homes—doubling up with relatives or friends), a contrasting picture emerges. There is no significant difference in the mental and physical health of homeless mothers and their poor but marginally housed peers (Burt et al., 1999).

Physical Health

Homeless people are subject to the same risk factors for physical illness as the general population, but they may be exposed to excessive levels of such risk and also experience risk factors unique to homelessness. Risk factors include excessive use of alcohol, illegal drugs, and cigarettes; sleeping in an upright position (resulting in venous stasis and its consequences); extensive walking in poor-fitting shoes; and inadequate nutrition (Brickner et al., 1985).

Further, homelessness itself is physically dangerous. The homeless are at risk for assault and victimization, as well as exposure to the elements. Homeless people are at great risk of being victimized for lack of personal security, whether they live in a shelter or outdoors. Moreover, they are exposed to communicable diseases such as tuberculosis and common illnesses such as asthma and flu in the shelter environment (Fischer, Shapiro, Breakey, Anthony, & Kramer, 1986).

Consequently, the homeless have a much higher rate of physical illness than the general population. About 37 percent of homeless persons report having poor health, compared to 10 percent in the general population (Gallagher, Andersen, Koegel, & Gelberg, 1997). Among homeless persons, those who are older, women, people with less education, and those who indicate a physical or mental health condition are more likely to report their health status as fair or poor. Length of time homeless is negatively associated with perceived health status by homeless persons. One-third to one-half of homeless adults have at least one chronic condition (Burt et al., 1999). Thus, illness appears to be taking its toll, preventing some of the homeless from escaping their predicament. For example, one-quarter of homeless adults report that their poor health prevented them from working or going to school (Robertson & Cousineau, 1986).

Age-adjusted mortality is very high for homeless persons (Hwang, 2000). In Philadelphia, homeless men and women who were living in shelters or outdoors had 3.5 times the age-adjusted mortality rate as the general population. Among sheltered homeless families, who tend to exit the homeless condition quicker than single homeless adults, both homeless adults and children in these families experience higher rates of mortality than the general and low-income housed population (Kerker et al., 2011). However, of any homeless subgroup, white men were most likely to die (Hibbs et al., 1994). In New York City, homeless men and women living in shelters had two to three times the age-adjusted mortality rate as the general population of that city.

Contagious Diseases

Contagious diseases, such as tuberculosis (Brickner et al., 1985) and HIV infection (Zolopa et al., 1994), are much more common among the homeless than the general population. Prevention, diagnosis, and treatment of these diseases among homeless populations must be a high priority for health care, housing, and social service providers.

Tuberculosis. The prevalence of positive tuberculosis (TB) skin testing (test for lifetime exposure to tuberculosis) among homeless adults ranges from 21 percent in Palo Alto (Cheung et al., 2002) to 32 percent in San Francisco (Zolopa et al., 1994) and Los Angeles (Gelberg et al., 1997), to 43 percent in New York (McAdam et al., 1990). These rates of latent TB prevalence are three to six times greater than the 5 to 10 percent prevalence of TB infection among the general population (Des Prez & Heim, 1990). Active tuberculosis among the homeless aged twenty-five to forty-four may be as high as twenty times that of the general population (Brewer et al., 2001). The rate of active tuberculosis among men in a New York shelter clinic is 6 percent (McAdam, Brickner, & Glicksman, 1985); more than half of it is due to primary tuberculosis and not reactivation of old disease (Barnes et al., 1996).

Positive tuberculosis skin tests have been found to be related to duration of homelessness, living in crowded shelters or single-room occupancy hotels, and increasing age. Homeless persons with active tuberculosis were more likely than housed persons with this infection to be located in western and southern states; to be born in the United States; to be incarcerated at the time of diagnosis; to have alcohol abuse, injection, or noninjection drug use; and to be coinfected with HIV (34 percent). Further, they were more likely to be infectious, resulting in great risk to other homeless as well as housed persons (Haddad et al., 2005). Tuberculosis is harder to treat among the homeless because of the difficulty of screening, following, and maintaining tuberculosis treatment among this population and because many have multidrug-resistant organisms. However, several measures have been successful in curbing the spread of tuberculosis: annual screening of all homeless people to identify and treat cases with active disease and to reduce transmission to homeless as well as other persons; screening to identify and treat cases with latent disease to prevent reactivation disease; directly observed therapy to ensure completion of therapy and prevention of multidrug-resistant tuberculosis; and use of electronic medical records across systems of care to identify outbreaks of tuberculosis and to identify and treat those who have moved or were lost to follow-up whose tuberculosis treatment has not been completed.

Hepatitis C and B. Hepatitis C virus (HCV) is a serious infectious disease emerging in the homeless population with a frequency much greater than in the general population. Estimated lifetime rates of hepatitis C for the homeless are 22 percent in a convenience sample of homeless and impoverished adults in Los Angeles (Nyamathi, Robbins, et al., 2002a), 26 percent in a probability sample of homeless adults in the Skid Row of Los Angeles (Gelberg et al., 2012; Strehlow et al., 2012) 32 percent in a mobile medical clinic in Manhattan (Rosenblum et al., 2001), 42 percent (Cheung et al., 2002) to 44 percent (Desai, Rosenheck, & Agnello, 2003) among homeless veterans in VA domiciliary programs, and 50 percent among homeless male clinic patients in Los Angeles (Stein & Nyamathi, 2004). This is in contrast to the 1.8 percent prevalence of HCV infection in the United States (Alter et al., 1999). Among those who tested positive for HCV in a community epidemiological sample, 72 percent had no previous knowledge that they were positive (Stein, Andersen, Robertson, & Gelberg, 2012). Compared to homeless persons that did not test positive, those who were positive were more likely to be less educated, to not have a regular source of care, to not have case management, and had greater perceived bad health (Stein et al., 2012).

The major risk factor for HCV among the homeless is drug use, particularly injection drug use (Cheung et al., 2002). Other correlates of HCV in homeless male patients include sharing razors and toothbrushes, and receipt of tattoos (Stein & Nyamathi, 2004). Sexual transmission has not been found to be a risk factor for hepatitis C (Nyamathi, Dixon, et al., 2002b).

The homeless also inordinately experience hepatitis B (Klinkenberg et al., 2003), another serious disease affecting the liver. Rates of lifetime hepatitis B range from 23 percent in a Palo Alto (Cheung et al., 2002) and 34 percent in a Los Angeles VA domiciliary program (Gelberg, Robertson, et al., 2001b) to 47 percent in a mobile medical clinic in Manhattan (Rosenblum et al., 2001). Few homeless persons are vaccinated for hepatitis B, suggesting that immunization programs to cover adults are necessary.

HIV. HIV infection among the homeless is much more common than in the housed population. Studies reveal an HIV infection rate of 9 to 10.5 percent among San Francisco's homeless and marginally housed adults (Zolopa et al., 1994). Among the homeless in that city, HIV seroprevalence was 6.3 percent among women (Robertson, 2004), similar to the rate of 6.2 percent among homeless persons with comorbid mental illness and substance abuse (Klinkenberg et al., 2003). Risk factors for HIV infection include being black, injection drug use, and chronic homelessness (Robertson, Zlotnick, & Westerfelt, 1997). In contrast, HIV in the general population nationally is estimated at between 0.3 percent and 0.4 percent (McQuillan et al., 1997). The rate of HIV in homeless clinic populations varies greatly: 0.9 percent (1.3 percent for men and 0.1 percent for women) (Shlay et al., 1996) in a treatment sample of homeless clients of a primary care clinic in Denver, 15 percent among patients of a mobile medical clinic in Manhattan (Rosenblum et al., 2001), and 1.8 percent among homeless veterans in a VA domiciliary program (Cheung et al., 2002).

HIV is the major cause of death among the adult homeless population. In a treatment sample of 17,292 homeless adult clients of the Boston Health Care for the Homeless Program, AIDS was the leading cause of death among those age twenty-five to forty-four (Hwang, O'Connell, & Brennan, 1997). Not only does homelessness increase a person's risk for HIV ninefold, but HIV increases the risk for homelessness by three times. This suggests that both HIV prevention and homeless prevention programs must continue to target homeless populations with high-risk behaviors for HIV (Culhane, Golub, Kuhn, & Shpaner, 2001). Given their high risk factors for HIV, there need to be enhanced efforts to mass-screen homeless populations for HIV. Current (past twelve months) HIV testing rates range from 52 percent among homeless youths (DeRosa et al., 2001) and 57 percent among homeless persons with serious mental illness (Desai & Rosenheck, 2004) to 68 percent among homeless women (Herndon et al., 2003). Homeless persons must have screening for HIV and continuity of care that maximizes sustained antiretroviral therapy, thus reducing the risk of death for homeless persons with HIV (Riley et al., 2005).

Women's Health

Homeless women are severely lacking in health services. However, pregnancy and recent births are risk factors for becoming homeless (Weitzman, 1989). Despite their lack of a home, many homeless women have children; yet only 29 percent of homeless women with children under eighteen years of age had their children living with them. Substance abusers and the chronic homeless were least likely to have their children living with them (Zlotnick, Robertson, & Tam, 2003a).

Whereas many homeless women wish to have children, those interested in contraception often experienced significant barriers in their effort to prevent pregnancy. Among homeless women interviewed in Los Angeles, 41 percent had used no contraceptive method of any kind during the past year, although the average reported frequency of vaginal intercourse during that time was once per week (Gelberg, Leake, et al., 2001a). Fewer than 10 percent use condoms regularly, despite lifestyles that place them at great risk for AIDS and other sexually transmitted diseases (Shuler, Gelberg, & Davis, 1995). Many are willing to use long-term forms of birth control such as Depo-Provera. Fewer than 5 percent had ever used a female condom, but 38 percent of all homeless women and 73 percent of homeless youths said they were willing to try them (Gelberg, Leake, et al., 2001a). This suggests that the female condom might be an alternative to the male condom for homeless women in STD and pregnancy prevention. The most commonly cited deterrents to contraceptive use (mentioned by 20 to 27 percent of women) were side effects, fear of potential health risks, and partner's dislike of contraception and cost (Gelberg et al., 2002). Still, the opportunities for some kind of prevention are great. Among homeless family planning clinic users, 60 percent had a history of a sexually transmitted disease and 28 percent had a history of pelvic inflammatory disease (PID) (Brickner et al., 2011); among homeless women in the community 48 percent had a history of an STD and 22 percent had a history of PID (Gelberg, 2000; Gelberg, Leake, et al., 2001a).

Homeless women receive little cancer screening. Half of homeless women age forty or older received a clinical breast exam in the past year

(Long et al., 1998), compared to 77 percent of the general population. Further, 32 to 47 percent (Long et al., 1998) of homeless women age forty or older living in California received a mammogram in the past year, compared to 73 percent of housed women (Chau et al., 2002). Further, 54 percent (Long et al., 1998) to 55 percent (Chau et al., 2002) of homeless women in California received a Pap smear in the past year, compared to 77 percent of women in the U.S. general population and 67 percent in the California general population (Chau et al., 2002). Lower use of Pap smears is alarming given that a history of abnormal Pap smears was reported by 23 percent of homeless family planning clinic users (Shuler, 1991) and 26 percent of homeless women sampled from the community (Lim et al., 2002).

Violence

Homeless persons in the United States suffer disproportionately from violent and abusive behavior. More than half of homeless individuals report having been criminally victimized while homeless (Burt et al., 1999), in contrast to 37 percent of the general population who have been victimized in the past year. Homeless men experience somewhat more recent physical victimization than homeless women (20 percent versus 18 percent, respectively). However, homeless women experience considerably more recent sexual violence (9 percent versus 1 percent, respectively) (Burt et al., 1999). In one study, 13 percent of homeless women report being sexually assaulted or raped in the past year, compared to 2.7 percent of women in the general population (Wenzel, Leake, & Gelberg, 2000). Having housing, even marginal housing, reduced sexual violence among impoverished women (Kushel et al., 2003).

Homeless Youths

Current estimates of the number of homeless youths range from 100,000 to 500,000 (Dietz & Coburn, 1991). The 1999 Second National Incidence Studies of Missing, Abducted, Runaway, and Thrownaway Children (NISMART-2), a national household and juvenile facility probability survey, found that 1,682,900 youths had a runaway or throwaway episode in that year (Molina, 2005). Eight percent of adolescents in a nationally representative sample of youths reported they were homeless at least one night in the past twelve months (Ringwalt, Greene, Robertson, & McPheeters, 1998).

Youths become homeless largely as a result of persistent family dysfunction and conflict, specifically parental neglect, physical or sexual abuse, family substance abuse, and family violence (MacLean, Embry, & Cauce, 1999). However, many homeless youths are still in contact with their families. A large proportion of their social network is made up of family and friends, and they are receiving social support from their family and friends from home. The majority (65 percent) of newly homeless youths do return home within their first year of homelessness, usually to live with a parent (Milburn et al., 2005).

Given their homelessness and other life problems, it is not surprising that homeless youths suffer from mental health problems (Whitbeck et al., 2004). They include poor coping skills, suicidal tendencies, substance abuse (Van Leeuwen, Hopfer, & Hooks, 2004), depression, and other mental health problems that result in a high rate of psychiatric hospitalization (Roy et al., 2001). Mental disorder and victimization are especially high for LGBTU (lesbian, gay, bisexual, transgender, or unsure) homeless youths (Whitbeck et al., 2004). The rate of LGBTU persons among homeless youths is about 20 percent or higher in larger cities (Whitbeck et al., 2004). Many have experienced self-mutilation (69 percent) (Tyler, Cauce, & Whitbeck, 2004) and suffer from a high level of dissociative behavior (Tyler et al., 2004). Moreover, 28 percent of street youths and 10 percent of shelter youths have participated in survival sex (sold sex for food, clothing, or shelter) (Greene, Ennett, & Ringwalt, 1999).

Homeless youths also suffer from victimization and health problems that largely extend from their homeless condition. They experience an extremely high frequency of psychological maladjustment and victimization while homeless. Assault and robbery are reported by one-fourth to one-half of homeless youths, and rape in the past three months is reported by one in ten of these youths (MacLean et al., 1999).

Mental Illness and Substance Abuse

Alcohol, drug abuse, and mental health problems among the homeless dominate the research on homeless inquiry. More than three-quarters (86 percent) of the homeless have experienced at least one alcohol, drug, or mental health problem in their lifetime, with 57 percent having mental health problems, 62 percent having alcohol problems, and 58 percent having drug problems. Some evidence, albeit slight, suggests that early homeless experiences are predictive of drug use behavior (Johnson &

Fendrich, 2007). Psychiatric problems are also very common. Two-thirds of homeless individuals have experienced at least one alcohol problem (38 percent), drug problem (26 percent), or mental health (39 percent) problem during the past month (Burt et al., 1999). It appears that the prevalence of lifetime mood and substance use disorders (especially cocaine abuse among women) has increased since the 1980s (North, Eyrich, Pollio, & Spitznagel, 2004).

One-third of homeless adults suffer from current *serious mental illnesses* (SMIs)—schizophrenic disorders, affective disorders, personality or character disorders, and cognitive disorders—according to diagnostic data (Fischer, Shapiro, et al., 1986). Further, one-third have a substance abuse disorder (Fischer, Shapiro, et al., 1986). About 11 percent have schizophrenia, fewer than half of whom are currently receiving treatment (Folsom & Jeste, 2002). About 17 percent have a dual diagnosis of chronic mental illness and chronic substance use (Koegel & Burnam, 1988). These individuals pose a challenge to developing services that successfully address both aspects of their illness (Koegel, Burnam, & Farr, 1988). In addition to intrinsic illness processes, environmental stresses and homeless appearance must be considered so as to avoid inaccurate diagnosis of mental illness. These individuals may experience chronic isolation, geographical mobility, disturbed sleep, and fear of victimization; they may appear disheveled and show signs of lacking self-care, each of which could result in symptoms that might be taken for mental illness.

Suicide

Given the high frequency of suicide within the homeless population, there is evidence suggestive of a high prevalence of inadequately treated mental illness within this population: 25 percent of homeless adults considered committing suicide, and 7 percent attempted suicide during the preceding year (Robertson, Ropers, & Boyer, 1985). In a sample of veterans in an inpatient substance abuse rehabilitation program, women were more likely than homeless men to have suicidal ideation or to have made a suicide attempt (Benda, 2005).

Neuropsychological Impairment

Homeless persons commonly have *neuropsychological impairment,* some of which is related to a history of traumatic brain injury, mental illness, or substance abuse. Eighty percent of the homeless suffer cognitive impairment, and 20 percent suffer mental retardation (Solliday-McRoy et al., 2004). Both conditions can have a negative impact on treatment outcomes, especially for usual treatments, which are cognitively demanding. Further, nearly one-third had reading abilities at or below the fifth-grade level, suggesting that they lack sufficient basic skills to function in society (Solliday-McRoy et al., 2004).

Use of Physical Health Services

During the past year, 63 percent of homeless persons had an ambulatory care visit, 32 percent visited an emergency room, and 23 percent were hospitalized (Kushel, Vittinghoff, & Haas, 2001). However, 24 percent report they needed to see a doctor in the last year but were not able to (Burt et al., 1999), and 32 percent reported being unable to obtain prescribed medication (Kushel, Vittinghoff, & Haas, 2001). Moreover, their sources of health care use suggest inappropriate health care delivery. For example, more than half (57 percent) lack a regular source of care (a "medical home" has been acknowledged as an important indicator of access to medical care), compared to 24 percent of the poverty population in the United States and 19 percent of the general population (Gallagher et al., 1997). Homeless people with a regular source of care were two-thirds less likely to have gone without needed medical care than those without (Lewis, Andersen, & Gelberg, 2003), and homeless women with a regular source of care had more outpatient visits and preventive health screens (Lim et al., 2002).

The majority of the homeless seek care at places that do not offer continuous quality care. Of those who sought care in the past year, 32 percent report receiving medical care at a hospital emergency room, 27 percent at a hospital outpatient clinic, 21 percent at a community health center, 20 percent at a hospital as an inpatient, and 19 percent at a private doctor's office (Burt et al., 1999). Some hospitalizations and emergency room visits are appropriate, but the high rate of emergency room use and hospitalization in this young population suggests substitution of inpatient and emergency room care for outpatient ambulatory care services.

Homeless adults are more likely than the general population to have had a medical hospitalization during the preceding year. For example, a Hawaiian study found that their age- and sex-adjusted acute care hospitalization rate was 542 per 1,000 person-years compared to the general population rate of 96 per 1,000 person-years. In this study, homeless adults were admitted to acute care hospitals for 4,766 days compared to a predicted 640 days, resulting in costs of $2.8 million per year for excess hospitalization (Martell et al., 1992). Further, if hospitalized, homeless adults are most likely to be admitted to a general county hospital (Robertson & Cousineau, 1986).

Preventive Care

Homeless adults also have fewer preventive visits than the general population. For example, despite having greater risks for cancer, their screening rate was typically much lower than for the general population (Chau et al., 2002). Regarding colon cancer screening, homeless adults fifty years and older were less likely to have ever had a lower endoscopy (23 percent versus 47 percent for the general population), though they had a similarly low rate for fecal occult blood testing in the past year (19 percent versus 16 percent). As for prostate cancer screening, despite the fact that the majority of homeless men are African American and thus at higher risk for prostate cancer, homeless men fifty and older were much less likely to have had screening with a prostate-specific antigen blood test in the past year (11 percent versus 54 percent). In addition, very few homeless persons had ever been screened for skin cancer with a skin exam (24 percent ever; 15 percent past year). Homeless women have less breast and cervical cancer screening as well. This suggests that the homeless may delay seeking medical attention at a stage when severe illness could have been prevented.

Children and Youth

Even though sheltered youths are more likely to have a regular source of care than street youths (64 percent versus 50 percent), the rate is much lower than for their housed counterparts (85 percent) (Klein et al., 2000). Homeless adolescents use considerable emergent services that possibly could have been avoided with early primary care; one-quarter visited an emergency room and one-fifth were hospitalized in the preceding year. Only half have ever been tested for HIV.

We need to design health service programs that facilitate health access and health promotion for homeless adolescents. All are at risk for multiple health problems, but only 28 percent used medical care services in a year (McGuire, 2000). Compared to their poor but housed counterparts, homeless children are more likely to use ambulatory medical services (two or more emergency department visits during the past year and more outpatient visits for well and sick care), but they are also more likely to have been hospitalized in the past year (Almeida, Dubay, & Ko, 2001). These findings highlight not only the poor health status of young homeless persons, but also the need for programs for them that increase outreach efforts and improve the availability of and access to ongoing primary care services.

Use of Mental Health and Substance Abuse Services

As we have noted, mental illness and substance abuse are more prevalent among homeless people than the general population. Consequently, the majority (52 percent) of hospital admissions for homeless people were for treatment of substance abuse or mental illness, compared to 20 percent for other low-income patients (Salit et al., 1998). A large number (15 percent to 44 percent) of homeless adults report having had a previous psychiatric hospitalization (Koegel, Burnam, & Farr, 1988). The age- and sex-adjusted rate of admission of homeless persons to state psychiatric hospitals in Hawaii was 105 per 1,000 person-years, compared to the general population rate of 0.8 per 1,000 person-years (Martell et al., 1992).

Despite the high prevalence of current mental illness and prior psychiatric hospitalization, most of the homeless use existing outpatient mental health and substance abuse systems infrequently. Only 18 percent of homeless people in Baltimore's shelters had used outpatient mental health services during a six-month period (Fischer, Shapiro, et al., 1986), and the majority of those with a previous mental hospitalization had not made an outpatient mental health visit in the past five years (Gelberg, Linn, & Leake, 1988). Although 51 percent of homeless persons with chronic mental illness had used outpatient mental health services at some time in their life, only 14 percent had used these services in the past two months (Koegel et al., 1988). Seventy-three percent of homeless clients who report inpatient treatment for mental health problems received this treatment before they became homeless (Burt et al., 1999). These data suggest that homeless individuals who are mentally ill are in need of continuity of mental health services (Lamb & Bachrach, 2001), but are not receiving these services in an outpatient setting.

The data on lack of outpatient treatment are even more striking for outpatient substance abuse services. Only 26 percent of homeless persons with recent substance abuse problems (within the past six months) used outpatient services at some time in their life, compared to 43 percent who used inpatient services (Koegel et al., 1988). Moreover, about half (52 percent) of those with recent substance abuse dependence had received treatment from the formal substance abuse treatment delivery system (Koegel et al., 1988). Recent residential treatment (past two months) for substance abuse problems was far more common than recent outpatient treatment. Only 7 percent of homeless people with substance abuse problems used outpatient substance abuse services in the past two months, compared to 16 percent who used inpatient services during this time period (Koegel et al., 1988). Even when they did use inpatient or residential services, retention was difficult for those with the greatest need for treatment. Limited use of outpatient treatment, as well as lack of any treatment use among recent substance abusers, suggests that system-level characteristics may interfere with the homeless receiving the services they need. Outreach of mental health and substance abuse professionals to shelter settings is a start at improving access to care in dealing with mental illness and substance abuse problems among homeless persons (Bradford et al., 2005).

Barriers to Health Care

Compounding their increased risk for disease is evidence that homeless people encounter major obstacles to obtaining needed medical and psychiatric services. About 73 percent of homeless persons reported at least one past-year unmet need for health care, and 49 percent reported two or more unmet needs (Baggett, O'Connell, Singer, & Rigotti, 2010). Overall, 32 percent of homeless persons reported an unmet need for medical or surgical care in the preceding year, 36 percent reported an unmet need for prescription medications, 21 percent reported an unmet need for mental health care or counseling, 41 percent reported an unmet need for eyeglasses, and 41 percent reported an unmet need for dental care (Baggett et al., 2010).

More than half did not have a regular source of care (Gallagher et al., 1997). Among homeless women, one-third stated they had not obtained needed medical care during the past year (Lewis et al., 2003). Some homeless people do seek care for their health problems, but certain segments of the population are less likely to obtain care even if they are sick or have a regular source of care. Those living on the streets are the least likely of all the homeless to obtain outpatient visits and preventive health screens, and even hospital inpatient care, although they are most in need (Lim et al., 2002). Their situation is similar to the pre-Medicaid and Medicare era, when impoverished populations with acute illness had difficulty getting inpatient hospital care. Further, homeless adults with little education (Stein, Andersen, Koegel, & Gelberg, 2000) and without health insurance are less likely to seek care even if they are sick (Lim et al., 2002). People who are less likely to have a regular source of care are young, Hispanic, and do not have health insurance; they are long-term homeless (five or more years since last housed), have subsistence difficulties, and are socially isolated (Gallagher et al., 1997). The homeless with mental health problems were less likely to seek mental health services if they had not received mental health advice or a referral from a service provider outside the mental health system, or if they had an affective disorder (such as depression) (Koegel et al., 1988). Homeless persons with substance abuse problems were less likely to seek treatment for them if they did not get help accessing these services, spent more time in places that were not meant for sleeping, and lived in a service-poor environment (Koegel et al., 1988).

Homeless individuals face numerous problems in obtaining appropriate health care: cost, transportation, competing needs, mental illness, the homeless lifestyle, personal barriers, lack of availability of health services, medical provider bias, insufficient discharge planning from hospitals, lack of recuperative care, and so on.

Future Directions

Any policy response to the health of the homeless must consider an approach that combines structural factors (situational context in which health is influenced and occurs) and individual factors (risk factors and vulnerabilities, such as risky behavior, that influence health). The persistent and widening gap in health disparities among the homeless is largely the result of health policies that have been traditionally based on altering individual behavior as a means of improving the health circumstances of the homeless. However, this approach ignores the environmental and economic structures, social and cultural norms, and institutions that shape decision-making processes to facilitate and perpetuate patterns of behavior. An integrative approach combines individual and structural factors to probe beyond myopic models to broader motivational assumptions. This approach would examine such factors as refinement of housing codes to reflect current knowledge of healthful housing, adding measures of housing quality and satisfaction in local health department reports, the collaboration of public health representatives in local urban planning processes, and encouraging neighborhood collective efficacy and organizational participation to mobilize communities around issues of neighborhood and health conditions. In this sense, the *integrative model* can take a leading role in setting priorities for social, economic, and health policy to better promote health among society's most vulnerable members.

The National Institutes of Health (NIH) have been the largest funder of research on the homeless. For more than two decades, the NIH has invested millions of dollars in research that has amassed information on the composition, health needs, and health service use of the homeless population. The ultimate intent of this research has been to improve the health of the homeless. However, available research has not been translated into practice. Issues such as the large volume of conflicting research results, constraints on physicians' time, and lack of policies to foster implementation have served as barriers to translating research results into practical and sustaining practice.

The NIH Roadmap outlines translation of research advances using expanded research partnerships and integrated research networks in the context of a patient-centered approach, consistent with recent recommendations from the Institute of Medicine. The NIH Roadmap marks a paradigm shift in health research, from one that traditionally focused on homogeneous clinical and biological questions about the human organism to population-based interventions that deal with human behaviors, health priorities, economic and social structures, laws, and cultures that are heterogeneous across settings. The paradigm shifts largely resulted from research results that lacked relevance in the community setting and remain unaccepted by the communities that might benefit from them. Traditional terms of funding supports forced researchers to focus on generalizable research questions and results and then move onto the next project. Community engagement has become a strategic imperative within the new dominant paradigm of health research. The new paradigm requires community stakeholder involvement in the entire research process, which enables research priorities and research results to become more relevant and actionable in local situations for those who would apply them.

The integrative approach (structural and individual) to addressing issues of the health of the homeless effectively accommodates the new NIH paradigm for health research. The integrative approach offers a framework in which to focus research questions on the health of homeless persons, while the new NIH research paradigm imparts the structure for which answers to these research questions will be translated into practice within the community. Both the integrative model on homeless health issues and the new NIH research paradigm focus on a population health approach. These complementary models allow individuals from the community—clinical practitioners, policymakers, urban planners, and homeless people themselves—to (1) come together around a common purpose; (2) examine research questions about the homeless that involve individual behaviors and the political, environmental, economic, and social context; and (3) make decisions and develop confidence in their ability to solve their own problems. Ultimately, these complementary models will help develop much-needed information on which services work, for which homeless groups, in which communities, and at what costs—all critical elements for effective and economically efficient public policies regarding the homeless.

SUMMARY

According to Meyer and Schwartz (2000), "the study of social and economic factors in public health may have unintended consequences that, paradoxically, serve to preserve disparities rather than eliminate them. This can occur because public health research transports social issues into the health domain, where they are examined through the narrow prism of health relevance instead of within their political, social, and economic contexts. We refer to this as the 'public healthification' of social problems, akin to the 'medicalization' and 'healthism' that have occurred with the advance of biomedicine in the last century."

Perhaps of greatest concern is that our nation seems to have come to accept homelessness as just another negative aspect of modern life, similar in this way to violent crime. It is difficult for health policymakers to address the problems of the homeless population when public support for homeless people is weak at best. Perhaps advocates for the homeless have done a disservice by focusing on homeless people's medical, mental health, and substance abuse problems and needs, rather than on the core issues of lack of low-income housing and the breakdown of social cohesiveness and community relations in this country.

KEY TERMS

Integrative model combines individual and structural factors to address the challenges of the homeless. This approach incorporates such structural factors as refining housing codes, using measures of housing quality and satisfaction in local health department reports, promoting collaboration of public health representatives with local urban planning processes, and encouraging neighborhood collective action.

Neuropsychological impairment among the homeless, such impairment is often related to a history of traumatic brain injury, mental illness, or substance abuse. The homeless suffer high rates of cognitive impairment and mental retardation.

Serious mental illnesses (SMIs) schizophrenic disorders, affective disorders, personality or character disorders, and cognitive disorders.

DISCUSSION QUESTIONS

1. The homeless are subject to the same risk factors for physical illness as the general population, but they may be exposed to excessive levels of such risk and also experience risk factors unique to homelessness. Discuss some of the rates of physical illness and communicable disease among the homeless as compared to the general population. Apply the individual limitations perspective and the structuralist perspective to explain why the homeless have harbored physical illness and communicable diseases at such high rates.

2. The socioeconomic gradient in health—where even marginally higher socioeconomic position equates to better health—has historical underpinnings and is found for almost all diseases and many health risk behaviors. What does the evidence reveal about the gradient in health among the homeless and their poor but housed peers? Discuss the gradient in health within the homeless population.

3. The homeless are heavy users of health services, as compared to the general population, reflecting their substantial need for health care. Why is a preoccupation with health services serving as a magic bullet that prevents or cures the homeless of myriad adverse health conditions misguided? What are some of the structural (ecological and sociological) factors that affect health conditions and health outcomes that policymakers should consider?

FURTHER READING

Burt, M., Aron, L. Y., Lee, E., & Valente, J. (2001). *Helping America's homeless: Emergency shelter or affordable housing?* Washington, DC: The Urban Institute. http://www.urban.org/pubs/homeless/chapter1.html

This book examines the structural conditions and individual characteristics that affect homelessness and describes homeless people and homeless service systems across America toward the end of the 1990s. It is based on data from the National Survey of Homeless Assistance Providers and Clients (NSHAPC), conducted in 1996.

National Health Care for the Homeless Council. http://www.nhchc.org

This website provides research, training and education, and clinical resources for agencies, individuals, clinicians, and advocates who work to improve the health of homeless people.

The United States Interagency Council on the Homeless. http://www.ich.gov

The Interagency Council on the Homeless is responsible for creating the federal strategy and realize the president's commitment to end chronic homelessness in ten years. The council, which comprises twenty cabinet secretaries and agency heads, has forged a strategy of intraagency, interagency, intragovernmental, intergovernmental, and intercommunity collaborations to end homelessness. The website gives an overview of the council's policy efforts both locally and nationally to end homelessness.

REFERENCES

Almeida, R. A., Dubay, L. C., & Ko, G. (2001). Access to care and use of health services by low-income women. *Health Care Financing Review, 22,* 27–47.

Alter, M., Kruszon-Moran, D., Nainan, O. V., McQuillan, G. M., Gao, F., ... Margolis, H. S. (1999). The prevalence of hepatitis C virus infection in the United States, 1988 through 1994. *New England Journal of Medicine, 341,* 556–562.

Arangua, L., Andersen, R., & Gelberg, L. (2005). The health circumstances of homeless women in the United States. *International Journal of Mental Health, 34,* 62–92.

Baggett, T. P., O'Connell, J. J., Singer, D. E., & Rigotti, N. A. (2010). The unmet health care needs of homeless adults: A national study. *American Journal of Public Health, 100*(7), 1326–1333.

Barnes, P. F., El-Hajj, H., Preston-Martin, S., Cave, M. D., Jones, B. E., Otaya, M., ... Eisenach, K. D. (1996). Transmission of tuberculosis among the urban homeless. *Journal of the American Medical Association, 275,* 305–307.

Bauman, K. (1999). Shifting family definitions: The effect of cohabitation and other nonfamily household relationships on measures of poverty. *Demography, 36,* 315–325.

Benda, B. B. (2005). Gender differences in predictors of suicidal thoughts and attempts among homeless veterans that abuse substances. *Suicide and Life Threatening Behavior, 35,* 106–116.

Bradford, D. W., Gaynes, B. N., Kim, M. M., Kaufman, J. S., & Weinberger, M. (2005). Can shelter-based interventions improve treatment engagement in homeless individuals with psychiatric and/or substance misuse disorders? *Medical Care, 43,* 763–768.

Brewer, T., Heymann, S. J., Krumplitsch, S. M., Wilson, M. E., Colditz, G. A., & Fineberg, H. V. (2001). Strategies to decrease tuberculosis in U.S. homeless populations: A computer simulation model. *Journal of the American Medical Association, 286,* 834–842.

Brickner, P. W., Scanlan, B. C., Conanan, B., Elvy, A., McAdam, J., Scharer, L. K., . . . Vicic, W. J. (1985). *Health care of homeless people.* New York: Springer.

Brickner, P. W., Scharer, L., Conanan, B., Savarese, M., & Scanlan, B. (Eds.). (2011). *Under the safety net: The health and social welfare of the homeless in the United States.* New York: Norton.

Burt, M. R., Aron, L. Y, Douglas, T., Valente, J., Lee, E., & Iwen, B. (1999). *Homelessness: Programs and the people they serve—summary report.* Washington, DC: Interagency Council on Homelessness.

Chau, S., Chin, M., Chang, J., Luecha, A., Cheng, E., Schlesinger, J., . . . Gelberg, L. (2002). Cancer risk behaviors and screening rates among homeless adults in Los Angeles County. *Cancer Epidemiology, Biomarkers and Prevention, 11,* 431–438.

Cheung, R. C., Hanson, A. K., Maganti, K., Keeffe, E. B., & Matsui, S. M. (2002). Viral hepatitis and other infectious diseases in a homeless population. *Journal of Clinical Gastroenterology, 34,* 476–480.

Cortes, A., Leopold, J., Rothschild, L., Buron, L., Khadduri, J., & Culhane, D. (2011). *The 2010 annual homeless assessment report to Congress.* Washington, DC: U. S. Department of Housing and Urban Development, Office of Community Planning and Development.

Cousineau, M. (2001). Comparing adults in Los Angeles County who have and have not been homeless. *Journal of Community Psychology, 29,* 693–701.

Culhane, D. P., Gollub, E., Kuhn, R., & Shpaner, M. (2001). The co-occurrence of AIDS and homelessness: Results from the integration of administrative databases for AIDS surveillance and public shelter utilization in Philadelphia. *Journal of Epidemiology and Community Health, 55,* 515–520.

Culhane, D., & Kuhn, R. (1998). Patterns and determinants of public shelter utilization among homeless adults in New York City and Philadelphia. *Journal of Policy Analysis and Management, 17,* 23–43.

DeRosa, C. J., Montgomery, S. B., Hyde, J., Iverson, E., & Kipke, M. D. (2001). HIV risk behavior and HIV testing: A comparison of rates and associated factors among homeless and runaway adolescents in two cities. *AIDS Education and Prevention, 13,* 131–148.

Des Prez, R., & Heim, C. (1990). Mycobacterium tuberculosis. In G. Mandell, G. Douglas, & J. Bennett (Eds.), *Principles and practices of infectious diseases.* New York: Churchill Livingstone.

Desai, M. M., & Rosenheck, R. A. (2004). HIV testing and receipt of test results among homeless persons with serious mental illness. *American Journal of Psychiatry, 161*(12), 2287–2294.

Desai, R. A., Rosenheck, R. A., & Agnello, V. (2003). Prevalence of hepatitis C virus infection in a sample of homeless veterans. *Social Psychiatry and Psychiatric Epidemiology, 38,* 396–401.

Dietz, P., & Coburn, J. (1991). *To whom do they belong? Runaway, homeless and other youth in high-risk situations in the 1990s.* Washington, DC: National Network for Runaway and Youth Services.

Fischer, P., & Breakey, W. (1986). Homelessness and mental health: An overview. *International Journal of Mental Health, 14,* 6–41.

Fischer, P. J., Shapiro, S., Breakey, W. R., Anthony, J. C., & Kramer, M. (1986). Mental health and social characteristics of the homeless: A survey of mission users. *American Journal of Public Health, 76*(5), 519–524.

Folsom, D., & Jeste, D. (2002). Schizophrenia in homeless persons: A systematic review of the literature. *Acta Psychiatrica Scandinavica, 105,* 404–413.

Gallagher, T., Andersen, R., Koegel, P., & Gelberg, L. (1997). Determinants of regular source of care among homeless adults in Los Angeles. *Medical Care, 35,* 814–830.

Gamache, G., Rosenheck, R., & Tessler, R. (2001). The proportion of veterans among homeless men: A decade later. *Social Psychiatry and Psychiatric Epidemiology, 36,* 481–485.

Gamache, G., Rosenheck, R., & Tessler, R. (2003). Overrepresentation of women veterans among homeless women. *American Journal of Public Health, 93,* 1132–1135.

Gelberg, L. (2000, June 25). *Homeless women's use and endorsement of contraceptive methods.* Association for Health Services Research annual meeting, Los Angeles.

Gelberg, L., Leake, B., Lu, M., Andersen, R., Nyamathi, A., Morgenstern, H., & Browner, C. (2002). Chronically homeless women's perceived deterrents to contraception. *Perspectives on Sexual and Reproductive Health, 34,* 278–285.

Gelberg, L., Leake, B. D., Lu, M. C., Andersen, R. M., Wenzel, S. L., Morgenstern, H., . . . Browner, C. H. (2001a). Use of contraceptive methods among homeless women for protection against unwanted pregnancies and sexually transmitted diseases: Prior use and willingness to use in the future. *Contraception, 63,* 277–281.

Gelberg, L., Linn, L., & Leake, B. (1988). Mental health, alcohol and drug use, and criminal history among homeless adults. *American Journal of Psychiatry, 145,* 191–196.

Gelberg, L., Panarites, C. J., Morgenstern, H., Leake, B., Andersen, R. M., & Koegel, P. (1997). Tuberculosis skin testing among homeless adults. *Journal of General Internal Medicine, 12,* 25–33.

Gelberg, L., Robertson, M. J., Arangua, L., Leake, B. D., Sumner, G., Moe, A., . . . Nyamathi, A. (2012). Prevalence, distribution, and correlates of hepatitis C virus infection among homeless adults in Los Angeles. *Public Health Reports, 127*(4), 407–421.

Gelberg, L., Robertson, M. J., Leake, B., Wenzel, S. L., Bakhtiar, L., Hardie, E. A., . . . Getzug, T. (2001b). Hepatitis B among homeless and other impoverished U.S. military veterans in residential care in Los Angeles. *Public Health, 115,* 286–291.

Greene, J., Ennett, S., & Ringwalt, C. (1999). Prevalence and correlates of survival sex among runaway and homeless youth. *American Journal of Public Health, 89,* 1406–1409.

Haddad, M. B., Wilson, T. W., Ijaz, K., Marks, S. M., & Moore, M. (2005). Tuberculosis and homelessness in the United States, 1994–2003. *Journal of the American Medical Association, 293,* 2762–2766.

Herndon, B., Asch, S. M., Kilbourne, A. M., Wang, M., Lee, M., Wenzel, S. L., . . . Gelberg, L. (2003). Prevalence and predictors of HIV testing among a probability sample of homeless women in Los Angeles County. *Public Health Reports, 118,* 261–269.

Hibbs, J. R., Benner, L., Klugman, L., Spencer, R., Macchia, I., Mellinger, A., . . . Fife, D. K. (1994). Mortality in a cohort of homeless adults in Philadelphia. *New England Journal of Medicine, 331,* 304–309.

Hwang, S. (2000). Mortality among men using homeless shelters in Toronto, Ontario. *Journal of the American Medical Association, 283*, 2152–2157.

Hwang, S., O'Connell, J., & Brennan, T. (1997). Causes of death in homeless adults in Boston. *Annals of Internal Medicine, 126*, 625–628.

Johnson, T. P., & Fendrich, M. (2007). Homelessness and drug use: Evidence from a community sample. *American Journal of Preventative Medicine, 32*(6 Suppl), S211–S218.

Kerker, B. D., Bainbridge, J., Kennedy, J., Bennani, Y., Agerton, T., Marder, D., . . . Thorpe, L. E. (2011). A population-based assessment of the health of homeless families in New York City, 2001–2003. *American Journal of Public Health, 101*(3), 546–553.

Klein, J. D., Woods, A. H., Wilson, K. M., Prospero, M., Greene, J., & Ringwalt, C. (2000). Homeless and runaway youths' access to health care. *Journal of Adolescent Health, 27*, 331–339.

Klinkenberg, W. D., Casyln, R. J., Morse, G. A., Yonker, R. D., McCudden, S., Ketema, F., . . . Constantine, N. T. (2003). Prevalence of human immunodeficiency virus, hepatitis B, and hepatitis C among homeless persons with co-occurring severe mental illness and substance use disorders. *Comprehensive Psychiatry, 44*, 293–302.

Koegel, P. (1992). Through a different lens: An anthropological perspective on the homeless mentally ill. *Culture, Medicine and Psychiatry, 16*, 1–22.

Koegel, P., & Burnam, A. (1991). *The course of homelessness study: Aims and designs.* Rockville, MD: National Institute of Mental Health.

Koegel, P., & Burnam, M. (1988). Alcoholism among homeless adults in the inner city of Los Angeles. *Archives of General Psychiatry, 45*, 1011–1018.

Koegel, P., Burnam, A., & Farr, R. (1988). The prevalence of specific psychiatric disorders among homeless individuals in the inner-city of Los Angeles. *Archives of General Psychiatry, 45*, 1085–1092.

Koegel, P., Sullivan, G., Burnam, A., Morton, S. C., & Wenzel, S. (1988). Utilization of mental health and substance abuse services among homeless adults in Los Angeles. *Medical Care, 37*, 306–317.

Kushel, M. B., Evans, J. L., Perry, S., Robertson, M. J., & Moss, A. R. (2003). No door to lock: Victimization among homeless and marginally housed persons. *Archives of Internal Medicine, 163*, 2492–2499.

Kushel, M. B., Vittinghoff, E., & Haas, J. S. (2001). Factors associated with the health care utilization of homeless persons. *Journal of the American Medical Association, 285*, 200–206.

Lamb, H. R., & Bachrach, L. L. (2001). Some perspectives of deinstitutionalization. *Psychiatric Services, 52*, 1039–1045.

Lewis, J., Andersen, R., & Gelberg, L. (2003). Health care for homeless women. *Journal of General Internal Medicine, 18*, 921–928.

Lim, Y. W., Andersen, R., Leake, B., Cunningham, W., & Gelberg, L. (2002). How accessible is medical care for homeless women? *Medical Care, 40*, 510–520.

Link, B. G., Susser, E., Stueve, A., Phelan, J., Moore, R. E., & Struening, E. (1994). Lifetime and five-year prevalence of homelessness in the United States. *American Journal of Public Health, 84*, 1907–1912.

Long, H. L., Tulsky, J. P., Chambers, D. B., Alpers, L. S., Robertson, M. J., Moss, A. R.,...Chesney, M. A. (1998). Cancer screening in homeless women: Attitudes and behaviors. *Journal of Health Care for the Poor and Underserved, 9*, 276–292.

MacLean, M., Embry, L., & Cauce, A. (1999). Homeless adolescents' paths to separation from family: Comparison of family characteristics, psychological adjustment, and victimization. *Journal of Community Psychology, 27*, 179–187.

Martell, J. V., Seitz, R. S., Harada, J. K., Kobayashi, J., Sasaki, V. K., & Wong, C. (1992). Hospitalization in an urban homeless population: The Honolulu urban homeless project. *Annals of Internal Medicine, 116*, 299–303.

McAdam, J., Brickner, P., & Glicksman, R. (1985). Tuberculosis in the SRO/homeless population. In P. W. Brickner, L. K. Scharer, A. E. Conanan, & A. E. Savarese (Eds.), *Health care for homeless people*. New York: Springer.

McAdam, J. M., Brickner, P. W., Scharer, L. L., Crocco, J. A., & Duff, A. E. (1990). The spectrum of tuberculosis in a New York City men's shelter clinic (1982–1988). *Chest, 97*, 798–805.

McGuire, J. (2000). Hoptel equalizes length of stay for homeless and domiciled inpatients. *Medical Care, 38*, 1003–1010.

McQuillan, G. M., Khare, M., Karon, J. M., Schable, C. A., & Vlahov, D. (1997). Update on the seroepidemiology of human immunodeficiency virus in the United States household population: NHANES III, 1988–1994. *Journal of Acquired Immune Deficiency Syndrome and Human Retrovirology, 14*, 355–360.

Metraux, S., & Culhane, D. (1999). Family dynamics, housing and recurring homelessness among women in New York City homeless shelters. *Journal of Family Issues, 20*, 371–396.

Meyer, I. H., & Schwartz, S. (2000). Social issues as public health: promise and peril (Editorial). *American Journal of Public Health, 90*, 1189–1191.

Milburn, N. G., Rotheram-Borus, M. J., Batterham, P., Brumback, B., Rosenthal, D., & Mallett, S. (2005). Predictors of close family relationships over one year among homeless young people. *Journal of Adolescence, 28*, 263–275.

Mojtabai, R. (2005). Perceived reasons for loss of housing and continued homelessness among homeless persons with mental illness. *Psychiatric Services, 56*, 172–178.

Molina, B. S. (2005). High risk adolescent and young adult populations: Consumption and consequences. *Recent Developments in Alcoholism, 17*, 49–65.

North, C. S., Eyrich, K. M., Pollio, D. E., & Spitznagel, E. L. (2004). Are rates of psychiatric disorders in the homeless population changing? *American Journal of Public Health, 94*, 103–108.

Nunez, R., & Cox, C. (1999). A snapshot of family homelessness across America. *Political Science Quarterly, 114*, 289–299.

Nyamathi, A. M., Dixon, E. L., Robbins, W., Smith, C., Wiley, D., Leake, B.,...Gelberg, L. (2002b). Risk factors for hepatitis C virus infection among homeless adults. *Journal of General Internal Medicine, 17*, 134–144.

Nyamathi, A., Robbins, W. A., Fahey, J. L., Wiley, D., Pekler, V. A., Longshore, D.,...Saab, S. (2002a). Presence and predictors of hepatitis C virus in the semen of homeless men. *Biological Research for Nursing, 4*, 22–30.

O'Connell, J. J., Roncarati, J., Reilly, E. C., Kane, C. A., Morrison, S. K., Swain, S. E.,...Jones, K. (2004). Old and sleeping rough: Homeless persons on the streets of Boston. *Care Management Journals, 5*, 101–106.

Phelan, J., & Link, B. (1999). Who are "the homeless"? Reconsidering the stability and composition of the homeless population. *American Journal of Public Health, 89,* 1334–1338.

Quigley, J., Raphael, S., & Smolensky, E. (2001). *Homelessness in California.* San Francisco: Public Policy Institute of California.

Riley, E. D., Bangsberg, D. R., Guzman, D., Perry, S., & Moss, A. R. (2005). Antiretroviral therapy, hepatitis C virus, and AIDS mortality among San Francisco's homeless and marginally housed. *Journal of Acquired Immune Deficiency Syndrome 38,* 191–195.

Ringwalt, C., Greene, J., Robertson, M., & McPheeters, M. (1998). The prevalence of homelessness among adolescents in the United States. *American Journal of Public Health, 88,* 1325–1329.

Robertson, M. J. (2004). HIV seroprevalence among homeless and marginally housed adults in San Francisco. *American Journal of Public Health, 94*(7), 1207–1217.

Robertson, M., & Cousineau, M. (1986). Health status and access to health services among the urban homeless. *American Journal of Public Health, 76,* 561–563.

Robertson, M., Ropers, R., & Boyer, R. (1985). *The homeless of Los Angeles County: An empirical evaluation.* Los Angeles: UCLA School of Public Health.

Robertson, M., Zlotnick, C., & Westerfelt, A. (1997). Drug use disorders and treatment contact among homeless adults in Alameda County, California. *American Journal of Public Health, 87,* 221–228.

Rosenblum, A., Nuttbrock, L., McQuistion, H. L., Magura, S., & Joseph, H. (2001). Hepatitis C and substance use in a sample of homeless people in New York City. *Journal of Addictive Diseases, 20,* 15–23.

Rosenheck, R., Frisman, L., & Chung, A. (1994). The proportion of veterans among homeless men. *American Journal of Public Health, 84,* 466–469.

Roy, E., Haley, N., Leclerc, P., Boivin, J., Cédras, L., & Vincelette, J. (2001). Risk factors for hepatitis C virus infection among street youths. *Canadian Medical Association Journal, 165,* 557–560.

Salit, S., Kuhn, E. M., Hartz, A. J., Vu, J. M., & Mosso, A. L. (1998). Hospitalization costs associated with homelessness in New York City (Special article). *New England Journal of Medicine, 338,* 1734–1740.

Schanzer, B., Dominguez, B., Shrout, P. E., & Caton, C. L. (2007). Homelessness, health status, and health care use. *American Journal of Public Health, 97*(3), 464–469.

Shinn, M., Weitzman, B. C., Stojanovic, D., Knickman, J. R., Jimenez, L., Duchon, L., ... Krantz, D. H. (1998). Predictors of homelessness among families in New York City: From shelter request to housing stability. *American Journal of Public Health, 88,* 1651–1657.

Shlay, J., Blackburn, D., O'Keefe, K., Raevsky, C., Evans, M., & Cohn, D. L. (1996). Human immunodeficiency virus seroprevalence and risk assessment of a homeless population in Denver. *Sexually Transmitted Diseases, 23,* 304–311.

Shuler, P. A. (1991). *Homeless women's holistic and family planning needs: An exposition and test of the nurse practitioner model* (Dissertation). University of California, Los Angeles.

Shuler, P. A., Gelberg, L., & Davis, J. E. (1995). Characteristics associated with the risk of unintended pregnancy among urban homeless women. *Journal of the American Academy of Nurse Practitioners, 7,* 13–22.

Solliday-McRoy, C., Campbell, T. C., Melchert, T. P., Young, T. J., & Cisler, R. A. (2004). Neuropsychological functioning of homeless men. *Journal of Nervous and Mental Disease, 192*, 471–478.

Stein, J., Andersen, R., Koegel, P., & Gelberg, L. (2000). Predicting health services utilization in homeless adults: A prospective analysis. *Journal of Health Care for the Poor and Underserved, 11*, 212–230.

Stein, J. A., Andersen, R. M., Robertson, M., & Gelberg, L. (2012). Impact of hepatitis B and C infection on health services utilization in homeless adults: A test of the Gelberg-Andersen Behavioral Model for Vulnerable Populations. *Health Psychology, 31*(1), 20–30.

Stein, J. A., & Nyamathi, A. (2004). Correlates of hepatitis C virus infection in homeless men: A latent variable approach. *Drug and Alcohol Dependence, 75*, 89–95.

Strehlow, A. J., Robertson, M. J., Zerger, S., Rongey, C., Arangua, L., Farrell, E.,...Gelberg, L. (2012). Hepatitis C among clients of health care for the homeless primary care clinics. *Journal of Health Care for the Poor and Underserved, 23*(2), 811–833.

Tyler, K., Cauce, A., & Whitbeck, L. (2004). Family risk factors and prevalence of dissociative symptoms among homeless and runaway youth. *Child Abuse and Neglect, 28*, 355–366.

U.S. Interagency Council on Homelessness. (2010). *Opening doors: Federal strategic plan to prevent and end homelessness.* Washington, DC: U.S. Interagency Council on Homelessness.

Van Leeuwen, J. M., Hopfer, C, & Hooks, S. (2004). A snapshot of substance abuse among homeless and runaway youth in Denver, Colorado. *Journal of Community Health, 29*, 217–229.

Vangeest, J., & Johnson, T. (2002). Substance abuse and homelessness: Direct or indirect effects? *Annals of Epidemiology, 12*, 455–461.

Weitzman, B. C. (1989). Pregnancy and childbirth: Risk factors for homelessness? *Family Planning Perspectives, 21*(4), 175–178.

Wenzel, S., Leake, B., & Gelberg, L. (2000). Health of homeless women with recent experience of rape. *Journal of General Internal Medicine, 15*, 265–268.

Whitbeck, L. B., Chen, X., Hoyt, D. R., Tyler, K. A., & Johnson, K. D. (2004). Mental disorder, subsistence strategies, and victimization among gay, lesbian, and bisexual homeless and runaway adolescents. *Journal of Sex Research, 41*, 329–342.

Wood, D., Valdez, R. B., Hayashi, T., & Shen, A. (1990). Homeless and housed families in Los Angeles: A study comparing demographic, economic, and family function characteristics. *American Journal of Public Health, 80*(9), 1049–1052.

Zlotnick, C., Robertson, M. J., & Tam, T. (2003a). Substance use and separation of homeless mothers from their children. *Addictive Behavior, 28*, 1373–1383.

Zlotnick, C., Tam, T., & Robertson, M. J. (2003b). Disaffiliation, substance use, and exiting homelessness. *Substance Use and Misuse, 389*, 577–599.

Zolopa, A., Hahn, J. A., Gorter, R., Miranda, J., Wlodarczyk, D., Peterson, J.,...Moss, A. R. (1994). HIV and tuberculosis infection in San Francisco's homeless adults: Prevalence and risk factors in a representative sample. *Journal of the American Medical Association, 272*, 455–461.

PART FIVE

DIRECTIONS FOR CHANGE

CHAPTER TWENTY

CHANGING THE HEALTH CARE DELIVERY SYSTEM

Nadereh Pourat
Hector P. Rodriguez

Learning Objectives

- Clarify how health care market failures result in the fragmentation of patient care and an overemphasis on treatment of medical problems, rather than preventing them in the first place
- Summarize the contemporary efforts to change the U.S. health care delivery system
- Analyze the most prominent delivery system reform strategies aimed at (1) patients, (2) health care professionals, and (3) payers and insurers
- Assess the trade-offs associated with using intrinsic versus extrinsic motivators for changing provider behavior
- Compare the promises and challenges of current delivery system strategies to improve performance
- Through discussion, develop strategic priorities for the implementation of delivery system change in different health care delivery settings

The movement to improve the U.S. health care delivery system has intensified and accelerated with the passage of the 2010 Patient Protection and Affordable Care Act. It is widely recognized that past market-based efforts to reform the health care delivery system have generally failed to reduce costs and improve the population health. The primary reason is that health care markets function very differently from other types of markets. Free-market principles such as having many buyers and many sellers, symmetric information between buyers and sellers, and voluntary exchange are often violated in health care markets. Frequently, health care prices are set administratively, rather than by the free market. For example, the Medicare program often will make coverage and price decisions that will affect coverage decisions and prices in the commercial market. Moreover, critical patient information is not efficiently exchanged across the care continuum and between patients and providers, and patients have limited choices when selecting their health care arrangements. Importantly, some aspects of free markets such as supplier-induced demand and subsequent growth of the market are less desirable outcomes in health care markets because of the societal costs incurred by investing in health care versus other important social services or goods. The incentives that drive providers to provide more care and unnecessarily aggressive therapies for patients work against national efforts to reduce overall health care expenditures.

Market failures in health care also have resulted in the fragmentation of patient care, an overemphasis on treatment of medical problems rather than preventing them in the first place, limited focus on providing care in a manner that is centered on patient preferences and needs, and high administrative complexity. The United States has high administrative costs as a proportion of overall health care spending, yet patients' experiences of care coordination and access to care are worse in the United States compared to other industrialized countries. Major differences in these important outcomes stem from the fragmentation in organization and financing of health care in the United States, where multiple payers and providers may be involved in delivery of care for a given patient even in one illness episode, resulting in errors and duplication of services. A vast body of research comparing integrated and network health care organizations underscores the benefits of integrated health care delivery on patient care experiences, quality of patient care, and costs of care. For example, 27 percent of chronically ill patients in the United States reported that their test results or records were not available during appointments or that duplicate tests were ordered during the previous two years, compared to only 11 percent, 13 percent, and 15 percent in Switzerland, the United Kingdom, and New Zealand, respectively (Schoen, et al., 2011). Within the U.S. health care system, integrated physician organizations and large multispecialty physician organizations have been found to provide higher quality of care (Mehrotra, Epstein, & Rosenthal, 2006) and foster more positive patient care experiences (Rodriguez, von Glahn, Elliott, Rogers, & Safran, 2009) at a lower cost (Weeks et al., 2010). Nevertheless, fully integrated delivery systems are outnumbered by network health care organizations due to consumer demand for provider choice, flexibility for organizations to grow and shrink nimbly with changes in demand for services, and lack of incentives to realize system-level savings.

Numerous policy proposals and strategies are aimed at remedying the problems described here. This chapter summarizes *current* health care delivery system organization and financing reforms, including those targeting specific elements such as patients or providers and those targeting systemwide delivery system redesign.

Conceptual Framework: Intervention and Innovations to Correct System Failures

The conceptual framework presented in Figure 20.1 depicts the past and current efforts to change the U.S. health care delivery system. These efforts have targeted patients, providers, and payers and insurers either separately or conjointly.

Patients have been targeted by traditional public health education campaigns at the population level. These efforts raise awareness of disease risk factors, highlight importance of preventive care, and promote healthy behaviors including healthy diets and physical exercise. At the individual level, primary care providers have also provided health education on the same topics, as well as training patients in self-care to varying degrees and levels of success. Payers and insurers have become increasingly involved in providing wraparound services to patients in response to escalating health care costs and lack of improvement in patient outcomes and quality of care. These interventions range from health education efforts undertaken by managed care organizations (MCOs) and employers (such as enrollee or employee mailings to promote smoking prevention and encourage physical exercise), prepaid or in-house programs (such as gym memberships and exercise classes at place of employment), financial incentives (such as for participation in online health assessments), disease management (to teach self-care for specific chronic conditions, for example), and intensive case management (to provide one-on-one guidance and help to high service utilizers).

FIGURE 20.1. CONCEPTUAL FRAMEWORK FOR ASSESSING CHANGES IN THE HEALTH CARE DELIVERY SYSTEM

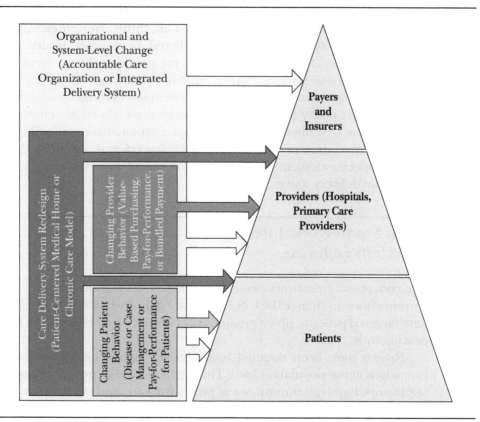

Providers have also been targeted to reduce costs and improve patient outcomes and quality of care. These efforts have varied by type of provider. The interventions targeting *hospitals* include a range of payment reform policies such as prospective payment systems (such as diagnosis-related groups, or DRGs), uncompensated care reimbursement (Disproportionate Share Hospital Payments), teaching allocations (Graduate Medical Education Payments), value-based purchasing, and penalties for iatrogenic diseases or thirty-day readmissions. Interventions to improve quality of care include a broad range of clinical guidelines (such as for diabetes care) and administrative guidelines (such as advance directives) to improve delivery of care, as well as addition of specific staff and services (such as for discharge planning and posthospitalization case management).

Interventions targeting *other providers* such as physicians, nurse practitioners, and physician assistants can also be divided into reimbursement and quality-of-care interventions. Reimbursement interventions range from targeted incentives for specific activities (such as pay-for-performance) to broad and systematic payment reform (such as capitation, prospective payment systems, and bundled payment). Quality-of-care interventions can include dissemination of clinical practice guidelines, decision support systems, referral management, and targeted training (such as diabetes care management, antihypertensive medication prescriptions, or lab testing for primary care providers). Interventions to develop new allied health care professions (such as community health care workers) or training existing allied providers to deliver new services (such as medical assistants) don't directly target physicians, but nevertheless lead to changes in delivery of primary care such as delegation of routine services to midlevel providers and provision of more complex care by physicians.

Providers may be in independent practice or organized under managed care organization, medical groups, community clinics, or other arrangements. Thus, the various provider interventions can be delivered by these organizations, directly through payers and insurers, or from a combination of these sources.

The preceding interventions can be bundled in a more comprehensive approach to simultaneously target both *providers and patients*. Primary care delivery redesign implemented under the Chronic Care Model and the Patient-Centered Medical Home bring together multiple elements of various interventions to change patient and provider behaviors with the goals of improving quality of care and patient outcomes. These models are also assumed to reduce health care expenditures for patients with chronic conditions and frequent utilizers of health care because of increased efficiencies that lead to better management of care and elimination of duplicate services.

Payers and insurers include private (such as employers, MCOs, PPOs) and public entities (such as Medicare and Medicaid) as well as organizations that serve as both insurer and provider (such as Kaiser and Veterans Affairs). Past efforts that target this part of the U.S. health care system are frequently focused on changing provider payment policies (such as Medicare diagnostic related groupings, relative value scales, and capitation). Increasingly, more systematic approaches have been implemented at the organizational level including creation of integrated delivery systems (IDSs), and accountable care organizations (ACOs). IDSs are health care systems that provide a comprehensive array of health and support services, while taking on financial risk as an MCO. ACOs are the latest effort at systematic change and require the integration of providers to develop IDS or MCO type organizations that take on financial risk as well as additional responsibility for improving patient health, improving quality and access to care, and reducing costs.

The initiators of these efforts to reform the system are diverse organizations with diverse goals. Initiators include governmental agencies, academic and private research organizations, foundations, and professional and advocacy organization. Examples of governmental organizations include Centers for Medicare and Medicaid Services that sets reimbursement policies and designs demonstration projects to test the impact of specific interventions; Centers for Disease Control and Prevention that monitors health and develops public health policies and disease prevention guidelines; and Agency for Health Care Research and Quality that supports research on quality and effectiveness of health care and develops care delivery guidelines. Foundations fund research and interventions to test the impact of methods of cost saving or care delivery, and they affect policy by disseminating their findings (such as Robert Wood Johnson's Aligning Forces for Quality and the Commonwealth Fund's Safety Net Medical Home Initiative: Transforming Primary Care). Professional organizations may endorse or develop measurement standards and accreditations programs (such as the National Committee for Quality Assurance and the National Quality Forum), or influence policy by advocating and promoting specific perspectives (such as the American Medical Association and the American College of Physicians).

Interventions Targeting Patients

Chronic conditions account for more than 75 percent of the $1.6 trillion spent annually on medical care with asthma, diabetes, heart disease, hypertension, and mood disorders accounting for nearly half of U.S. health care spending (Bernstein, Chollet, & Peterson, 2010; Tsai, Morton, Mangione, Keeler, 2005). Managing chronic disease, as a strategy to contain costs and change health care use patterns, has been employed by MCOs historically but is increasingly adopted by employers and safety net providers in nonmanaged care settings.

Efforts to manage chronic disease may be referred to as disease management, care management, or case management services. The programs may be integrated or coordinated with delivery of medical care by physicians or delivered as supplemental services independently with limited or no involvement from primary care providers. Chronic care management services are delivered along a continuum of intensity of care and comprehensiveness of services. At the lowest intervention level, programs may target a specific disease and low-risk patients, contact them periodically by mail, and focus on patient education on how to manage self-care. At the highest intervention level, high-risk patients with multiple chronic and behavioral conditions and high levels of inappropriate use of medical care are identified to receive services on an "as needed" basis. Patient education services may be combined with medical care coordination plus social and support services. The primary providers of chronic care management services are often specially trained registered nurses, but care teams sometimes include social workers, pharmacists, psychologists, community health workers, and other personnel.

Disease management (DM) programs primarily focus on changing patients' health behaviors by developing evidence-based and guideline concordant individualized care plans, educate patients about proper self-care, and coordinate care for patients (Bernstein, Chollet, & Peterson, 2010). Some, though not all, DM programs may also share the patients' care plans with their providers and send reminder and prompts on delivery of evidenced based care (Goetzel, Ozminkowski, Villagra, & Duffy, 2005).

DM programs are usually provided at periodic intervals and maybe delivered in-person in a group setting or individually, on the phone, or through mailings depending on the severity of the illness being managed. In contrast, *case management* services are delivered when and as frequently as needed with direct and intensive supervision of patients, in-person and by telephone. Case management services often go beyond DM services to accompanying patients to medical visits and arranging for social and support services such as transportation and housing. The intensity and range of services covered under these programs depends on the organization's goals. DM programs target populations of patients with specific disease and use risk stratification to determine the intensity of the intervention to be provided. Case management programs target individuals with multiple physical and behavioral health or substance abuse problems that have excessive use of services particularly emergency room visits (Kominski, Morisky, Abdelmomem, Kotlerman, 2008; Welch, Bergsten, Cutler, Bocchino, & Smith, 2002).

The National Committee for Quality Assurance (NCQA) uses the following criteria for Accreditation of DM programs, including (1) using evidence-based guidelines or standards of care in developing program content for patients and practitioners with practitioner oversight; (2) identifying and engaging eligible participants with risk stratification using administrative and claims data and providing self-management support (such as information, coaching, reminders, and referrals) and encouraging patient participation in care (such as financial incentives); (3) interacting collaboratively with providers by providing evidence-based information and feedback on care opportunities to providers including provider education and reminders (Weingarten et al., 2002); (4) providing feedback to patients and providers on patients' progress towards their care plans and coordinating referrals to case management programs or other resources; (5) assessing financial outcomes, quality of care delivered, and patient and provider experiences and including such information in quality improvement efforts; (6) assessing and improving program operations by insuring access to DM services, employing and training personnel, responding to complaints, insuring patient safety and privacy of patient information; and (7) regular assessment of organizational performance according to accreditation criteria (National Committee for Quality Assurance, 2010). Health information technology, though not a criteria, is essential in insuring the success of DM programs to allow identification and rapid real-time assessment of patients' health and service use, improving communication with patients and providers, and capturing additional patient information (Demiris et al., 2008; Horswell et al., 2008; Villagra & Ahmed, 2004; Welch et al., 2002).

Evaluations of success of DM programs have focused on success in reducing costs and return-on-investment, but also include assessment of improvements in quality of care delivered and patient outcomes. The evidence of success of these programs is inconsistent to date, partly due to significant variation in program design, measurement, setting, and rates of engagement or active participation (Bernstein, Chollet, & Peterson, 2010; Mattke, Seid, & Ma, 2007). Nevertheless, DM programs have been found to improve quality of care processes for a number of chronic conditions (Goetzel et al., 2005; Mattke, Seid, Ma, 2007; Ofman et al., 2004). Provision of counseling, information feedback, education, and other patient support mechanisms are found to be correlated with improved health outcomes in DM programs (Institute of Medicine, 2001a). Also, DM has been shown to improve quality of care and health outcomes in diabetes, congestive heart failure, chronic obstructive pulmonary disease, and asthma (Goetzel et al., 2005; Tsai et al., 2005). Success in these programs has been measured in terms of compliance with clinical practice guidelines (such as increased retinal and neuropathy screening among diabetes patients), medication compliance, and improved self-management (Dall et al., 2010; Gillespie & Rossiter, 2003; Knight et al., 2005; Mangione et al., 2006; Zhang, Wan, Rossiter, Murawski, & Patel, 2008). But evidence of improvements in patients' quality of life is sparse (Smith et al., 2005).

The success of DM programs in reducing utilization of health services and net reduction of costs remains inconclusive, particularly for underserved populations (Kominski et al., 2008; Mattke, Seid, & Ma, 2007; Ofman et al., 2004). Cost savings have been realized in the TRICARE program, in some Medicaid programs, in Medicare Advantage for diabetes patients, but not for the Medicare program in general (Dall et al., 2010; Gillespie & Rossiter, 2003; Holmes et al., 2008; McCall & Cromwell, 2011; Rosenzweig et al., 2010). Programs focusing on severely ill enrollees have shown impact on cost among these enrollees or for more intensive intervention (Krause, 2005). Also, DM programs concentrating on congestive heart failure reduced use of emergency room and inpatient services and returned a positive return-on-investment but those aimed at asthma, diabetes, and depression produced mixed results (Afifi, Morisky, Kominski, Kotlerman, 2007; Villagra, 2004).

Interventions Targeting Providers

Given the historically strong influence of the dominant fee-for-service provider payment system, changing provider behavior has been a major challenge for health care delivery and financing organizations. Strategies aimed at improving provider behavior (1) extrinsically motivate providers to improve performance by use of performance-based financial and non-financial incentives, or (2) intrinsically motivate providers to improve performance, or by enhancing the quality of the work environment to support patient-centered care and teamwork.

Extrinsic Provider Motivation Strategies

Another method of motivating providers to make changes in their practices to improve the quality of patient care and patients' experiences of care is through the use of *performance-based financial incentives*, or paying doctors and health care systems for achieving quality targets. Performance-based financial incentives can improve the provision of evidence-based care rather than providing more care or types of care that will generate the most financial benefit (Frolich, Talavera, Broadhead, & Dudley, 2007). Using financial incentives to induce meaningful and lasting improvements in health care quality is a strategy that is gaining rapid and widespread appeal in the United States. To date, *pay-for-performance (P4P)* has been employed in select markets in the United States and most extensively implemented in the United Kingdom (Campbell, Reeves, Kontopantelis, Sibbald, & Roland, 2009). Recent efforts by the Centers for Medicare and Medicaid Services (CMS) to implement P4P in the Medicare program, however, have catapulted the approach into high prominence in the United States.

The state of California has the largest and most long-standing experience with P4P. The Integrated Health Association's (IHA) statewide initiative, launched in 2004, is the nation's largest and longest standing multi-stakeholder P4P program. IHA improves clinical care processes and patient care experiences for a large number of hospitals and physician organizations by standardizing performance measures and reporting requirements. Broad efforts such as IHA are an important strategy for reducing the burden of disconnected payer reporting initiatives for medical groups. Achieving the cooperation of commercial competitors, however, has been a major challenge for many communities in the United States (Damberg, Raube, Williams, & Shortell, 2005). Some statewide initiatives manage to attain the consensus of commercial health plan and medical groups to support physician practice-level performance measurement and improvement. These large-scale performance improvement efforts, however, have failed to produce breakthrough quality improvements (Damberg, Raube, Teleki, & Dela Cruz, 2009; Pearson, Schneider, Kleinman, Coltin, & Singer, 2008). Observers are skeptical that a natural evolution toward multipayer collaborations will emerge (McMahon, Hofer, & Hayward, 2007; Rosenthal, 2007). Most P4P programs in the United States continue to be organized and implemented by single insurers and payers. Single insurer P4P programs, however, run a high risk of misclassifying organizational performance due to small sample sizes per group in a single insurer's population of patients (Rodriguez et al., 2011). Nevertheless, multistakeholder efforts to improve quality have not naturally evolved, underscoring the challenge for reliable physician and group performance measurement in the context of P4P initiatives.

The successes and challenges of improving clinical care processes have been well documented following the introduction of public reporting and/or financial incentives (Felt-Lisk, Gimm, & Peterson, 2007; Pearson, Schneider, Kleinman, Coltin, & Singer, 2008). Reviews of the literature indicate that there is a very weak empirical basis for P4P in health care (Scott et al., 2011). Lack of an effect may be due to poor study design or inconsistent results related to the impact of P4P in most studies that have examined the effect of P4P on quality of health care. Nevertheless, it is clear that P4P initiatives have placed health care quality measurement and improvement at the forefront of the industry's implementation priorities.

Bundled payment for an episode of care is another financial incentive strategy increasingly implemented to influence provider behavior. Bundled payment is an effort to counter the incentives created by FFS payment to give patients more care, rather than the most cost-effective care. Bundled payments are fixed reimbursement for an episode of care rather than reimbursement for specific services provided within a care episode. The objective of bundled payment systems is for providers to focus on providing the most effective care in order to prevent hospital readmissions or other health care charges associated with the episode of care. For example, under a FFS arrangement, a patient with acute lower back pain might receive aggressive and costly treatment for higher reimbursement even if it carries a high risk of complications. By contrast, under a bundled payment system, the same patient will receive a fixed amount for an acute back pain episode, irrespective of the intensity of treatment. As a result, health care providers will consider other factors in their clinical decision making, including patients' preferences and concerns and provide the most efficient and cost-effective service. Pilot tests of bundled payment systems are currently conducted in many U.S. health care markets. However, a key measurement challenge is how to define an "episode of care," a barrier to the wide dissemination of bundled payment systems.

Value-based purchasing (VBP) is another financial strategy aimed at improving the provision of cost-effective, evidence-based health care. VBP differs from P4P in that VBP programs are led by employers and other purchasers of health care as opposed to single insurers and payers. In addition, VBP programs aim to reduce unnecessary care and waste and include quality and cost criteria in the performance measurement and reward systems, while P4P programs are designed largely to address underuse of specific health care services and intermediate outcomes of care. VBP programs reward top performing health plans and delivery systems by agreeing to larger contracts and assuring continued patient volume. The goal behind VBP is to stimulate improvement among lower performing providers through selective contracting, payment withholds, and eliminating existing contractual relationships with underperforming providers. While VBP holds tremendous promise for improving quality and reducing health care costs, many barriers have prevented the widespread adoption of VBP initiatives. For example, VBP has largely focused on health plan performance and not individual providers. There is strong evidence that health plan comparisons are challenged because of overlapping physician networks or physicians contracting with multiple health plans, thereby masking performance differences among medical groups, practice sites, and individual physicians (Solomon, Zaslavsky, Landon, & Cleary, 2002). Without integrated and standardized reporting across diverse payers and providers, VBP initiatives have limited ability to stimulate quality' improvements within individual practice environments.

A non-financial method used to improve the quality of care and improve patient care experiences is transparent *public reporting* of performance of providers in medical group and health plans. Current large-scale efforts aimed at publicly sharing information on quality of care and patient experiences include statewide programs in Massachusetts and California and a national program called Aligning Forces for Quality Program to stimulate quality improvement in whole communities. Public reporting programs differ tremendously in their level of transparency and reporting frequency. Most initiatives collect and report information annually, post results via the internet, and report on medical group or health plan performance. Most public reporting efforts do not report physician-level results due to challenges with small numbers of patients who qualify for specific clinical quality measures (Holmboe et al., 2010; Kaplan, Griffith, Price, Pawlson, & Greenfield, 2009; Rodriguez, von Glahn, Chang, Rogers, & Safran, 2009; Sequist, Schneider, Li, Rogers, & Safran, 2010). In the late 1990s, before the Institute of Medicine called attention to the importance of patient-centered care (Institute of Medicine, 2001b), there were few efforts to measure and publicly report clinical quality measures. Moreover, there were no statewide or other large-scale efforts to measure patient care experiences. Most public reporting programs focused entirely on clinical quality measures, and if improvement was observed ("Health plans bear down on quality," 2001). Patients' experiences of primary care, however, deteriorated in both commercially-insured adult and Medicare-insured elderly patient populations during this same period (Montgomery et al., 2004; Murphy, Chang, Montgomery, Rogers, & Safran, 2001), indicating lack of focus on improving patient care experiences. Recent evaluations of public reporting efforts (Damberg, Raube, Williams, & Shortell, 2005; Williams, Raube, Damberg, & Mardon, 2006) show the heightened salience of patient-centered care nationally during recent years. Addition of specific measurement and accountability activities for patient care experiences, in California for example, are thought to account for improvements in commercially-insured primary care patients' experiences of care (Rodriguez, von Glahn, Elliott, Rogers, & Safran, 2009) in recent years.

Intrinsic Provider Motivation Strategies

Over the past decade, there has been increasing evidence of physician dissatisfaction with work (Landon et al., 2002), especially among primary care physicians. Compared to other industrialized countries, the average U.S. physician is more burdened by the administrative complexity of the health care system, reports substantially greater burnout and low work control, and experiences frustrations with coordinating care across the fragmented delivery system. These challenges have generated a sense of urgency among policy makers and practitioners to restructure the health care delivery system to better support primary care physicians and their practices. New initiatives such as the Patient-Centered Medical Home and the Chronic Care Model utilize approaches to improve patient self-care and engagement and prioritize the use of inter-professional care teams for leveraging primary care time and to reduce physician burnout (Reid et al., 2010).

Interventions Targeting Patients and Providers

Two dominant approaches have emerged to change the dynamics of care delivery between providers and patients. This is based on the realization that significant change is unlikely if system reform targets only one participant in the health care delivery interaction. These approaches include the Chronic Care Model (CCM) and the Patient-Centered Medical Home (PCMH). They vary somewhat in perspective but espouse related constructs and have significant overlap.

These models are propelled to the forefront of desirable approaches to address the failures of the U.S. health care in part due to the Institute of Medicine report *Crossing the Quality Chasm: A New Health System for the 21st Century* (Institute of Medicine, 2001c). The report identifies a significant lag in delivery of high quality health care given advances in scientific knowledge and technology as well as changes in public health needs. The report highlights the system's failures in care of the increasingly prevalent chronic conditions and calls for a sweeping system redesign while keeping the following aims for improvement in focus: safe, effective, patient-centered, timely, efficient, and equitable health care. The IOM report refrained from defining a road map for system redesign, leaving room for innovation and flexibility in approach.

Around the same time, the *Chronic Care Model* was developed and proposed to redesign the delivery of primary care to chronically ill patients (Bodenheimer, Wagner, & Grumbach, 2002; Wagner, 2001). CCM identifies five essential elements that are required to improve patient outcomes. These elements include: (1) availability of community level resources and policies such as self-management support for patients; (2) appropriate organization of the health care system including design of the delivery system and availability of decision support and clinical information systems; (3) informed patients that are involved in their care; (4) a prepared practice team that is proactive; and (5) productive interactions between patients and doctors. CCM argues that medical practice has to be restructured to deliver care by a practice teams in which the non-physician personnel provide the planned routine services for chronically ill patients. Training patients and their families to learn skills and confidence to manage their chronic conditions is an important element of CCM. The other essential aspects of CCM are providing evidence-based clinical practice guideline to providers to aid in effective management of chronic conditions as well as information systems that aid physicians in adhering to guidelines by sending reminders, providing feedback on their performance, and contain disease registries to help plan patient care. Linkages with community-based resources are also required to expand the availability of supportive care to patients such as case-managers and patient education classes. According to CCM, the innovations and change outlined in the elements above would not be possible in the absence of a commitment to prioritize management of chronic conditions by the health care organization.

The concept of medical home was first introduced by the American Academy of Pediatrics in 1967 as an appropriate model of care delivery to children with special needs (Backer, 2007). In 2004, a coalition of seven national family medicine organizations expanded on this concept and recommended that everyone have a "personal medical home" to receive primary, chronic, and preventive care services (Future of Family Medicine Project Leadership Committee, 2004). In 2007, the American Academy of Family Physicians, the American Academy of Pediatrics, the American College of Physicians and the American Osteopathic Association, released the Joint Principles of the Patient-Centered Medical Home (American Academy of Family Physicians [AAFP], 2007). The principals of PCMH included broader concepts that were previously called for in CCM or other competing models such as the Advanced Medical Home (American College of Physicians, 2006).

Seven PCMH principles are identified including (1) personal physician, (2) physician directed medical practice, (3) whole person orientation, (4) coordinated and/or integrated care, (5) quality and safety, (6) enhanced access, and (7) payment (see Figure 20.2). Collectively, these principals are aimed at redesigning the delivery of health care by putting the primary care physician in a central role as the first point of contact and as the leader of a team of providers to provide all the patient's health care needs or to coordinate the delivery of needed care with other providers and across the patient's life span. Primary care physicians are also responsible for ensuring quality, safety and timely access using electronic and phone communication and should receive adequate compensation for providing care that is more convenient for patients. Achieving PCMH principals requires infrastructure and a myriad of support services including health information technology and health information exchange. The availability of key support services is greater in integrated systems of care and more difficult to achieve in the absence of organizational support and infrastructure. Equally important is the alignment of payments and financial incentives with goals of PCMH such as quality and care coordination to achieve systematic and lasting change in practice redesign.

Multiple pathways exist to achieve the ideal principals of PCMH and practice redesign. Depending on perspective, the desired focus of PCMH may be on care coordination, health information technology, shared decision making, or whole-person care (Fontaine, Flottemesch, Solberg, & Asche, 2011). Among efforts to measure PCMH status, those undertaken by NCQA are arguably most widely known, and recognition as a PCMH is increasingly sought after and received by numerous providers. NCQA has identified a maximum of 149 standards and elements by 2011, spanning six main categories of (1) enhanced access and continuity, (2) identifying and managing patient populations, (3) planning and managing care, (4), providing self-care and community support, (5) tracking and coordinating care, and (6) measuring and improving performance. Acknowledging the effort required in redesigning primary care practice, NCQA accredits practices on a three tier basis and requires achieving all six basic elements and a minimum of thirty-five total elements to be recognized as a level 1 PCMH, and a minimum of eighty-five points to achieve level three recognition (National Committee for Quality Assurance, 2011). NCQA standards may not be applicable to all practice settings or difficult to achieve in the absence of supportive services and infrastructure provided by an integrated delivery system. However, complementary attempts to

FIGURE 20.2. JOINT PRINCIPLES OF THE PATIENT-CENTERED MEDICAL HOME

Personal physician: each patient has an ongoing relationship with a personal physician trained to provide first-contact, continuous, and comprehensive care.

Physician-directed medical practice: the personal physician leads a team of individuals at the practice level who collectively take responsibility for the ongoing care of patients.

Whole-person orientation: the personal physician is responsible for providing for all the patient's health care needs or taking responsibility for appropriately arranging care with other qualified professionals. This includes care for all stages of life: acute care, chronic care, preventive services, and end-of-life care.

Care is coordinated and/or integrated across all elements of the complex health care system (such as subspecialty care, hospitals, home health agencies, and nursing homes) and the patient's community (family, public, private, and community-based services). Care is facilitated by registries, information technology, health information exchange, and other means to ensure that patients get the indicated care when and where they need and want it in a culturally and linguistically appropriate manner.

Quality and safety are hallmarks of the medical home:

- Practices advocate for their patients to support the attainment of optimal, patient-centered outcomes that are defined by a care planning process in a compassionate, robust partnership among physicians, patients, and the patient's family.
- Evidence-based medicine and clinical decision-support tools guide decision making.
- Physicians in the practice accept accountability for continuous quality improvement through voluntary engagement in performance measurement and improvement.
- Patients actively participate in decision making, and feedback is sought to ensure that patients' expectations are being met.
- Information technology is utilized appropriately to support optimal patient care, performance measurement, patient education, and enhanced communication.
- Practices go through a voluntary recognition process by an appropriate nongovernmental entity to demonstrate that they have the capabilities to provide patient-centered services consistent with the medical home model.
- Patients and families participate in quality improvement activities at the practice level.

Enhanced access to care is available through systems such as open scheduling, expanded hours, and new options for communication between patients, their personal physician, and practice staff.

Payment appropriately recognizes the added value provided to patients who have a Patient-Centered Medical Home.

address shortcomings of the current health care system such as accountable care organizations can provide the additional resources required to achieve PCMH status in a variety of practice settings.

Perhaps the most significant challenge to delivery of care according to CCM or PCMH models is the level of effort required to reorganize practices and retrain providers towards a team-based approach to care delivery (Berenson et al., 2008). A cultural and practical shift in practice patterns is required to implement changes such as delegating certain routine patient care from physicians to other staff such as medical assistants, establishing regular meetings to plan the care of complex patients, proactively managing patient populations with chronic conditions, coordinating care through referrals and following up with a broad array of medical, behavioral and social services. A cultural shift is most effectively achieved by realigning financial and non-financial incentives that currently reward urgent and episodic care (Barr, 2010; Berenson et al., 2008; Bodenheimer et al., 2002). Additional challenges to delivery of care according to CCM or PCMH models include availability of a trained workforce and information technology among others (Berenson et al., 2008). The required information technology is not limited to availability of electronic patient records and disease registries in a given practice but extends to exchange of such information across providers, patients, and payers. Content, functionality, and interoperability of electronic data are essential criteria needed for successful implementation of practice redesign under the PCMH and CCM models (Finkelstein, Barr, Kothari, Nace, & Quinn, 2011).

Evidence of implementation of PCMH and CCM and the subsequent impact on individual and population health, quality of care, and costs are slowly emerging. Extensive variation in implementation and evaluation of PCMH and CCM models exist, leading to difficulties in meaningful comparisons and conclusions about the elements that have produced the desired results (Bitton, Martin, & Landon, 2010; Sidorov, 2008). Arguably, identifying specific elements, such as having a personal physician and using team-based approach, may be difficult to distinguish from the overall practice redesign activities. In addition, studies of impact of PCMH and CCM that incorporate all elements of these models are rare and not systematic in their approach, although some effective programs have been identified.

A prospective quasi-experimental evaluation of a PCMH demonstration identified better patient experiences, enhanced access to care, more specialist visits, fewer emergency services, high emotional exhaustion among providers, and no significant differences in overall costs after one year of implementation (Reid et al., 2009). Other studies have found improvements in quality of care and reductions in hospital admissions, emergency room visits, outpatient visits, and pharmacy services with PCMH implementation (Paulus, Davis, & Steele, 2008; Roby et al., 2010; Steiner et al., 2008). Consistent attendance within PCMH was also associated with fewer primary care and specialist visits and lower professional fees (Fontaine et al., 2011). Studies of PCMH implementation for children with special health care needs have also identified evidence of better health, timely care, family functioning, and family centeredness (Homer et al., 2008). Studies of CCM implementation have also found reductions in HgA1c and lipid levels and increases in patients with self-management goals, and increases in eye and foot examinations (Bodenheimer et al., 2002; Tsai et al., 2005).

Interventions Targeting Insurers, Payers, Providers, and Patients

Recent approaches to address market failures in the United States and change the health care delivery system include *integrated delivery systems (IDSs)* and *accountable care organizations (ACOs)*. Both these approaches address gaps in quality as well as the fragmentation in financing and delivery of care by creating systems of care.

In the 1990s health care reform debates, Alan Enthoven and colleagues proposed a restructuring of the U.S. health care system and coined the phrase "managed competition," which proposed that integrated delivery systems (IDSs) should be developed and rewarded over time to enable more comprehensive, patient-centered care. Given the challenges with passing reform at the time, the health care market continued to move away from integrated delivery systems to virtual integration, or contractual relationships between physician organizations, hospitals and health plans with a high level of overlapping contractual relationships among organizations. By the end of the 1990s, a clear managed care backlash ensued and created even fewer organizational incentives to transition into IDSs. Patients demanded choice of providers and managed care organizations were perceived to restrict patient choice and skimp on appropriate care because of managed care payment incentives.

In 2009, Enthoven described an IDS as an organized and coordinated network of providers that is vertically integrated to provide coordinated care along the continuum of care and is clinically and fiscally accountable for quality of care and health of the enrolled population (Enthoven, 2009). In recent years various entities have embarked on a wide range of virtual organizational relationships with varying levels of integrated administrative systems and care integration. Evidence suggests that IDSs provide higher quality care compared to network physician organizations, or independent practice associations.

The more recent concept of an ACO is described as "provider groups that accept responsibility of the cost and quality of care delivered to a specific population of patients cared for by the groups' clinicians" (Shortell, Casalino, & Fisher, 2010). While the ACO concept encompasses IDS as a form of ACO, other formations based on multispecialty group practices, physician-hospital organizations, independent practice associations, or virtual physician organizations can also become ACOs (Shortell et al., 2010).

In 2012, the Centers for Medicaid and Medicare Services (CMS) funded large ACO demonstration projects around the United States with the goal of creating integrated systems across the health care delivery continuum. Central to the ACO demonstration projects is the goal to deliver cost-effective patient care. The ACO demonstration projects are required to demonstrate cost savings for continued renewal of the projects. To achieve this goal, ACO demonstrations are turning to VBP and the implementation of PCMHs as strategies to improve cost-effective and patient-centered care. The challenge of delivery system integration cannot be understated. ACO partners are challenged by disconnected health information systems and existing financial incentives that impede system change, and they often experience professional collaboration growing pains. The evaluation of ACO demonstration projects will be instrumental for demonstrating the potential gains achieved through focused care delivery system integration across diverse stakeholders and partners.

Future Directions

The passage of ACA has increased the pressure to reduce costs and improve quality of care and patient outcomes. Many of the strategies in changing the delivery of care and systemic incentives that lead to inefficiencies and poor patient outcomes that are described in this chapter are in early stages of implementation, or are implemented inconsistently and sporadically. The rapid implementation of strategies such as PCMH, VBP, P4P, IDS, and ACOs in the coming years will be coupled with further evidence of whether these strategies are effective in achieving the triple aims of reduced cost, better quality, and better outcomes. The barriers to broad implementation of the ideals of PCMH, IDS, and ACOs are likely to lead to further refinement and standardization of essential elements of each model that are most effective. Further hybrid models are also likely to emerge and payers and providers will selectively implement various strategies. Despite the uncertainty in which of the strategies described in this chapter are likely to be most effective in the long run, the concept of accountability is here to stay.

SUMMARY

Numerous attempts to correct the deficiencies and failures of the health care system in the United States are undertaken to various levels of success. These interventions and innovations have targeted patients, providers, insurers, and payers either separately or simultaneously. Recent interventions targeting patients include disease management programs primarily designed to change patient behaviors. Evidence of success of these programs is inconsistent, but points to reduction of health care utilization and limited success in savings. Interventions that target providers include attempts to motivate physicians to improve quality of care through financial or other means. The evidence of the success of financial and nonfinancial motivators is either unavailable or inconsistent with some improvements in quality indicators. System-level interventions such as integrated delivery systems and accountable care organizations are either infrequent or too recent to assess success in addressing the shortcomings they aim to correct.

The success of these innovations in the long term remains to be identified in future years. In the meantime, policymakers and various organizations are engaging in rapid deployment of these strategies, counting on the promises of reducing costs and improving quality and patient outcomes.

KEY TERMS

Accountable care organization (ACO) is a group of providers that can accept responsibility for the cost and quality of care delivered to a specific population of patients. An ACO may be an integrated delivery system, a multispecialty group practice, a physician-hospital organization, or an independent practice association.

Bundled payment refers to payment for an entire episode of care, rather than for each visit related to the same health condition. Bundled payment can be a single payment to all the providers engaged in delivery of care for an episode of illness and imparts financial and performance accountability to these providers.

Case management services often go beyond disease management services and include more intensive interventions such as accompanying patients to medical visits and arranging for social and support services such as transportation and housing.

Chronic Care Model (CCM) is a redesign of methods of care delivery for chronic conditions and focuses on delivery of guideline concordant with evidence-based care, proactive patient management, and improved patient-provider interaction.

Disease management (DM) programs are often implemented by health plans or public programs to improve the health of their respective patient populations with specific chronic conditions by providing wraparound care management services. DM is designed to assess patients' health, develop management goals and treatment plans, teach patients self-care skills and encourage behavior change, engage patients in decision making with their providers, and provide care coordination services. DM services are intended to be based on evidence-based and guideline-concordant care, provide individualized care plans, educate patients about proper self-care, and coordinate care of patients.

Integrated delivery system (IDS) is defined as an organized and coordinated network of providers that is vertically integrated to provide coordinated care along the continuum of care and is clinically and fiscally accountable for the quality of care and the health of the enrolled population.

Patient-Centered Medical Home (PCMH) focuses on redesign of delivery of primary care to a proactive care delivery model that is focused on patients' needs and values, is comprehensive, is coordinated with all other providers, is easily accessible, and focuses on quality and safety.

Pay-for-performance (P4P) is a type of performance-based financial incentive that uses payment to provide a specific service or achieve a quality indicator.

Performance-based financial incentives generally refer to payments to physicians and health care providers for achieving meaningful improvements in health care quality in addition to payment for services provided.

Value-based purchasing (VBP) is a strategy employed by public and private purchasers of health care to reward the best-performing providers with enhanced payment, market share, and recognition. VBP rewards are frequently based on standardized and comparative performance indicators such as costs, patient health status, and patient experiences.

DISCUSSION QUESTIONS

1. Health care delivery system leaders are faced with many demands from employers and other purchasers, payers, and the public to improve quality and patient-centered care. Imagine that you are the quality improvement director of a network of independent primary care practices that has been struggling with achieving high performance on clinical performance and patient experience measures. Considering the diverse strategies outlined in this chapter, which strategies for improving the quality of health care would you consider? What information would you need to decide which strategies would be most advantageous for your small, independent primary care practice?

2. As the director of a county department of health, you are charged with implementing a pilot program to provide health coverage to the safety net users in your county. Your provider network consists of county facilities, federally qualified health centers, and physicians in private practice. The pilot requires that all program enrollees should be enrolled in a Patient-Centered Medical Home. The network providers vary in their ability to deliver care according to PCMH principles in several areas. What elements of the PCMH should the county ideally require from the network providers? Since private practice physicians do not have sufficient infrastructure to deliver the "must-pass" elements of PCMH, what infrastructure and support services can the county provide for these physicians to incorporate these elements?

3. Past and current approaches to reform the health care system in the United States have not addressed important market failures or are too recent for their impact to be assessed. The failure of some approaches is due in part to their implementation in limited sectors of the health care market such as Medicare or to their targeting only patients or providers. Of the more recent approaches discussed in this chapter, which has the greatest potential to address the failures of the health care market? Discuss your reasons. Of the approaches with limited success to date,

what changes might improve their effectiveness in improving health care quality and reducing costs?

4. The Medicaid program in your state is requiring all contracted Medicaid managed care organizations (MCOs) to participate in identifying and selecting a new payment model to achieve the triple aims of reduced costs and improved quality of care and patient outcomes. As the CEO of the largest Medicaid MCO in the state, you and your board of directors are concerned about the impact of the change in payment method on your ability to contract with providers. You are tasked with a study of the various payment methods and have to recommend which one holds the greatest promise to achieve the triple aims set by Medicaid. Discuss various payment methods and their pros and cons. Propose one of the methods to your board and provide an argument why you have chosen this method.

FURTHER READING

Pourat, N., Davis, A. C., Salce, E., Hilberman, D., Roby, D. H., & Kominski, G. F. (2012). In ten California counties, notable progress in system integration within the safety net, although challenges remain. *Health Affairs, 31*(8), 1717–1727.

Pourat, N., Reifman, C., Roby, D. H., Meng, Y. Y., Diamant, A. L., & Kominski, G. F. (2009). *Health coverage in the safety net: How California's coverage initiative is providing a medical home to low-income uninsured adults in ten counties—interim findings.* Los Angeles: UCLA Center for Health Policy Research.

Volpp, K. G., Pauly, M. V., Loewenstein, G., & Bangsberg, D. (2009). P4P4P: An agenda for research on pay-for-performance for patients. *Health Affairs, 28*(1), 206–214.

REFERENCES

Afifi, A. A., Morisky, D. E., Kominski, G. F., & Kotlerman, J. B. (2007). Impact of disease management on health care utilization: Evidence from the Florida: A Healthy State (FAHS) Medicaid program. *Preventive Medicine, 44*(6), 547–553.

American Academy of Family Physicians, American Academy of Pediatrics, American College of Physicians, & American Osteopathic Association. (2007). *Joint principles of the Patient-Centered Medical Home.* Retrieved from http://www.medicalhomeinfo.org/joint Statement.pdf

American College of Physicians. (2006). *The advanced medical home: A patient-centered, physician-guided model of health care.* Retrieved from http://www.acponline.org/advocacy/current_policy_papers/assets/adv_med.pdf

Backer, L. (2007). The medical home: An idea whose time has come . . . again. *Family Practice Management, 14*(8), 38–41.

Barr, M. S. (2010). The patient-centered medical home: Aligning payment to accelerate construction. *Medical Care Research and Review, 67*(4), 492–499.

Berenson, R. A., Hammons, T., Gans, D. N., Zuckerman, S., Merrell, K., Underwood, W. S., & Williams, A. F. (2008). A house is not a home: Keeping patients at the center of practice redesign. *Health Affairs, 27*(5), 1219–1230.

Bernstein, J., Chollet, D., & Peterson, G. G. (2010). Disease management: Does it work? *Mathematica Policy Research, 4,* 1–5.

Bitton, A., Martin, C., & Landon, B. (2010). A Nationwide survey of patient centered medical home demonstration projects. *Journal of General Internal Medicine, 25*(6), 584–592.

Bodenheimer, T., Wagner, E. H., & Grumbach, K. (2002). Improving primary care for patients with chronic illness. *Journal of the American Medical Association, 288*(14), 1775–1779.

Campbell, S. M., Reeves, D., Kontopantelis, E., Sibbald, B., & Roland, M. (2009). Effects of pay for performance on the quality of primary care in England. *New England Journal of Medicine, 361*(4), 368–378.

Dall, T. M., Askarinam Wagner, R. C., Zhang, Y., Yang, W., Arday, D. R., & Gantt, C. J. (2010). Outcomes and lessons learned from evaluating TRICARE's disease management programs. *American Journal of Managed Care, 16*(6), 438–446.

Damberg, C. L., Raube, K., Teleki, S. S., & Dela Cruz, E. (2009). Taking stock of pay-for-performance: A candid assessment from the front lines. *Health Affairs (Millwood), 28*(2), 517–525.

Damberg, C. L., Raube, K., Williams, T., & Shortell, S. M. (2005). Paying for performance: Implementing a statewide project in California. *Quality Management in Health Care, 14*(2), 66–79.

Demiris, G., Afrin, L. B., Speedie, S., Courtney, K. L., Sondhi, M., Vimarlund, V., . . . Lynch, C. (2008). Patient-centered applications: Use of information technology to promote disease management and wellness. A white paper by the AMIA knowledge in motion working group. *Journal of American Medical Informatics Association, 15*(1), 8–13.

Enthoven, A. C. (2009). Integrated delivery systems: The cure for fragmentation. *American Journal of Managed Care, 15*(10 Suppl), S284–S290.

Felt-Lisk, S., Gimm, G., & Peterson, S. (2007). Making pay-for-performance work in Medicaid. *Health Affairs, 26*(4), w516–w527.

Finkelstein, J., Barr, M. S., Kothari, P. P., Nace, D. K., & Quinn, M. (2011). Patient-centered medical home cyberinfrastructure: Current and future landscape. *American Journal of Preventive Medicine, 40*(5), S225–S233.

Fontaine, P., Flottemesch, T. J., Solberg, L. I., & Asche, S. E. (2011). Is consistent primary care within a patient-centered medical home related to utilization patterns and costs? *Journal of Ambulatory Care Management, 34*(1), 10–19.

Frolich, A., Talavera, J. A., Broadhead, P., & Dudley, R. A. (2007). A behavioral model of clinician responses to incentives to improve quality. *Health Policy, 80*(1), 179–193.

Future of Family Medicine Project Leadership Committee. (2004). The future of family medicine: A collaborative project of the family medicine community. *Annals of Family Medicine, 2*(Suppl 1), S3–S32.

Gillespie, J., & Rossiter, L. (2003). Medicaid disease management programs: Findings from three leading US state programs. *Disease Management Health Outcomes, 11*(6).

Goetzel, R. Z., Ozminkowski, R. J., Villagra, V. G., & Duffy, J. (2005). Return on investment in disease management: A review. *Health Care Financing Review, 26*(4), 1–19.

Health plans bear down on quality, HEDIS scores improve dramatically. (2001). Managed *Care, 10*(10), 34–35.

Holmboe, E. S., Weng, W., Arnold, G. K., Kaplan, S. H., Normand, S. L., Greenfield, S., . . . Lipner, R. S. (2010). The comprehensive care project: Measuring physician performance in ambulatory practice. *Health Services Research, 45*(6 Pt 2), 1912–1933.

Holmes, A. M., Ackerman, R. D., Zillich, A. J., Katz, B. P., Downs, S. M., & Inui, T. S. (2008). The net fiscal impact of a chronic disease management program: Indiana Medicaid. *Health Affairs, 27*(3), 855–864.

Homer, C. J., Klatka, K., Romm, D., Kuhlthau, K., Bloom, S., Newacheck, P., . . . Perrin, J. M. (2008). A review of the evidence for the medical home for children with special health care needs. *Pediatrics, 122*(4), e922–e937.

Horswell, R., Butler, M. K., Kaiser, M., Moody-Thomas, S., McNabb, S., Besse, J., & Abrams, A. (2008). Disease management programs for the underserved. *Disease Management, 11*(3), 145–152.

Institute of Medicine. (2001a). *Crossing the quality chasm: A new health system for the 21st century.* Washington, DC: National Academy Press.

Institute of Medicine. (2001b). *Crossing the quality chasm: A new health system for the 21st century* (Vol. 6). Washington, DC: National Academy Press.

Institute of Medicine. (2001c). *Crossing the quality chasm: A new health system for the 21st century.* Washington DC: Author.

Kaplan, S. H., Griffith, J. L., Price, L. L., Pawlson, L. G., & Greenfield, S. (2009). Improving the reliability of physician performance assessment: Identifying the "physician effect" on quality and creating composite measures. *Medical Care, 47*(4), 378–387.

Knight, K., Badamgarav, E., Henning, J. M., Hasselblad, V., Gano, A. D., Jr., Ofman, J. J., & Weingarten, S. R. (2005). A systematic review of diabetes disease management programs. *American Journal of Managed Care, 11*(4), 242–250.

Kominski, G. F., Morisky, D. E., Abdelmomem, A. A., & Kotlerman, J. B. (2008). The effect of disease management on utilization of services by race/ethnicity: Evidence from the Florida Medicaid Program. *The American Journal of Managed Care, 14*(3).

Krause, D. S. (2005). Economic effectiveness of disease management programs: A meta-analysis. *Disease Management, 8*(2), 114–134.

Landon, B. E., Aseltine, R., Jr., Shaul, J. A., Miller, Y., Auerbach, B. A., & Cleary, P. D. (2002). Evolving dissatisfaction among primary care physicians. *American Journal of Managed Care, 8*(10), 890–901.

Mangione, C. M., Gerzoff, R. B., Williamson, D. F., Steers, W. N., Kerr, E. A., Brown, A. F., . . . Selby, J. V. (2006). The association between quality of care and the intensity of diabetes disease management programs. *Annals of Internal Medicine, 145*(2), 107–116.

Mattke, S., Seid, M., & Ma, S. (2007). Evidence for the effect of disease management: Is $1 billion a year a good investment? *American Journal of Managed Care, 13*(12), 670–676.

McCall, N., & Cromwell, J. (2011). Results of the Medicare health support disease-management pilot program. *New England Journal of Medicine, 365*(18), 1704–1712.

McMahon, L. F., Jr., Hofer, T. P., & Hayward, R. A. (2007). Physician-level P4P—DOA? Can quality-based payment be resuscitated? *American Journal of Managed Care, 13*(5), 233–236.

Mehrotra, A., Epstein, A. M., & Rosenthal, M. B. (2006). Do integrated medical groups provide higher-quality medical care than individual practice associations? *Annals of Internal Medicine, 145*(11), 826–833.

Montgomery, J. E., Irish, J. T., Wilson, I. B., Chang, H., Li, A. C., Rogers, W. H., & Safran, D. G. (2004). Primary care experiences of Medicare beneficiaries, 1998 to 2000. *Journal of General Internal Medicine, 19*(10), 991–998.

Murphy, J., Chang, H., Montgomery, J. E., Rogers, W. H., & Safran, D. G. (2001). The quality of physician-patient relationships: Patients' experiences, 1996–1999. *Journal of Family Practice, 50*(2), 123–129.

National Committee for Quality Assurance. (2010). *2010 DM standards overview.* Retrieved from http://www.ncqa.org/tabid/1108/Default.aspx

National Committee for Quality Assurance. (2011). *Draft standards for patient-centered medical home, 2011.* Retrieved from http://www.ncqa.org/Portals/0 /PublicComment/PCMH2011_draft_standards_527.pdf

Ofman, J. J., Badamgarav, E., Henning, J. M., Knight, K., Gano, A. D., Levan, R. K., . . . Weingarten, S. R. (2004). Does disease management improve clinical and economic outcomes in patients with chronic diseases? A systematic review. *American Journal of Medicine, 117*(3), 182–192.

Paulus, R. A., Davis, K., & Steele, G. D. (2008). Continuous innovation in health care: Implications o the Geisinger experience. *Health Affairs, 27*(5), 1235–1245.

Pearson, S. D., Schneider, E. C., Kleinman, K. P., Coltin, K. L., & Singer, J. A. (2008). The impact of pay-for-performance on health care quality in Massachusetts, 2001–2003. *Health Affairs (Millwood), 27*(4), 1167–1176.

Reid, R. J., Coleman, K., Johnson, E. A., Fishman, P. A., Hsu, C., Soman, M. P., . . . Larson, E. B. (2010). The group health medical home at year two: Cost savings, higher patient satisfaction, and less burnout for providers. *Health Affairs, 29*(5), 835–843.

Reid, R. J., Fishman, P. A., Yu, O., Ross, T. R., Tufano, J. T., Soman, M. P., & Larson, E. B. (2009). Patient-centered medical home demonstration: A prospective, quasi-experimental, before and after evaluation. *American Journal of Managed Care, 15*(9), e71–e87.

Roby, D. H., Pourat, N., Pirritano, M. J., Vrungos, S. M., Dajee, H., Castillo, D., & Kominski, G. F. (2010). Impact of patient-centered medical home assignment on emergency room visits among uninsured patients in a county health system. *Medical Care Research and Review, 67*(4), 412–430.

Rodriguez, H. P., Perry, L., Conrad, D. A., Maynard, C., Martin, D. P., & Grembowski, D. E. (2011). The reliability of medical group performance measurement in a single insurer's pay for performance program. *Medical Care, 50*(2), 117–123.

Rodriguez, H. P., von Glahn, T., Chang, H., Rogers, W. H., & Safran, D. G. (2009). Measuring patients' experiences with individual specialist physicians and their practices. *American Journal of Medical Quality, 24*(1), 35–44.

Rodriguez, H. P., von Glahn, T., Elliott, M. N., Rogers, W. H., & Safran, D. G. (2009). The effect of performance-based financial incentives on improving patient care experiences: A statewide evaluation. *Journal of General Internal Medicine, 24*(12), 1281–1288.

Rosenthal, M. B. (2007). P4P: Rumors of its demise may be exaggerated. *American Journal of Managed Care, 13*(5), 238–239.

Rosenzweig, J. L., Taitel, M. S., Norman, G. K., Moore, T. J., Turenne, W., & Tang, P. (2010). Diabetes disease management in Medicare Advantage reduces hospitalizations and costs. *American Journal of Managed Care, 16*(7), e157–e162.

Schoen, C., Osborn, R., Squires, D., Doty, M., Pierson, R., & Applebaum, S. (2011). New 2011 survey of patients with complex care needs in eleven countries finds that care is often poorly coordinated. *Health Affairs (Millwood), 30*(12), 2437–2448.

Scott, A., Sivey, P., Ait Ouakrim, D., Willenberg, L., Naccarella, L., Furler, J., & Young, D. (2011). The effect of financial incentives on the quality of health care provided by primary care physicians. *Cochrane Database of Systematic Reviews, 9*, CD008451.

Sequist, T. D., Schneider, E. C., Li, A., Rogers, W. H., & Safran, D. G. (2010). Reliability of medical group and physician performance measurement in the primary care setting. *Medical Care, 49*(2), 126–131.

Shortell, S. M., Casalino, L. P., & Fisher, E. S. (2010). How the Center for Medicare and Medicaid Innovation should test accountable care organizations. *Health Affairs (Millwood), 29*(7), 1293–1298.

Sidorov, J. E. (2008). The patient-centered medical home for chronic illness: Is it ready for prime time? *Health Affairs, 27*(5), 1231–1234.

Smith, B., Forkner, E., Zaslow, B., Krasuski, R. A., Stajduhar, K., Kwan, M., . . . Freeman, G. L. (2005). Disease management produces limited quality-of-life improvements in patients with congestive heart failure: Evidence from a randomized trial in community-dwelling patients. *American Journal of Managed Care, 11*(11), 701–713.

Solomon, L. S., Zaslavsky, A. M., Landon, B. E., & Cleary, P. D. (2002). Variation in patient-reported quality among health care organizations. *Health Care Financing Review, 23*(4), 85–100.

Steiner, B. D., Denham, A. C., Ashkin, E., Newton, W. P., Wroth, T., & Dobson, L. A., Jr., (2008). Community care of North Carolina: improving care through community health networks. *Annals of Family Medicine, 6*(4), 361–367.

Tsai, A. C., Morton, S. C., Mangione, C. M., & Keeler, E. B. (2005). A meta-analysis of interventions to improve care for chronic illnesses. *American Journal of Managed Care, 11*(8), 478–488.

Villagra, V. (2004). Strategies to control costs and quality: A focus on outcomes research for disease management. *Medical Care, 42*(4 Suppl), III24–30.

Villagra, V. G., & Ahmed, T. (2004). Effectiveness of a disease management program for patients with diabetes. *Health Affairs (Millwood), 23*(4), 255–266.

Wagner, E. H. (2001). Meeting the needs of chronically ill people. *British Medical Journal, 323*(7319), 945–946.

Weeks, W. B., Gottlieb, D. J., Nyweide, D. E., Sutherland, J. M., Bynum, J., Casalino, L. P., . . . Fisher, E. S. (2010). Higher health care quality and bigger savings found at large multispecialty medical groups. *Health Affairs (Millwood), 29*(5), 991–997.

Weingarten, S. R., Henning, J. M., Badamgarav, E., Knight, K., Hasselblad, V., Gano, A., Jr., & Ofman, J. J. (2002). Interventions used in disease management programmes for patients with chronic illness: Which ones work? Meta-analysis of published reports. *British Medical Journal, 325*(7370), 925.

Welch, W. P., Bergsten, C., Cutler, C., Bocchino, C., & Smith, R. I. (2002). Disease management practices of health plans. *American Journal of Managed Care, 8*(4), 353–361.

Williams, T. R., Raube, K., Damberg, C. L., & Mardon, R. E. (2006). Pay for performance: Its influence on the use of IT in physician organizations. *Journal of Medical Practice Management, 21*(5), 301–306.

Zhang, N. J., Wan, T. T., Rossiter, L. F., Murawski, M. M., & Patel, U. B. (2008). Evaluation of chronic disease management on outcomes and cost of care for Medicaid beneficiaries. *Health Policy, 86*(2–3), 345–354.

CHAPTER TWENTY ONE

MEDICARE REFORM

Gerald F. Kominski
Jeanne T. Black
Thomas H. Rice

Learning Objectives

- Explain the history of failed attempts to enact national health insurance in the United States
- Examine the strategy and philosophy behind the compromise that led to a more limited approach focused on the elderly
- Explain the evolution of Medicare since enactment in 1965
- Understand future challenges facing Medicare, including the nature of the often-discussed "crisis" in Medicare
- Enumerate the recent efforts and proposals to reform Medicare, including efforts to further privatize Medicare through premium support

Medicare was enacted in 1965 as a compromise on the road toward a comprehensive system of national health insurance. Like most great compromises, its original design reflected prevailing concepts about health benefits and health care delivery that have changed substantially in the last fifty years. As the second largest social insurance program in the United States after Social Security, Medicare continues to bestow tremendous benefit to beneficiaries and their families, who might otherwise individually bear the entire health care costs associated with aging. More than a safety net, Medicare gives seniors and the disabled access to the highest-quality health care. But in the second decade of the twenty-first century, nearly fifty years after its enactment, Medicare is facing several significant challenges that threaten the very principles on which the program was originally based.

This chapter begins with a review of the origins of Medicare as an alternative, incremental strategy developed after decades of failed attempts to enact comprehensive national health insurance (Marmor, 2000; Hirshfield, 1970). We then discuss how Medicare has evolved, including its benefit structure and payment mechanisms, to meet various challenges since its enactment in 1965. Next we review the current challenges facing Medicare, including the demographic threat to its long-term solvency. We describe significant changes to Medicare enacted as part of the Medicare Prescription Drug, Improvement, and Modernization Act of 2003. Finally, we review key elements of the Affordable Care Act of 2010, as well as ongoing efforts to transform Medicare from a defined benefits program to one based on defined contributions.

Origin and Philosophy of Medicare

The United States stands alone among developed nations in not providing universal health coverage to its population. Proposals for national health insurance in the United States were first made before World War I. Following the Great Depression, every decade of the twentieth century saw major proposals put forward that failed to win approval in the U.S. Congress. At the root of these failures are fundamental ideological differences between liberal and conservative policymakers. Historically, liberals have advocated a system of social insurance, while conservatives have favored a welfare approach that extends assistance only to those who cannot fend for themselves in the private market.

The theory of social insurance recognizes that the benefits and costs of capitalism are not equally distributed within society and that in a democracy government has a role in tempering the impact of a competitive market economy on individuals (Dionne, 1998). Thus, the United States has social insurance programs to cushion the financial impact of occupational injuries, unemployment, and poverty in old age. In general, social insurance programs share three principles:

1. Pooled risk, because serious illness, injury, or job loss is unpredictable
2. Redistribution of income through the tax system, to achieve affordable coverage for all
3. National administration, to ensure universal access

Although the United States has failed to adopt a system of universal coverage for all residents, it does have a program of social health insurance for its elderly population. The Medicare program, enacted on July 30, 1965, as Title XVIII of the Social Security Act, is the most important piece of health insurance legislation in U.S. history. Its passage raises a fundamental question: Why was Medicare enacted rather than universal health insurance? To answer this question, and to understand how Medicare evolved along with current proposals for its reform, requires a brief review of the history of national health insurance initiatives in the United States.

The first efforts to promote national health insurance in the United States grew out of the Progressive Movement that emerged during the first decade of the twentieth century. Those efforts were based on European models of compulsory social insurance, first enacted into law by Chancellor Otto von Bismarck of Germany in 1883. The leaders of the American Medical Association (AMA), having positive views of the German and British systems, initially were supportive of the Progressives' efforts (Ball, 1998). However, the AMA soon found that local medical societies were vehemently opposed. By 1920, the medical profession solidified its opposition to comprehensive health reform, a position that it maintained throughout the remainder of the twentieth century. Conversely, organized labor, which initially feared that government programs such as compulsory social insurance would lessen workers' need to join labor unions, later became an outspoken advocate of national health insurance.

Calls for health reform to address rising medical costs are not a recent phenomenon. In 1927, eight private foundations established the Committee on the Costs of Medical Care. The committee's final report, published in 1932, called for reorganizing health care delivery into prepaid medical group practice and for promoting experiments in voluntary health insurance. Voicing its opposition, the *Journal of the American Medical Association* editorialized against "the forces representing the great foundations, public health officialdom, social theory—even socialism and communism" that were threatening the "sound practice of medicine" (Fishbein, 1932).

Following the Great Depression, President Franklin Delano Roosevelt established the Committee on Economic Security. Its recommendations formed the basis for the package of social legislation known as the

New Deal, which included the Social Security Act of 1935. However, the committee's consideration of health insurance brought an immediate storm of criticism from the AMA. As a result, Roosevelt did not publicly support national health insurance, fearing that passage of his entire program—and his reelection—could be jeopardized by its inclusion. At the same time, the AMA, suspicious of future government involvement in health care, began to support the private, voluntary hospital insurance programs begun by Blue Cross and commercial insurance companies, and state Blue Shield programs for surgical and medical expenses (Marmor, 2000).

Despite the failure to enact a national health insurance program as part of the New Deal, support for such a program remained strong in Congress. Every year between 1939 and 1951, a comprehensive health insurance bill sponsored by Sen. Robert Wagner (D-N.Y.), Sen. James Murray (D-Mont.), and Rep. John Dingell, Sr. (D-Mich.) was introduced into Congress. Over this thirteen-year period, the Murray-Wagner-Dingell bills never received enough support to be reported out of committee, and thus these bills never reached a vote on the floor of the House or Senate. In 1948, Harry Truman campaigned for president on a Fair Deal platform that included national health insurance. Once elected, however, he was unable to overcome the opposition of a coalition of Republicans and Southern Democrats. The AMA mounted a nationwide campaign promoting the horrors of "socialized medicine," and several supporters of national health insurance failed to win reelection in 1950 (Marmor, 2000).

By the early 1950s, Truman's advisors in the Federal Security Agency (now the Department of Health and Human Services) were convinced that a new strategy was necessary. They concluded that progress toward national health insurance required a more limited, incremental approach. Popular support for the Social Security program meant that a health insurance program for the elderly stood the greatest chance of approval. Linking a program of Medicare to Social Security had the added benefit of avoiding the stigma associated with a welfare program and portraying Medicare as analogous to private insurance for which the beneficiary has paid.

A program to address the needs of the elderly was also more difficult for the AMA to oppose. In the words of Robert M. Ball, who worked on the initial Medicare proposals and later became a Social Security Commissioner:

> The elderly were an appealing group to cover first in part because they were so ill suited for coverage under voluntary private insurance. They used on average more than twice as many hospital days as younger

people but had only about half as much income. Private insurers, who set premiums to cover current costs, had to charge them much more, and the elderly could not afford the charges. Group health insurance, then as today, was mostly for the employed and was just not available to the retired elderly. The result of all this was that somewhat less than half of the elderly had any kind of health insurance, and what they had was almost always inadequate . . . So the need was not hard to prove, nor was it difficult to prove that voluntary individual insurance was not only not meeting the need, but that it really could not meet the need (Ball, 1998, p. 31).

To win political support, it also was crucial for Medicare not to be viewed as a threat to the existing health care delivery or financing system. The program was positioned as a solution to the financial difficulties of the elderly that resulted from use of medical services, particularly costly hospitalization, rather than one that would comprehensively address their health needs. As a strategy to temper the AMA's opposition, physician services were not included in the initial Medicare proposals.

Between 1958 and 1963, numerous Congressional hearings and intense lobbying took place on the subject of Medicare. Although it was now generally accepted that there was strong public support for a program of health insurance for the elderly, there was vociferous debate between social insurance and welfare advocates regarding the benefits and structure of the program and whether it should be administered by the federal government or by the states. President John F. Kennedy strongly supported providing hospital insurance for the elderly through the Social Security program. However, he was unable to obtain the support of the majority on the House Ways and Means Committee, which had authority for proposed legislation requiring new federal expenditures and whose members included a conservative coalition of Republicans and Southern Democrats opposed to expansion of federal programs. Finally, the landslide Democratic victories in the 1964 elections led President Lyndon Johnson to make hospital insurance for the elderly the first piece of legislation introduced into both houses of Congress as part of his Great Society program.

Competing bills were submitted and considered by the Ways and Means Committee. Under the chairmanship of Rep. Wilbur Mills (D-Ark.), a surprising compromise was reached. The Medicare program would provide hospital insurance to all Social Security beneficiaries on the basis of the Blue Cross model and voluntary insurance for physician services along the lines of the health plan for federal employees offered by Aetna Life

Insurance. Conservatives had hoped to limit Medicare to state programs serving the very poor elderly. However, in the final bill, benefits for the poor were expanded to cover all ages, to be administered as a joint federal-state program known as Medicaid.

In summary, Medicare emerged out of frustrated efforts to pass national health insurance that began in the early part of the twentieth century. Its proponents conceived it as a social insurance program, and they hoped and expected that it would be the foundation for incremental expansion to other populations and additional benefits. But the compromises that led to its passage masked these philosophical underpinnings and sowed the seeds for many of the conflicts over Medicare's design and financing that continue into the present.

Evolution of Medicare

Medicare has evolved significantly since its enactment in 1965, even though its core elements remain essentially unchanged. This section discusses the four major components of the program: Medicare Parts A and B, known as traditional Medicare, and Parts C and D, which have been added within the past two decades.

Medicare Parts A (Facility-Based Care) and B (Physician and Outpatient Care)

The original Medicare program included two parts, Hospital Insurance (Part A) and Supplementary Medical Insurance (Part B). The major benefits covered under Part A were ninety days of hospital care per *episode of care* plus sixty *lifetime reserve days*, one hundred days of posthospital care per episode in a skilled-nursing facility (SNF) if preceded by an inpatient admission, one hundred posthospital home health visits per year, and 190 lifetime days of inpatient psychiatric care. Hospice benefits were added later, and home health care was shifted to Part B. Part B covered most physician services, outpatient hospital services, and durable medical equipment. There was no coverage for outpatient prescription drugs, nor any limit on a beneficiary's out-of-pocket expenses. The original Medicare benefits package remains essentially unchanged, with the exception of a new outpatient prescription drug benefit, discussed below that began in 2006, and some changes in coverage for preventive services enacted in 2003 and 2010.

Medicare is financed by a combination of payroll taxes, general revenues, and beneficiary contributions. *Part A* is a true social insurance program, with eligibility based on payment of payroll taxes that are mandatory for all workers. In 1966, the Medicare payroll tax was 0.35 percent from both the employee and employer on the first $6,600 of wages or salary. Since 1986, workers pay 1.45 percent of total wages or salary into Medicare Part A, with an equal contribution from their employer. The withholding rate remained unchanged from 1986 until 2013, when an additional 0.9 percent tax was imposed on earnings above $200,000 for individuals or above $250,000 for married couples filing jointly. Since 1993, there is no limit on wages or salary subject to Medicare Part A payroll deductions.

Part B intentionally diverges from the social insurance model; it is voluntary and is financed in part by current beneficiary premiums. The political opponents of social insurance for physician services (primarily the American Medical Association) accepted their inclusion in a separate voluntary insurance plan to preempt future efforts to expand the social insurance component of Part A. All beneficiaries eligible for Part A are also eligible for Part B. In addition, seniors 65 and older who not eligible for Part A can enroll in Part B. Part B requires enrollees to pay monthly premium payments, which are deducted directly from Social Security checks for those receiving government retirement benefits. These premiums are set to be approximately 25 percent of Part B costs, with the remainder contributed by federal general revenues.

Both Part A and Part B require beneficiary cost sharing. For Part A, this includes a deductible for the first day of hospital care plus coinsurance for hospital care beyond sixty days, and coinsurance for SNF care beyond twenty days as well as for durable medical equipment provided by a home health agency. Part B has an annual deductible and requires 20 percent coinsurance for most services.

Medicare copayments and deductibles are updated annually. For 2013, the Part A deductible for inpatient hospital care was $1,184 per episode and coinsurance was $296 per day for the sixty-first through ninetieth days and $592 per day for hospital stays beyond ninety days. Skilled-nursing facility coinsurance was $144.50 per day for the twenty-first through the hundredth days. The Part B premium was $104.90 per month, and the deductible was $147 per year. Since 2007, Part B monthly premiums have been income-related, so that high-income beneficiaries pay more; up to $335.70 per month in 2013 for those with incomes above $214,000 (CMS, 2013a).

Medicare's framers also knew that political support for the program required that it be modeled on the existing system of health care delivery and financing. As a result, hospital reimbursement followed the existing form of cost-based agreements with the Blue Cross system, and insurance companies served as payment intermediaries. Similarly, fearing physician refusal to participate in the program, Part B did not establish a fee schedule. Instead, it established payments based on a modified version of the physician's "usual, customary, and reasonable (UCR)" fees charged to privately insured patients; Medicare's version was known as "customary, prevailing, and reasonable (CPR)" charges. To reassure physicians that the physician-patient relationship would remain intact, Part B allowed physicians to bill patients directly, with the patient to seek payment from the government. In addition, physicians could bill patients for the difference between Medicare's allowed charge for a service and the physician's usual charge, a practice known as balance billing.

Once Medicare had been enacted, implementing it was an enormous task. To ensure passage and smooth implementation, Medicare's developers made accommodations to a wide range of interest groups. One result of these compromises was rapid growth in Medicare expenditures. The cost-based hospital reimbursement system and CPR physician payment system were predictably inflationary, and both hospital charges and physician fees increased sharply in the program's early years. However, the program's initial emphasis was on removing financial barriers to care, not on changing the delivery or financing of the health care system. In 1972, Medicare was expanded to cover individuals with end-stage renal disease and disabled people under age sixty-five who had been receiving Social Security disability benefits for two years.

During the 1970s, the rising cost of health care was a growing national concern, and it shaped concerns about the future of Medicare for the next two decades. National health expenditures as a percent of gross domestic product (GDP) rose from 7.2 percent in 1970 to 9.2 percent in 1980 (CMS, 2013b). Medicare's share of national health care costs grew from 10.3 percent to 14.6 percent over the same period (CMS, 2013b). Following the failure of various national health insurance proposals in the 1970s and of legislative and voluntary efforts to control hospital costs, the Medicare program began to adopt a new stance toward provider payment beginning in the mid-1970s. Medicare sponsored several demonstration projects during this period to develop incentive reimbursement programs for hospitals that would encourage greater efficiency and cost containment. Beginning in the 1980s, Medicare received increased Congressional scrutiny because of the growing federal budget deficit. The stage was thus set for Medicare to adopt new policies aimed at restraining costs.

In 1983, the Health Care Financing Administration (the federal agency responsible for Medicare and Medicaid, now the Centers for Medicare and Medicaid Services) implemented an inpatient prospective payment system (PPS) for hospitals. Rather than paying hospitals according to their retrospective costs, PPS paid them a fixed amount related to the patient's reason for admission, categorized according to a classification system known as diagnosis-related groups (DRGs). PPS had an immediate effect on hospital utilization; length of stay decreased more than 10 percent between 1983 and 1985, and admissions declined as hospitals shifted procedures to the outpatient setting (Moon, 1996).

Medicare also implemented price controls and global expenditure targets for payment of physician services beginning in 1992. The Medicare fee schedule (MFS), based on the resource-based relative value scale (RBRVS) developed at Harvard University, initially had as explicit goals redistribution of payments from surgical to primary care services as well as from urban to rural practitioners. Both the DRG and RBRVS approaches subsequently were adopted by many commercial insurance plans as successful cost-containment measures (Carter, Jacobson, Kominski, & Perry, 1994).

When the MFS schedule was adopted in 1992, Medicare adopted volume performance standards to control total Part B expenditures, because the incentives under Part B's fee-for-service payments still encouraged overutilization of services. Because Part B expenditures continued to grow rapidly in the 1990s, in 1997 Medicare replaced volume performance standards with the Sustainable Growth Rate (SGR) method to control the growth of Part B expenditures. This method are been plagued with problems, which will be discussed further in the Future Directions section.

Medicare Part C (Managed Care)

Despite successful implementation of hospital and physician price controls, Medicare continued to face challenges in the 1990s, since expenditures continued to grow at a faster rate than revenues. This led to concerns about the long-term solvency of the program, which according to projections in the mid-1990s would be in a deficit position by the year 2001. To address this impending financing crisis, the Balanced Budget Act (BBA) of 1997 was enacted with strong bipartisan support. The BBA included a number of measures aimed at controlling Medicare spending as well as creation of *Medicare Part C* (called Medicare+Choice, later renamed

Medicare Advantage) to offer more options for Medicare beneficiaries to join health plans. In 1998, the growth rate in Medicare expenditures fell to an unprecedented 1.5 percent (Pear, 1999a), and Medicare costs actually decreased in the six months ending in March 1999 (Pear, 1999b). However, by 2000, lawmakers were facing political pressure to return some of these savings from several key stakeholders, including providers seeking higher payments, health plans seeking higher capitation rates, and beneficiaries seeking expanded benefits. The Medicare Prescription Drug, Improvement, and Modernization Act (MMA) of 2003 addressed many of these stakeholder demands. In addition to adding a long-overdue prescription drug benefit to Medicare, the MMA increased payments to hospitals and health plans and introduced an improved risk-adjustment system for payments to health plans to further encourage them to enroll high-risk beneficiaries. Enrollment in private Medicare Advantage plans more than doubled between 2005 and 2012, to 13.1 million, or 27 percent of all Medicare beneficiaries, including a 10 percent increase from the prior year (Gold, Jacobson, Damico, Neuman, 2012).

Medicare Part D (Prescription Drug Coverage)

The Medicare Prescription Drug, Improvement, and Modernization Act (MMA) was signed into law in 2003. Although it included a number of provisions, the key component was an outpatient prescription drug benefit, beginning in January 2006. Along with lack of long-term care coverage, most observers viewed this as the program's major coverage gap—one that had become especially conspicuous with the surge in drug spending among seniors.

A previous Medicare prescription drug benefit was enacted in 1988 but repealed the next year before being implemented. The passage and then almost immediate repeal of the Medicare Catastrophic Coverage Act (MCCA) of 1988 represented a major shock to supporters of program reform. It is therefore not surprising that a full fifteen years passed before another major reform bill, the MMA, was able to attain sufficient support. Perhaps the major reason for repeal of the MCCA was that the bill's entire cost was borne by Medicare beneficiaries, much of it through a supplemental income tax payment on seniors with higher income. Because many of these beneficiaries already had subsidized prescription drug coverage through a former employer, they tended to view the legislation as providing little in the way of new benefits but at a substantial cost (Rice, Desmond, & Gabel, 1990).

MMA, although ultimately approved by Congress in 2003, followed a most contentious debate. In general, Republican supporters favored a benefit that would be administered through the private insurance system on the basis of market forces, whereas Democratic detractors called for a government-administered benefit based on the federal government negotiating drug prices. Under the legislation that was approved, those beneficiaries wishing drug coverage obtain it either through a Medicare Advantage plan or through a stand-alone prescription drug plan. Interestingly, the latter had not been marketed previously, largely because insurers were concerned about adverse selection into such a product. The drug benefit is voluntary, like Part B coverage, but it differs in that one must explicitly choose to purchase the benefit rather than the benefit being the default. Dual-eligible beneficiaries who received drug coverage from state Medicaid programs are automatically eligible for, and enrolled in, a prescription drug plan.

Because the Part D premiums are subsidized on the order of 75 percent through federal general revenues, it is generally a good investment. About 90 percent of Medicare beneficiaries now have some form of prescription drug coverage, through such sources Part D, a Medicare Advantage Plan, dual-eligibility with Medicaid, or an employer or former employer. Adverse selection has not been much of a problem because the vast majority of Medicare beneficiaries have obtained some form of prescription drug coverage.

The legislation is perhaps most noted for its unusual benefit structure including what has been dubbed the "doughnut hole." After paying a monthly premium estimated to be about $40 per month in 2013 (Hoadley, Cubanski, Hargrave, Summer, & Huang, 2012), the 2013 benefit looks like this (with the doughnut analogy in parentheses):

- A $325 annual deductible before the benefit kicks in (the person has not begun to eat the doughnut)
- Insurance coverage with a beneficiary copayment until the cost of covered prescription drugs, the deductible, and the copayments equal $2,970 (the part of the doughnut before the hole is consumed)
- A $3,985 gap in coverage; that is, no coverage for annual prescription drug spending between $2,970 and $6,955 per year (the doughnut hole)
- 95 percent coverage for annual spending in excess of $6,955 (the part of the doughnut after the hole is consumed)

These numbers may seem odd; it is because in 2006 somewhat "rounder" numbers were used but they have been adjusted for medical care inflation in the meantime.

This benefit may be unlike any other in the annals of insurance, so an explanation is order. Because drug costs are so high, and because Congress did not want to spend more than $400 billion over the first ten years of the benefit (although current cost estimates turn out to be much higher), it needed a way to contain costs but at the same time ensure that most enrollees would enjoy some of the benefits. The solution was to have a low deductible so that most would see some of the benefits in the second bullet point above. However, it was too expensive to provide that level of coverage for all spending over the deductible; hence the doughnut hole. Near-full coverage then recommences once annual expenses reach the truly catastrophic level of $6,955 annually in 2013. As part of the Affordable Care Act, the doughnut hole is being reduced every year until 2020, after which it is scheduled to be permanently removed.

Health plans and insurers selling the benefit must conform to certain rules, including provision of a minimum of two or more drugs in a particular therapeutic class. They are allowed to establish formularies of covered drugs and use their purchasing power to negotiate lower prices with drug manufacturers. Government is not allowed to negotiate prices, in sharp contrast to other programs such as the Veterans Administration and Medicaid. In addition, in order to try to ensure that a cross section of seniors (rather than a group of predominantly sicker ones) sign up for the benefit, those who do not enroll during an open enrollment period will face a 1 percent increase in premiums every month they wait.

A final key provision concerns subsidies for low-income beneficiaries. Individuals who have income below 150 percent of the federal poverty level and who meet certain asset restrictions will receive substantial discounts with respect to both premiums and cost-sharing requirements. For example, a person dually eligible for Medicare and Medicaid with income below 100 percent of the poverty level would pay no premiums, and just $1 per prescription for generic drugs and $3 per prescription for brand-name drugs. Conversely, beneficiaries with income above specified levels must pay an extra amount in addition to their drug plan premium. In 2013, this amount ranged from $11.60 per month for individuals with 2011 annual income between $85,000 and $107,000 (double these amounts for joint tax returns) to an additional $66.60 per month for individuals with 2011 annual income above $214,000 or filing a joint tax return with income above $428,000 (CMS, 2013a).

Part D has been in effect for over half a dozen years now, so some preliminary conclusions can be drawn. The benefit is a popular one—hardly a surprise given the reliance so many seniors have on prescription drugs and the fact that 75 percent of the cost is subsidized by the federal government. This is also evidenced by the dramatic increase in prescription drug coverage compared to the period before the legislation went into effect in 2006. In 2003, the year in which Part D was passed by Congress, it was estimated that 27 percent of seniors lacked drug coverage (Safran et al., 2005); while the current figure is only 10 percent (Kaiser Family Foundation, 2012). One other encouraging note is that premium costs are lower than projected. There is, however, some disagreement as to why this is the case. Proponents point to effective competition among competing insurers, while opponents note that the last few years has seen a fall in the number of new, expensive "blockbuster" drugs and a greater than expected reliance on generic drugs (Center on Budget and Policy Priorities, 2012).

Curiously, in spite of the fact that premiums are lower than predicted, it appears that beneficiaries are not making cost-effective drug plan choices. It has been estimated that only six percent are choosing the lowest cost plan available, costing the average person $300—$500 more per year than necessary (Gruber, 2009). While people are given the option to switch drug plans each year, only about five percent voluntarily choose to do so. It appears that seniors are subject to "status quo bias"; once they pick a drug plan the first time, they are very reluctant to change. Part of the reason is the sheer number of plans. When the program began, the typical person had a choice of fifty plans, with those in urban areas often having several dozen other Medicare Advantage choices. The Obama Administration has worked to reduce the number, but there are still, on average, over thirty Part D plan choices. The other reason is that choosing the best plan is difficult. There is a Medicare website available (https://www.medicare.gov/find-a-plan/questions/home.aspx), but it is cumbersome to enter all of the details of each prescription drug accurately to obtain information on what constitutes the cheapest plan. It remains to be seen what, if anything, the federal government can (or is willing to do) do to better facilitate good drug plan choices in the future.

Is Medicare Facing a Crisis?

There is no question that the Medicare program faces formidable challenges in the coming decades. As with U.S. health care costs overall, Medicare expenditures have risen steadily as a proportion of GDP. The aging of the Baby Boom generation will create enormous additional demands. The Medicare benefit package, envisioned initially as just a first step toward comprehensive coverage, has become increasingly inadequate to meet beneficiaries' health needs. The Affordable Care Act of 2010 (ACA) made only incremental changes in traditional Medicare benefits, but it included a number of approaches intended to reduce the fragmentation inherent in the fee-for-service system. The policy question is whether the ACA can succeed in "bending the cost curve" sufficiently to preserve the viability of traditional Medicare, or whether a more radical change is required. This section discusses the demographic and utilization factors that contribute to rising Medicare costs, forecasts of Medicare insolvency, and the rising financial burden on beneficiaries.

Demographics

The most significant threat to the future of the Medicare program is the aging of the U.S. population. The Baby Boom generation (those born between 1946 and 1964) began to reach the age of 65 in 2011, and this demographic bulge will continue until 2029, creating a tremendous financial burden on Medicare. The number of beneficiaries is estimated to rise from nearly forty million in 2000 to eighty million in 2030 (Cubanski, Huang, Damico, Jacobson, & Neuman, 2010). Though the population age sixty-five to seventy-nine is projected to increase by 82 percent between 2011 and 2050, those eighty-five and older will be the fastest-growing segment of the elderly, increasing as much as 227 percent (U.S. Census Bureau, 2013).

Demographic changes have political and social implications for the Medicare program in addition to their economic impact (Friedland & Summer, 2004). Population projections depend on assumptions regarding mortality, fertility, and immigration. Average life expectancy in the United States increased throughout the twentieth century as a result of improved standards of living as well as advances in medical care. Key questions here are whether historical improvement in mortality will continue, whether there is a genetically determined limit to the human life-span, and whether increasing income inequality will lead to a rise in mortality rates in the U.S. population. Whatever the answer to these questions, further improvement in average life expectancy would increase the number of years individuals are dependent on the Medicare program.

Fertility and immigration rates are important because they affect population growth, the proportion represented by the elderly, and the ratio of tax-paying workers to the number of Medicare beneficiaries. However, the Great Recession of 2008 makes both of these components particularly challenging to forecast. U.S. fertility rates in the last decade of the twentieth century were slightly below replacement level (Hollmann, Mulder, & Kallan, 2000), but had begun to increase due to higher fertility rates among immigrants (Dye, 2010; Grieco et al., 2012). These children of immigrants will contribute to an increase in the proportion of younger workers in the population. However, the combined effects of U.S. immigration policy and economic conditions have led to a decrease in total immigration (Passel & Cohn, 2011). It is also notable that as of 2011, births to members of ethnic groups currently identified as "minorities" represented more than half of all births (Passel, Livingston, & Cohn, 2012). Despite recent concerns about the long-term sustainability of Medicare in light of the rapidly aging population, the combined number of children and the elderly relative to the size of the working age population (that is, the dependency ratio) is forecast to be lower in 2060 than it was in 1960, suggesting that the long-term sustainability is more favorable than portrayed in political discussions (Board of Trustees, OASDI, 2012).

Because Medicare is a public program for a targeted population group, it is subject to unique political pressures not experienced by universal health care programs. In countries with national health insurance, the risk pool includes the entire population, of which the elderly are a relatively small proportion. Expenditures for individuals under age sixty-five are already counted in the system, so the effect of a growing number of individuals reaching age sixty-five is simply the incremental cost of health care for sixty-five-year-olds versus sixty-four-year-olds. In contrast, the baby boom generation will create a huge budgetary impact in the United States, because most beneficiaries transition from private insurance (or no coverage) to public insurance when they become eligible for Medicare. The European countries and Japan have already absorbed the health costs of a population that aged more rapidly than that of the United States. Though there have been signs of strain and incremental reforms in their health systems, these countries continue to furnish universal coverage, and cost pressures have not resulted in radical restructuring (Ikegami & Anderson, 2012; Reinhardt, Hussey, & Anderson, 2004).

Costs

A generally accepted means of assessing trends in health care expenditures is to examine their relationship to national GDP. Between 1975 and 1995, Medicare expenditures exceeded GDP growth by 3.5 to 4.0 percent per year (Fuchs, 1999). Consequently, the Medicare program became an ever larger proportion of the national economy. The Trustees of the Part A and Part B trust funds are required by law to make an annual report to Congress that forecasts future expenditures and revenue. The addition of the Part D drug benefit and increased payments to Medicare Advantage plans under the MMA of 2003 increased forecasts of Medicare spending relative to the economy. The latest Trustees' report forecasts that Medicare expenditures will increase from 3.7 percent of GDP in 2012 to 6.0 percent in 2040—but that the Part A Trust Fund would be exhausted in 2024 (Board of Trustees, Medicare, 2012).

Price, volume, and intensity of service all play a role in medical expenditures. Both the PPS and MFS were mechanisms to limit provider payment and reduce utilization. These approaches to price controls have been partially effective, but they do not address other underlying determinants of continuing expenditure growth—that is, the diffusion of medical technology and the increasing intensity of services. One factor driving growth in health care costs of the elderly has been technology increasing the intensity of services consumed per capita (Moon, 1996; Fuchs, 1999). Analysts differ in their assumptions about how individuals will use services in the future, and the evidence is contradictory. Factors that would increase costs include the oldest old being far more likely to be institutionalized or to require assistance with activities of daily living.

In addition, utilization rates for procedures such as angioplasty and hip replacement among Medicare beneficiaries have increased dramatically over the past ten years, with some of the largest increases in the population age eighty-five and older. Will the average eighty-five-year-old consume fewer resources because she will be healthier? Or will she consume the same or more because she will have transcatheter aortic valve implantation and a hip replacement to continue playing tennis?

Finally, many chronic conditions are not strongly associated with mortality, so that increased longevity will mean more people living with chronic and costly conditions such as dementia (Zilberberg & Tjia, 2011; Bynum et al., 2004). On the other hand, several factors support the notion that per capita use of services may decline as the population ages. For example, a large proportion of Medicare costs are incurred in the last year of a beneficiary's life; thus, increased longevity means that the cost of dying will be spread over a longer period of time. In addition, the cost of dying is lower for the oldest old (Levinsky et al., 2001). The costs for a ninety-three-year-old who dies of pneumonia in a nursing home are less than those for a sixty-eight-year-old who dies in the intensive care unit of complications from open heart surgery. In addition, advances in treatment and improved understanding of risk factors can delay the onset of some chronic conditions (Wolfe, 1993).

Efforts to reduce growth in the price and volume of services, whether through regulation or competition, were the focus of Medicare reform efforts in the 1980s and 1990s. The Sustainable Growth Rate (SGR) method was adopted in 1997, replacing the volume performance standard (VPS) method, to control the growth of Part B expenditures. The SGR approach of tying Part B expenditure growth to growth in overall GDP is widely viewed as a failed policy at this point, but an effective alternative has yet to be adopted by Congress. With the addition of a prescription drug benefit as part of the MMA of 2003, controlling program expenditures will continue to be a challenge facing the Medicare program during the next decade, because Part B and Part D expenditures are growing much faster than the other components of Medicare.

Forecasts of Insolvency

The Medicare Part A Trust Fund has been forecast to become insolvent many times during its history. The frequent declarations of a crisis in Medicare can be explained in part by the nature of economic forecasts. Forecasting requires assumptions about demographics, economic growth, worker productivity, health care costs, and other important variables. Small differences in assumptions compound over time, with the result that analysts' forecasts can vary significantly and change dramatically from year to year. Nevertheless, the Medicare trustees are required by law to project the funds' status seventy-five years into the future. Considering the changes that have occurred since the 1930s in medicine, in technology generally, in society, and in the world economy, it is obviously absurd to expect long-term forecasts to be reliable.

Reliable short-term estimates are also difficult to produce. In 1996, the Part A Trust Fund was projected to be bankrupt in 2001 (Moon, 1996). However, the reimbursement changes mandated by the BBA of 1997 were more successful than anticipated in restraining Medicare costs, and by the time of the 1999 Trustees' report bankruptcy of the trust fund had been put off until 2015 (Boards of Trustees, Social Security and Medicare, 1999). The 2011 and 2012 annual reports both estimate that the trust fund will remain solvent until 2024, although the 2012 report emphasizes the added uncertainty associated with the Affordable Care Act (Board of Trustees, OASDI, 2012). These continually changing forecasts illustrate just how sensitive the projections are to assumptions about changes in the economy as well as expenditure patterns among Medicare beneficiaries.

Benefit Gaps and Rising Out-of-Pocket Expenditures

The Medicare benefit package was modeled after the private health plans of the 1960s, with Part A analogous to Blue Cross hospital coverage and Part B to Aetna coverage of physicians' services. The private "Medigap" market developed to offer supplementary insurance, similar to major medical policies sold by many private insurers. Medicare as originally designed was not intended to cover all the medical expenditures of the elderly. Early estimates were that it would pay about 40 percent (Marmor, 2000). In 2006, it was estimated to cover 48 percent of medical and long-term care costs (Cubanski et al., 2010). The program has always required beneficiaries to contribute a significant amount toward their covered medical benefits in the form of the part B premium as well as deductibles and coinsurance. In 2007, beneficiaries with traditional fee-for-service Medicare spent a median $3,138 out-of-pocket, or 16.6 percent of income. Prescription drugs accounted for the largest proportion of out-of-pocket spending for covered services, while long-term care represented the largest component of spending on non-covered services, with median spending of $7,069 (Noel-Miller, 2012).

In 1965, the medical profession, which fought so strenuously against the passage of Medicare, also considered prepaid group practice to be socialized medicine and ostracized physicians who practiced in what are now called group-model HMOs. However, rising health care costs stimulated many changes in the structure of private health plans. As discussed in Chapter Seven, by the 1990s HMOs and other forms of managed care had replaced indemnity fee for service (FFS) as the predominant type of health plan design. Managed care plans eliminated the distinctions between hospital and physician benefits, which had become unwieldy as health care delivery moved increasingly into ambulatory care. They also included benefits for preventive services. Many employers also added prescription drug coverage to managed care plans as an inducement for their employees to switch from costly indemnity plans. Meanwhile, the basic structure of Medicare remained unchanged. What began as a program that mirrored private health insurance in 1965 became one with a distinctly different benefit structure by the end of the twentieth century.

As of 2000, the traditional Medicare program lacked two important benefits found in most employer-sponsored health plans: prescription drugs and catastrophic coverage. Although prescription drugs are increasingly important in treating the chronic illnesses suffered by the elderly, their cost has been rising more rapidly than that of health care overall. National health spending on prescription drugs almost tripled between 1995 and 2003. In contrast, total national health expenditures increased by only 70 percent (National Center for Health Statistics [NCHS], 2005). Although 89 percent of beneficiaries in 2001 had supplemental coverage (through privately purchased Medigap policies, Medicare HMOs, employer-sponsored plans, or Medicaid) (Laschober, 2004), 27 percent had no coverage for prescription drugs (Safran et al., 2005). The burden of prescription drug expenses for the elderly has been exacerbated by the fact that the retail pharmacy prices paid by the elderly and others without prescription drug coverage are substantially higher than the prices negotiated by managed care plans. This gap in Medicare coverage led to enactment of Medicare Part D, discussed earlier in this chapter.

Even after the addition of Part D drug coverage, the coverage provided by traditional Medicare is somewhat less generous than large employer health plans. According to a study by the Kaiser Family Foundation and Aon Hewitt, for an age person age sixty-five or older, Medicare would cover 97 percent of the amount covered by the Blue Cross/Blue Shield Standard Option (a PPO) in the Federal Employees Health Benefit Plan (FEHBP) and 93 percent of the amount covered by a typical large employer PPO (McArdle, Stark, Levinson, & Neuman, 2012). The gap between traditional Medicare and employer plans has shrunk in recent years due to a provision of the Affordable Care Act that added a brand name drug discount of 50 percent for beneficiaries in the Part D "doughnut hole" and an increase in the out-of-pocket spending limit in the FEHBP.

Medicare has no limitation on beneficiaries' out-of-pocket costs, whereas the typical private insurance plan covers all expenses after the enrollee has incurred a specified amount of co-insurance payment, up to the policy's lifetime maximum. Nor does Medicare cover long-term nursing home care, which also is not generally covered by private employer-sponsored health insurance. Although there is a small private market for long-term care insurance, most nursing home costs are paid by the Medicaid program (for those who are poor or who spend down their assets), or out of pocket by the elderly or their families. Although the need is great, there are currently no viable reform proposals to include nursing home care as part of the basic Medicare benefit package.

The poverty rate among the elderly has dropped from 28.5 percent in 1966 to 8.7 percent in 2011 (DeNavas-Walt, Proctor, & Smith, 2012).

However, health care costs have risen much faster than the incomes of the elderly. Therefore out-of-pocket costs represent an increasing proportion of income—the very condition Medicare was enacted to ameliorate. In 2006, out-of-pocket costs for Medicare beneficiaries represented 16 percent of median income, with this proportion projected to rise to 26 percent by 2020, including expenditures for long-term care (Neuman, Cubanski, Huang, & Damico, 2011a).

Future Directions

During the 1990s, the Clinton administration consistently supported use of the private market to achieve cost savings and promote innovation in delivering health services. The Medicare+Choice program was established as part of the BBA of 1997 to expand private sector health plan options for Medicare beneficiaries. Managed care plans participating in Medicare+Choice (renamed Medicare Advantage as part of the MMA of 2003) must cover the basic package of Medicare benefits. They compete within a given market on the basis of supplemental benefits such as prescription drugs, provider networks, and customer service. But there is no evidence of significant competition on price, leading to lower premiums. Beneficiaries continue to pay the same basic Part B premium, and their total cost sharing cannot be greater than that of traditional Medicare. All plans within a county are paid the same rate per beneficiary, with adjustment for health status and other risk factors. As the name implied, Medicare+Choice gave many beneficiaries the choice between traditional Medicare and a managed care plan similar to that offered by employers in the private sector, while preserving the basic entitlements of the original Medicare program. The use of private markets and choice was further expanded with the enactment of Part D prescription drug coverage during the next decade.

Since the passage of Medicare in 1965, the political values of the United States have shifted fundamentally. Whereas government was once viewed as a positive force for social change, the prevailing climate holds that government is inefficient and that markets can better meet the desires of individual consumers. This orientation, coupled with cyclic forecasts of trust fund insolvency, has led some policymakers to assert that the Medicare program requires radical restructuring if it is to survive in the new century. Supporters of the role of government, on the other hand, argue that continued innovation in payment systems, improvement in chronic disease management (particularly among dually eligible Medicare and Medicaid beneficiaries), taking advantage of the federal government's purchasing power, and other incremental steps can both reform Medicare and preserve its function as a social insurance program. Below, we discuss two potentially large reform proposals: increasing the age of eligibility for Medicare, and moving to a "premium support" system.

Increasing the Age of Eligibility

One of the surest ways to improve Medicare's fiscal prospects is to increase the age of eligibility. When Medicare was enacted, eligibility for benefits was pegged at age sixty-five, the same age as Social Security. Since that time, life expectancy has increased a great deal. In 1960, the average sixty-five-year old lived 14.3 more years. By 2007, this had increased more than four years, to 18.6 (NCHS, 2011). In response to this trend, Social Security raised its eligibility age to sixty-seven, and many have suggested that Medicare do the same. The Congressional Budget Office (CBO) estimates that enacting such a proposal would save the federal government about $150 billion over a ten-year period, reducing program expenditures by about 5 percent (Congressional Budget Office [CBO], 2012).

CBO concluded that many seniors between ages sixty-five and sixty-seven would have to pay more in premiums by being forced to purchase private coverage. Moreover, if such coverage were less generous than Medicare's, then cost-sharing requirements would go up as well. These impacts would probably not be as great as they would have been otherwise with the implementation of the ACA because insurers are not allowed to charge those with a history of illness more in premiums than others (Neuman, Cubanski, Waldo, Eppig, & Mays, 2011b). They may charge older individuals up to three times as much as younger people, however.

Since 1965 when Medicare was enacted, the average retirement age decreased from about sixty-five to sixty-two as of 2000 (Gendell, 2001), although more recent data from the Bureau of Labor Statistics shows that average retirement age stayed relatively constant during the 2000 to 2010 period. Seniors do not show a tendency to want to work longer so there is little doubt that raising the age of Medicare eligibility will face a great deal of political opposition. If such a change is adopted, it is likely to be one of many elements of a much larger reform package aimed at improving the financial viability of Medicare.

Privatizing Medicare: Premium Support

Traditional fee-for-service Medicare is a defined benefits program in which all beneficiaries are guaranteed a defined set of benefits regardless of ability to pay or health status. As health care costs rise and the beneficiary population increases, this system creates an open-ended financial obligation for the federal government. Policymakers who seek to limit this obligation have proposed replacing the current program with a defined contribution (sometimes called "voucher") or "premium support" approach.

In its purest form, defined contribution would limit the obligation of the federal government by giving beneficiaries a fixed dollar amount with which they would purchase their own health insurance in the private market. One of the choices could include traditional Medicare coverage along with an array of private plans. The amount of the government contribution could be adjusted for inflation using a standard economic indicator such as the Consumer Price Index (CPI) or GDP. Thus federal Medicare expenditures would be fixed at a targeted level, equal to the government's contribution multiplied by the number of eligible beneficiaries, and beneficiaries would pay any difference between the cost of the plan they chose and the federal contribution. If health care costs continue their historical pattern of rising faster than GDP, the financial risk for these increased costs would be shifted to beneficiaries because Medicare's contribution would be fixed.

Noting that a strict voucher approach would not be viable either politically or programmatically, economists Henry Aaron and Robert Reischauer proposed a version of the defined contribution approach termed *premium support* (Aaron & Reischauer, 1995). There are two crucial assumptions underlying this approach: private sector competition is the best means to restrain the rate of cost increases in the Medicare program; and the federal government's financial obligation should be limited in order to impose fiscal discipline on the program and avoid the need for future tax increases to support Medicare.

Premium support differs from defined contribution in that the federal government and beneficiaries would share the risk of rising health care costs. As originally conceived, the federal contribution would not be tied to an external economic indicator but would instead be based on bids submitted by private sector health plans seeking to participate in the Medicare program. The traditional Medicare program would be retained, but it would be required to compete with private health plans. Recent proposals, however, have hedged reliance on competition to control costs. At time of writing, the proposal receiving the most attention, which was proposed jointly by Democratic Senator Ron Wyden and Republican Congressman Paul Ryan, would raise the federal contribution by no more than one percentage point above the growth in GDP (Wyden &

Ryan, 2011). While this is more in line with the way in which defined contribution is defined, it is still being called a premium support proposal, so we use that terminology here.

In theory, premium support would offer beneficiaries greater choice, enabling them to select the health plan that best meets their needs. Because they would pay the difference between the premium support contribution and the cost of their chosen plan, beneficiaries would have a financial incentive to choose a plan that offered the best value in terms of cost and quality. There have been a number of criticisms expressed as well. It is not clear if premium support, as originally envisaged, would save much money because most health care costs are borne by those with expensive chronic illnesses—premium support, in itself, does not affect how care for this population is delivered. Moreover, if federal contributions are limited to a formula like GDP plus one percentage point, then costs are likely to be shifted over time to beneficiaries since health care costs are likely to continue growing faster than that. There are also concerns that Medicare will attract a sicker group of enrollees (not fully accounted for by current risk-adjustment formulas) and become more expensive than private plans, further segmenting coverage and making it difficult for unhealthy and low-income populations to afford care.

During 2012, nearly all Republicans in Congress expressed support for premium support. Most Democrats opposed it, although it is perhaps significant that one of the authors of the Wyden-Ryan proposal is a Democrat. With President Obama's reelection in November 2012, premium support would appear to be on hold for the foreseeable future. However, the ultimate decision on whether to transform Medicare into a premium support program is likely to hinge not only on election results but also whether other means are found to make the Medicare program more financially viable in the long run.

SUMMARY

Medicare was implemented in 1965 as an incremental step toward national health insurance in the United States. Fifty years later, it survives as the country's second largest social insurance program and is likely to continue well into the twenty-first century as a separate program. The fundamental challenges facing the future of Medicare are how to finance the projected growth in enrollment and the increased costs of technology, and whether ongoing efforts to privatize the program will stabilize it financially.

When Medicare was enacted, a founding principle was that it was supposed to reflect mainstream medicine and health insurance, including mainstream delivery and payment methodologies. One obvious question regarding the future of Medicare is whether various reform proposals are consistent with this original principle. Despite the substantial movement during the past two decades toward defined contributions for pension benefits in the private sector, defined contribution plans for health benefits are still not common, although recent developments to encourage Health Savings Accounts may fundamentally change the nature of employment-based coverage during the next decade. Before beginning a grand experiment with the future of Medicare, however, perhaps policymakers should wait until the private market fully embraces consumer-directed health plans. Enrollment in health savings accounts and high-deductible health plans rose to 13.5 million by January 2012, with 82 percent of that in employer-sponsored plans (America's Health Insurance Plans [AHIP], 2012). At the same time, the proportion of the U.S. population under age sixty-five covered by employer-sponsored health insurance decreased by 10.6 percentage points between 2000 and 2010, to 58.6 percent (Gould, 2012).

In the meantime, incremental efforts to expand benefits and offer additional subsidies to low-income beneficiaries are likely to reduce existing disparities within the program and improve the health and financial stability of those who are most vulnerable. Congress may also need to revisit the MMA of 2003 to address its costs, which are already projected to far exceed the original estimates of about $400 billion over its first ten years, as well as other aspects of the legislation, which shortly after implementation appeared to be both poorly understood and problematic.

KEY TERMS

Episode of care Under Medicare Part A, an episode starts with an inpatient admission and ends sixty days after discharge from a hospital or skilled-nursing facility. Thus, beneficiaries can have multiple episodes per year.

Lifetime reserve days A pool of sixty days that can be used if a beneficiary has an inpatient episode exceeding ninety days. Lifetime reserve days cannot be replaced once used.

Medicare Part A Coverage for hospital and other facility-based services. Originally based on Blue Cross insurance.

Medicare Part B Coverage for physician and other outpatient care services. Originally based on Aetna insurance.

Medicare Part C Also known as Medicare Advantage; provides coverage for managed care by combining Medicare Parts A and B with approved health plans. Allows beneficiaries to select a health plan, which is paid a monthly premium by Medicare. Generally provides Medicare benefits, as well as additional benefits, with lower or no copayments or deductibles.

Medicare Part D Prescription drug benefit; like Medicare Part B, it is financed through a combination of beneficiary monthly premiums and government general tax revenues.

Premium support Proposal first developed in the 1990s to transform Medicare from a defined benefits program to a defined contribution program, thus limiting government contributions.

DISCUSSION QUESTIONS

1. The United States stands alone among developed nations in not providing universal health coverage to its population. Why?
2. Does the intergenerational nature of Medicare (in which current workers pay the bills for current retirees) weaken the value of the program to the current generation, because they won't directly benefit until the future? What if Medicare did not exist and the burden of health care costs fell onto the elderly and their families? Do you and your family have a stake in Medicare and its future?
3. Is Medicare in need of fundamental reform, or can the program survive with incremental changes in benefits and financing?
4. If you were designing a government health insurance program for the elderly today, what would it look like? What elements of Medicare would you retain? What elements would you change?

FURTHER READING

Kaiser Family Foundation. (2005). *Medicare at 40.* http://www.kff.org/medicaid/40yearsvideo.cfm

The Kaiser Family Foundation has produced an online documentary on Medicare at its fortieth anniversary that includes interviews with some of the key members of the Johnson administration as well as supporters and opponents of this historic legislation enacted in 1965.

Kaiser Family Foundation. (2010). *Medicare chartbook 2010* (4th ed.). http://facts.kff .org/chartbook.aspx?cb=58

Excellent overview of beneficiary characteristics, spending, benefits, utilization, MedicareAdvantage, and prescription drug benefit under Medicare Part D. This chartbook is updated periodically. In the interim, annual fact sheets on Medicare can be found on the Kaiser Family Foundation website.

Marmor, T. R. (2000). *The politics of Medicare* (2nd ed.). New York: Aldine de Gruyter.

Definitive analysis of the politics leading to the enactment of the Medicare program.

Neuman, P., & Cubanski, J. (2013). *Policy options to sustain Medicare for the future.* Menlo Park, CA: Kaiser Family Foundation.

This report provides in-depth analysis of options for sustaining Medicare without fundamentally dismantling the program by converting it into a fixed-contribution voucher system.

REFERENCES

Aaron, H. J., & Reischauer, R. D. (1995). The Medicare reform debate: What is the next step? *Health Affairs, 10*(4), 8–30.

America's Health Insurance Plans (AHIP). (2012). *Census shows 13.5 million people covered by health savings account/high-deductible health plans (HSA/HDHPS).* Washington, DC: America's Health Insurance Plans, Center for Policy and Research.

Ball, R. M. (1998). Medicare's social contract: Reflections on how Medicare came about. In R. D. Reischauer, S. Butler, & J. R. Lave (Eds.), *Medicare: Preparing for the challenges of the 21st century.* Washington, DC: National Academy of Social Insurance.

Board of Trustees, Medicare. (2012). 2012 Annual report of the board of trustees of the Federal Hospital Insurance and Federal Supplementary Health Insurance Trust Funds. Retrieved from http://www.cms.hhs.gov/ReportsTrustFunds/downloads /tr2012.pdf

Board of Trustees, OASDI. (2012). *2012 Annual report of the board of trustees of the Federal Old-Age and Survivors Insurance and Disability Insurance Trust Funds.* Table V.A.2. Washington, DC: U.S. Government Printing Office. Retrieved from http://www.ssa .gov/OACT/TR/2012/tr2012.pdf

Boards of Trustees, Social Security and Medicare. (1999). *Status of the Social Security and Medicare programs: A summary of the 1999 annual reports.* http://www.ssa .gov/history/pdf/tr99summary.pdf

Bynum, J. P., Rabins, P.V., Weller, W., Niefeld, M., Anderson, G. F., & Wu, A. W. (2004). The relationship between a dementia diagnosis, chronic illness, Medicare expenditures, and hospital use. *Journal of the American Geriatrics Society, 52,* 187–194.

Carter, G. M., Jacobson, P. D., Kominski, G. F., & Perry, M. J. (1994). Use of diagnosis-related groups by non-Medicare payers. *Health Care Financing Review, 16,* 127–158.

Center on Budget and Policy Priorities. (2012). *Lower-than-expected Medicare drug costs mostly reflect lower enrollment and slowing of overall drug spending, not reliance on private plans.* Retrieved from http://www.cbpp.org/cms/index.cfm?fa=view&id=3775

Centers for Medicare and Medicaid Services (CMS). (2013a). *Medicare costs at a glance.* Retrieved from http://www.medicare.gov/your-medicare-costs/costs-at-a-glance/costs-at-glance.html

Centers for Medicare and Medicaid Services (CMS). (2013b). *National health expenditures, 1960–2011.* Retrieved from http://www.cms.gov/Research-Statistics-Data-and-Systems/Statistics-Trends-and-Reports/NationalHealthExpendData/Downloads/tables.pdf

Congressional Budget Office (CBO). (2012). *Raising the ages of eligibility for Medicare and Social Security.* Retrieved on from http://www.cbo.gov/sites/default/files/cbofiles/attachments/01–10–2012-Medicare_SS_EligibilityAgesBrief.pdf

Cubanski, J., Huang, J., Damico, A., Jacobson, G., & Neuman, T. (2010). *Medicare chartbook 2010* (4th ed.). Menlo Park, CA: Kaiser Family Foundation. Retrieved from http://www.kff.org/medicare/upload/8103.pdf

DeNavas-Walt, C., Proctor, B. D., & Smith, J. C. (2012). *Income, poverty, and health insurance coverage in the United States: 2011* (Current Population Reports, P60-239). Washington, DC: U.S. Census Bureau. Retrieved from http://www.census.gov/prod/2012pubs/p60–243.pdf

Dionne, E. J. (1998). Medicare's social contract: Social insurance commentary. In R. D. Reischauer, S. Butler, & J. R. Lave (Eds.), *Medicare: Preparing for the challenges of the 21st century.* Washington, DC: National Academy of Social Insurance.

Dye, J. L. (2010). *Fertility of American women: June 2008* (Current Population Reports, P20–563). Washington, DC: U. S. Census Bureau. Retrieved from http://www.census.gov/prod/2010pubs/p20–563.pdf

Fishbein, M. (1932). The committee on the costs of medical care. *Journal of the American Medical Association, 99,* 1950–1952.

Friedland, R. B., & Summer, L. (2004). *Demography is not destiny, revisited.* Washington, DC: Georgetown University Center on an Aging Society.

Fuchs, V. (1999). Health care for the elderly: How much? Who will pay for it? *Health Affairs, 18,* 11–21.

Gendell, M. (2001). Retirement age declines again in the 1990s. *Monthly Labor Review, 124,* 12–21.

Gold, M., Jacobson, G., Damico, A., & Neuman, T. (2012). *Medicare Advantage 2012 data spotlight: Enrollment market update* (Publication No. 8323). Menlo Park, CA: Kaiser Family Foundation. Retrieved from http://www.kff.org/medicare/upload/8323.pdf

Gould, E. (2012). *A decade of declines in employer-sponsored health insurance coverage* (Briefing Paper No. 337). Washington, DC: Economic Policy Institute. Retrieved on from http://www.epi.org/files/2012/bp337.pdf

Grieco, E. M., Acosta, Y. D., de la Cruz, G. P., Gambino, C., Gryn, T., Larsenet, L. J., . . . Walter, N. P. (2012). *The foreign-born population in the United States: 2010.* Washington, DC: U.S. Census Bureau American Community Survey Reports.

Gruber, J. (2009). *Choosing a Medicare Part D plan: Are Medicare beneficiaries choosing low-cost plans?* Menlo Park, CA: Kaiser Family Foundation. Retrieved from http://www.kff.org/medicare/upload/7864.pdf

Hirshfield, D. S. (1970). *The lost reform: The campaign for compulsory health insurance in the United States from 1932 to 1943.* Cambridge, MA: Harvard University Press & Commonwealth Fund.

Hoadley, J., Cubanski, J., Hargrave, E., Summer, L., & Huang, J. (2012). *Medicare Part D: A first look at Part D plan offerings in 2013* (Publication No. 8375). Menlo Park, CA: Kaiser Family Foundation. Retrieved from http://www.kff.org/medicare/upload/8375.pdf

Hollmann, F. W., Mulder, T. J., & Kallan, J. E. (2000). *Methodology and assumptions for the population projections of the United States: 1999 to 2100* (Population Division Working Paper No. 38). Washington, DC: U. S. Census Bureau. Retrieved from http://www.census.gov/population/www/documentation/twps0038/twps0038.html#B1

Ikegami, N., & Anderson, G. F. (2012). In Japan, all-payer rate setting under tight government control has proved to be an effective approach to contain costs. *Health Affairs, 31,* 1049–1056.

Kaiser Family Foundation. (2012). *The Medicare prescription drug benefit: Fact sheet.* Retrieved from http://www.kff.org/medicare/upload/7044–13.pdf

Laschober, M. (2004). *Trends in Medicare supplemental insurance and prescription drug benefits, 1996–2001.* Washington, DC: Kaiser Family Foundation.

Levinsky, N. G., Yu, W., Ash, A., Moskowitz, M. Gazelle, G., Saynina, O., & Emanuel, E. J. (2001). Influence of age on Medicare expenditures and medical care in the last year of life. *Journal of the American Medical Association, 286,* 1349–1355.

Marmor, T. R. (2000). *The politics of Medicare* (2nd ed.). New York: Aldine de Gruyter.

McArdle, F., Stark, I., Levinson, Z., & Neuman, T. (2012). *How does the benefit value of Medicare compare to the benefit value of typical large employer plans? A 2012 update* (Issue Brief). Menlo Park, CA: Kaiser Family Foundation. Retrieved from http://www.kff.org/medicare/7768.cfm

Moon, M. (1996). *Medicare now and in the future.* Washington, DC: Urban Institute Press.

National Center for Health Statistics (NCHS). (2005). *Health, U.S., 2005.* Table 122. Hyattsville, MD: National Center for Health Statistics.

National Center for Health Statistics (NCHS). (2011). *Health, U.S., 2010.* Retrieved from http://www.cdc.gov/nchs/data/hus/hus10.pdf

Noel-Miller, C. (2012). *Medicare beneficiaries' out-of-pocket spending for health care.* Washington, DC: AARP Public Policy Institute.

Neuman, T., Cubanski, J., Huang, J., & Damico, A. (2011a). *How much "skin in the game" is enough? The financial burden of health spending for people on Medicare* (Data Spotlight, Publication No. 8170). Menlo Park, CA: Kaiser Family Foundation. Retrieved from http://www.kff.org/medicare/upload/8170.pdf

Neuman, T., Cubanski, J., Waldo, D., Eppig, F., & Mays, J. (2011b). *Raising the age of Medicare eligibility: A fresh look following implementation of health reform.* Menlo Park, CA: Kaiser Family Foundation. Retrieved from http://www.kff.org/medicare/upload/8169.pdf

Passel, J., & Cohn, D. (2011). *Unauthorized immigrant population: National and state trends, 2010.* Washington, DC: Pew Research Center. Retrieved from

http://www.pewhispanic.org/2011/02/01/unauthorized-immigrant-population
-brnational-and-state-trends-2010

Passel, J., Livingston, G., & Cohn, D. (2012). *Explaining why minority births now outnumber white births*. Washington, DC: Pew Research Center. Retrieved from http://www.pewsocialtrends.org/2012/05/17/explaining-why-minority-births
-now-outnumber-white-births/?src=hispanic-footer

Pear, R. (1999a, January 12). '98 Medicare growth slowest since program began in '65. *New York Times*, p. A1.

Pear, R. (1999b, May 4). With budget cutting, Medicare spending fell unexpectedly. *New York Times*, pp. A20, A24.

Reinhardt, U., Hussey, P., & Anderson, G. (2004). U.S. health care spending in an international context. *Health Affairs, 23*, 10–25.

Rice, T., Desmond, K., & Gabel, J. (1990). The Medicare Catastrophic Coverage Act: A post-mortem. *Health Affairs, 9*, 75–87.

Safran, D. G., Neuman, P., Schoen, C., Kitchman, M. S., Wilson, I. B., Cooper, B., . . . Rogers, W. H. (2005). Prescription drug coverage and seniors: Findings from a 2003 national survey. *Health Affairs (Web Exclusives)*, W5-152–W5-166.

U.S. Census Bureau. (2013). *2012 National population projections: Summary tables*. Table 2. Retrieved from http://www.census.gov/population/projections/data/national/2012/summarytables.html

Wolfe, J. R. (1993). *The coming health care crisis: Who will pay for care for the aged in the twenty-first century?* Chicago: University of Chicago Press.

Wyden, R., & Ryan, P. (2011, December 15). *Guaranteed choices to strengthen Medicare and health security for all*. Retrieved from http://budget.house.gov/uploadedfiles/wydenryan.pdf

Zilberberg, M. D., & Tjia, J. (2011). Growth in dementia-associated hospitalizations among the oldest old in the United States: Implications for ethical health services planning. *Archives of Internal Medicine, 171*, 1850–1851.

CHAPTER TWENTY TWO

PUBLIC HEALTH AND CLINICAL CARE

Jonathan E. Fielding
Lester Breslow
Steven M. Teutsch

Learning Objectives

- Understand the role of public health related to the clinical care system from a population-health perspective
- Understand how the clinical care system can advance the public's health by advancing prevention
- Learn how public health agencies have traditionally provided clinical care services and how this role may decrease with health reform
- Understand the *core functions of public health*: assessment, policy development, and assurance

In our current effort to reform the organization, delivery, and financing of clinical care, the broad question of how these services contribute to the health of our country receives little consideration. Much discussion about clinical care has focused on the Affordable Care Act: how to control the enormous and escalating costs of medical, physician, pharmaceutical, hospital, and other services and how to overcome the access barriers that arise from lack of health insurance and other challenges to obtaining needed care, including ethnic discrimination, stigma, and poor distribution of providers. More recently, considerable discussion has also focused on issues of patient safety and quality of care. This chapter addresses the appropriate role of governmental public health agencies in addressing the medical care system.

Neglect of this issue probably derives from inadequate funding of the public health system and the myth that public health is concerned only with disease control by such measures as epidemiological investigation, immunization, health education, and attention to health hazards in the physical environment. Compounding the problem is the common public misperception is that if public health agencies have any role in medical care delivery, it should be providing or financing care for the economically disadvantaged segment of the population, as the safety net.

Public Health's Mission and Scope

A perspective on appropriate roles for public health derives from its mission. According to the Institute of Medicine, National Academy of Sciences, the mission is "fulfilling society's interest in assuring conditions in which people can be healthy" (Institute of Medicine, 1988). Public health thus concerns itself with the health of the entire population and how it may be enhanced by improving the health-related conditions in which people live. It includes all the ways in which a society organizes to protect and advance the health of its members: through governmental agencies, voluntary associations, professional societies, and community groups devoted to health.

Public health efforts aim at improving three conditions that can contribute to population health: the physical environment; the social environment, including its effect on behavior; and the system of delivery of clinical care services. The *physical environment*, all those physical aspects of people's natural and built surroundings, profoundly affects their health. The well-known impact of working conditions, water safety, and food handling—among myriad other living circumstances—illustrates the point. Therefore modern public health has directed substantial effort toward ensuring a healthful physical environment, at first mainly focusing on ways to reduce microbial threats to health but increasingly aiming more broadly at the whole physical milieu such as our transportation infrastructure and housing. Historically, physical environmental control measures have been public health's most fundamental way of carrying out its mission because, once in place and maintained, they do not require specific behaviors on the part of individuals to protect their health from that source. A good example is ensuring a safe water supply.

With the twentieth-century transition from communicable to non-communicable diseases as the predominant group of health problems, evidence has grown that people's behavior (for example, with respect to tobacco and alcohol) has a strong and often definitive influence on the disease mechanisms that cause death, disability, and the timing of disease development. In analyzing the underlying causes of death rather than the disease mechanisms involved, Mokdad, Marks, Stroup, and Gerberding (2004) found that almost two-fifths are attributable to tobacco, diet or activity patterns, and alcohol (see Table 22.1).

The behavior of both individuals and groups is shaped by the broader *social environment*, including such factors as the laws, enforcement, media, strength of family and other social relationships, sense of shared responsibility for the quality of life in the community, and beliefs. Thus the social environment strongly influences patterns of health and ill health in the population overall and in subgroups defined by gender, age, race, ethnicity, and other factors (Evans, Barer, & Marmor, 1994).

TABLE 22.1. ACTUAL CAUSES OF DEATH IN THE UNITED STATES, 2000

Cause	Estimates of Total Deaths	
	Number	Percentage
Tobacco	435,000	18
Diet and activity patterns	365,000	15
Alcohol	85,000	4
Microbial agents	75,000	3
Toxic agents	55,000	2
Motor vehicles	43,000	2
Firearms	29,000	1
Sexual behavior	30,000	1
Illicit use of drugs	20,000	1
Total	1,137,000	47

Source: Mokdad, Marks, Stroup, & Gerberding, 2004.

The third major influence on the health of the population is the availability and quality of medical care. Extensive achievements in this field during recent decades—in biochemistry, pharmacology, noninvasive testing procedures, surgical techniques, and other areas—have increased the possibility of longer and healthier lives. The often-dramatized impact of these innovations on the health of an individual or small group of individuals, however, creates a tendency for society to overestimate their overall health significance. Bunker, Frazier, and Mosteller (1994) attribute only five years of the thirty-year increase in life expectancy of Americans during the twentieth century to the work of the medical care system.

Public health has generally operated inconspicuously, identifying and implementing means to improve all three conditions that can advance health. Credit is rarely given for what has been accomplished through public health initiatives, in part because their success is often measured by health problems that do not occur, or whose impact is mitigated but not eliminated and because of the dominance of commercial interests in health care. Hence we take for granted that pasteurized milk is safe to drink, and that individuals with tuberculosis are identified quickly and appropriately treated so they are not a threat to the public.

There are, then, a number of reasons for public health involvement in clinical care:

1. Clinical care is an effective means of improving a population's health, and thereby a legitimate concern of public health.
2. A substantial proportion of the population in the United States either does not have financial access to a minimum set of medical care services or may lose access with change in government programs or in living circumstances such as a job move or job loss.
3. A considerable portion of the clinical care services currently delivered suffer from overuse and misuse, and a deficiency in quality, often adversely affecting health outcomes.
4. The recent spiral in medical care costs has absorbed a disproportionate share of social resources, limiting investment to improve access to health services as a whole, and preventing investment in other *sectors* (transportation, social services, housing, environmental protection, and so forth) that could potentially yield higher dividends in health at the population level.

Examination of public health's role in clinical care services is therefore timely and important. Public health represents society's interest, but how should society's interests be advanced? What are the leverage points to effect change?

Prevention In Clinical Care Services

Because public health's hallmark is prevention, it has traditionally emphasized this aspect of clinical care services. Historically, the medical care system has operated mainly in a complaint-response mode; people with a complaint of being sick seek a physician (or other health care provider), who responds with diagnosis and therapy. It has not proactively assured delivery of the clinical services their patients need. The public health perspective is different; it focuses on the entire population, with or without symptoms of being sick, and aims at maintaining health and preventing disease.

Prevention is often divided into three categories: primary, secondary, and tertiary. Primary prevention consists of preventing disease onset through efforts to maximize positive and minimize negative health effects of the physical and social environments, as well as to advance the application of specific preventive medical measures of proven effectiveness. For example, public health seeks to control air pollution as an environmental source of disease and to diminish excessive consumption of fatty foods, a behavior that can lead to cardiovascular and other diseases.

Medical care can, and increasingly does, incorporate substantial primary prevention services. Perhaps the most obvious is immunization. Vaccination against the communicable diseases of childhood, and more recently those of adults as well, such as against influenza and pneumonia, has drastically curtailed the burden for these diseases. Public health works with the medical care system, including provision of some direct public health services, to ensure protection of people against communicable diseases that can be avoided by immunization. These include evidence-based guidelines for immunizations, patient and professional education, enhancing access to services, monitoring of delivery of immunizations, implementation of immunization requirements in schools, and providing incentives for delivery of those services.

Because certain behavioral practices have been clearly identified as causing disease (lack of exercise, tobacco use, excessive alcohol consumption, and so on), public health seeks to minimize these behavior patterns. One way has been to seek incorporation of advice on such matters into a medical practice. Two problems, however, have deterred physicians from using their opportunity to help patients adopt healthful behaviors. One is the common belief among physicians that their efforts in this regard do not yield much benefit; the second is the failure of the payment system to compensate clinicians adequately for the time involved in providing the service. Further, the benefit of physician advice on behavioral issues has not been shown for some key behaviors. However, there is good evidence indicating that physician advice for smoking cessation can have a useful effect and obesity counseling is effective when combined with intensive follow up services (Glynn & Manley, 1993; U.S. Preventive Services Task Force, n.d.).

Secondary prevention consists of detecting and treating disease or its clear precursors at a time when an intervention to reduce the risk level can be most effective. Cervical cancer in situ is almost universally curable. Hypertension, although asymptomatic, greatly increases the risk for stroke and other cardiovascular disease if not effectively treated. Public health has therefore advocated screening to find health risk factors and disease itself as promptly after onset as possible, before adverse health effects have advanced. The number of tests to detect important risk factors or early stages of treatable conditions has expanded in the recent past. The U.S. Preventive Services Task Force has codified the evidence for them and makes evidence-based recommendations for clinical practice. Along with the recommendations of the Advisory Committee on Immunization Practices, these have become the recommended standard for clinical care and are ensconced in the Affordable Care Act as services that need to be provided with no copayment (U.S. Preventive Services Task Force, n.d.).

Managing disease that has already occurred so as to minimize the likelihood of its progressing to further damage, disability, and other possible adverse consequences, or to mortality, is sometimes called tertiary prevention. Many companies that now sell health insurance, so-called health plans, offer encouragement and assistance by specialized personnel (deemed coaches or care coordinators) to patients with selected chronic diseases, because they have discovered that such coaching lowers the cost of providing services to their beneficiaries and improves health outcomes (J. E. Wennberg, personal communication, 2004). Increasingly many major companies in the United States have established work-site health promotion and disease prevention programs (Pelletier, 1999). External vendors often provide these services, but some companies use their own staff. The rationale for broad adoption of these company-sponsored programs is to reduce the cost of medical services and to improve productivity.

Prevention may be considered in individual clinical situations and in community endeavors. The former involve physicians and other health care professionals in their practice with their particular patients. Increasingly, however, various disease prevention services are being offered to groups outside of the main medical care setting. For example, campaigns are undertaken to screen those at high risk for HIV with the intent of finding people with early stages of the condition and, with follow-up treatment to them, reducing the progression to AIDS. Other population-oriented programs may target schools, worksites, religious organizations, or entire communities. The Guide to Community Preventive Services (Community Preventive Services Task Force, n.d.) provides numerous evidence-based recommendations for systems changes that improve the delivery of *clinical preventive services.*

Preventive services have been effective in reducing some disease burdens. Probably the most obvious is seen in advances against vaccine-preventable diseases, of which worldwide smallpox eradication is the most notable example. Table 22.2, however, reveals the great success in recent decades against the acute communicable diseases that were formerly so prominent—in large part accomplished through immunization programs. Progress has occurred with respect to diphtheria, influenza, and other conditions, but much remains to be done with immunization, as a 2010 epidemic of pertussis in California illustrates. In addition to notable achievements in children's health, the former major chronic communicable diseases of adult life, syphilis and tuberculosis, have also declined substantially as a result of active case finding by public health agencies and

TABLE 22.2. DECLINE OF SELECTED ACUTE COMMUNICABLE DISEASE CASES, UNITED STATES, 1920–2000

Year	Smallpox	Diphtheria	Poliomyelitis	Measles
1920	102,128	147,991	2,338	469,924
1940	2,795	15,536	9,804	291,102
1960	0	918	3,190	442,000
1980	0	3	9	13,506
2000	0	1	0	176
2010	0	0	0	63

Source: U.S. Department of Health Education and Welfare, 2012, cited in Mechanic, 1983 (for 1920 registration area only); National Center for Health Statistics, 2012.

medical treatment. The resurgence of tuberculosis during the late 1980s and early 1990s, however, underscores the importance of maintaining surveillance of diseases that have declined in frequency.

Less widely recognized chronic noncommunicable disease death rates have likewise been yielding to control efforts. Table 22.3 indicates that heart disease mortality dropped by more than 60 percent between 1950 and 2000, and cerebrovascular disease even more sharply. Cancer mortality, though increasing until about 1990, has since declined to below the rate prevailing in 1950. These advances probably reflect the combined influence of both more effective clinical care and the broader public health activities. The latter include, first, epidemiological investigations that have disclosed the role of tobacco, obesity, increased fat consumption, excessive alcohol consumption, use of illicit drugs, and increased sedentary lifestyles; and then initiation of educational and other efforts to control these factors.

Public health agencies have also been extensively involved with clinical preventive services in seeking secondary prevention for cervical, colorectal, and breast cancer, and hypertensive heart disease among other conditions, through promotion and sometimes actual provision of screening for these and other noncommunicable diseases (Community Preventive Services Task Force, n.d.). Health departments, voluntary health agencies, community clinics, and concerned physician groups have often collaborated in such endeavors.

Disease control accomplishments during the twentieth century have yielded substantively longer lives, from an average of forty-seven years in 1900 to seventy-seven years in 2000 (National Center for Health Statistics, 2003). Not only are people routinely surviving into their eighties and

TABLE 22.3. DEATH RATES FROM MAJOR NONCOMMUNICABLE DISEASES, UNITED STATES, 1950–2000, SELECTED YEARS

Disease	Years				
	1950	1970	1990	2000	2010
Heart disease	587	493	322	258	178
Cancer	194	199	216	200	172
Cerebrovascular disease	181	148	65	61	39

Note: Age-adjusted rates.

Source: Murphy, Xu, & Kochanek, 2012.

nineties; they are doing so with reasonably good health. In 2002, more than 90 percent of the American people assessed their health as excellent or good, not fair or poor; 78 percent of persons sixty-five to seventy-four years of age rated their health as excellent or good, as did 69 percent of those over seventy-five (National Center for Health Statistics, 2004). Thus, it is no longer appropriate to identify aging with infirmity, although the frequency of the latter does increase with age.

We are now entering what some have called a third era of health in the modern world, as distinguished from a first era when communicable diseases dominated the health scene, and a second era when chronic noncommunicable diseases prevailed (Breslow, 2004). We have by no means completely overcome these two sets of diseases (and never will!), but thinking about health must no longer be restricted to its opposite, that is, disease occurrence and how to deal with it. Now we can move onto considering *health* in the sense of the WHO Ottawa Charter definition: "a resource for everyday life" (Ottawa Charter for Health Promotion, 1986). People increasingly regard health as the capacity to do what they want to do in life: the fitness to climb a mountain, the cognition and memory to play bridge, the vision and hearing to enjoy an opera, and so forth. They seek health to permit them to live life as they want to, not merely to overcome diseases. Public health, including the assurance of clinical care, must now turn attention to this third era of health: to advance and maintain health in a positive sense.

Public Health and Provision of Clinical Care Services

As the principal governmental agencies for public health, local and sometimes state health departments have long administered certain clinical services directed toward health promotion and disease prevention. They have often provided prenatal care and childhood immunization services directly, particularly for those segments of the population that the private health care system seldom reaches effectively. In many locales the health department has served as planner, convener, and facilitator, helping to mobilize community resources to extend services to the economically disadvantaged. Also, in many states and communities public health departments have assumed responsibility for a broader array of clinical services for people with low income. For example, some local public health agencies carry responsibility for Medicaid and local indigent care programs.

These responsibilities are exercised in several forms. Some jurisdictions operate medical care plans for Medicaid eligibles and other low-income individuals, contracting with physicians, hospitals, clinics, and other providers and performing the other required functions of a managed care organization. Other jurisdictions have comprehensive clinical care delivery systems, including both inpatient and outpatient activities. In some jurisdictions the local health agency has been given statutory responsibility for medical care for the indigent. The responsibility to furnish clinical services to a substantial population without other access to medical care has become so burdensome in some jurisdictions, however, that it jeopardizes the conduct of other public-health-sponsored activities with a potentially greater impact on population health. This trend has therefore favored the tendency to separate public health departments from agencies concerned primarily with indigent medical care and, with passage of the Affordable Care Act, to further reduce the delivery of clinical care services as coverage increases for these populations (Institute of Medicine, 2012).

Historically, actual involvement in clinical services emerged initially as a critical aspect of public health's original task: communicable disease control. During the early part of the century, when the struggle against infectious diseases extended beyond environmental action to include developing personal immunity in individuals, health departments undertook mass smallpox vaccinations (and subsequently other immunizations). More substantial engagement in clinical services by public health agencies expanded into maternal and child health during the 1920s, as a result of the growing conviction that such services could reduce the excessively high maternal and infant death rates prevailing at that time. Then came certain diagnostic procedures, especially as technology for communicable disease control advanced. For example, tuberculin testing of tuberculosis patients' contacts and then x-raying positive reactors became an accepted public health practice. Further, health department laboratories offered communicable disease diagnostic services to physicians in their communities. Subsequently, these services expanded into other realms such as screening for diseases having genetic and environmental causes.

Advances in clinical science and corresponding improvements in medical care have been accompanied with the problems of overuse, underuse, and misuse of clinical care services and causes significant harms, necessitating greater involvement of public health in quality improvement, monitoring, and oversight (Institute of Medicine, 2001).

Direct Medical Service Delivery by Government

Direct delivery of clinical care by government in the United States started with the U.S. Marine Hospital Service, which was established to offer care for merchant seamen in support of the nation's entry into international commerce, and to the country's early military medical services. These two agencies, for merchant seamen and military forces, have evolved into the current U.S. Public Health Service and the Armed Forces Medical System.

Over the years the federal government has assumed responsibility for directly supplying medical services to other substantial segments of the population. The Department of Veterans Affairs operates an array of medical centers, nursing units, domiciliary care units, and outpatient clinics for its beneficiaries, many of which are affiliated with academic medical centers, both to enhance the quality of care and to give training opportunities to young physicians (U.S. Department of Veterans Affairs, 1994). The Indian Health Service operates (or funds the operation by Indian tribal government of) hospitals, health centers, and other types of ambulatory care unit on tribal lands throughout the country (U.S. Department of Health and Human Services, 1994).

State governments historically have provided hospital services, not for such specific segments of the population but rather for people suffering from particular conditions, such as mental illness and tuberculosis. Beds for these purposes have declined substantially over the last quarter century as tuberculosis cases fell and were also treated increasingly on an ambulatory basis, and as state hospitalization for mentally ill patients was curtailed with the notion that they would be better served in community centers. Unfortunately, the latter have not materialized to the extent needed.

Many county and city governments have offered both inpatient and outpatient general hospital services for the indigent, and emergency and some other medical services, often with financial support from state and federal sources. However, funding for these operations in recent years has usually been precarious, with financial crises common. Overall, indigent care, regardless of who provides it, tends to be uneven in extent and quality, reflecting the lack of nationally ensured services in the United States.

From 1975 to 2008, the total number of hospitals in the United States dropped 19 percent and the number of beds more than one-third; beds under federal governmental auspices fell by more than one-half, reducing the proportion from 10 to 5 percent of the total (see Table 22.4). The proportion of beds operated by state and local governments remained quite

TABLE 22.4. HOSPITALS, BEDS, AND OCCUPANCY RATES, ACCORDING TO TYPE OF HOSPITAL, UNITED STATES, SELECTED YEARS, 1975–2008

	1975	1990	2008
Hospitals			
Total	7,156	6,649	5,815
Federal	382	337	213
State and local government	1,761	1,444	1,105
Community, nonprofit	3,339	3,191	2,923
For-profit	775	749	982
Beds (in thousands)			
Total	1,073	1,025	951
Federal	132	98	46
State and local government	210	169	131
Community, nonprofit	658	657	557
For-profit	73	101	121
Occupancy rate (percentage)			
Total	76.7	69.5	68.2
Federal	80.7	72.9	67.9
State and local government	70.4	65.3	68.4
Community, nonprofit	77.5	69.3	57.8
For-profit	65.9	52.8	59.0

Note: Excluded are long-term hospitals and hospital units in institutions such as prisons and college dormitories, facilities for the mentally retarded, and alcoholism and chemical dependency hospitals.

Source: National Center for Health Statistics, 2010.

steady, about one-seventh of the total. Meanwhile community nonprofit hospitals expanded their proportion of beds, now over one-half of the total; and community for-profit hospitals had doubled their share, from 5 to 11 percent. The former increase largely reflects services of community hospitals that were previously undertaken by specialized rather than general hospitals.

Future Directions

The public health care system delivers substantial amounts of medical care, particularly for the economically disadvantaged, the severely mentally ill, and the developmentally impaired. But this role is only one expression of the public health mission. Unfortunately, local fiscal authorities have often diverted what resources are appropriated for the traditional public health core functions focused on protecting and improving the health of all residents of their jurisdiction into clinical care for the poor. This reflects the strain of fifty million Americans being without health insurance in 2010 (U.S. Census Bureau, 2010), a number that should decrease but not be eliminated with the implementation of the Affordable Care Act. However, the other consequence of allocating money to what appears to be the most pressing priority (sick people without other access to urgently needed medical services) is that these funds are not available for community-oriented prevention activities. Consequently, public health suffers a diminished ability to respond to serious public health threats such as the resurgence of tuberculosis, or the emergence of HIV/AIDS and new forms of influenza or to adequately address the pressing problems of obesity and health literacy.

The growing perception that our nation had lost sight of its public health goals, allowing the public health infrastructure to fall into disarray, led to the previously cited Institute of Medicine recommendation that the *public health mission* be defined as "fulfilling society's interest in assuring conditions in which people can be healthy." On the basis of this mission, the report identified three principal core functions for public health: assessment, assurance, and policy development.

Assessment

An indispensable role for a governmental public health agency is to assess the opportunities to improve the health of the population it serves. In so doing, the public health agency needs sophistication in assessing the contributions of the various determinants of health to the burden imposed on the population by ill health. An essential initial step is to collect (directly or through access to external databases) a health-and-disease profile of the population. Traditionally, assessments have targeted the major causes of morbidity, mortality, and more recently disability. In addition, health can be measured as a set of positive attributes based on the more recent definitions of health adopted by public health bodies nationally and internationally.

At the state and local levels, an ideal assessment would be to array the major causes of morbidity, disability, mortality, and lack of well-being for major segments of the population defined by age, gender, and geography, and also by race or ethnic identity. Traditionally, ill health has been arrayed according to disease (cancer, heart disease, arthritis, and so on). However, as McGinnis and Foege (1993) have proposed, a better way to consider health improvement opportunities might be to focus on the common factors that underlie many of the most burdensome health conditions (see Table 22.1). These factors have in common that they can be considerably ameliorated through behavior change. A recent IOM report (2011) has emphasized the need to assess the health of the community as a whole, not merely the sum of the health of the individuals in the community. Such an assessment should include an assessment of the social and environmental conditions to create healthy community.

In analogous fashion, how might we judge the potential contribution of clinical services to health improvement in the overall population of a defined area and in population subgroups? The point of departure for such an exercise is to determine the proportion of the population variance in key health measures that is associated with those services. To take as a hypothetical example acquired heart disease, clinical care services might be found to account for 10 percent of the variance in mortality and disability rates. The next step would be to determine, on the basis of the best evidence, the characteristics of health service systems and specific diagnostic and therapeutic modalities that are reproducibly associated with the best and worst outcomes.

To the degree possible, differences between the best and worst outcomes would be partitioned into problems of access to services, overuse and underuse of appropriate services, poor coordination of care, and poor technical quality of services. Developing databases that would permit this degree of problem definition remains at an early stage for most health conditions. However, a substantial investment in quality indicators, practice guidelines, and outcomes measurement should in time produce sufficient tools for public health departments to assume leadership in helping solve the problems in organizing and delivering clinical care on the part of both private and public providers.

A related role is to identify the characteristics of populations that are not receiving adequate care by virtue of diminished access, poor quality, or lack of financial resources. Traditionally, public health organizations have taken the lead in pointing out that there is a substantial segment of our population, including 9.8 percent (7.3 million) of children, who do not have access to any organized source of continuing medical care or payment for such care (U.S. Census Bureau, 2010; Trevino & Jacobs, 1994), though that proportion should drop substantially with implementation of the Affordable Care Act. They are largely dependent on so-called emergency services that state or local governments may provide or require other local institutions to provide. In addition, many millions work in precarious job situations where they are at risk of both job loss and loss of health insurance benefits offered by or through their employer.

Most striking, during the 1990s—a period of unprecedented economic growth in the United States—the number of uninsured continued to grow and the proportion of Americans covered by employer-related health benefits declined; this problem has continued during the first decade of the twenty-first century, exacerbated by the recession of 2008. Public health agencies should become the most trusted source for information on unmet service needs, the quality assurance practices used by providers, health outcomes, and the health status of subpopulations within their territory. They should also systematically assess the degree of integration of health services with other governmental and private-sector services, such as education, social services, and welfare.

Tools have been developed to help public health agencies in the overall assessment and planning process. APEX (Assessment Protocol for Excellence in Public Health) and PATCH (Planned Approach to Community Health) are among these guides for assessing community health needs (National Association of County Health Officials, 1992). Many health departments are using Healthy Communities 2000: Model Standards, a guidebook to marrying the national objectives in Healthy People 2000 with local needs and priorities (American Public Health Association, 1991). The quality of public health departments should be further enhanced by codification of standards as part of the accreditation process for which one requirement is a comprehensive community health assessment (by the Public Health Accreditation Board: www.phaboard.org).

Assurance

The Institute of Medicine report stressed "assurance" that services necessary to achieve agreed-on goals are made available, whether by encouraging action on the part of other entities (private or public sector), or by requiring such action through regulation, or by supplying services directly. Public health agencies should involve key policymakers and the general public in determining a set of high-priority personal and communitywide health services that governments will guarantee to every member of the community. This guarantee should include subsidization or direct provision of necessary clinical care for those unable to afford them (Institute of Medicine, 2012; Booske, Athens, Kindig, Park, & Remington, 2010).

Assurance of appropriate services for appropriate health care is a central function of public health. In proposing plans to improve the health of its population, a department of public health should ensure that all groups have access to a minimum set of high-quality clinical care services. The plans should also set expectations for the performance of health care systems and health care providers.

Developing large managed care organizations with broad responsibility for the health care of defined, enrolled populations is a natural point of leverage in assuring the nation of adequate performance of the health care system. Large managed care organizations such as Kaiser Permanente are developing clinical data systems that generate databases amenable to analysis of care outcomes and of the types of service furnished to individuals and groups defined by disease (for example, adult onset diabetes mellitus), age group (such as infants from zero to one year), income level, or geography. In addition, quality has become a basis for competition in the market for clinical care. Therefore, health department leadership should include helping to define the kinds of outcome an organization should be able to show, according to best practices as recorded in the literature and ensuring dissemination of this information to consumers as well as health professionals in understandable form.

Health departments should have special expertise in setting expectations for outcomes in clinical preventive services (such as age-specific immunization rates and mammography rates by age) and in monitoring them. However, monitoring the results of services administered when a disease state is present is of equal importance. For this reason, public health agencies should also participate in setting expectations for disease and procedure outcomes, such as the mortality rate for cardiovascular disease, or frequency of complications for endoscopy, angioplasty, or joint replacement. They may also suggest the specifications and dissemination plans for report cards that are increasingly required of health care providers, because these reports can identify problems with access and quality and yield helpful relevant information to those deciding among health plan or provider groups.

Currently, most health departments have no jurisdiction over the organizations delivering comprehensive care, except for licensing health care institutions and sometimes other provider groups. In some areas, particularly large cities, the health department may also deliver clinical services; this presents a potential conflict of interest in setting standards or expectations for results. Nonetheless, there are existing levers that can be used to help ensure good outcomes in delivering personal health care services. The public health department can help to establish a local coalition of private and public medical service purchasers that sets requirements for both the services to be provided and the service data that plans and providers must make available in a standard format. The health department can also champion the important quality assurance work of AHRQ and the Joint Commission and of voluntary national and statewide groups focused on improving quality care. Additionally, the health department can take the lead in disseminating information on a required core of preventive services, such as those developed by the U.S. Preventive Services Task Force (n.d.). Further, the department can publicize the evidence-based practice guidelines that are being developed through public and private processes, and it can urge consumers to ask questions about treatment outcomes, both in general and for specific conditions about which they are especially concerned, before selecting choices under an employer-sponsored health benefit plan.

Public health agencies should make it a central function to receive, analyze, and report on the results of quality assurance efforts in clinical care delivery. This should become progressively more feasible as electronic health records become more commonly used and health information exchanges become more robust. They can use their role as guardian of the public's health to publicize problems and progress alike to the public, as well as to inform providers and professional organizations about opportunities for improvement in both access and quality. Ensuring that the public has objective information on the performance of alternative health care purchasing organizations and physician groups is increasingly important as more employers adopt a passive purchaser role vis-à-vis health plans, giving employees a fixed amount of money and letting them choose among a number of locally available plans.

Public Policy

A number of assurance functions are accomplished through participating in development of public policy. Some access data and quality-assessment requirements are being incorporated into laws or administrative regulations. Public health, as an agent of the public with the responsibility of "fulfilling society's interest in assuring conditions in which people can be healthy," should be proactive in suggesting where and what regulation is appropriate, and in commenting on proposals advanced by others.

An important public policy role is to underscore the large number of people uninsured for medical and hospital services, and the fact that these groups often have below average health outcomes. In addition to preventable deaths, lack of health insurance can lead to reduced productivity of workers, affecting both individual employers and our national competitiveness. Policymakers need to be shown that the uninsured population is much less likely to receive preventive care, seek care for serious symptoms, and have continuing sources of care. This results in failure to have problems diagnosed at an early and more treatable stage. They need to understand that making public medical services available directly to the uninsured is even more challenging as public systems are buffeted by competition from the private sector that is able to secure payment for services to specific subgroups under Medicaid and Medicare.

Identifying the opportunity to improve health outcomes through broader benefit coverage is part of a larger need to educate the public and policymakers on the key determinants of health, and on how policy options can affect these factors. In this context, almost all careful studies of determinants of health have found that personal health care services make a difference in health, but this difference accounts for a small fraction of the variance in health among populations and for most specific health conditions (Booske, Athens, Kindig, Park, & Remington, 2010). Determinants with a generally larger total contribution to variance include income distribution, social factors, environmental exposure, and health behavior.

Among these items, health habits have received the most attention in recent years, but the other contributors to common diseases often display strong effects. For example, in cardiovascular disease the degree of social isolation presents risk gradients about equal in magnitude to behavioral risk factors. For most disease categories, and certainly for quality of well-being, poverty is a quantitatively more important risk factor than access to health care services or the quality of those services. In addition, economic, community, social, and political factors are the primary contributors to such major societal problems of ill health as child abuse, spousal abuse, other violence, and poor birth outcomes.

As part of this educational effort, public health departments can generate data showing that the current level of investment in medical services is disproportionate to the ability of those services to diminish the population burden of ill health. Whether the argument is for additional resources or for reallocation of existing resources to address other causal factors, the rhetoric is not likely to strike a responsive chord unless the health department can make a convincing case for what type of investment is likely to achieve greater societal returns. For example, would after-school programs for youth in areas of high risk of school dropout and gang membership be a better investment than a higher density of MRI machines, or increasing the Medicare payment for erythropoietin? Would a prenatal and postnatal home visiting program for lower-income pregnant women yield a better health return than routinely offering amniocentesis as a covered medical service benefit? Would a social marketing campaign to encourage youths to drink nonalcoholic beverages have more impact on alcoholism than more or better rehabilitation facilities?

Although there are not unequivocal answers to most of these questions, showing the effects of well-evaluated model programs is a useful initial step in this educational process.

Improvements in health will require greater integration of the clinical and public health systems, particularly for the systematic delivery of population health services to address the social and environmental determinants of health. This will not only lead to a healthier population, but decrease the demand for costly clinical care services. The Affordable Care Act is an important first step in that direction.

SUMMARY

What is the interest and capacity of public health agencies at the state and local levels to assume the set of responsibilities we have outlined? The Institute of Medicine reports and strong efforts by the CDC, the American Public Health Association, and national and local health officer associations to define core public health functions have raised consciousness of the role public health should play in health promotion at the community level. Barriers to assuming these important roles include restricted flexibility in use of funds (which are often channeled from categorical programs), mismatch of skills and interests between existing personnel and new priorities, and some outsiders' perception that a more limited role for public health agencies is advisable. For example, a survey of thirty-two health departments and districts in Washington state found that the self-assessed strengths of most were program management and direct provision of service. They felt that the major deficiencies were assessment functions and use of data to guide community and program planning and policy.

If public health is to ensure the health of populations, then establishing its expertise and credibility as the path-finding organizer and lead planner in achieving goals in this area must be accorded a high priority.

KEY TERMS

Clinical preventive services Chemoprevention (such as aspirin prophylaxis), screening (such as colorectal cancer screening), and counseling (such as tobacco cessation) services that should be delivered in clinical settings to otherwise healthy individuals.

Core functions of public health Assessment, policy development, and assurance

Health "A resource for everyday life" (Ottawa Charter for Health Promotion, 1986)

Health system The intersectoral, multistakeholder system whose core is the government public health infrastructure but also includes business, the clinical care delivery system, communities, schools, and nonprofit organizations (Institute of Medicine, 2011)

Physical environment People's natural and built surroundings

Public health mission The mission of public health is to "fulfill society's interest in assuring conditions in which people can be healthy" (Institute of Medicine, 1988).

Sectors Parts of the economy, such as transportation, criminal justice, housing, agriculture, or the environment

Social environment The combination of social and cultural institutions, norms, patterns, beliefs, and processes that influence the life of an individual or community (Secretary's Advisory Committee, 2010).

DISCUSSION QUESTIONS

1. The term *preventive medicine* is often used in many senses, from the extremely limited to the general and vague. Outline the three specific categories of prevention, with examples of each.
2. Big industry has recently begun to show substantial interest in health maintenance and prevention services. Why has that occurred?
3. Public health agencies have long provided selected clinical services. In doing so, on what aspects of health have they concentrated, and why?
4. What is the role of public health in assessing the need for and performance of the medical care system?

5. What should public health be doing in developing policy for chronic disease control?

6. What can public health do to assure access of all people to good medical care?

FURTHER READING

Fielding, J. E., & Teutsch S. M. (2013). *Public health practice: What works.* New York: Oxford University Press.

Case studies in public health.

LaLonde, M. (1974). *New perspective on the health of Canadians.* Ottawa: Canadian Department of Health and Welfare.

A seminal report on the definition and determinants of health.

Scutchfield, F. D., & Keck, C. W. (Eds.). (2009). *Principles of public health practice* (3rd ed.). Independence, KY: Cengage Learning.

An excellent standard textbook on public health.

REFERENCES

American Public Health Association. (1991). *Healthy Communities 2000: Model standard* (3rd ed.). Washington, DC: American Public Health Association.

Booske, B. C., Athens, J. K., Kindig, D. A., Park, H., & Remington, P. L. (2010). *County health rankings working paper: Different perspectives for assigning weights to determinants of health.* University of Wisconsin. Retrieved from http://www.county healthrankings.org/sites/default/files/differentPerspectivesForAssigningWeights ToDeterminantsOfHealth.pdf

Breslow, L. (2004) Perspectives: The third revolution in health. In J. F. Fielding, R. C. Brownson, & N. M. Clark (Eds.), *Annual review of public health.* Palo Alto, CA: Annual Reviews.

Bunker, J. P., Frazier, H. S., & Mosteller, F. (1994). Improving health: Measuring effects of medical care. *Milbank Quarterly, 72,* 225–258.

Centers for Disease Control and Prevention. (2012). Notifiable diseases and mortality tables. *Morbidity and Mortality Weekly Report, 60*(51), 1762–1775. Retrieved from http://cdc.gov/mmwr/preview/mmwrhtml/mm6052md.htm?s_cid =mm6052md_w

Community Preventive Services Task Force. (n.d.). *The Guide to community preventive services.* http://thecommunityguide.org/index.html

Evans, R. G., Barer, M. L., & Marmor, T. R. (1994) *Why are some people healthy and others not?* New York: Aldine de Gruyter.

Glynn, T. J., & Manley, M. W. (1993). *How to help your patients stop smoking: A National Cancer Institute manual for physicians* (45 DHHS PHS NIH NCI NIH Publication 93-3064). Bethesda, MD: National Cancer Institute.

Institute of Medicine. (1988). *The future of public health.* Washington, DC: National Academy Press.

Institute of Medicine. (2001). *Crossing the quality chasm: A new health system for the 21st century.* National Academies Press.

Institute of Medicine. (2011). *For the public's health: The role of measurement in action and accountability.* Washington, DC: National Academies Press.

Institute of Medicine. (2012). *For the public's health: investing in a healthier future.* Washington, DC: National Academies Press.

McGinnis, J. M., & Foege, W. H. (1993). Actual cases of death in the United States. *Journal of the American Medical Association, 270,* 2207–2212.

Mechanic, D. (Ed.). (1983). *Handbook of health, health care, and the health professions.* New York: Macmillan.

Mokdad, A. H., Marks, J. S., Stroup, D. F., & Gerberding, J. L. (2004). Actual causes of death in the United States, 2000. *Journal of the American Medical Association, 291,* 1238–1245.

Murphy, S. L., Xu, J., & Kochanek, K. D. (2012). *Deaths: preliminary data for 2010. National Vital Statistics Reports.* Retrieved from http://www.cdc.gov/nchs/data/nvsr/nvsr60/nvsr60_04.pdf

National Association of County Health Officials. (1992). Assessment Protocol for Excellence in Public Health (APEX/PH). Washington, DC: Author.

National Center for Health Statistics. (2003). *Health, United States, 2003.* Hyattsville, MD: Author.

National Center for Health Statistics. (2004). *Health, United States, 2004.* Hyattsville, MD: Author.

National Center for Health Statistics. (2010). *Health, United States, 2010.* Table 113. Hyattsville, MD: Author. Retrieved from http://www.cdc.gov/nchs/data/hus/hus10.pdf

Ottawa Charter for Health Promotion. (1986). *Canadian Journal of Public Health, 77,* 425–436.

Pelletier, K. (1999). A review and analysis of the clinical and cost-effectiveness studies of comprehensive health promotion and disease management programs at the worksite, 1995–1998: Update (IV). *American Journal of Health Promotion, 13,* 333–345.

Secretary's Advisory Committee on National Health Promotion and Disease Prevention Objectives for 2020. (2010). *Healthy people 2020: An opportunity to address societal determinants of health in the United States.* Washington, DC: Author.

Trevino, F. M., & Jacobs, J. P. (1994). Public health and health care reform: The American Public Health Association's perspective. *Journal of Health Policy, 15,* 397–406.

U.S. Census Bureau. *Health insurance: Highlights, 2010.* Retrieved from http://www.census.gov/hhes/www/hlthins/data/incpovhlth/2010/highlights.html

U.S. Department of Health and Human Services. (1994). *Trends in Indian health.* Washington, DC: U.S. Government Printing Office.

U.S. Department of Veterans Affairs. (1994). Annual report of the secretary of Veterans Affairs/Department of Veterans. Washington, DC: U.S. Government Printing Office.

U.S. Preventive Services Task Force. (n.d.). Retrieved from http://www.uspreventive servicestaskforce.org

CHAPTER TWENTY THREE

STRENGTHENING THE SAFETY NET

Dylan H. Roby

Learning Objectives

- Understand the funding sources, patient populations, and services provided by safety-net providers
- Analyze the impact of health reform, specifically the Affordable Care Act, on public hospitals, community health centers, and other safety-net providers
- Understand how safety-net hospitals and clinics contribute to access, quality of care, and the cost of health care
- Explain the changing role of safety-net providers in the context of health insurance expansions, given their current patient population and sources of payment

Previous chapters underscored the important relationships among access, quality, and cost in the U.S. health care system. While the U.S. health care system and reform efforts often focus on providing insurance coverage to the uninsured or underserved to facilitate access to essential health care services, the "safety net" has developed over the years to help meet the needs of those who cannot easily afford or obtain care due to geography, poverty, language needs, disabilities, and other factors (Redlener & Grant, 2009). This safety net is made up of a mix of providers and programs funded through various sources. Historically, the health care safety net has responded by providing care for people with an episode of illness or injury. However, the ability for the spectrum of safety-net providers to proactively manage preventive and primary care, reduce unnecessary emergency room use and hospitalizations, and coordinate care for high-need or high-risk individuals has been a challenge. The relatively loose system can be difficult to navigate for patients and their families, and equally difficult for clinicians and payers to coordinate effectively (Hoffman & Sered, 2005).

In this chapter, you will learn about the main health care providers and programs that make up the safety net, the individuals who seek care through these providers, and how the safety net is likely to change and expand under the Patient Protection and Affordable Care Act (ACA). While some health care experts consider public insurance payers (Medicaid, Medicare, and CHIP) a component of the safety net, for the purposes of this discussion we will focus on the providers of care who commonly contribute to caring for vulnerable populations. However, we will discuss the important role of public insurance reimbursement in supporting our health care safety net and the new opportunities for safety-net providers after the full implementation of the ACA.

Defining the Safety Net

The safety net is ill defined in the U.S. health care system. In the most limited definition, the term is used to describe the "core" safety-net providers: community health centers, local health departments and public hospitals that uninsured and Medicaid patients use in order to access health care (Hoffman & Sered, 2005; Lewin & Altman, 2000). These provider groups typically receive financial support from federal, state, and county governments in the form of grants, budget allocations and subsidies to support the provision of care to patients who need it, regardless of insurance status.

In broader and potentially more accurate terms, the safety net represents a loosely defined set of providers in private practice, privately and publicly owned rural and urban community clinics, free clinics, federally supported community and migrant health centers, acute care hospitals, mental health clinics, psychiatric hospitals, and public health departments that deliver direct services to low-income or vulnerable patients with and without insurance coverage (Lewin & Altman, 2000). The broader set of providers listed previously do not necessarily have the distinguishing characteristics of "core" safety-net providers as described by the IOM:

1. Either by legal mandate or explicitly adopted mission, they offer care to patients regardless of their ability to pay for those services; and
2. A substantial share of their patient mix are uninsured, Medicaid, and other vulnerable patients (Lewin & Altman, 2000).

Regardless, it is important to understand the disparate providers that make up the safety net by examining the magnitude of their contribution, the level of their involvement, and the unique ways that they may enhance access to care, improve the quality of health care, and change the underlying trends in health care spending.

Ensuring Access to Care for the Poor, Uninsured, and Underserved

For many of the uninsured and underserved in the United States, the sole gateway to access necessary, affordable health care is through the safety net. This safety net, which is admittedly filled with numerous holes and gaps, is made up of a mix of health care providers and programs designed to improve access to high quality health care for vulnerable populations (disabled, limited English–proficient, poor, and undocumented residents), the uninsured, and the underinsured (Felt-Lisk, McHugh, & Howell, 2001). A series of federal laws gradually expanded safety-net programs and funding over the past century, as well as the expectations around caring for the uninsured and underserved (Hawkins & Rosenbaum, 1998; Gage, 1998). Now, faced with the implementation of the ACA, safety-net providers will be better integrated into our health care system than ever before. However, despite being an indispensible cornerstone of our flawed system, safety-net providers will face challenges navigating the post-ACA world.

There is substantial evidence that having a usual source of care (a place where you can go when you feel sick or need health care) is helpful to patients in improving access to care and reducing the likelihood of expensive acute illnesses that result in emergency room visits or inpatient hospital stays (Fryer, Dovey, & Green, 2000; Roby et al., 2010). Having comprehensive primary care through a safety-net clinic can certainly improve access to primary health care services, but there are still problems for uninsured patients who need specialty care, diagnostic screening, elective or necessary surgeries, ongoing treatment, pharmaceuticals, and follow-up care (Cook et al., 2007). Recent work has underscored the potential for reductions in episodic care, emergency room visits and other unnecessary and expensive service use through coordination and medical home assignment in the safety net for the uninsured (Roby et al., 2010; Ku et al., 2012).

The safety net is built around caring for the 48.6 million uninsured in the United States. However, an additional 50.8 million people are low income and have Medicaid (DeNavas-Walt, Proctor, & Smith, 2012). Approximately 60 million people are considered medically disenfranchised because of physician shortages in their communities, despite insurance coverage. These barriers vary based on geographic location, low payment rates that discourage provider participation in Medicaid, CHIP and Medicare, or provider shortages or maldistribution of specialists (National Association of Community Health Centers [NACHC], 2009).

Financing the Safety Net

The definitional differences in characterizing the safety net spill over into understanding the financing of the loose "meshwork" of providers that comprise our health care system for the poor, uninsured, and underserved (Hoffman & Sered, 2005). The funding and support for "core" safety-net providers, as defined by the Institute of Medicine, appears to be clearer than that available for the varied providers that make up a substantial, but perhaps smaller, portion of the care for the uninsured and underserved in the United States.

The core support for community health centers comes from the Health Resources and Services Administration's (HRSA) Bureau of Primary Health Care (BPHC) in the form of direct grants to fund operations of existing clinics, expand to new sites, and add services (Hawkins & Rosenbaum, 1998). Specifically, BPHC awards Section 330 grants to community, migrant, homeless, urban housing, and school-based health centers. The National Association of Community Health Centers (NACHC, 2012) estimates the mandatory and discretionary federal support for these health centers to be approximately $3.1 billion per year. To differentiate these clinics, those receiving federal funding are often referred to as federally qualified health centers (FQHCs). FQHC status not only indicates grant support from the federal government, but also guarantees a cost-related prospectively calculated reimbursement rate developed by each state for Medicaid services. FQHC status also carries with it other benefits, including Federal Tort Claims Act protection, and requirements, such as charging uninsured patients based on their ability to pay.

Funded by states, cities, and counties with grants and annual budget allocations, local health departments have had to expand from disease surveillance, education, and immunization programs into full-fledged providers of primary care (Donaldson, Yordy, Lohr, & Vanselow, 1996). Public hospitals are supported by local and state government funds to provide care for the area's residents, in addition to federal support from the Medicare and Medicaid Disproportionate Share Hospital (DSH) payment programs (Gage, 1998).

Safety-net providers may receive insurance reimbursement from Medicare, Medicaid, or state and local indigent care programs to pay for the care they deliver to their insured or uninsured patients. In addition, many safety-net providers provide free or uncompensated care, negotiate discounted prices with their patients based on their ability to pay, use payment plans, or charge for services on a sliding fee schedule based on patient income. Other providers with significant uncompensated care burdens will engage in their own cross-subsidization of uncompensated care, called "cost shifting." In this case, hospitals and other providers will charge their paying patients and commercial insurance companies more to offset the losses from providing Medicaid and uninsured care (Dobson, DeVanzo, & Sen, 2006).

Size and Scope of the Safety Net

The safety net is not only limited to the providers willing to take care of Medicaid beneficiaries and the uninsured, but also those who provide care to low-income Medicare beneficiaries, dual-eligible Medicare-Medicaid beneficiaries, and even families with commercial insurance or high-deductible health plans who cannot go to conventional private physicians and private hospitals due to inability to pay or geographic location.

The variety of safety-net providers that make up our system of care for the uninsured, underinsured, and Medicaid beneficiaries vary in capacity, financial support, available services, and coordination with other providers across the continuum of care. Previous research indicates that expansion of community health centers and encouraging physician offices to take on uninsured and Medicaid populations would improve the access to appropriate care in the safety net more than investing in outpatient hospital clinics. Patients who received primary care in outpatient hospital settings were more likely to have poorer health status and experience less continuity of care, in addition to using more diagnostic imaging, minor surgeries, and specialty referrals than their counterparts in community health centers and private physician offices (Forrest & Whelan, 2000).

While our understanding of the safety net has improved over the past ten years, there are certainly gaps in information related to the number of patients in the U.S. health care system who use discounted fees, free clinics, and other sources of health care. In the next section, we will catalog the various types of providers that contribute to the safety net.

Community Health Centers

In 2011, there were 1,128 Section 330 Health Center organization grantees operating over 8,500 clinic sites through the United States. These health centers had $13.7 billion in total operating costs in 2011, approximately $2.3 billion of which were provided through federal BPHC grants. Less than one-quarter of revenue collected by health centers was provided through the federal BPHC grant designed to support the core mission of the organization to provide care to the uninsured and Medicaid beneficiary population (Bureau of Primary Health Care [BPHC], 2012). The ACA included approximately $9.5 billion in funding for new community health centers and $1.5 billion to modernize and expand health center sites over five years to serve forty million patients by 2015 (NACHC, 2010).

In fiscal year 2013, the federal budget contained a $1.5 billion mandatory appropriation to support community health centers and an additional $1.58 billion in discretionary funding. However, with the volatile federal budget situation, there is no guarantee that the funding allocated in current budget projections will be maintained in upcoming budget cycles.

Community health centers are required to be located in medically underserved areas (MUAs) or health professional shortage areas (HPSAs) to ensure that they are reaching the populations that are most in need of safety-net services. As federally-qualified health centers, they also benefit from cost-related Medicaid reimbursement rates, protection under the Federal Tort Claims Act (FTCA) for malpractice liability and other lawsuits, and from National Health Service Corps (NHSC) physician placements to help provide adequate supply of primary care providers. In addition to these benefits, FQHCs are also subject to certain terms and conditions of their federal grant, such as being governed by a majority community board of health center patients, providing services to low-income patients using a sliding fee scale based on their ability to pay, and maintaining a set of services including comprehensive primary care. The patient-friendly policies and requirements, coupled with federal support and prospective cost-related reimbursement, make FQHCs one of the most important components of the health care safety net.

While community health centers provide 25 percent of all primary care visits for low-income individuals in the country, there are still significant gaps in access for people without insurance coverage (NACHC, 2011). Community health centers provide services to over twenty million people per year, but only 7.4 million (36 percent) of them are uninsured. Another 7.8 million (39 percent) are on Medicaid, while 2.9 million (14 percent) have private insurance (BPHC, 2012). Despite the investment over the past half-century, only 15 percent of the uninsured and 15 percent of Medicaid beneficiaries obtain care through community health centers. Compared to the U.S. population, it is clear that health center patients are more likely to be poor, uninsured, Medicaid recipients, Latino, African American, and rural residents (see Table 23.1).

As mentioned, low levels of Medicaid reimbursement have been blamed for driving community physicians in small private practices and medical groups from accepting Medicaid patients (Decker, 2012). Because community health centers and other safety-net clinics have a stated mission to provide care for anyone, regardless of their ability to pay, they are often tasked with taking care of the uninsured and Medicaid patients who cannot access community-based primary care due to lack of ability to pay or lack of acceptance of their insurance coverage.

The Public Health Service Act of 1975 created a special category for federally qualified health centers that protected their status, funding, and ability to be reimbursed based on their reported costs for Medicaid visits for comprehensive primary care services. The Medicare, Medicaid, and SCHIP Benefits Improvement and Protection Act (BIPA) in 2000, required health centers to be paid a Prospective Payment System-based rate that is cost-related or accept an alternative payment method (APM) proposed by their state. Typically, this means that community health centers avoid the relatively poor Medicaid reimbursement for outpatient primary care that is available in most states. However, because the PPS rate is cost-related instead of cost-based, there may be more pressure on FQHCs to deliver very efficient care. The cost-related PPS rate is designed to include services that may not occur in a traditional physician's office, including enabling

TABLE 23.1. CHARACTERISTICS OF COMMUNITY HEALTH CENTER USERS AND THE OVERALL U.S. POPULATION, 2011

	Health Center Users	U.S. Population
Income		
100% of poverty or below	72%	20%
Under 200% of poverty	93%	39%
Insurance		
Uninsured	36%	16%
Medicaid	39%	16%
Medicare	8%	13%
Race or Ethnicity		
Latino	35%	17%
African American	25%	13%
Asian or Pacific Islander	5%	5%
White	2%	1%
Location		
Rural area	49%	16%

Source: National Association of Community Health Centers, 2012.

services like child care and education, some dispensing of prescription drugs, and case management.

Other Community Clinics

Several other community-based clinic providers contribute to the safety net as well, by providing care in rural and urban areas to various types of patients. There are approximately 3,800 Rural Health Clinics (RHC) certified by the Centers for Medicare and Medicaid Services in the United States, with a focus on providing care to underserved Medicare and Medicaid beneficiaries in rural areas with underservice and health professional shortage problems. Like their FQHC counterparts, RHCs also benefit from a prospectively identified cost-related Medicaid reimbursement rate (Medicare Learning Network, 2007). However, they do not receive federal grant support like the community health center grantees.

There are four other major clinic providers of comprehensive primary care in the safety net: hospital-based outpatient primary care clinics, stand-alone hospital-owned outpatient primary care clinics, stand-alone community clinics, and state or county health department primary care clinics. Some of these stand-alone clinics have met federal standards to become an FQHC look-alike clinic, which entitles them to the same prospective payment rate that their community health center counterparts are paid. However, they are not technically a Section 330 grantee and do not receive any funding directly from the Bureau of Primary Health Care. The other stand-alone clinics that are hospital, county, or state-owned usually do not have FQHC or FQHC look-alike status, making them reliant on the lower fee-for-service or capitated Medicaid reimbursement that other private practice or outpatient hospital clinics receive to care for their Medicaid patients. The lack of grant money or other subsidies also makes it difficult for them to care for uninsured or underinsured patients who do not have the ability to pay for their own care.

There are other disease-specific clinics that are important to consider when understanding the scope of the safety net. HIV/AIDS clinics, women's health clinics, family planning clinics, and other providers with defined missions make up an important component of our health care safety net. However, the services these clinics can provide is often limited and is based on the funding situation and their main goals as an organization. HIV/AIDS and women's health clinics are often part of managed care networks for Medicaid plans and continue to see patients once they obtain insurance. However, much of the care delivered is focused on the uninsured and those who cannot afford care on their own.

Free Clinics

A vital part of the safety net has been historically overlooked as a source of comprehensive primary care. Free clinics began operating in the 1960s to provide services based on the specific needs of local communities. However, over the years they have grown due to local needs for primary care and the donation of time and money by physicians, local communities, and philanthropists. One of the major common characteristics of free clinics is the reliance on volunteer staff and clinicians, donations of goods, community support, and local fundraising to provide the resources and revenue to operate (National Association of Free and Charitable Clinics, 2013).

A recent survey, the first census of free clinic providers in over forty years, found that there are over one thousand free clinics in the United States and that they provide care to 1.8 million people nationwide (Darnell, 2010). Unlike community health centers and ambulatory care clinics that are part of public hospitals, the majority receive no government revenue

(58.7 percent). One unique characteristic of free clinics relates to their operating hours: the free clinics surveyed were open an average of eighteen hours per week. This is partially due to seasonality (as some free clinics are open for only part of the year) or to limited hours year-round.

Free clinics are reliant on donated physician time, grants, donations, limited patient out-of-pocket collections, and other sources of revenue to supply patient care. While a vital part of the safety net, their focus is on primary care and like many other comprehensive primary care clinics, they do not have the ability to provide specialty care on-site, pay for patients to receive referrals to specialists, or have the ability to circumvent emergency and inpatient care delivered through safety-net hospitals.

Public and Private Hospitals

Ambulatory safety-net providers like hospital-based clinics, community health centers, free clinics, and county or state-owned public health clinics provide substantial primary care to the uninsured, underserved, and underinsured. However, emergency rooms are also considered a significant source of care for the uninsured or underinsured because of a federal law passed in 1986 called the Emergency Medical Treatment and Active Labor Act (EMTALA). EMTALA applies to hospitals that receive federal Medicare and Medicaid payments and have emergency departments to conduct a medical screening examination for all patients presenting in the emergency department and stabilize emergent patients without regard for the patient's ability to pay and insurance status. Violating EMTALA could result in a loss of Medicaid and Medicare reimbursement, which is a large source of revenue for most inpatient acute care facilities, and fines (Zibulewsky, 2001).

EMTALA results in a de facto expansion of the safety net to include any hospital that has an emergency room, regardless of public or private ownership, nonprofit or for-profit status, and existing insurance contracts and negotiated rates. Every patient that presents in the emergency room must be triaged, even if the diagnosis is limited in scope and represents little more than a primary care visit. In addition, hospitals that face significantly higher-risk populations will often need to provide resource intensive emergency and inpatient services to individuals in an emergency room setting, despite the relative efficiency and effectiveness of sending the patient to see a primary care physician in a medical office.

In larger states like California and Texas, the safety net is often anchored by a public hospital system owned and operated by counties or hospital districts. In smaller states, the main public hospitals are owned by the state. However, many localities do not have public hospitals to absorb the needs of the uninsured or underserved. Instead, these areas are reliant on community nonprofit hospitals, for-profit hospitals, and academic medical centers to provide uncompensated or discounted acute inpatient and ambulatory care to patients without an ability to pay. While EMTALA requires these facilities to triage and stabilize patients who come to the emergency room, as soon as patients are stabilized they are legally allowed to transfer patients to other facilities or to discharge them from the hospital. In areas without a dedicated safety-net hospital with a mission to provide care to the poor, uninsured and underserved, patients are far more likely to receive episodic emergency care with limited or no follow-up care.

Nonprofit hospitals are required by federal and state laws to provide community benefit programs to maintain their nonprofit status, such as providing free services to the uninsured through organized indigent care programs or forgiving medical debts, but these programs are often fragmented and focused on providing episodic care (Barnett & Somerville, 2012). For the most part, private, non-safety-net hospitals have not used their uncompensated care funds to develop comprehensive primary care capacity and coverage for a variety of services (Jones & Sajid, 2010).

According to the National Association of Public Hospitals and Health Systems (now called America's Essential Hospitals), their member hospitals provided five times the nonemergency outpatient visits as other acute care hospitals in the United States during 2010 (Zaman, Cummings, & Laycox, 2012). Similarly to community health centers, NAPH hospitals reported substantial proportions of outpatient visits and inpatient discharges provided to uninsured patients and Medicaid beneficiaries (see Figure 23.1).

The ninety-six public hospitals in the United States that responded to the NAPH survey in Figure 23.1 were responsible for an average of 78,743 emergency department visits, 573,720 outpatient visits (both primary and specialty care), and 21,300 inpatient discharges in 2010. The provision of uncompensated care and Medicaid services by public hospitals dwarfs that provided by the typical community or private hospital, based on comparisons with American Hospital Association data.

Children's hospitals are also an important part of the safety net, due to the population they care for. Children's hospitals are typically nonprofit, and some are affiliated with academic medical centers, like Mattel Children's Hospital at the Ronald Reagan UCLA Medical Center. Children with significant acute care needs often qualify for Medicaid, CHIP, and other programs for children with special health care needs.

FIGURE 23.1. PAYER MIX FOR NAPH MEMBER HOSPITALS, 2010

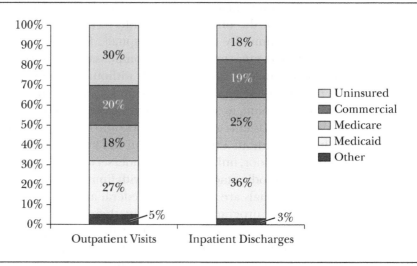

Source: Zaman, Cummings, & Laycox, 2012.
Note: Columns may not sum to 100 due to rounding error

While these public payers are often not able to pay commercial rates for services, the level of uncompensated care is usually quite low in Children's hospitals due to the categorical eligibility criteria used by Medicaid and the fact that CHIP programs cover many children with family incomes up to 250 percent of FPL. However, if Medicaid payment is very low in specific states, it can create serious financial barriers for children's hospitals that have to provide a high level of care to Medicaid beneficiaries. For example, in Ohio, where the average Medicaid caseload is 12 percent in most adult acute care facilities, 43 percent of children seeking care at children's hospitals were enrolled in Medicaid (Ohio Children's Hospital Association, 2010).

Private Physician Offices

Private providers represent a substantial, difficult to estimate, contributor to the health care safety net. In 2001, it was estimated that more than $5 billion in free and discounted care was provided by private office-based physicians (Jones & Sajid, 2010). An older study in Florida found that 26 percent of all cases were voluntarily reduced below the usual customary charge, but only a little more than half were attributed to charity care.

In addition, although 31 percent of cases were self-pay patients, they represented 52 percent of uncollected revenue (Kilpatrick, Miller, Dwyer, & Nissen, 1991). Unlike FQHCs, private practice physicians seeing uninsured patients are not able to receive federal grant money and are often faced with reductions in Medicaid and Medicare reimbursements that make it difficult to provide care to the low-income, underserved population. In a recent study comparing community health centers to office-based physicians, health centers were 31 percent more likely to accept new Medicaid patients than office-based practices (97 percent versus 66 percent). Surprisingly, although only 66 percent of office-based practices were willing to take new Medicaid patients, 93 percent of them were open to take new commercial patients (Hing, Hooker, & Ashman, 2011).

While the ACA might provide some relief with newly insured patients and a short-term increase in primary care visits for Medicaid providers, we are likely to see a continued recession of private physicians from providing care to uninsured patients and Medicaid beneficiaries.

Reducing Costs

One of the arguments behind investment in comprehensive primary care has been the potential savings the system can achieve by preventing expensive, inappropriate use of emergency rooms and inpatient hospital beds. Several studies have demonstrated that having a health center as your usual source of care can lead to improvements in control of chronic disease, avoiding ambulatory care sensitive condition–based hospitalizations and emergency room use (Rust et al., 2009; Ku et al., 2010). The community health center model, and any clinic model that incentivizes coordinated primary care and access to basic services can help to achieve that goal of efficiency for the system, even for low-income, underserved, previously uninsured patients that have been forced to seek care through episodic, uncoordinated safety-net programs and providers. Ku and colleagues (2010) at the George Washington University estimated that the ACA's investment in community health center expansion could ultimately save $181 billion by 2019, including $52 billion in federal Medicaid savings and another $33 billion in state Medicaid savings.

A recent study by John Snow International (2013) found that FQHC patients had 64 percent lower rates of multiple-day admissions, only one-quarter of the total inpatient bed days, 18 percent lower emergency department visits, and 5 percent lower readmission rates than non-FQHC patients in the same health plan. These findings confirm the value that FQHC and other coordinated clinic models may provide, even for insured populations.

For public hospitals, one of the most contentious provisions of the ACA relates to reductions in Disproportionate Share Hospital (DSH) payments. While private and public hospitals both receive DSH funding from Medicare and Medicaid, public hospitals receive the most on average because of their very high levels of low-income, uninsured, and Medicaid patients (see Figure 23.1). The ACA proposes to reduce Medicare DSH payments by 75 percent and Medicaid DSH payments by $18.1 billion by 2020, based on the idea that newly insured Medicaid and health insurance exchange beneficiaries will offset the losses of subsidies for the uninsured (Graves, 2012). The NAPH reported that the average hospital margin for its member facilities in 2010 was 2.3 percent, in contrast with a 7.2 percent average operating margin for all hospitals in the country. Without Medicaid DSH, NAPH forecasted that their average member's margin would sink to −6.1 percent, a drastic 8.4 percent reduction.

Although public hospitals could experience a surge in new patients with insurance coverage, their continued involvement as a safety-net provider for ambulatory primary and specialty, emergency, and inpatient care could make it difficult to replace lost DSH subsidies with new revenue, while also fulfilling their mission to provide care to those without the ability to pay.

Safety-net providers have historically been successful in delivering high-quality care to their patient population while also managing their spending effectively. Efficiency will be a key component of strengthening the safety net after ACA implementation, along with continuing to develop systems and strategies that will allow the disparate providers that make up the safety net to change roles and adapt to the new markets for health insurance and the remaining uninsured who are left out of the reforms.

Improving Quality

Community health centers and public hospitals have been involved in significant long-term improvements to the safety-net system—not just related to expanding access, but to quality improvement and care coordination. The BPHC gathers information on birth weight outcomes, services delivered, and basic clinical process measures of quality as part of its annual

Uniform Data System submissions for each clinic organization. This dedication to quality improvement relates to early efforts by advocates and community health centers to take on a leadership role as a high quality provider of primary care services. The Institute for Healthcare Improvement/Wagner Chronic Care Model was deployed in 1999 as part of the HRSA/IHI Health Disparities Collaboratives in community health center sites. Evaluations of this quality improvement and disparities reduction effort demonstrated that the collaboratives improved process measures for asthma and diabetes, although they did not necessarily change clinical outcomes or reduce disparities (Landon et al., 2007).

Throughout the past ten years, community health centers and public hospitals were engaged in quality improvement and system redesign activities at the local and state level to implement electronic health records (EHR), develop patient-centered medical home (PCMH) models, and use care coordination to improve chronic illness care. However, efforts were sporadic and there were concerns about sustainability.

In 2009, the passage of the American Recovery and Reinvestment Act (ARRA) and its Health Information Technology for Economic and Clinical Health (HITECH) provisions enabled community health centers, private practices, and hospital systems to improve their information systems using federal subsidies and incentives. Advocates for adoption of the PCMH model by physicians, clinics, and hospitals rightly see a connection between the HITECH provisions and the capacity needed to operate a successful medical home, despite needed additional steps (Moreno, Peikes, & Krilla, 2010). The investment in infrastructure for safety-net clinics and hospitals to develop health information technology systems and engage in meaningful use of data to improve patient care, achieve integration, and reduce fragmentation will be a vital step in strengthening our health care safety net.

Further support for improving quality within safety-net providers came in the form of the ACA in 2010. Multiple provisions call for care coordination, use of care transition models, medical or health home implementation, and team-based approaches to care in community health centers and other safety-net providers. Some community health centers will directly benefit from the FQHC Advanced Practice Demonstration, which incentivizes participating providers to save money for Medicare while developing and strengthening their PCMH model. Others will participate in state options to develop a set of health home services that will be paid for largely by the federal government through Medicaid matching (90 percent).

Many of the cost savings in the ACA are dependent on changes to Medicare payments for readmissions, value-based purchasing, and controlling year-to-year spending growth through Accountable Care Organizations and the Independent Payment Advisory Board. However, the majority of direct quality improvement reforms were focused on developing capacity in community health centers to manage chronic illness, coordinate care for costly Medicare patients, and invest in staff, systems, and clinic sites that would expand access to high-quality care to millions of the remaining uninsured, Medicaid, and low-income exchange beneficiaries.

The ACA is expected to facilitate insurance coverage through Medicaid expansion at the state level and affordable insurance coverage throughout the county via health insurance exchanges. However, even the most generous estimates assume that roughly eighteen million of the uninsured will remain without care. These residually uninsured will include undocumented immigrants, people with very low incomes (under the federal tax filing threshold) who are exempt from the minimum essential coverage requirements, people with breaks of fewer than three months without insurance coverage, those with religious objections or membership in a recognized American Indian tribe, and those who cannot afford coverage due to financial hardship because it represents over 8 percent of their household income. These eighteen million individuals will use a variety of services, despite not actively seeking out insurance coverage options due to the ACA.

In addition, the ACA is expected to increase Medicaid enrollment by twelve million by 2020, resulting in millions of new patients and additional revenue for community health centers. The law also allowed states to temporarily increase primary care payments for Medicaid providers to 100 percent of the Medicare rate from 2013 to 2014 (Congressional Budget Office, 2013).

The ACA may cover a majority of the currently uninsured in new programs. However, the safety net will still be needed to care for the residually uninsured population and the newly insured low-income population that will face challenges accessing care through more traditional providers. Efforts to expand Medicaid and the exchanges are likely to generate revenue for safety-net providers through services purchased by newly insured patients, but the level of need for continually uninsured individuals will be significant as well. Safety-net facilities will need to be aware of the availability of new programs, attempt to enroll people in the appropriate coverage options, and join networks for Medicaid and exchange plans in order to retain their current patients, develop relationships with new ones, and continue to care for the uninsured who cannot or will not buy insurance coverage. Providing high-quality, patient-centered care will be highly effective in becoming a provider of choice for their patient population.

Future Directions

The safety net in the United States will be in flux for the next decade or two as the ACA is implemented and providers figure out the role they can play in caring for the low-income, uninsured, or underserved population in their areas. Although many providers will benefit from the insurance expansions and can offset losses in DSH payments or federal grant support, others will still need to take care of a substantial portion of low-income uninsured, undocumented, or otherwise disenfranchised members of society. This tension could alter the development and goals of different health centers and clinics, hospitals, and physicians, depending on their unique situation. Despite these tensions, the various safety-net providers are facing unprecedented opportunities to contribute to the health of the previously underserved and uninsured in 2014 and beyond.

SUMMARY

The health care safety net is a loosely affiliated mesh of providers that provide some level of care for the uninsured, underserved, low-income, and vulnerable individuals and families in the United States. While some safety-net facilities, like community health centers and public hospitals, are driven by a mission to provide the best care possible to their patients despite lack of resources, others care for the uninsured and Medicaid out of obligation and regulation.

The safety-net system will undergo a significant transformation over the next decade. As the ACA is fully implemented, thirty million currently uninsured patients will enroll in coverage through Medicaid and commercial insurance products. At the same time, the undocumented and those who are still unable to afford or enroll in coverage will become further disenfranchised by our health care system. As safety-net providers, our community health centers, public health clinics, private physicians, hospitals, free clinics, and indigent care programs will have to effectively plan and develop strategies for coordinating and delivering care for all of their patients. The challenges may be different, but we still must strengthen the safety net by supporting DSH funding and Section 330 Health Center grants, training primary care physicians, encouraging reasonable Medicaid reimbursement, engaging in innovations to deliver high-quality care, and making efforts to enroll people in the affordable coverage to which they are entitled.

KEY TERMS

Community health centers A term used to describe the Section 330 grantee clinics that receive partial funding from the Health Resources and Services Administration (HRSA) Bureau of Primary Health Care and receive cost-related reimbursement from state Medicaid programs. Often referred to as federally qualified health centers (FQHC). Some clinics, called FQHC look-alikes, do not receive grant funding from BPHC, but do benefit from enhanced cost-related Medicaid reimbursement.

Disproportionate Share Hospital (DSH) Pronounced "dish," DSH refers to actual subsidies provided to hospitals through Medicaid and Medicare to compensate facilities that see a high proportion of low-income uninsured or Medicaid patients. Medicaid DSH recipients must have either (1) a low-income utilization rate (LIUR) of 25 percent or more or (2) a Medicaid utilization rate over one standard deviation above the mean Medicaid utilization in the state. Medicare DSH recipients are typically identified based on their ratio of low-income costs to overall costs. Often, DSH is used to refer to a specific type of hospitals that receive these subsidy payments ("DSH hospitals").

Indigent care Health care services provided to uninsured and low-income individuals (typically earning 200 percent of the federal poverty level [FPL] or below) by state and local governments and providers. In some states, indigent care may be funded by hospital fees aggregated into an uncompensated care pool or by county appropriations from property taxes and state support. The organization, application process, eligibility criteria, and services covered vary by state and locality. Often these programs provide emergency episodic care for the uninsured without an ability to pay for services, but do not provide comprehensive coverage for a wide variety of services.

Public hospitals Hospitals owned and operated by state or county governments, with a specific mission to care for the residents of an area. In California, public hospitals are county-owned and provide care to all residents of the county, regardless of their ability to pay, insurance status, or citizenship status. Examples include San Francisco General Hospital and Riverside County Regional Medical Center. In other states, like Massachusetts, public hospitals are state-owned and operated (such as Massachusetts General Hospital). Typically, university-owned hospitals are not considered "public" hospitals, even if they are state university–affiliated (such as UCLA's Ronald Reagan Medical Center or UCSF Medical Center).

Uncompensated care Services delivered by hospitals, physicians, clinics, and other providers to uninsured or underinsured patients that are not paid by patients or insurers. These uncompensated care bills are often paid for by local or state indigent care programs or are reported as bad debt or charity care by the provider.

Underinsured Insurance coverage that does not cover specific benefits, caps annual or lifetime spending, contains high deductibles, or other limitations that result in patients having uncovered out-of-pocket expenses.

Underserved Individuals and families facing barriers to accessing care, sometimes due to being uninsured, not having a place to go when they get sick, or being unable to afford care despite having insurance. Many rural residents and people living in impoverished urban areas are underserved because of the lack of available primary care, specialty physicians, or hospital facilities operating in their area.

DISCUSSION QUESTIONS

1. In considering the impact of the ACA on safety-net facilities like community health centers and public hospitals, do you think their business model will need to change? If so, how?
2. In Chapter One, you learned about the goals of the Affordable Care Act related to expansion of insurance coverage. Identify groups that you think will continue to rely on the health care safety net and explain why they are "left out" of the benefits provided through the ACA.
3. Cost shifting due to underpayment and uncompensated care is a significant problem in our health care system. Do you think that safety-net hospitals will now have a more stable, paying customer base, or will they continue to rely on shifting costs to provide services to the uninsured, low-income populations in their area?

4. Medicaid has often been considered a safety-net program, because it has typically covered children, pregnant women, low-income mothers, the aged, and the disabled. With the expansion of Medicaid due to the ACA, do you think that Medicaid should still be considered a safety-net program? Why or why not?

FURTHER READING

Websites

Kaiser Commission on Medicaid and the Uninsured: www.kff.org/about/kcmu
National Association of Community Health Centers: www.nachc.com
America's Essential Hospitals (formerly the National Association of Public Hospitals and Health Systems): essentialhospitals.org

Video

Kaiser Family Foundation Tutorial on America's Health Care Safety Net: www.kaiseredu .org/Tutorials-and-Presentations/Americas-Health-Care-Safety-Net.aspx

Books

Lewin, M. E., & Altman, S. E. (Eds.). (2000). *America's health care safety net: Intact, but endangered.* Washington, DC: National Academy Press. http://iom.edu/Reports /2000/Americas-Health-Care-Safety-Net-Intact-but-Endangered.aspx
Summer, L. (2011). *The impact of the Affordable Care Act on the safety net.* Washington, DC: AcademyHealth. http://www.academyhealth.org/files/FileDownloads/AHPolicy brief_Safetynet.pdf

Articles

Cunningham, P. (2007). The healthcare safety net: What is it, what good does it do, and will it still be there when you need it? *Harvard Health Policy Review, 8*(2), 5–15.
Wilensky, S., & Roby, D. H. (2005). Health centers and health insurance: Complements, not alternatives. *Journal of Ambulatory Care Management, 28*(4), 348–356.

REFERENCES

Barnett, K., & Somerville, M. H. (2012). *Hospital community benefits after the ACA: Schedule H and Hospital Community Benefit—Opportunities and challenges for the states.* Baltimore, MD: The Hilltop Institute.
Bureau of Primary Health Care. (2012). 2011 National Uniform Data System. Bethesda, MD: Health Resources and Services Administration. Retrieved from http://bphc .hrsa.gov/uds/doc/2011/National_Universal.pdf

Congressional Budget Office. (2013). *Effects of the Affordable Care Act on health insurance coverage: February 2013 Baseline.* Retrieved from http://www.cbo.gov /sites/default/files/cbofiles/attachments/43900_ACAInsuranceCoverageEffects .pdf

Cook, N. L., Hicks, L. S., O'Malley, J., Keegan, T., Guadagnoli, E., & Landon, B. (2007). Access to specialty care and medical services in community health centers. *Health Affairs, 26*(5), 1459–1468.

Darnell, J. S. (2010). Free clinics in the United States: A nationwide survey. *Archives of Internal Medicine, 170*(11), 946–953.

Decker, S. L. (2012). In 2011 nearly one-third of physicians said they would not accept new Medicaid patients, but rising fees may help. *Health Affairs, 31*(8), 1673–1679.

DeNavas-Walt, C., Proctor, B. D., & Smith, J. C. (2012). Income, poverty, and health insurance coverage in the United States: 2011 *(U.S. Census Bureau Current Population Report P60-243).* Washington, DC: U.S. Government Printing Office.

Dobson, A., DaVanzo, J., & Sen, N. (2006). The cost-shift payment "hydraulic": Foundation, history, and implications. *Health Affairs, 25*(1), 22–33.

Donaldson, M. S., Yordy, K. D., Lohr, K. N., & Vanselow, N. A. (Eds.). (1996). *Primary care: America's health in a new era.* Washington, DC: National Academy Press.

Felt-Lisk, S., McHugh, M., & Howell, E. (2001). *Study of safety net provider capacity to care for low-income uninsured patients.* Washington, D.C.: Mathematica Policy Research. Retrieved from http://www.mathematica-mpr.com/PDFs/safetynet.pdf

Forrest, C. B., & Whelan, E. M. (2000). Primary care safety-net delivery sites in the United States: A comparison of community health centers, hospital outpatient departments, and physicians' offices. *Journal of the American Medical Association, 284*(16), 2077–2083.

Fryer, G. E., Dovey, S. M., & Green, L. A. (2000). The importance of having a usual source of care. *American Family Physician, 62,* 477.

Gage, L. S. (1998). The future of safety-net hospitals. In S. H. Altman, U. E. Reinhardt, & A. E. Sheilds (Eds.), *The future healthcare system: Who will care for the poor and uninsured?* (pp. 123–149). Chicago: Health Administration Press.

Graves, J. (2012). Medicaid expansion opt-outs and uncompensated care. *New England Journal of Medicine, 367,* 2365–2367.

Hawkins, D. R., & Rosenbaum, S. (1998). The challenges facing health centers in a changing healthcare system. In S. H. Altman, U. E. Reinhardt, & A. E. Sheilds (Eds.), *The future healthcare system: Who will care for the poor and uninsured?* (pp. 99–122). Chicago: Health Administration Press.

Hing, E., Hooker, R. S., & Ashman, J. J. (2011). Primary health care in community health centers and comparison with office-based practice. *Journal of Community Health, 36*(3), 406–413.

Hoffman, C., & Sered, S. S. (2005). *Threadbare: Holes in America's health care safety net.* Washington, DC: Kaiser Commission on Medicaid and the Uninsured. Retrieved from http://www.kff.org/uninsured/upload/Threadbare-Holes-in-America-s -Health-Care-Safety-Net-report.pdf

John Snow International. (2013). *Value of community health centers study.* Sacramento: California Primary Care Association. Retrieved from http://www.cpca.org/cpca /assets/File/Announcements/2013–01–29-ValueofCHCStudy.pdf.

Jones, A. S., & Sajid, P. S. (2010). *A primer on health care safety nets*. Princeton, NJ: Robert Wood Johnson Foundation. Retrieved from http://www.rwjf.org/content/dam /supplementary-assets/2010/06/49869.pdf

Kilpatrick, K. E., Miller, M. K., Dwyer, J. W., & Nissen, D. (1991). Uncompensated care provided by private practice physicians in Florida. *Health Services Research, 26*(3), 277–302.

Ku, L., Regenstein, M., Shin, P., Mead, H., Levy, A., Buchanan, K. & Byrne, F. (2012). Coordinating and integrating care for safety net patients: Lessons from six communities. Washington, DC: The George Washington University. Retrieved from http:// sphhs.gwu.edu/departments/healthpolicy/dhp_publications/pub_uploads/dhp Publication_618A2D24–5056–9D20–3D475D756ACE11FB.pdf

Ku, L., Richard, P., Dor, A., Tan, E., Shin, P., & Rosenbaum, S. (2010). *Strengthening primary care to bend the cost curve: The expansion of community health centers through health reform* (Policy Research Brief No. 19). Washington, DC: Geiger Gibson/RCHN Community Health Foundation Research Collaborative.

Landon, B. E., Hicks, L. S., O'Malley, A. J., Lieu, T. A., Keegan, T., McNeil, B. J., & Guadagnoli, E. (2007). Improving the management of chronic disease at community health centers. *New England Journal of Medicine, 356*(9), 921–934.

Lewin, M. E., & Altman, S. E. (Eds.). (2000). *America's health care safety net: Intact, but endangered*. Washington, DC: National Academy Press.

Medicare Learning Network. (2007). *Rural health clinic fact sheet*. Baltimore, MD: Centers for Medicare and Medicare Services. Retrieved from http://www.hsagroup.net /images/rhcfactsheet.pdf

Moreno, L., Peikes, D., & Krilla, A. (2010). *Necessary but not sufficient: The HITECH Act and health information technology's potential to build medical homes* (Agency for Healthcare Research and Quality Publication No. 10-0080-EF). Washington, DC: Mathematica Policy Research.

National Association of Community Health Centers. (2009). *Primary care access: An essential building block of health reform*. Retrieved from http://www.nachc.com /client/documents/pressreleases/PrimaryCareAccessRPT.pdf

National Association of Community Health Centers. (2010). *Expanding health centers under health care reform*. Retrieved from http://www.nachc.com/client/HCR_ New_Patients_Final.pdf

National Association of Community Health Centers. (2011). *Access endangered: Profiles of the medically disenfranchised*. Retrieved from http://www.nachc.com /client//NACHC__Access_Endangered_2011.pdf

National Association of Community Health Centers. (2012). *United States Health Center Fact Sheet*. Retrieved from https://www.nachc.com/client//US121.pdf

National Association of Free and Charitable Clinics. (2013). *What is a free or charitable clinic?* Retrieved from http://www.nafcclinics.org/about-us/what-is-free-charitable-clinic

Ohio Children's Hospital Association. (2010). *Ohio Children's Hospitals Medicaid funding fact sheet*. Retrieved from http://www.ohiochildrenshospitals.org/doc /Childrens_HC_funding_fact_sheet%20051011.pdf

Redlener, I., & Grant, R. (2009). America's safety net and health care reform: What lies ahead? *New England Journal of Medicine, 361*, 2201–2204.

Roby, D. H., Pourat, N. Pirritano, M. J., Vrungos, S. M., Dajee, H., Castillo, D., & Kominski, G. F. (2010). Impact of patient-centered medical home assignment on emergency room visits among uninsured patients in a county health system. *Medical Care Research and Review*, *67*(4), 412–430.

Rust, G., Baltrus, P., Ye, J., Daniels, E., Quarshie, A., Boumbulian, P., & Strothers, H. (2009). Presence of a community health center and uninsured emergency department visit rates in rural counties. *Journal of Rural Health*, *25*(1), 8–16.

Zaman, O. S., Cummings, L. C., & Laycox, S. (2012). *America's safety net hospitals and health systems, 2010*. Washington, DC: National Association of Public Hospitals and Health Systems. Retrieved from http://www.naph.org/Main-Menu-Category /Publications/Safety-Net-Financing/2010-NAPH-Characteristics-Report.aspx? FT=.pdf

Zibulewsky, J. (2001). The Emergency Medical Treatment and Active Labor Act (EMTALA): What it is and what it means for physicians. *Baylor University Medical Center Proceedings*, *14*(4), 339–346.

CHAPTER TWENTY FOUR

ETHICAL ISSUES IN PUBLIC HEALTH AND HEALTH SERVICES

Pauline Vaillancourt Rosenau
Ruth Roemer
Frederick J. Zimmerman

Learning Objectives

- List the three cardinal principles of public health ethics
- Discuss ethical issues in the allocation of resources to health care and within the health care industry
- Discuss ethical issues related to the distribution of and access to health care utilization
- Analyze the institutional factors required to ensure that medical and public health research are ethical
- Apply the principles of public health ethics to a discussion of how health care is financed
- Outline ethical issues in the management and delivery of health care services
- List some of the methods for resolving ethical issues in health care

The cardinal principles of medical ethics—autonomy, beneficence, and justice (Beauchamp & Childress, 1989; Beauchamp & Walters, 1999b)—apply in public health ethics but in somewhat altered form.

Personal *autonomy* and respect for autonomy are guiding principles of public health practice as well as of medical practice. In medical ethics, the concern is with the privacy, individual liberty, freedom of choice, and self-control of the individual. From this principle flows the doctrine of informed consent. In *public health ethics*, autonomy, the right of privacy, and freedom of action are recognized insofar as they do not result in harm to others. Thus, from a public health perspective, autonomy may be subordinated to the welfare of others or of society as a whole (Burris, 1997).

Beneficence, which includes doing no harm, promoting the welfare of others, and doing good, is a principle of medical ethics. In the public health context, beneficence is the overall goal of public health policy and practice. It must be interpreted broadly, in light of societal needs, rather than narrowly, in terms of individual rights.

Justice—whether defined as equality of opportunity, equity of access, or equity in benefits—is the core of public health. Serving the total population, public health is concerned with *equity* among various social groups, with protecting vulnerable populations, with compensating persons for suffering disadvantage in health and health care, and with surveillance of the total health care system. As expressed in the now-classic phrase of Dr. William H. Foege, "Public health is social justice" (Foege, 1987).

This chapter concerns public health ethics as distinguished from medical ethics. Of course, some overlap exists between public health ethics and medical ethics, but public health ethics, like public health itself, applies generally to issues affecting populations, whereas medical ethics, like medicine itself, applies to individuals. Public health involves a perspective that is population-based, a view of conditions and problems that gives preeminence to the needs of the whole society rather than exclusively to the interests of single individuals (Annas, 2005).

To illustrate the concept of public health ethics, we raise several general questions to be considered within three overarching themes:

- What tensions exist between protection of the public health and protection of individual rights?
- As we transition from a society that can, as a whole, pay for all efficacious care to one that has both political and economic difficulty in doing so, *how should scarce resources be allocated and used?* In particular,
  - What should the balance be between expenditures and quality of life in the case of chronic and terminal illness?
  - What are appropriate limits on using expensive medical technology?
  - What obligation exists for government to protect the most vulnerable sectors of society?

- What responsibility exists for the young to finance health care for older persons?
- *What obligations do health care insurers and health care providers have* in meeting the right to know of patients as consumers?

We cannot give a clear, definitive answer that is universally applicable to any of these questions. Context and circumstance sometimes require qualifying even the most straightforward response. In some cases, differences among groups and individuals may be so great and conditions in society so diverse and complex that no single answer to a question is possible. In other instances, a balance grounded in a public health point of view is viable. Sometimes there is no ethical conflict at all because one solution is optimal for all concerned—for the individual, the practitioner, the payer, and society. For example, few practitioners would want to perform an expensive, painful medical act that is without benefit and might do damage. Few patients would demand it, and even fewer payers would reimburse for it. But in other circumstances, competition for resources poses a dilemma. How does one choose, for example, between a new, effective, but expensive drug of help to only a few, or use of a less expensive but less effective drug for a larger number of persons? The necessity for a democratic, open, public debate about rationing in the future seems inevitable.

The goal of public health ethics is not to definitively resolve these issues, but rather to provide a framework within which they can be productively discussed. The fundamental principles of this framework are beneficence, justice, and respect for persons. Evidence can be brought to bear on these issues and it can support one view rather than another. But evidence rarely convinces everyone when the ethical issue in question is a matter of personal values or preferences. Even in the absence of agreement on ethical assumptions, and facing diversity and complexity that prohibit easy compromises, we suggest mechanisms for resolving the ethical dilemmas in health care do exist. We explore them in the concluding section of this chapter.

A word of caution: space is short and our topic complex. We cannot explore every dimension of every relevant topic to the satisfaction of all readers. We offer here, instead, an introduction whose goal is to awaken readers—be they practitioners, researchers, students, patients, or consumers—to the ethical dimension of public health. We hope to remind them of the ethical assumptions that underlie their own public health care choices. This chapter, then, is limited to considering selected ethical issues in public health and provision of personal health services. We examine our topic by way of components of the health system: (1) development of health resources, (2) economic support, (3) organization of services, (4) management of services, (5) delivery of care, and (6) assurance of the quality of care.

Overarching Public Health Principles: Our Assumptions

We argue for these general principles of a public health ethic:

- Equity and nondiscrimination in distribution of resources, giving due regard to vulnerable groups in the population (ethnic minorities, migrants, children, pregnant women, the poor, the handicapped, and others), and without regard to race, religion, gender, or sexual orientation. Equity demands that a certain set of basic needs be provided to all without regard to ability to pay, even though the identification of the set of basic needs is contentious.
- Respect for human rights—including autonomy, privacy, liberty, and well-being.
- Determination of need for health care services should be evidence-based and not influenced by the self-interest of care providers or their suppliers.

Central to the solution of ethical problems in health services is the role of law, which sets forth the legislative, regulatory, and judicial controls of society. The development of law in a particular field narrows the discretion of providers in making ethical judgments. At the same time, law sets guidelines for determining policy on specific issues or in individual cases. (For examples of the symbiotic relationship between ethics and law, see Annas, 1998, and Annas, 2005.)

Ethical Issues in the Allocation of Resources

When we talk about allocating resources, we mean health personnel, facilities, drugs and equipment, and knowledge. Choices among the amount and kinds of personnel trained, the facilities made available, and the commodities produced are not neutral. Producing and acquiring each of these involve trade-offs, and therefore ethical assumptions, and they in turn have public health consequences. Questions about the allocation of resources involve questions of:

The amount of resources to allocate to health care as opposed to other functions in the economy

The allocation of resources across different uses within the health care sector

The distribution of resources to different types of people who use health care

These questions are interrelated in ways that are ethically complex.

The Allocation of Resources to Health Care

Ethical public health dilemmas are confronted with respect to health facilities. From a public health point of view, the need for equitable access to quality institutions and for fair distribution of health care facilities may be in competition with an individual real estate developer's ends or the preferences of for-profit hospital owners. Offering a range of facilities to maximize choice suggests the need for both public and private hospitals, community clinics and health centers, and inpatient and outpatient mental health facilities, as well as long-term care facilities and hospices. At the same time, not-for-profit providers, on several performance variables, do a better job than the for-profit institutions. Overall, studies since 1980 suggest that nonprofit providers outperform for-profit providers on cost, quality, access, and charity care (Rosenau, 2003; Rosenau & Linder, 2003a, 2003b). For example, the medical loss ratio is much higher in nonprofit health care providers compared to for-profit health care providers. The higher the medical loss ratio, the greater the proportion of revenue received that goes for health care, rather than administration and management. In 1995, for example, Kaiser Foundation Health Plan in California "devoted 96.8 percent of its revenue to health care and retained only 3.2 percent for administration and income" (Bell, 1996). Nonprofits have lower disenrollment rates (Dallek & Swirsky, 1997), offer more community benefits (Claxton, Feder, Shactman, & Altman, 1997), and feature more preventive services too (Himmelstein, Woolhandler, Hellander, & Wolfe, 1999). How long this can continue to be the case in the highly competitive health care market is unknown because not-for-profits may have to adopt for-profit business practices to survive (Melnick, Keeler, & Zwanziger, 1999).

The financial crisis facing public hospitals throughout the nation poses an ethical problem of major proportions. At stake is the survival of facilities that handle an enormous volume of care for the poor, that train a large number of physicians and other health personnel, and that make available specialized services—trauma care, burn units, and others—for the total urban and rural populations they serve. As a result of the Patient Protection and Affordable Care Act, many public hospitals are now in the position of having to provide more care within their financial allotment, while at the same time improving quality to retain and attract patients.

Rationing medical care is not always ethically dubious; rather, it may conform to a public health ethic. In some cases, too much medical care is counterproductive and may produce more harm than good. All nations, including the United States, have rationing of one sort or another. Canada, Sweden, the United Kingdom, and the state of Oregon, among others, have chosen to ration care by making a basic set of health care a universal right and by making more expensive the care that evidence has shown to be not clinically useful (Maynard & Bloor, 1998). By contrast, in the United States, virtually all health care is very inexpensive (at the margin) to those with health insurance, while virtually all health care is extremely expensive to consumers without insurance. These different types of rationing matter to outcomes. For example, Canada quantity-rations health care, pays one-third less per person than the United States, and offers universal coverage; yet health status indicators do not suggest that Canadians suffer. In fact, on several performance indicators Canada surpasses the United States (Anderson & Poullier, 1999). With better information about medical outcomes and the efficacy of many medical procedures, rationing would actually benefit patients if it discouraged the unneeded and inappropriate treatment that plagues the U.S. health system (Schuster, McGlynn, & Brook, 1998).

Rationing organ transplants, similarly, is a matter of significant ethical debate because fewer organs are available for transplant than needed for the eighty-five thousand people on waiting lists. Rationing must therefore be used to determine who is given a transplant. Employing tissue match makes medical sense and also seems ethically acceptable. But to the extent that ability to pay is a criterion, ethical conflict is inevitable. It may, in fact, go against scientific opinion and public health ethics if someone who can pay receives a transplant even though the tissue match is not so good as it would be for a patient who is also in need of a transplant but unable to pay the cost. Rationing on this basis seems ethically unfair and medically ill advised. It is no surprise, then, that the National Organ Transplant Act, adopted in 1984, made it illegal to offer or receive payment for organ transplantation. Yet the sale of organs for transplantation still exists. It has even been advocated as a market-friendly, for-profit solution to the current supply problems, although it is a solution that raises enormous ethical issues of its own because it discriminates against the poor (Kaserman & Barnett, 2002).

One way to resolve some of these ethical dilemmas would be to make more organs available through mandatory donation from fatal automobile accidents, without explicit consent of individuals and families. A number of societies have adopted this policy of presumed consent because the public health interest of society and the seriousness of the consequences are so great for those in need of a transplant that it is possible to justify ignoring the individual autonomy (preferences) of the accident victim's friends and relatives. Spain leads other nations regarding organ donation, with 33.8 donors per million in 2003, by interpreting an absence of prohibition to constitute a near-death patient's implicit authorization for organ transplantation (Bosch, 1999). This has not been the case in the United States to date (Council of Europe: National Transplant Organization in Parliamentary Office of Technology, 2004).

The Allocation of Resources across Different Uses within Health Care

The numbers and kinds of personnel required and their distribution are critical to public health (Gebbie, Merrill, & Tilson, 2002). We need to have an adequate supply of personnel and facilities for a given population in order to meet the ethical requirements of providing health care without discrimination or bias. The proper balance of primary care physicians and specialists is essential to the ethical value of beneficence so as to maximize health status. The ethical imperative of justice requires special measures to protect the economically disadvantaged, such as primary care physicians working in health centers. Specialty physician compensation in the United States is strongly influenced by the Specialty Society Relative Value Scale Update Committee, a committee of the American Medical Association, which is primarily staffed by specialty physicians. This self-dealing has resulted in low pay for primary care physicians and far too many specialists relative to generalists. Other modern western countries have achieved better balance, but this has involved closely controlling compensation, medical school enrollments, and residency programs.

At the same time, the ethical principle of autonomy urges that resource development be diverse enough to permit consumers some choice of providers and facilities. Absence of this choice results in part from the limited range of personnel. Patients should have some freedom—though not unlimited—to choose the type of care they prefer. Midwives, chiropractors, and other effective and proven practitioners should be available if health resources permit without sacrificing other ethical considerations. The ethical principle of autonomy here might conflict with that of equity, which would limit general access to specialists in the interest of better distribution of health care access to the whole population. The need for ample public health personnel is another ethical priority, necessary for the freedom of all individuals to enjoy a healthful, disease-free environment.

Physician assistants and nurses are needed, and they may serve an expanded role, substituting for primary care providers in some instances to alleviate the shortage of primary care physicians, especially in underserved areas. But too great a reliance on these providers might diminish quality of care if they are required to substitute entirely for physicians, particularly with respect to differential diagnosis (Roemer, 1977). The point of service is also a significant consideration. For example, effective and expanded health care and dental care for children could be achieved by employing the school as a geographic point for monitoring and providing selected services.

The Distribution of Resources across Different Patient Populations

Distribution of scarce health resources is another subject of debate. The principle of first come, first served may initially seem equitable. But it also incorporates the "rule of rescue," whereby a few lives are saved at great cost, and this policy results in the "invisible" loss of many more lives. Cost-benefit or cost-effectiveness analysis of health economics attempts to apply hard data to administrative decisions. This approach, however, does not escape ethical dilemmas either, because the act of assigning numbers to years of life, for example, is itself value-laden. If administrative allocation is determined on the basis of the number of years of life saved, then the younger are favored over the older, which may or may not be equitable. If one factors into such an analysis the idea of "quality" years of life, other normative assumptions must be made as to how important quality is and what constitutes quality. Some efforts have been made to assign a dollar value to a year of life as a tool for administering health resources. But here too, we encounter worrisome normative problems. Does ability to pay deform such calculations (Hillman et al., 1991)?

Similarly, in the United States an individual medical provider's free choice as to where to practice medicine has resulted in underserved areas, and ways to develop and train health personnel for rural and central city areas are a public health priority. Foreign medical graduates are commonly employed in underserved urban centers and rural areas in the United States today, but this raises other ethics questions. Is it just to deprive the citizens of the country of origin of these practitioners of their services (McMahon, 2004)?

An important issue in educating health professionals is the need to ensure racial and ethnic diversity in both the training and practice of health professionals. A series of court decisions and state initiatives have, with one exception, seriously limited admissions of minority students to professional schools.

Interrelations among Types of Allocations

These distribution and allocation issues are deeply intertwined, with important ethical implications. For example, solving the ethical distributional problems above has been understood to require additional compensation for rural providers, and those in other underserved areas.

Loan forgiveness and expansion of the National Health Service Corps, rural preceptorships, creating economic incentives for establishing a practice in a rural area, and employing physician assistants and nurse practitioners are all solutions to inequitable access to care, but they are not free and in general rely on greater resources being allocated to the health care system as a whole (Lewis, Fein, & Mechanic, 1976). Telemedicine may make the best medical consultants available to rural areas in the near future (Smothers, 1992; Wheeler, 1994), but the technology involves initial start-up costs that are not trivial. Higher Medicare payments to rural hospitals also ensure that they will remain open (Moscovice, Wellever, & Stensland, 1999).

In another example of knotty ethical trade-offs, the advantages of staff-model managed care are clear: team practice, emphasis on primary care, generous use of diagnostic and therapeutic outpatient services, and prudent use of hospitalization. All contribute to cost containment. At the same time, managed care systems have the disadvantage of restricted choice of provider. Today's for-profit managed care companies run the risk of underserving; they may achieve cost containment through cost shifting and risk selection (Rice, 1998).

The ethical issues in managed care are illustrated most sharply by the question of who decides what is medically necessary: the physician or patient, the disease management program, the insurer, the employer, or the state legislature (Bodenheimer, 1999; Mariner, 1994; Rosenbaum,

Frankford, Moore, & Borzi, 1999). This question is not unique to managed care; it has also arisen with respect to insurance companies and Medicaid, and will become an issue in Accountable Care Organizations as currently conceived. On the one hand, the physician has a legal and ethical duty to adhere to the standard of care that a reasonable physician in the same or similar circumstances would. On the other hand, insurers have traditionally specified what is covered or not covered as medically necessary in insurance contracts. The courts have sometimes reached contrasting results, depending on the facts of the case, the character of the treatment sought (whether generally accepted or experimental), and the interpretation of medical necessity. With the rise of managed care, the problem becomes an ethical dilemma because, as even those highly favorable to managed care agree, there is a risk of too little health care (Danzon, 1997).

As more and more integrated health care delivery systems are formed, as more mergers of managed care organizations occur, as pressure for cost containment increases, ethical issues concerning conflict of interest, quality of care choices, and patients' rights attain increasing importance. The principles of autonomy, beneficence, and justice are severely tested in resolving the ethical problems facing a complex corporate health care system.

If medicine is for-profit, as seems to be the case today and for the near future in the United States, then the ethical dilemma between patients' interests and profits will be a continuing source of conflict of interest (Emanuel, 1999). Sometimes the two can both be served, but it is unlikely to be the case in all instances. Publicly traded for-profit providers have to balance accountability to stockholders against their client-patients' interests. They bear an ethical responsibility to both. Surveys of business "executives admit and point out the presence of numerous generally accepted practices in their industry which they consider unethical" (Baumhart, 1961). As Fisher and Welch conclude, "Stakeholders in the increasingly market-driven U.S. health care system have few incentives to explore the harms of the technologies from which they stand to profit" (Deyo, Psaty, Simon, Wagner, & Omenn, 1997; Fisher & Welch, 1999). That both consumers and employers are concerned about quality of care is clear from Paul Ellwood's statement expressing disappointment in the evolution of HMOs because "they tend to place too much emphasis on saving money and not enough on improving quality—and we now have the technical skill to do that" (Noble, 1995). Yet overuse of care continues to be a substantial ethical problem, even if the exact amount of overuse is a matter of ongoing debate.

Ethical Issues in Research

Research serves a public health purpose too, and attempts by parties with a financial interest to distort research (Goldacre, 2010; Rosenstock & Lee, 2002) are ethically perilous, because they distort the information available to decision makers at all levels. Research has advanced medical technology, and its benefits in new and improved products should be accessible to all members of society. Public health ethics also focuses on the importance of research in assessing health system performance, including equity of access and medical outcomes. Only if what works and is medically effective can be distinguished from what does not work and what is medically ineffective are public health interests best served. Health care resources need to be used wisely and not wasted. Health services research can help ensure this goal. This is especially important in an era in which market competition appears, directly or indirectly, to be exerting a negative influence on research capacity (Moy, Mazzaschi, Levin, Blake, & Griner, 1997).

Research is central to developing public health resources. Equity mandates a fair distribution of research resources among the various diseases that affect the public's health because research is costly, resources are limited, and choices have to be made. Research needs both basic and applied orientation to ensure quality. There is a need for research on matters that have been neglected in the past (Gross, Anderson, & Powe, 1999), as has been recognized in the field of women's health. Correction of other gross inequities in allocating research funds is urgent. Congress regularly subverts the peer-review process to prioritize research on its favored causes and defund research in politically unpopular areas. While this problem may be ethically defended as the proper working of democracy (Deyo et al., 1997; Luo, 2011), it is only as democratic—and therefore as ethical—as the political system itself. When interested parties are able to push research agendas away from sensitive areas, there are ethical problems of failure to protect beneficence and non-maleficence. Ethical implications involving privacy, informed consent, and equity affect targeted research grants for AIDS, breast cancer, and other special diseases. The legal and ethical issues in the human genome project, and now stem cell research, involve matters of broad scope—wide use of genetic screening, information control, privacy, and possible manipulation of human characteristics. It is no surprise that Annas has called for "taking ethics seriously" (Annas, 1989).

An overarching problem is the conflict of interest of scientists who are judging the effectiveness of treatments and drugs and may be, at the same time, employed by or serving as consultants to a pharmaceutical or biotechnology firm. In 2005, several scientists at the National Institutes of Health resigned in the wake of a new regulation banning NIH scientists from accepting funding from pharmaceutical firms (Rosenwald & Weiss, 2005).

Correction of fraud in science and the rights of subjects are important ethical considerations in developing knowledge. Ethical conflict between the role of the physician as caregiver and as researcher is not uncommon inasmuch as what is good for the research project is not always what is good for the patient. Certainly, in some instances society stands to benefit at the expense of the research subject, but respect for the basic worth of the individual means that he or she has a right to be informed before agreeing to participate in an experiment. Only when consent is informed, clear, and freely given can altruism, for the sake of advancing science and humanity, be authentic.

Ethical Issues in Economic Support

Nowhere is the public health ethical perspective clearer than on issues of economic support. Personal autonomy and respect for privacy remain essential, as does beneficence. But a public health orientation suggests that the welfare of society merits close regard for justice. It is imperative that everyone in the population have equitable access to essential health care services with dignity, so as not to discourage necessary utilization. The ethical issues arise in how to define essential health services, and how to design access to them. As the other chapters in this book make clear, universal health insurance coverage is one efficient way of ensuring access. It is also ethical, as it satisfies the criteria of justice and beneficence, with the minimal necessary infringement on autonomy.

The PPACA stipulates the use of mandatory, privately purchased health insurance, which, it is clear, many consider to be an infringement on autonomy. It is ethically interesting that many of these same people do not perceive Medicare to involve the same infringement on autonomy. Perhaps the distinction arises because Medicare is fee for service, which allows extensive autonomy over choice of providers, while limiting choice of insurance mechanism, while, by contrast, the PPACA affords wider choice over insurance mechanism, with potentially much more limited choices over providers. This distinction neatly articulates the ethical difference between autonomy and choice.

At the same time, others consider it to be an infringement on autonomy to provide publicly financed or legally required charity care to those who have refused to purchase insurance. However this debate is resolved, it is ethically obvious that it must be resolved, as the denial of needed care to fifty million Americans who lack health insurance is a clear violation of the ethical principles of equity and beneficence.

Lack of health insurance makes for poorer medical outcomes even though individuals without health insurance do receive some care in hospital emergency rooms and community clinics. In particular, the uninsured do not get the care they need, even when some of their emergency-medical problems are treated. Most of the uninsured are workers in small enterprises whose employers do not offer health insurance for their workers or dependents (Schauffler, Brown, Rice, & Levan, 1997).

From a public health perspective, financial barriers to essential health care are inappropriate. Yet they exist to a surprising degree. Witness the fact that the cost reached $7,538 per person in the United States in 2008 (Kaiser Family Foundation, 2011). If each and every human being is to develop to his or her full potential, to participate fully as a productive citizen in our democratic society, then preventive health services and alleviation of pain and suffering due to health conditions that can be effectively treated must be available without financial barriers. Removing economic barriers to health services does not mean that the difference in health status between rich and poor will disappear. But it is a necessary (if not sufficient) condition for this goal.

From a public health point of view, the economic resources to support health services should be fair and equitable. Any individual's contribution should be progressive, based on ability to pay. Although some individual contribution is appropriate—no matter how small—as a gesture of commitment to the larger community, it is also ethically befitting for the nation to take responsibility for a portion of the cost. The exact proportion may vary across nation and time, depending on the country's wealth and the public priority attributed to health services (Roemer, 1991).

Similarly, justice and equity suggest the importance of the ethical principle of social solidarity in any number of forms (Bellah, Madsen, Sullivan, Swidler, & Tipton, 1996; Etzioni, 2004).

By definition, social insurance means that there is wisdom in assigning responsibility for payment by those who are young and working to support the health care of children and older people no longer completely independent. A public health orientation suggests that social solidarity forward and backward in time, across generations, is ethically persuasive. Those in the most productive stages of the life cycle today were once dependent children, and they are likely one day to be dependent older persons.

In 1983, the President's Commission for the Study of Ethical Problems in Medicine and Biomedical and Behavioral Research made as its first and principal recommendation on ethics in medicine that society has an obligation to ensure equitable access to health care for all its citizens (President's Commission for the Study of Ethical Problems in Medicine and Biomedical and Biobehavioral Research, 1983). This recommendation has stood the test of time, at the same time that inequality has increased in the United States. Equitable access, the commission said, requires that all citizens be able to secure an adequate level of care without excessive burden.

Ethical Issues in Management of Health Services

Management involves planning, administration, regulation, and legislation. The style of management depends on the values and norms of the population. Planning involves determining the population's health needs (with surveys and research, for example) and then ensuring that programs are in place to supply these services. A public health perspective suggests that planning is appropriate to the extent that it makes available efficient, appropriate health care (beneficence) to all who seek it (equity and justice). Planning may avoid waste and contribute to rational use of health services. But it is also important that planning not be so invasive as to be coercive and deny the individual any say in his or her health care, unless such intervention is necessary to protect public health interests. The ethical principle of autonomy preserves the right of the individual to refuse care, to determine his or her own destiny, especially when the welfare of others is not involved. A balance between individual autonomy and public health intervention that affords benefit to society is not easy to achieve. But in some cases the resolution of such a dilemma is clear, as with mandatory immunization programs. Equity and beneficence demand that the social burdens and benefits of living in a disease-free environment be shared. Therefore, for example, immunization requirements should cover all those potentially affected.

Health administration has ethical consequences that may be overlooked because they appear ethically neutral: organization, staffing, budgeting, supervision, consultation, procurement, logistics, records and reporting, coordination, and evaluation (Roemer, 1991). But all these activities involve ethical choices. Cost cutting, for example, places tremendous pressure on nurse-staffing ratios, yet adequate staffing has been shown to prevent mortality (Needleman et al., 2011). Denial of appropriate needed health care is an ethical problem related to beneficence.

Crucial to management of health services are legal tools—legislation, regulations, and sometimes litigation—necessary for fair administration of programs. Legislation and regulations are essential for authorizing health programs; they also serve to remedy inequity and to introduce innovation into a health service system. Effective legislation depends on a sound scientific base, and ethical questions are especially troubling when the scientific evidence is uncertain.

Enactment of legislation and issuance of regulations are important for management of a just health care system, but these strategies are useless if they are not enforced. For example, state legislation has long banned the sale of cigarettes to minors, but only recently have efforts been made to enforce these statutes rigorously through publicity, "stings" (arranged purchases by minors), and penalties on sellers, threats of license revocation, denial of federal funds under the Synar Amendment, and banning cigarette sales from vending machines (Roemer, 1993; U.S. Department of Health and Human Services, 1989). A novel case of enforcement involves a Baltimore ordinance prohibiting billboards promoting cigarettes in areas where children live, recreate, and go to school, enacted in order to enforce a law banning tobacco sales to minors. The Baltimore ordinance has not been overturned despite the fact that a Massachusetts regulation restricting advertising of tobacco and alcohol near schools was struck down as unconstitutional by the U.S. Supreme Court on the ground of preemption (Garner, 1996).

Thus management of health services involves issues of allocating scarce resources, evaluating scientific evidence, measuring quality of life, and imposing mandates by legislation and regulation. Although a seemingly neutral function, management of health services must rely on principles of autonomy, beneficence, and justice in its decision-making process.

Ethical Issues in Delivery of Care

Delivery of health services—actual provision of health care services—is the end point of all the other dimensions just discussed. The ethical considerations of only a few of the many issues pertinent to delivery of care are explored here.

Delivery of services raises conflict-of-interest questions for providers that are of substantial public health importance. Criminal prosecution of fraud in the health care sector increased threefold between 1993 and 1997 (DeFino, 1999). In today's market-driven health system, about half of all doctors report that they have "exaggerated the severity of a patient's condition to get them care they think is medically necessary" (Kaiser Family Foundation and Harvard University School of Public Health, 1999). Hospitals pressed by competitive forces strain to survive and in some cases do so only by less-than-honest cost shifting—or even direct fraud. A recent survey of hospital bills found that more than 99 percent included "mistakes" that favored the hospital (Kerr, 1992; Rosenthal, 1993).

Class action suits claim that HMOs are guilty of deceiving patients because they refuse to reveal financial incentives in physician payment structures (Pear, 1999). Physicians have been found to refer patients to laboratories and medical testing facilities that they co-own to a far greater extent than can be medically justified (Hillman et al., 1992). As the trend to make medicine a business develops, the AMA's Council on Ethical and Judicial Affairs has adopted guidelines for the sale of nonprescription, health-related products in physicians' offices, but problems remain (Krimsky & Nader, 2004). The purpose is to "help protect patients and maintain physicians' professionalism" (Prager, 1999). The public health ethic of beneficence is called into question by unnecessary products and inappropriate medical tests.

The practice of medicine and public health screening presents serious ethical dilemmas. Screening for diseases for which there is no treatment, except where such information can be used to postpone onset or prevent widespread population infection, is difficult to justify unless the information is explicitly desired by the patient for personal reasons (life planning and reproduction). In a similar case, screening without provision to treat those discovered to be in need of treatment is unethical. Public health providers need to be sure in advance that they can offer the health services required to care for those found to be affected. These are the ethical principles of beneficence and *social justice*.

Many other important ethical issues in delivering health care have not been discussed extensively in this chapter because of space limitations. There are three such issues that we want to mention briefly.

First, the end-of-life debate is generally considered a matter of medical ethics involving the patient, his or her family, and the physician. But this issue is also a matter of public health ethics because services at the end of life entail administrative and financial dimensions that are part of public health and management of health services. The Terri Schiavo case is an example where the potential alternative use of societal resources brings to mind the contradictions involved in end-of-life issues (Annas & Miller, 1994; Kitzhaber, 2005).

Second, in the field of mental health, the conflict between the health needs and legal rights of patients on the one hand and the need for protection of society on the other illustrates sharply the ethical problems facing providers of mental health services. This conflict has been addressed most prominently by reform of state mental hospital admission laws to make involuntary admission to a mental hospital initially a medical matter, with immediate and periodic judicial review as to the propriety of hospitalization—review in which a patient advocate participates.

The Tarasoff case presents another problem in providing mental health services: the duty of a psychiatrist or psychologist to warn an identified person of a patient's intent to kill the person, despite the rule of confidentiality governing medical and psychiatric practice (Beauchamp & Walters, 1999a). In both instances, a public health perspective favors protection of society as against the legal rights of individuals.

Third, basic to public health strategies and effective delivery of preventive and curative services are records and statistics. The moral and legal imperative of privacy to protect an individual's medical record gives way to public health statutes requiring reporting of gunshot wounds, communicable diseases, child abuse, and AIDS (Grad, 1990). More generally, the right to keep one's medical records confidential conflicts with society's need for epidemiological information to monitor the incidence and prevalence of diseases in the community and to determine responses to this information. At the same time, it is essential, for example, that an individual's medical records be protected from abuse by employers, marketers, and so on (Starr, 1999). A common resolution of this problem is to make statistics available without identifying information.

Congress adopted HIPAA (the Health Insurance Portability and Accountability Act) in 1996 to protect the privacy of medical records. Only in 2003 did these aspects of the law take effect. HIPAA limits who may see medical records, how the records are stored, and even how they are disposed of when no longer needed. Compliance costs have been enormous (Conkey, 2005).

Beneficence and justice are involved in full disclosure of information about quality to patients. Health plan report cards and quality ratings aim to fulfill this role. Employers, too, could use report cards to choose health plans for their employees, though some studies suggest that many employers are interested far more in cost than quality (McLaughlin & Ginsburg, 1998). How well reports actually measure quality is itself subject to debate (Hofer et al., 1999). PPACA has gone a long way toward increasing transparency of health information and making information about provider quality available to consumers. These matters are discussed in Part Three of this book.

Malpractice suits constitute one method of regulating the quality of care, although an erratic and expensive system. The subject is fully discussed elsewhere in this volume. Here we raise only the ethical issue of the right of the injured patient to compensation for the injury and the need of society for a system of compensation that is more equitable and more efficient than the current one.

The various mechanisms for ensuring quality of care all pose ethical issues. Peer review requires some invasion of privacy and confidentiality to conduct surveillance of quality, although safeguards have been devised. Practice guidelines involve some interference with physician autonomy but in return afford protection for both the patient and the provider. Malpractice suits raise questions of equity, since many injured patients are not compensated. In the process of developing and improving strategies for quality control, the public health perspective justifies social intervention to protect the population.

Future Directions

As the health care system continues to deal with state and federal budget cuts, the growing number of uninsured, and restructuring as a result of federal health insurance reform, ethical questions loom large. Perhaps their impact can be softened by imaginative and rational strategies to finance, organize, and deliver health care in accordance with the ethical principles of autonomy, beneficence, and justice.

Ethical issues in public health and health services management are likely to become increasingly complex in the future. New technology and advances in medical knowledge challenge us and raise ethical dilemmas. In the future they will need to be evaluated and applied in a public health context and submitted to a public health ethical analysis. Few of these developments are likely to be entirely new and without precedent, however. Already, current discussions such as those presented here may inform these new developments.

SUMMARY

Public health ethics embraces the triumvirate of ethical principles: justice, beneficence, and autonomy. Unlike in medical or bioethics, public health ethics places the emphasis not on individual transactions, but rather on the organizational and structural factors that determine the allocation of resources.

Even in the absence of agreement on ethical assumptions, and in the face of diversity and complexity that prohibit easy compromise, mechanisms for resolving ethical dilemmas in public health do exist. Among them are ombudsmen, institutional review boards, ethics committees, standards set by professional associations, practice guidelines, financing mechanisms, and courts of law. Some of these mechanisms are voluntary; others are legal. None is perfect. Some, such as financing mechanisms, are particularly worrisome.

Although ethics deals with values and morals, the law has been very much intertwined with ethical issues. In fact, the more that statutes, regulations, and court cases decide ethical issues, the narrower is the scope of ethical decision making by providers of health care (Grad, 1978). For example, the conditions for terminating life support for persons in a persistent vegetative state are clearer when the patient has an up-to-date living will. The scope of decision making by physicians and families is constrained. A court of law is therefore an important mechanism for resolving ethical issues in such cases.

The law deals with many substantive issues in numerous fields, including that of health care. It also has made important procedural contributions to resolving disputes by authorizing, establishing, and monitoring mechanisms or processes for handling claims and disputes. Such mechanisms are particularly useful for resolving ethical issues in health care because they are generally informal and flexible and often involve the participation of all parties. Administrative mechanisms are much less expensive than litigation and in this respect potentially more equitable.

Ombudsmen in health care institutions are a means of supporting patient representation and advocacy. They may serve as channels for expression of ethical concerns of patients and their families.

Ethics committees in hospitals and managed care organizations operate to resolve ethical issues involving specific cases in the institution. They may be composed solely of the institution's staff, or they may include an ethicist specialized in handling such problems.

Institutional review boards are required to evaluate research proposals for their scientific and ethical integrity.

Practice guidelines, also discussed earlier, offer standards for ethical conduct and encourage professional behavior that conforms to procedural norms generally recognized by experts in the field. The PRACA's Patient-Centered Outcomes Research Institute is a step in this direction.

Finally, financing mechanisms that create incentives for certain procedures and practices have the economic power to encourage ethical conduct. Perhaps the highest ethical priority in health care in the United States is achievement of universal coverage of the population by health insurance. At the same time, financing mechanisms may function to encourage the opposite behavior (Hillman et al., 1992).

KEY TERMS

Autonomy The ethical principle of respect for persons. In public health, autonomy, the right of privacy, and freedom of action are recognized insofar as they do not result in harm to others. Autonomy requires that we treat others as ends in themselves and never as means to our own ends.

Beneficence and nonmaleficence The ethical principles of doing good and not doing harm, respectively. In public health it is interpreted broadly, in light of a societal or population perspective.

Distribution Distribution may be defined over various dimensions, such as race, income, gender, sexual orientation, disability status, or geography. The distribution in an economy generally concerns the outcome of economic processes. Public health emphasizes fair distribution to vulnerable populations.

Equity The extent to which any given distribution conforms to ethical principles of fairness.

Justice The ethical principle of fairness. Justice can be defined as equality of treatment, equality of opportunity, equality of outcome, or in many other ways. Public health justice is concerned with equity among various social groups, with protecting vulnerable populations, with compensating persons for suffering disadvantage in health and health care, and with surveillance of the total health care system.

Public health ethics The study of ethical issues in population health and medical care delivery, with an emphasis on organizational, legal, and structural issues that influence the allocation of and access to resources. It gives preeminence to the needs of the whole society rather than focusing exclusively on the interests of single individuals.

Resource allocation The uses to which resources are put in the economy. Resources include money, labor time, equipment, education, natural resources, and other resources. The resource allocation in an economy generally concerns economic inputs but it has significant implications for public health.

Social justice The extent to which access to basic needs is distributed according to ethical principles of fairness.

DISCUSSION QUESTIONS

What would a public health understanding of autonomy, beneficence, and justice indicate to be an informed answer to the following questions?

1. What tensions exist between protection of the public health and protection of individual rights?
2. How should scarce resources be allocated and used?
3. What are appropriate limits on using expensive medical technology?
4. What obligations do health care insurers and health care providers have in meeting the right to know of patients as consumers?
5. What responsibility exists for the young to finance health care for older persons?
6. What obligation exists for government to protect the most vulnerable sectors of society?
7. Does the individual mandate represent an acceptable ethical compromise between the principles of autonomy and beneficence?

FURTHER READING

Bayer, R., & Fairchild, A. (2004). The genesis of public health ethics. *Bioethics, 18*(6), 473–492.

Callahan, D., & Jennings, B. (2002). Ethics and public health: Forging a strong relationship. *American Journal of Public Health, 92*(2), 169–176.

Childress, J. F., Faden, R. R., Gaare, R. D., Gostin, L. O., Kahn, J., Bonnie, R. J., ...Nieburg, P. (2002). Public health ethics: Mapping the terrain. *Journal of Law, Medicine, and Ethics, 30*(2), 170–178.

Darr, K. (2011). *Ethics in health services management* (5th ed.). Baltimore: Health Professions Press.

Gostin, L. O. (2010). Public health law and ethics: A reader *(revised and updated* 2nd ed.). Berkeley: UC Press.

Kass, N. (2001). An ethics framework for public health. *American Journal of Public Health, 91*(11), 1776–1782.

Lachman, V. (2009). *Developing your moral compass: Ethical challenges in health care* (1st ed.). New York: Springer.

Websites

Association of Schools of Public Health website with Ethics and Public Health: Model Curriculum—case studies in nine critical areas of public health ethics: http://www.asph.org/document.cfm?page=782

Public Health Leadership Society website (Principles of the Ethical Practice of Public Health: Code of Ethics): http://www.phls.org

School of Public Health modules on Public Health Ethics (four modules of thirty to forty minutes each): http://www.sph.unc.edu/oce/phethics—UNC

REFERENCES

Anderson, G. F., & Poullier, J. P. (1999). Health spending, access, and outcomes: trends in industrialized countries. *Health Affairs, 18*(3), 178–192.

Annas, G. J. (1989). At law: Who's afraid of the human genome? *Hastings Center Report, 19*(4), 19–21.

Annas, G. J. (1998). *Some choice: Law, medicine, and the market.* New York: Oxford University Press.

Annas, G. J. (2005). *American bioethics: Crossing human rights and health law boundaries.* New York: Oxford University Press.

Annas, G. J., & Miller, F. H. (1994). The empire of death: How culture and economics affect informed consent in the US, the UK, and Japan. *American Journal of Law and Medicine, 20*(4), 357–394.

Baumhart, R. C. (1961). How ethical are businessmen? *Harvard Business Review, 39*(4), 6–19.

Beauchamp, T. L., & Childress, J. F. (1989). *Principles of biomedical ethics.* New York: Oxford University Press.

Beauchamp, T. L., & Walters, L. (1999a). Ethical theory and bioethics. *Contemporary Issues in Bioethics, 1–32.*

Beauchamp, T. L., & Walters, L. R. (1999b). *Contemporary issues in bioethics.* Belmont: Wadsworth.

Bell, J. E. (1996). Saving their assets: How to stop plunder at Blue Cross and other nonprofits. *American Prospect, 26,* 60–66.

Bellah, R. N., Madsen, R., Sullivan, W. M., Swidler, A., & Tipton, S. M. (1996). *Habits of the heart: Individualism and commitment in American life.* Berkeley: University of California Press.

Bodenheimer, T. (1999). Disease management: Promises and pitfalls. *New England Journal of Medicine, 340*(15), 1202–1205.

Bosch, X. (1999). Spain leads world in organ donation and transplantation. *Journal of the American Medical Association, 282*(1), 17–18.

Burris, S. (1997). The invisibility of public health: Population-level measures in a politics of market individualism. *American Journal of Public Health, 87*(10), 1607–1610.

Claxton, G., Feder, J., Shactman, D., & Altman, S. (1997). Public policy issues in nonprofit conversions: An overview. *Health Affairs, 16*(2), 9–27.

Conkey, C. (2005, April 21). Doctors, hospitals act to safeguard medical data: Today is federal deadline for stepped-up security; compliance costs are high. *Wall Street Journal, p. D2.*

Council of Europe: National Transplant Organization in Parliamentary Office of Technology. (2004, October). *Legislation, practice, and donor rates (Postnote). 231,* 2.

Dallek, G., & Swirsky, L. (1997). *Comparing Medicare HMOs: Do they keep their members?* Washington, DC: Families USA Foundation.

Danzon, P. M. (1997). Tort liability: A minefield for managed care? *Journal of Legal Studies, 26*(2), 491–519.

DeFino, T. (1999). Mediscare. *Healthcare Business, 2*(3), 60–70.

Deyo, R. A., Psaty, B., Simon, G., Wagner, E. H., & Omenn, G. S. (1997). The messenger under attack: An occupational hazard for health researchers. *New England Journal of Medicine, 336*(16), 1176–1180.

Emanuel, E. J. (1999). Choice and representation in health care. *Medical Care Research and Review, 56*(Suppl 1), 113–140.

Etzioni, A. (2004). The responsive communitarian platform: Rights and responsibilities. In A. Etzioni, A. Volmert & E. Rothschild (Eds.), *The communitarian reader*. Oxford, U.K.: Rowman & Littlefield.

Fisher, E. S., & Welch, H. G. (1999). Avoiding the unintended consequences of growth in medical care. *Journal of the American Medical Association, 281*(5), 446–453.

Foege, W. H. (1987). Public health: Moving from debt to legacy. *American Journal of Public Health, 77*(10), 1276–1278.

Garner, D. W. (1996). Banning tobacco billboards. *Journal of the American Medical Association, 275*(16), 1263–1269.

Gebbie, K., Merrill, J., & Tilson, H. H. (2002). The public health workforce. *Health Affairs, 21*(6), 57–67.

Goldacre, B. (2010). *Bad science: Quacks, hacks, and Big Pharma flacks*. New York: Faber & Faber.

Grad, F. P. (1978). Medical ethics and the law. *Annals of the American Academy of Political and Social Science, 437*(1), 19–36.

Grad, F. P. (1990). *The public health law manual* (2nd ed.). Washington, DC: American Public Health Association.

Gross, C. P., Anderson, G. F., & Powe, N. R. (1999). The relation between funding by the National Institutes of Health and the burden of disease. *New England Journal of Medicine, 340*(24), 1881–1887.

Hillman, A. L., Eisenberg, J. M., Pauly, M. V., Bloom, B. S., Click, H., Kinosian, B., & Schwartz, J. S. (1991). Avoiding bias in the conduct and reporting of cost-effectiveness research sponsored by pharmaceutical companies. *New England Journal of Medicine, 324*(19), 1362–1365.

Hillman, B. J., Olson, G. T., Griffith, P. E., Sunshine, J. H., Joseph, C. A., Kennedy, S. D., . . . Bernhardt, L. B. (1992). Physicians' utilization and charges for outpatient diagnostic imaging in a Medicare population. *Journal of the American Medical Association, 268*(15), 2050–2054.

Himmelstein, D. U., Woolhandler, S., Hellander, I., & Wolfe, S. M. (1999). Quality of care in investor-owned vs. not-for-profit HMOs. *Journal of the American Medical Association, 282*(2), 159–163.

Hofer, T. P., Hayward, R. A., Greenfield, S., Wagner, E. H., Kaplan, S. H., & Manning, W. G. (1999). The unreliability of individual physician "report cards" for assessing the costs and quality of care of a chronic disease. *Journal of the American Medical Association, 281*(22), 2098–2105.

Kaiser Family Foundation. (2011). *Health care spending in the United States and selected OECD countries.* Menlo Park, CA: Author.

Kaiser Family Foundation and Harvard University School of Public Health. (1999). *Survey of physicians and nurses: Randomly selected verbatim descriptions from physicians and nurses of health plan decisions resulting in declines in patients' health status.* Menlo Park: Kaiser Family Foundation.

Kaserman, D. L., & Barnett, A. H. (2002). *The US organ procurement system: A prescription for reform.* Washington, DC: American Enterprise Institute.

Kerr, P. (1992, April 5). Wall Street; Glossing over health care fraud. *New York Times, p. F17.*

Kitzhaber, J. (2005, *April 4*). Congress' implicit healthcare rationing. Christian Science Monitor.

Krimsky, S., & Nader, R. (2004). *Science in the private interest: Has the lure of profits corrupted biomedical research?* Oxford, U.K.: Rowman & Littlefield.

Lewis, C. E., Fein, R., & Mechanic, D. (1976). *A right to health: The problem of access to primary medical care.* Hoboken: Wiley.

Luo, M. (2011, January 25). N.R.A. stymies firearms research, scientists say. *New York Times.*

Mariner, W. K. (1994). Patients' rights after health care reform: Who decides what is medically necessary? *American Journal of Public Health, 84*(9), 1515–1520.

Maynard, A., & Bloor, K. (1998). *Our certain fate: Rationing in health care.* London: Office of Health Economics.

McLaughlin, C. G., & Ginsburg, P. B. (1998). Competition, quality of care, and the role of the consumer. *Milbank Quarterly, 76*(4), 737–743.

McMahon, G. T. (2004). Coming to America: International medical graduates in the United States. *New England Journal of Medicine, 350*(24), 2435–2437.

Melnick, G., Keeler, E., & Zwanziger, J. (1999). Market power and hospital pricing: Are nonprofits different? *Health Affairs, 18*(3), 167–173.

Moscovice, I. S., Wellever, A., & Stensland, J. (1999). *Rural hospitals: Accomplishments and present challenges.* Minneapolis: Rural Health Research Center, School of Public Health, University of Minnesota.

Moy, E., Mazzaschi, A. J., Levin, R. J., Blake, D. A., & Griner, P. F. (1997). Relationship between National Institutes of Health research awards to US medical schools and managed care market penetration. *Journal of the American Medical Association, 278*(3), 217–221.

Needleman, J., Buerhaus, P., Pankratz, V. S., Leibson, C. L., Stevens, S. R., & Harris, M. (2011). Nurse staffing and inpatient hospital mortality. *New England Journal of Medicine, 364*(11), 1037–1045.

Noble, H. B. (1995, July 3). Quality is focus for health plans. *New York Times, pp. 1–7.*

Pear, R. (1999, October 9). Stung by defeat in house, H.M.O.s seek compromise. *New York Times*, p. A9.

Prager, L. O. (1999). Selling products OK—but not for profit. *American Medical News, p. 1.*

President's Commission for the Study of Ethical Problems in Medicine and Biomedical and Biobehavioral Research. (1983). *Securing access to health care: The ethical implications of differences in the availability of health services.* Washington, DC: U.S. Government Printing Office.

Rice, T. H. (1998). *The economics of health reconsidered.* Chicago: Chicago Health Administration Press.

Roemer, M. I. (1977). Primary care and physician extenders in affluent countries. *International Journal of Health Services, 7*(4), 545–555.

Roemer, M. I. (1991). National health systems of the world: The countries *(Vol. 1).* New York: Oxford University Press.

Roemer, R. (1993). *Legislative action to combat the world tobacco epidemic* (2nd ed.). Geneva: World Health Organization.

Rosenau, P. V. (2003). Performance evaluations of for-profit and nonprofit hospitals in the US. *Nonprofit Management and Leadership, 13*(4), 401–423.

Rosenau, P. V., & Linder, S. H. (2003a). A comparison of the performance of for-profit and nonprofit US psychiatric inpatient care providers since 1980. *Psychiatric Services, 54*(2), 183–187.

Rosenau, P. V., & Linder, S. H. (2003b). Two decades of research comparing for-profit and nonprofit health provider performance in the United States. *Social Science Quarterly, 84*(2), 219–241.

Rosenbaum, S., Frankford, D. M., Moore, B., & Borzi, P. (1999). Who should determine when health care is medically necessary? *New England Journal of Medicine, 340*(3), 229–232.

Rosenstock, L., & Lee, L. J. (2002). Attacks on science: The risks to evidence-based policy. *American Journal of Public Health, 92*(1), 14–18.

Rosenthal, E. (1993, *January 27).* Confusion and error are rife in hospital billing practices. New York Times.

Rosenwald, M. S., & Weiss, R. (2005, April 2). New ethics rules cost NIH another top researcher. *Washington Post, p. A1.*

Schauffler, H. H., Brown, E. R., Rice, T. H., & Levan, R. (1997). *The state of health insurance in California, 1996.* Los Angeles: UCLA Center for Health Policy Research.

Schuster, M. A., McGlynn, E. A., & Brook, R. H. (1998). How good is the quality of health care in the United States? *Milbank Quarterly, 76*(4), 517–563.

Smothers, R. (1992, September 16). 150 Miles away, the doctor is examining your tonsils. *New York Times, p. C14.*

Starr, P. (1999). Health and the right to privacy. *American Journal of Law and Medicine, 25,* 193–201.

U.S. Department of Health and Human Services. (1989). *Reducing the health consequences of smoking: 25 Years of progress. A report of the Surgeon General,* Washington, DC: Author.

Wheeler, S. V. (1994, Fall). TeleMedicine. *Biophotonics, 34–40.*

INDEX